O9-AHW-143

Quick Check
GUIDE TO
GLUTEN-
FREE
FOODS

Linda McDonald, M.S., R.D., L.D.
and the Editorial Staff
of Barron's Educational Series, Inc.

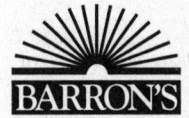

BARRON'S

Acknowledgments

The author and publisher gratefully acknowledge all the national gluten-free companies for assisting with the compilations of nutritional data for this edition. We also appreciate the additional information provided by the following companies: Amy's Kitchen, Andean Dream, LLC, Annie's Homegrown, Applegate Farms, Bakery on Main, Beanitos, Inc., Bigelow Tea, BiPRO USA, Bora Bora Ltd., Campbell Soup Company, Everybody Eats, Inc., French Meadow, General Mills, Idahoan, Jones Dairy Farm, Kellogg's, Lundberg Family Farms, Nana's Cookie Company, Nestlé USA, Perdue and Quinoa Corporation.

Thanks to all the restaurants that provided nutritional data for their menu items for this edition. The following also provided additional information: Arby's, Boston Market, Dunkin' Donuts, Jason's Deli, Old Spaghetti Factory, Red Robin International, Romano's Macaroni Grill, Red Mango, Rubios Mexican Grill, Sonic Drive-In, Ted's Montana Grill, and Wendy's.

© Copyright 2013 by Barron's Educational Series, Inc.

All Rights Reserved.
No part of this publication may be reproduced or distributed in any form or by any means without the written permission of the copyright owner.

All inquiries should be addressed to:
Barron's Educational Series, Inc.
250 Wireless Boulevard
Hauppauge, New York 11788
www.barronseduc.com

ISBN: 978-1-4380-0242-2

Library of Congress Control Number: 2012036723

Library of Congress Cataloging-in-Publication Data

McDonald, Linda.
  Food facts : guide to gluten-free foods / Linda McDonald, M.S., R.D. -- First edition.
     pages; cm. -- (Quick check)
  ISBN 978-1-4380-0242-2 (alk. paper)
1. Gluten-free diet--Popular works. 2. Nutrition--Popular works.
I. Title. II. Title: Guide to gluten-free foods.
  RM237.86.M3773 2012
  613.26--dc23

                                    2012036723
Printed in the United States of America

9 8 7 6 5 4 3 2

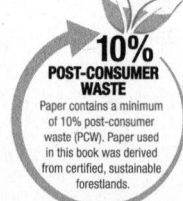

10%
POST-CONSUMER
WASTE
Paper contains a minimum
of 10% post-consumer
waste (PCW). Paper used
in this book was derived
from certified, sustainable
forestlands.

Contents

Preface   **vii**
Introduction   **ix**
    (Including Gluten-Free Healthy Eating and Shopping Tips)

Grains & Grain-Based Foods   **1**
  Baked Products
    (Including Mixes and Refrigerated Dough)   4
  Breads   21
  Cereals   29
  Cereal Bars   35
  Cookies   37
  Crackers   47
  Flours & Baking Ingredients   53
  Pasta & Pasta Products   58
  Rice / Grains   64

Vegetables   **71**
  Potatoes   73
  Spices / Seasonings / Herbs   74
  Vegetable Products (Including Canned Items)   76
  Vegetables   85

Fruits   **95**
  Fruit Juices   97
  Fruits   105

Dairy   **115**
  Cheeses   117
  Dairy   123
  Dairy Alternatives
    (Soy Milk & Yogurts, Coconut Milk, Almond Milk, etc.)   124
  Dairy Based Desserts
    (Puddings, Frozen Yogurts, Ice Cream)   139
  Milk   143
  Yogurt   148

Protein Foods   **165**

Beans, Peas & Legumes   167
Meats (Beef, Lamb, Pork)   171
Nuts & Seeds, Including Nut Butters   177
Poultry   185
Protein Alternatives, Including Vegetable Proteins
    (Soy & Tofu Products)   189
Sausages & Luncheon Meats   190
Seafood (Fish, Shellfish, Misc. Seafood)   208

Fats & Oils   **213**

Butter / Margarine   215
Oils   216
Olives   217
Salad Dressings   218
Spreads & Dips   224

Snacks & Sweets   **227**

Candies (Including Brand-name Bars)   229
Chips, Pretzels & Popcorn   232
Misc. Sweets (Gums, Jellies, etc.)   251
Snack Bars   254
Sugars, Syrups, Frostings & Toppings
    (See also *Dairy Based Desserts* under *Dairy*)   266

Beverages   **271**

Alcoholic Beverages   273
Coffees & Teas   274
Energy & Sports Drinks   285
Flavored Drinks & Drink Mixes   289
    (See also *Fruit Juice* under *Fruits*)

Mixed Dishes   **293**

Condiments   296
Entrées / Meal Products   299
Sauces & Gravies   312
Soups (Including Soup-related Products)   322

Baby Foods / Formulas   **335**
    Baby Foods / Baby Formulas   340

Restaurants & Dining   **347**
    Applebee's   351
    Bertucci's   354
    Boston Market   356
    Bugaboo Creek Steak House   357
    California Pizza Kitchen   359
    Carrabba's Italian Grill   361
    Carrow's   362
    Chick-Fil-A   366
    Chili's   369
    Chipotle Mexican Grill   373
    Claim Jumper   375
    Cold Stone Creamery   376
    Dairy Queen   388
    Denny's   396
    Don Pablo's   401
    Dunkin' Donuts   405
    First Watch   416
    Hardee's   420
    Jamba Juice   422
    Jason's Deli   431
    LongHorn Steakhouse   434
    Montana Mike's   439
    Noodles & Company   446
    Old Spaghetti Factory   448
    Olive Garden   450
    On the Border Mexican Grill & Cantina   451
    Outback Steakhouse   454
    P. F. Chang's   459
    Pei Wei Asian Diner   462
    Red Lobster   463
    Red Mango   465
    Red Robin   469
    Romano's Macaroni Grill   472

Rubio's Fresh Mexican Grill   477
Ruby Tuesday   479
SONIC, America's Drive-In   483
Ted's Montana Grill   515
Uno Chicago Grill   519
Wendy's   521
Additional restaurants with gluten-free menu items   526

Appendix   **529**
Product Manufacturers   529
Where to Find Gluten-Free Products   547
Resources / Organizations   550

Preface

The information in this book was provided by the food manufacturers either directly, from their web sites, or from package labels. Additional information is based on the *USDA National Nutrient Database for Standard Reference, Release 23*, published in computer-readable form by the U.S. Department of Agriculture. Restaurant information was provided directly by the restaurants included.

For each food or beverage, we list the serving size and then the amount per serving. The following abbreviations are used.

Cal	–	Total Calories (kcal)
Total Fat (g)	–	Total Fat (grams)
Sat. Fat (g)	–	Saturated fat (grams)
Chol. (mg)	–	Cholesterol (milligrams)
Carb. (g)	–	Carbohydrate (grams)
Fiber (g)	–	Total Fiber (grams)
Sug. (g)	–	Sugar (grams)
Prot. (g)	–	Protein (grams)
Sod. (mg)	–	Sodium (milligrams)

In some cases, a component of nutritional data for food products or restaurant menu items may not have been provided or available. If so, an NA appears to indicate that.

About the Author

Linda McDonald, M.S., R.D., L.D., owns SUPERMARKET SAVVY, an information and resource service focused on making healthy shopping easy. Her national newsletter, teaching tools, and website (*www.supermarketsavvy.com*) assist health professionals and consumers to shop healthy.

Mrs. McDonald is a graduate of the University of Houston with a Master of Science from the University of Texas Graduate School of Biomedical Sciences. She works with Dietetic Interns from the University of Houston, Texas Women's University, and University of Texas School of Public Health.

Disclaimer

Quick Check Guide to Gluten-Free Foods has been prepared for the gluten-free consumer in order to make gluten-free grocery shopping and eating out healthier, safer, easier, and more enjoyable.

The book should be used in choosing gluten-free food products in the supermarket and when selecting menu items in restaurants. The content of this book is not medical advice and should not take the place of consulting with a medical professional, a physician, or dietitian, including the diagnosis or treatment of any health condition. Neither the author, Linda McDonald, nor the editorial staff at Barron's Educational Series, Inc. shall be held liable or responsible to any person or entity with respect to gluten ingestion or any health consequences.

Nutrient information in this book was provided by the food companies and restaurants listed and was not confirmed to be gluten-free by lab analysis. Unfortunately, the USDA Food and Drug Administration (FDA) does not currently have a rule for gluten-free labeling although it is unlawful to make an inaccurate and misleading claim.

Food companies indicate that product and recipe ingredients may change periodically. Therefore, the consumer needs to always check the ingredients on the package label of food and beverage products to be certain they are gluten-free before consuming them. For specific questions or if you need further information on gluten-free products, manufacturer contact information has been provided on pages 529 to 546.

The restaurant chains in the book are nationally recognized. Restaurant menus items do change from time to time and adherence to gluten-free food preparation may possibly vary from one restaurant to another. Every effort has been made to make the gluten-free restaurant guide as accurate as possible. For the convenience of the reader, restaurant websites have also been provided to direct you to the latest information. Be sure to check with each restaurant you visit to make sure that they are adhering to the gluten-free recipes and using gluten-free preparation methods. For additional gluten-free eating out tips, please refer to page 347.

Introduction

If you or someone in your family is trying to follow a gluten-free diet, you may be frustrated with finding gluten-free foods and balancing these foods with a healthy diet. It is possible to eat a healthy gluten-free diet. Start by understanding the basics of gluten-free foods. Then use the tips and guidelines in this book to work gluten-free foods into a healthy diet.

Warning!

This book has been prepared for the gluten-free consumer in order to make gluten-free grocery shopping easier and healthier. The content of this book should not be considered medical advice. If you have a medical or health problem, you should consult your physician. The advice given is for general healthy, gluten-free eating.

Every effort has been made to make this gluten-free product guide as complete and accurate as possible. However, the food industry is a dynamic, changing industry with new and reformulated products hitting the supermarket shelves daily. Therefore this book should be used as a general guide, not as the ultimate source for gluten-free information. Always check the label and ingredients to make sure a food or beverage is gluten-free. If you have questions, contact the manufacturer. Find contact information for food and beverage manufacturers on page 529.

What is Gluten?

Gluten is the general name for one of the proteins found in wheat, rye, and barley. It gives elasticity to dough, helping it to rise and to keep its shape, and often gives the final product a chewy texture.

Why is avoiding Gluten important?

If you have celiac disease (CD) or dermatitis herpetiformis (DH), a skin form of celiac disease, even a small amount of gluten is harmful. In CD, gluten damages the small intestine resulting in poor absorption of nutrients. In DH, gluten causes skin rashes and itching and also damages the small intestine. A strict gluten-free diet (GFD) is the only treatment for CD and DH and requires the lifelong elimination of all foods containing wheat, barley, rye, and related cereal grains.

What is Gluten sensitivity?

Gluten sensitivity (also called gluten intolerance) is a range of disorders that go from life threatening celiac disease to the inconvenience of a wheat allergy, in which gluten has an adverse effect on the body. Until recently, the terms "gluten sensitivity" and "celiac disease" were used interchangeably. However, emerging research is beginning to identify the differences that exist between celiac disease and gluten sensitivity. Symptoms of gluten sensitivity may include bloating, abdominal discomfort, pain, or diarrhea; or it may present with a variety of symptoms outside of intestinal issues including headaches and migraines, lethargy and fatigue, attention-deficit disorder and hyperactivity, muscular disturbances, as well as bone and joint pain.

Common Misconceptions

You will lose weight on a gluten-free diet. Not necessarily! You may lose weight because you are eating differently, but gluten-free foods are not diet foods (low in calories). If weight is a concern, you will still need to watch your calories and exercise to lose weight.

It is impossible to eat a gluten-free diet. I hope that this book will show you that eating gluten-free is different, but not impossible. Just follow our tips and guidelines for successful gluten-free eating.

Gluten-free diets are nutritionally deficient. Gluten-free diets do not eliminate any food groups. You can include all the food groups in a gluten-free food plan. Eating gluten-free is as healthy or unhealthy as you make it.

You will feel better immediately on a gluten-free diet. If you have celiac disease or are gluten intolerant, you should feel better on a gluten-free diet—but it may not be immediate. Your body may need to adjust to eating gluten-free, and the damage done by gluten to your system may not be reversible. Be sure to communicate with your doctor and dietitian as you follow the gluten-free diet. There may be other issues that are causing symptoms such as lactose intolerance or other allergies.

Where is Gluten found?

Gluten is found in the grains wheat, barley, and rye, and derivatives of these grains such as bulgur, spelt, and kamut. Gluten may sound easy to avoid, but it is not! Many foods containing gluten ingredients don't use any of these terms and are hard to identify. Get familiar with the following list of gluten-containing, gluten-free, and questionable foods, beverages, and ingredients and learn to check the ingredients list on products. Use the list of gluten-free foods, brands, and restaurants in this book to help you achieve a healthy gluten-free diet.

Enjoy these Gluten-Free Foods, Beverages, and Ingredients:

Alcohol (distilled), Amaranth, Annatto, Arabic Gum, Arrowroot, Artificial Color, Baking Soda, Beans, BHA, BHT, Beta Carotene, Blue Cheese, Buckwheat, Calcium Carbonate, Calcium Caseinate, Calcium Chloride, Caramel Color, Carrageenan, Cellulose, Chickpeas, Citric Acid, Coloring, Corn, Cream of Tartar, Dextrose, Flax, Gelatin, Glucose Syrup, Gram Flour (chickpea flour), Grits, Guar Gum, Hemp, Herbs, Honey, Hydrolyzed Soy Protein, Inulin, Kasha, Legumes (dried peas, beans, lentils), Lecithin, Maize, Maltodextrin, Masa, Millet, Mono and Diglycerides, Monosodium Glutamate (MSG), Oats (pure, uncontaminated, labeled gluten-free), Polenta, Polysorbates, Potato Flour, Potato Starch, Psyllium, Quinoa, Rice, Sorghum, Soy, Spices, Sugar (brown, cane, white), Sulfites, Tapioca, Teff, Tumeric, Vanilla, Vanilla Extract, Vanilla Flavoring, Vanillin, Vinegars (Apple Cider, Balsamic, White, Wine), Wine, Xanthan Gum, Yeast (Autolyzed, Baker's, Torula), and Yogurt.

Avoid these Gluten-Containing Foods, Beverages, and Ingredients:

Ale (derived from barley), Atta, Barley, Barley Malt, Barley Malt Flavoring, Barley Malt Extract, Beer (derived from barley), Bran, Bread Flour, Brewer's Yeast, Bulgur, Couscous, Dinkel, Durum, Einkorn, Emmer, Farina, Farro, Graham Flour, Groats, Hydrolyzed Wheat Protein, Kamut, Lager (derived from barley), Malt, Malted Milk, Malt Vinegar, Matzoh, Oats (not labeled gluten-free), Rye, Seitan, Semolina, Spelt, Sprouted Wheat, Tabbouleh (made from wheat), Teriyaki Sauce, Textured Vegetable Protein (TVP), Udon, Wheat, Wheat Flour, Wheat Bran, Wheat Germ, Wheat Starch and Whole Wheat Flour.

Check out these Foods and Ingredients that may contain Gluten:

Bouillon, Broths, Dextrin, Baking Powder, Food Starch, Gravy Cubes, Maltose, Miso, Modified Food Starch, Mustard Powder, Processed Meats, Salad Dressing, Seasonings, Soba Noodles, Soup Bases, Soy Sauce, Starch, Stock Cubes, Tofu, and Vitamins.

Can't I just avoid products that list "Wheat" in the allergen statement?

Wheat is one of the eight major food allergens that must always be declared on food labels either in the list of ingredients or at the end of the list of ingredients in the allergen statement. Barley and rye, which also contain gluten, are not included in the eight major food allergens and although usually identified in the ingredient list, they are not required to be listed in the "allergen" statement. In addition, there are many derivatives of wheat, barley, and rye that have completely different names that are difficult to identify.

Tips for Gluten-Free Shopping

The good news is that all supermarkets carry gluten-free foods and beverages. You just need to identify the gluten-free products. The number and variety of gluten-free products may vary from store to store.

Check the Supermarket for Gluten-Free Information

Many supermarket chains provide some form of gluten-free information. Check to see if your supermarket has a Gluten-Free product list, a Gluten-Free aisle in the store, or Gluten-Free shelf tags. Check the store website or talk to the manager about gluten-free shopping tools available in the supermarket where you shop. Find a list of supermarkets and the gluten-free resources they provide on page 547.

Shop for Fresh Foods on a Gluten-Free Diet

Concentrate on buying fresh or whole foods that are naturally gluten-free. For example fresh fruit, vegetables, nuts, poultry, meat, and fish do not contain any gluten when they're unprocessed, so you can always buy these items knowing that they're safe.

Avoid Processed Foods

The more processed a food is, the greater the chance it contains gluten. Gluten-free foods often contain a thickening or stabilizing agent. Check the list of "Enjoy" and "Avoid" Gluten-Free ingredients on page xi. The food lists in this book will help you find processed foods that are gluten-free. If you are in doubt about any product, check the food manufacturers' website or call and ask specifically about the product. You can find manufacturers' contact information on the product package. Unfortunately, product formulations change occasionally so it is always a good idea to check for the most current information.

Look for Gluten-Free Labels

If you do decide to purchase processed products, look for labels that say "Gluten-Free." This is the best and safest way to ensure that a product contains no gluten. The "Gluten-Free" designation may be on the front of the package in bold print or provided by a Gluten-Free logo in an obscure spot like under the Nutrition Facts and Ingredient Statement. Your supermarket may also provide Gluten-Free shelf tags.

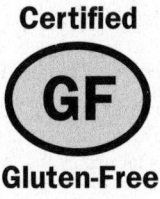

Certified

GF

Gluten-Free

Ask for Help to Find Gluten-Free Food

Ask for help from the store manager or clerks. Many are knowledgeable about gluten-free products. If a store doesn't carry something you really want, you can always ask if they would consider stocking it.

Buy Gluten-Free Grains as Substitutes

Know the names of gluten-free grains such as rice and rice flour, quinoa, and buck-wheat. When you first start eating a gluten-free diet, you might feel a bit restricted, but by adding these grains and grain-like foods into your diet, you'll really open up your options. You can also learn how to cook all your favorite foods using gluten-free grains. A gluten-free cookbook is a good investment and there are plenty of gluten-free recipes on food company websites.

Look for Sales on Gluten-Free Items

Don't forget to look online for non-perishable gluten-free items. Chances are, you'll find good deals on certain products and there's also the added bonus of being able to read other shopper's tips and reviews.

The Gluten-Free Kitchen

The goal of a gluten-free kitchen is to prevent cross-contamination where gluten-free food comes into contact with food that contains gluten. Unfortunately, there are many ways for cross-contamination to occur in your kitchen. Here are a few safety tips to help prevent cross-contamination:

Make sure all family members know about the Gluten-Free diet.

Everyone who uses the kitchen should be familiar with gluten-free guidelines to avoid cross-contamination.

Store Gluten-Free foods and flours away from Gluten-Containing foods.

Designate a gluten-free cupboard or shelf in the pantry and refrigerator.

Beware of sharing foods that could become contaminated with Gluten.

Don't spread crumbs in spreadable condiments such as jam, jelly, butter, margarine, mayonnaise, and peanut butter that are being shared. Purchase and label separate jars for use by the gluten intolerant individual(s) to avoid bread crumbs in shared jars.

Purchase a separate toaster.

Don't use the same toaster for gluten-free bread and regular bread. If you can only have one toaster, try to make it a toaster oven and get extra trays from the manufacturer or place aluminum foil on the rack to avoid contamination.

Clean countertops often to remove Gluten-Containing crumbs.

Don't prepare gluten-free foods on the same surface used to prepare foods with gluten unless the surface has been thoroughly cleaned.

Have separate cutting boards for wheat breads.

If possible, get a cutting board with a crumb-catcher underneath it, to limit the spread of gluten-containing crumbs. Wipe up any stray crumbs immediately.

Have separate sifters for Gluten-Free flours.

Handling wheat flour in a kitchen used to prepare gluten-free food is dangerous, as wheat flour can stay airborne for hours. If you must sift wheat flour, cover or remove all gluten-free food from the area.

Ideally, have separate cooking utensils, colanders, and pans.

Make sure utensils have been thoroughly cleaned after preparing gluten-containing foods. Even better, have separate sets of utensils for gluten-free food preparation and separate drawers and shelves to store them. Don't use the same sifter for gluten-free and regular flours. Clearly label the gluten-free sifter to avoid mistakes.

Gluten-Free & Healthy

Now that you know the basics of gluten-free living, you need to incorporate gluten-free foods into a healthy diet plan. Don't neglect other health needs while pursuing a gluten-free diet. Here are some basic tips that will help you choose healthy gluten-free foods. They are similar to general guidelines for any healthy eating plan.

Healthy Eating Tips

1. Think Variety

There are over 40 essential nutrients that you can only get from the foods you eat. Since each food contains only a few of these nutrients in limited amounts, you can see why eating a variety of foods is important. Not only do you need to eat foods from each of the food categories—grains, vegetables, fruits, dairy, proteins—but within each food category, you should eat a variety of foods. For instance, eating a rainbow of colors of fruits and vegetables will provide a variety of different nutrients—vitamins A, C, and other antioxidants. You can get all the nutrients you need in gluten-free foods.

2. Slash Sodium

The U.S. Dietary Guidelines for Americans and the American Heart Association recommend limiting sodium to less than 2,300 mg a day (the amount in 1 teaspoon of salt) for healthy adults and 1,500 mg per day for those who are sensitive to sodium's effects—individuals who have high blood pressure, are 40 years of age or older, or who are African-Americans. More than two-thirds of the adult population falls into one or more of these categories. Like all foods, gluten-free foods, especially processed foods, can be high in salt. It is important to be aware of the sodium content of all foods and choose those that are low in sodium.

3. Choose Healthy Fats

Research has shown that it is the type of fat, not the amount, that has the biggest effect on your health. Fats are necessary because they deliver essential fatty acids that your body can't manufacture, such as omega-3 fats. Also, certain vitamins are fat-soluble (vitamins A, D, E, and K), meaning they need fat to be digested and metabolized. However, fats are high in calories and should be enjoyed in moderation. The good fats are those that are poly or monounsaturated. The unhealthy fats include saturated and trans fats. Fats do not contain gluten, so choosing good-for-you fats is recommended.

4. Practice Portion Control

Eating gluten-free does not mean that you will lose weight. The calories in gluten-free foods and foods containing gluten are similar, so portion sizes matter. It is not just what you eat, but how much you eat that determines a healthy diet. Most people eat more than they need. Start by paying attention to the serving sizes recommended by the ChooseMyPlate program and those given in the Nutrition Facts on food labels. You may also want to measure foods and beverages with a scale, measuring cup, or spoon. Use the ChooseMyPlate recommendation to make half of your plate fruits and vegetables, a quarter of your plate gluten-free grains, and the final quarter protein. Use the suggested portion sizes given in this book to help you with portion control.

5. Go for Gluten-Free Whole Grains

The U.S. Dietary Guidelines recommend that you make half your grains whole. Research has shown that eating 2½ servings of grains per day is enough to lower your risk of heart disease. It appears that a greater whole grain intake is associated with reduced obesity, diabetes, high blood pressure, and high cholesterol. All grains contain three components—the germ, endosperm, and bran, but during processing one or more of these components are lost. The bran is full of fiber, while the germ and endosperm contain valuable phytonutrients. Eat the whole grain for the best nutrition. Gluten-free whole grains include brown rice, wild rice, corn, amaranth, millet, buckwheat, sorghum, teff, and quinoa.

6. Cut Added Sugar

We are drowning in sugar and the USDA recommends we get no more than 10 teaspoons a day—the average American downs about 34 teaspoons daily. In fact, the amount of sugar we eat and drink every year has soared nearly 30% since 1983 and is a major contributor to the soaring rates of overweight and obese Americans. Sugar often hides under several names and turns up in the most innocuous foods like bread, crackers, salad dressing, ketchup, and mustard—even gluten-free versions. Check the ingredient list on products for added sugars.

7. Go Fish

Seafood contains a variety of nutrients, most notably the omega-3 fatty acids EPA and DHA. The U.S. Dietary Guidelines recommend eating about 8 ounces of fish per week. Eating seafood contributes to the prevention of heart disease. Seafood varieties that are commonly consumed that are higher in EPE and DHA and lower in mercury include salmon, anchovies, herring, sardines, Pacific oysters, trout, and Atlantic and Pacific mackerel. All fresh fish and seafood is gluten-free unless it is breaded, marinated, or served with sauces that may not be gluten-free.

8. Use ChooseMyPlate

The U.S. Dietary Guidelines form the basis for the federal government's nutrition education program—ChooseMyPlate. This program uses a portioned plate logo to divide food choices into five food groups. This logo shows that half your plate should be fruits and vegetables, one quarter gluten-free grains, and the last quarter protein with a glass of milk. The ChooseMyPlate program provides recommended food plans, food lists, serving sizes, health benefits, nutrients, and tips for making wise choices. While ChooseMyPlate is intended for the general population, find suggestions in this book for eating gluten-free while following the USDA's food guidelines. Check out the healthy gluten-free recommendations, serving sizes, and tips throughout this book.

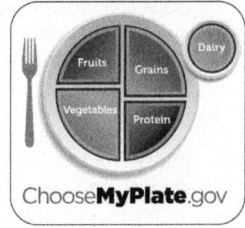

Choose**MyPlate**.gov

Healthy Shopping Tips

1. Shop with a List

Planning ahead is especially important not only for saving money, but for choosing gluten-free foods and healthy eating. Plan meals for a week at a time and keep a running grocery list in a central location where family members can add items as they are needed. Organize your list in categories based on the way you travel through the supermarket. If you are providing a mix of gluten-free and gluten-containing foods, you may find it useful to make separate lists.

2. Comparison Shop

Compare the prices of similar items. Most shelf tags have a total price and a price per unit that provides an easy way to compare apples to apples. Should you buy the bulk apples in a 3-lb bag for $4.99, or individual apples that are $0.99 each? Scan supermarket ads, circulars, and the internet for specials and coupons. Use coupons only for foods that are on your list.

3. Start on the Perimeter

Most gluten-free foods are fresh foods found on the perimeter of the supermarket—fresh fruits and vegetables; meats, poultry, and fish; and dairy products. This is where you can be assured of natural gluten-free nutrients without many preservatives or artificial ingredients. Some fresh items are in the interior—gluten-free grains and flours, rice, and nuts. Make the majority of your purchases from the perimeter before shopping the aisles.

4. Buy Seasonally and Locally

Seasonal and locally grown products are usually cheaper and healthier. They maintain more nutrients because they have not traveled as far from their origins to the store. They are cheaper because there are more available. Stay attuned to the season so that you can purchase fruits and vegetables that are the most economical, the freshest, and the cheapest. When produce is not in season, buy gluten-free canned or frozen versions without sauces and/or added salt.

5. Buy in Bulk

Buying foods in bulk can often save you money, but only if you can use the larger amount. Packaging costs money, so the less packaging the more you save. For instance, steel-cut oats in bulk are $0.89 a pound, while a tin runs $3.35 a pound. Other items you can save on by buying in bulk are gluten-free grains, lentils, dried beans, and rice. Check out the unit price to see how much you could save by buying the larger size.

6. Read Labels and Ingredient Lists

First look for a "Gluten-Free" certification logo or claim. You may also see claims like "Healthy," "Natural," and "Contains" on the front of a package, but the back or side of the package will give you the real scoop. Check out the Nutrition Facts box that gives you the amount of individual nutrients. Compare these nutrients between products to see which is healthier. Look for low amounts for calories, total fat, saturated fat, cholesterol, sodium, and sugar. Look for higher levels of protein, vitamins, and minerals. Read the Ingredient List to check for gluten-free ingredients and the allergen statement for wheat. Also check for other unhealthy terms like partially hydrogenated fats (that means trans fats) and added sugars.

7. Understand Health & Nutrition Claims

You'll find a variety of health and nutrition claims on labels. These can be a help to those who need to find foods that are heart healthy or low in sodium. But be sure to check the Nutrition Facts numbers to make sure the food fits into your diet plan.

8. Store Brands vs. National Brands

Some supermarket chains have gluten-free store brands that are usually cheaper than national brands. It used to be that store brands were cheaper and lower quality versions of national brands. Now, store brands are quality lines of products that can save you money. Statistics say that store brands can save 30% over nationally branded products. In some supermarkets, store brands account for as much as 35% of total sales. Check out the store brands and compare them to their national counterparts.

What Does "Healthy" Mean?

Food labeling allows manufacturers to make a "healthy" claim on a food or beverage label if it meets specific nutrient criteria. "Healthy" does not mean "gluten-free," just as "gluten-free" does not mean "healthy." The basic requirements for a "healthy" claim are:

- Low in fat (3g or less, or 30% or less fat calories)
- Low in sodium: 140 mg or less except for meal-type products (6 oz or more) that require 360 mg for individual foods and 480 mg for meal-type foods
- 10% or more of at least one of the following:

• Vitamin A	• Iron	• Protein
• Vitamin C	• Calcium	• Fiber

How To Use This Book

This book can help you plan your gluten-free menus and make a shopping list of healthy, gluten-free foods.

- Read the Gluten-Free Tips and ChooseMyPlate recommendations for each food category for number of servings, serving sizes, and recommended foods. The servings given are for an adult consuming 2,000 calories per day. For a personalized food plan based on your age, sex, weight, and activity level, go to *www.ChooseMyPlate.gov.*

- Make your shopping list of gluten-free foods by multiplying the number of people in your family by the recommended number of servings.

- Check the list of gluten-free foods in each category provided in this book and choose a variety of items.

- Compare nutrients within categories for the best food choices for positive nutrients, such as protein, fiber, calcium, vitamins, and minerals. Also check nutrients for foods with negative nutrients, such as total fat, saturated fat, cholesterol, and sodium.

- Read the Gluten-Free Shopping Tips and Shopping List Essentials for each category and include these suggestions into your meal planning and shopping list.

- Highlight the foods that are presently in your food plan and use a different color highlighter for the foods you want to try. Make a goal to try a new gluten-free food each week. Remember that variety is important for healthy eating.

- Take this book to the supermarket to find gluten-free foods and for a quick check on the nutrients in foods that may not have Nutrition Facts—fruits, vegetables, bulk items, meat, poultry, and fish.

Using Nutrition Facts

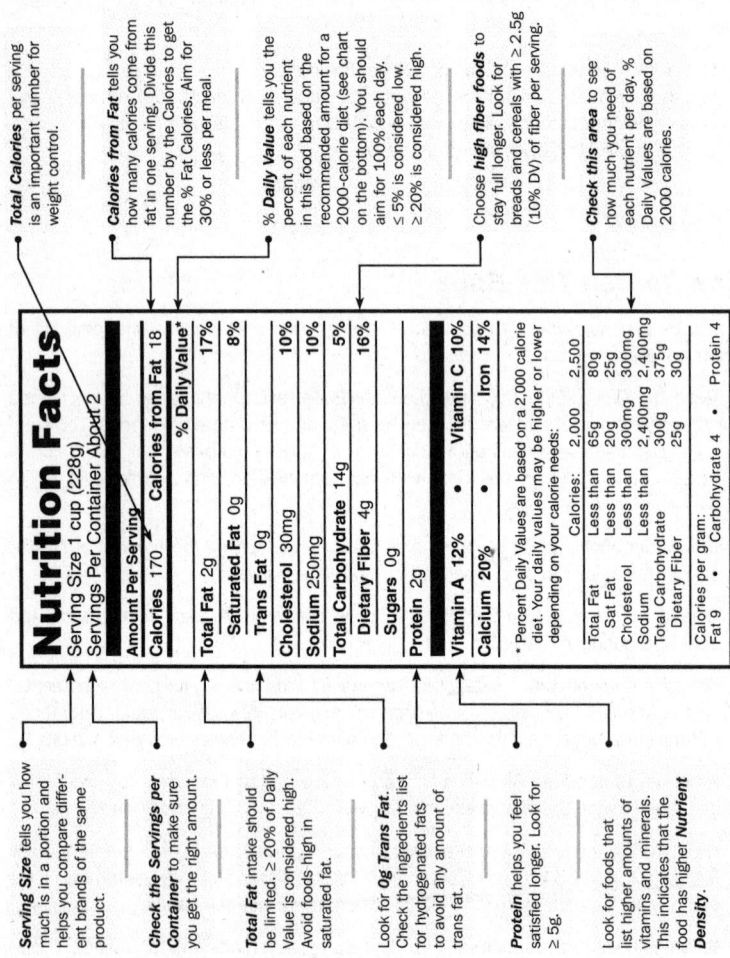

Total Calories per serving is an important number for weight control.

Calories from Fat tells you how many calories come from fat in one serving. Divide this number by the Calories to get the % Fat Calories. Aim for 30% or less per meal.

% **Daily Value** tells you the percent of each nutrient in this food based on the recommended amount for a 2000-calorie diet (see chart on the bottom). You should aim for 100% each day. ≤ 5% is considered low. ≥ 20% is considered high.

Choose **high fiber foods** to stay full longer. Look for breads and cereals with ≥ 2.5g (10% DV) of fiber per serving.

Check this area to see how much you need of each nutrient per day. % Daily Values are based on 2000 calories.

Serving Size tells you how much is in a portion and helps you compare different brands of the same product.

Check the Servings per Container to make sure you get the right amount.

Total Fat intake should be limited. ≥ 20% of Daily Value is considered high. Avoid foods high in saturated fat.

Look for **0g Trans Fat**. Check the ingredients list for hydrogenated fats to avoid any amount of trans fat.

Protein helps you feel satisfied longer. Look for ≥ 5g.

Look for foods that list higher amounts of vitamins and minerals. This indicates that the food has higher **Nutrient Density**.

Nutrition Facts

Serving Size 1 cup (228g)
Servings Per Container About 2

Amount Per Serving

Calories 170   Calories from Fat 18

	% Daily Value*
Total Fat 2g	17%
Saturated Fat 0g	8%
Trans Fat 0g	
Cholesterol 30mg	10%
Sodium 250mg	10%
Total Carbohydrate 14g	5%
Dietary Fiber 4g	16%
Sugars 0g	
Protein 2g	

Vitamin A 12%	•	Vitamin C 10%	
Calcium 20%	•	Iron 14%	

* Percent Daily Values are based on a 2,000 calorie diet. Your daily values may be higher or lower depending on your calorie needs:

	Calories:	2,000	2,500
Total Fat	Less than	65g	80g
Sat Fat	Less than	20g	25g
Cholesterol	Less than	300mg	300mg
Sodium	Less than	2,400mg	2,400mg
Total Carbohydrate		300g	375g
Dietary Fiber		25g	30g

Calories per gram:
Fat 9 • Carbohydrate 4 • Protein 4

©2011 Linda McDonald Associates, Inc., dba, SUPERMARKET SAVVY®, Houston, TX 77042, www.supermarketsavvy.com

ChooseMyPlate Key Messages

Take action on the Dietary Guidelines by making changes in these three areas. Choose steps that work for you and start today.

Balancing Calories

- Enjoy your food, but eat less.
- Avoid oversized portions.

Foods to Increase

- Make half your plate fruits and vegetables.
- Switch to fat-free or low-fat (1%) milk.
- Make at least half of your grains gluten-free whole grains.

Foods to Reduce

- Compare sodium in foods like soup, bread, and frozen meals—and choose foods with lower numbers.
- Drink water instead of sugary drinks.

Go to *ChooseMyPlate.gov* for a personalized food plan based on your age, sex, weight, and activity level. Find food lists and specific serving size photos.

Ideal Weight Chart

Height	Ideal Male Weight	Ideal Female Weight
4'6"	63–77 lbs.	63–77 lbs.
4'7"	68–84 lbs.	68–83 lbs.
4'8"	74–90 lbs.	72–88 lbs.
4'9"	79–97 lbs.	77–94 lbs.
4'10"	85–103 lbs.	81–99 lbs.
4'11"	90–110 lbs.	86–105 lbs.
5'0"	95–117 lbs.	90–110 lbs.
5'1"	101-123 lbs.	95–116 lbs.
5'2"	106–130 lbs.	99–121 lbs.
5'3"	112–136 lbs.	104–127 lbs.
5'4"	117–143 lbs.	108–132 lbs.
5'5"	122–150 lbs.	113–138 lbs.
5'6"	128–156 lbs.	117–143 lbs.
5'7"	133–163 lbs.	122–149 lbs.
5' 8"	139–169 lbs.	126–154 lbs.
5' 9"	144–176 lbs.	131–160 lbs.
5'10"	149–183 lbs.	135–165 lbs.
5'11"	155–189 lbs.	140-171 lbs.
6'0"	160–196 lbs.	144–176 lbs.
6'1"	166–202 lbs.	149–182 lbs.
6'2"	171–209 lbs.	153–187 lbs.
6'3"	176–216 lbs.	158–193 lbs.
6'4"	182–222 lbs.	162–198 lbs.
6'5"	187–229 lbs.	167–204 lbs.
6'6"	193–235 lbs.	171–209 lbs.
6'7"	198–242 lbs.	176–215 lbs.
6'8"	203–249 lbs.	180–220 lbs.
6'9"	209–255 lbs.	185–226 lbs.
6'10"	214–262 lbs.	189–231 lbs.
6'11"	220–268 lbs.	194–237 lbs.
7'0"	225–275 lbs.	198–242 lbs.

Grains & Grain-Based Foods

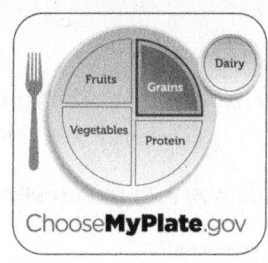

ChooseMyPlate.gov

Why Eat Grains?

Grains are important sources of many nutrients, including dietary fiber, several B vitamins (thiamin, riboflavin, niacin, and folate), and minerals (iron, magnesium, and selenium). Eating gluten-free whole grains as part of a healthy diet may reduce the risk of heart disease and help with weight management. Additionally, consuming foods containing fiber, such as whole grains, may reduce constipation and diverticulitis. B vitamins play a role in metabolism and are essential for a healthy nervous system. Folate (folic acid), a B vitamin, is important before and during pregnancy because it helps prevent birth defects.

Daily Goal

Six one-ounce servings for an adult on a 2000 calorie diet.
Forty-eight grams of gluten-free whole grains.
One-ounce equivalents:
   1 slice gluten-free bread
   1 cup gluten-free dry cereal
   ½ cup cooked rice or gluten-free pasta
   1 six-inch gluten-free tortilla

Gluten-Free Shopping Tips

- Make at least half your grains gluten-free whole grains—amaranth, buckwheat, corn, brown rice, wild rice, sorghum, teff, millet, quinoa, and oats* (must be designated gluten-free).
- Look for a gluten-free whole grain as the first ingredient—brown rice, oatmeal*, and corn meal are examples of gluten-free whole grains.
- Substitute gluten-free whole grain flour for up to half of regular gluten-free flour in baking.

Gluten-Free Shopping List Essentials

Gluten-Free Whole Grain Bread
Brown Rice
Wild Rice
Gluten-Free Whole Grain Flour
Gluten-Free Whole Grain Pasta (quinoa, brown rice)
Gluten-Free Whole Grain Cereal (oatmeal, corn, brown rice)

Oatmeal* (must be designated gluten-free)
Gluten-Free Whole Grain Crackers

Grain Foods Allowed and Those to Avoid on a Gluten-Free Diet

BREADS AND BAKED PRODUCTS

Gluten-Free

Items made with amaranth, arrowroot, buckwheat, corn bran, corn flour, corn-meal, cornstarch, flax, legume flours (bean, garbanzo or chickpea, lentil, pea), mesquite flour, millet, nut flours (almond, chestnut, hazelnut), potato flour, potato starch, and pure oat products*, quinoa, rice bran, rice flours (brown, glutinous, sweet, white), rice polish, sago, sorghum flour, soy flour, sweet potato flour, tapioca (cassava, manioc), taro, and teff.

Contain Gluten

Items made with wheat bran, wheat farina, wheat flour, wheat germ, wheat-based semolina, wheat starch, durum flour, gluten flour, graham flour, atta, bulgur, einkorn, emmer, farro (faro), kamut, spelt, barley, rye, triticale, and commercial oat products* (e.g., oat bran, oat flour, oat groats, oatmeal, and steel cut).

CEREALS — COLD

Gluten-Free

- Puffed or flaked amaranth, buckwheat, corn, millet, or rice.
- Rice crisps or corn flakes with no barley malt extract or barley malt flavoring.
- Rice flakes and soy cereal.

Contain Gluten

Cereal made with wheat or added barley malt extract or barley malt flavoring.

CEREALS — HOT

Gluten-Free

Cereal made with amaranth seed, cornmeal, cream of buckwheat, cream of rice (brown, white), hominy grits, pure oatmeal*, quinoa, rice flakes, soy flakes, and soy grits.

Contain Gluten

Cereals made from wheat, rye, triticale, barley and commercial oats*.

PASTAS

Gluten-Free

Macaroni, spaghetti, and noodles from beans, corn, lentils, peas, potato, quinoa, rice, soy, and wild rice.

Contain Gluten

Pastas made from wheat, wheat starch, and other ingredients not allowed (e.g., orzo).

RICE

Gluten-Free

Plain (e.g., basmati, brown, jasmine, white, wild).

Contain Gluten

Seasoned or flavored rice mixes.

Caution

*Oats are a gluten-free grain but because oats can be contaminated with gluten containing grains, you should not include oats in a gluten-free diet unless you are assured that they are gluten-free. Contamination can happen in the field, when oats are grown side-by-side with fields of wheat, or oats are often processed in facilities that also process wheat, barley, and rye. Look for oat products that claim "Gluten-Free."

"Corn starch" and "white rice" are not whole grains. If a product claims "whole grain" or sounds like it is made with whole grains, look for the amount of whole grains on the label or this Whole Grain Logo found on many, but not all, whole grain foods.

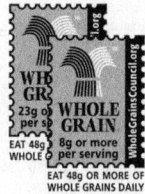

THE BASIC STAMP   THE 100% STAMP

Food Serving size	Cal.	(g) Total Fat	(g) Sat. Fat	(mg) Chol.	(g) Carb.	(g) Fiber	(g) Sug.	(g) Prot.	(mg) Sod.

Baked Products (Including Mixes and Refrigerated Dough)

Food Serving size	Cal.	Total Fat	Sat. Fat	Chol.	Carb.	Fiber	Sug.	Prot.	Sod.
1-2-3 Gluten Free, Buckwheat Pancake Mix 1/3 cup	150	0.5	0	0	35	0	6	2	840
1-2-3 Gluten Free, Sugar and Spice Pan Bars Mix 21.5g	80	0	0	0	20	0	12	0	160
Against the Grain, Gourmet Pesto Pizza 2 slices	475	30	8	98	33	<1	0	19	421
Against the Grain, Gourmet Pizza Shell 1 slice	158	2	5	37	17	1	0	3	110
Aleia's Gluten-Free Bakery, Classic Croutons 1/2 oz	80	4	1	15	10	1	2	1	55
Aleia's Gluten-Free Bakery, Italian Bread Crumbs 12 oz	60	2	0	10	9	1	2	1	70
Aleia's Gluten-Free Bakery, Original Real Panko 1/2 oz	35	0.5	0	0	7	1	1	1	65
Aleia's Gluten-Free Bakery, Parmesan Croutons 7g	60	3	0.5	10	6	1	1	1	35
Aleia's Gluten-Free Bakery, Plain Bread Crumbs 1/2 oz	60	2	0	10	10	1	2	1	55
Aleia's Gluten-Free Bakery, Plain Stuffing 1/2 oz	80	2.5	0	10	12	2	2	2	65
Aleia's Gluten-Free Bakery, Savory Stuffing 1/2 oz	80	2.5	0	10	12	2	2	2	75
Aleia's Gluten-Free Bakery, Sea Salt & Pepper Panko 1/2 oz	35	0.5	0	0	7	1	1	1	190
Amy's, Chocolate Cake 1.83 oz	190	6	0.5	0	26	1	15	2	200
Amy's, Gluten-Free Pound Cake 11 oz	180	7	3	15	27	1	14	2	230
Amy's, Gluten-Free Sandwich Rounds 1 round	90	4	0	0	13	1	1	2	135
Arrowhead Mills, Bake With Me Gluten-Free Chocolate Cupcake Mix, Prepared 1 cupcake	180	1	0	0	27	2	11	2	120

Food Serving size	Cal.	(g) Total Fat	(g) Sat. Fat	(mg) Chol.	(g) Carb.	(g) Fiber	(g) Sug.	(g) Prot.	(mg) Sod.
Arrowhead Mills, Bake With Me Gluten-Free Vanilla Cupcake Mix, Prepared									
1 cupcake	180	0	0	0	27	1	10	2	110
Arrowhead Mills, Gluten-Free All Purpose Baking Mix									
1/4 cup	140	0.5	0	0	32	<1	0	2	350
Arrowhead Mills, Gluten-Free Brownie Mix, Prepared									
1/20 of package	160	2	1.5	0	21	<1	13	1	40
Arrowhead Mills, Gluten-Free Chocolate Cake Mix									
1/12 cake	280	1	0	0	42	3	21	3	190
Arrowhead Mills, Gluten-Free Chocolate Chip Cookie Mix									
1 cookie	110	1	0.5	0	16	<1	8	<1	60
Arrowhead Mills, Gluten-Free Pizza Crust Mix, Prepared									
1 slice	150	0.5	0	0	33	<1	2	3	240
Arrowhead Mills, Gluten-Free Vanilla Cake Mix									
1/12 cake	180	0	0	0	41	0	17	2	170
Arrowhead Mills, Organic Gluten-Free Pancake and Baking Mix, Prepared									
1/4 cup	240	0	0	0	36	0	1	2	290
Authentic Foods, Gluten-Free Pancake and Baking Mix									
1/4 cup	130	1.5	0	0	24	2	1	5	170
Barkat, White Rice Gluten-Free Pizza Crust, 1 Per Pack									
1 crust	NA	4	0.4	NA	43.6	1.3	1.1	2	0.5
Better Batter, Gluten-Free Yellow Cake Mix									
1/12 dry mix	160	0	0	0	38	1	23	1	270
Betty Crocker, Bisquick Pancake and Baking Mix – Gluten Free									
1/3 cup	140	0.5	0	0	31	1	3	2	340
Betty Crocker, Bisquick, Gluten-Free									
1/3 cup	140	0.5	0	0	31	<1	3	2	340
Betty Crocker, Dessert Mixes, Gluten-Free Brownie Mix, Prepared									
1/16 package	150	2	1	0	24	1	18	1	60
Betty Crocker, Dessert Mixes, Gluten-Free Devil's Food Cake Mix									
1/10 pkg	160	1	0.5	0	36	1	20	1	240
Betty Crocker, Dessert Mixes, Gluten-Free Yellow Cake Mix									
1/10 pkg	150	0	0	0	37	0	17	1	230
Bob's Red Mill, Biscuit Mix, Prepared									
1 biscuit	180	1	0	0	21	1	0	3	450

Food Serving size	Cal.	(g) Total Fat	(g) Sat. Fat	(mg) Chol.	(g) Carb.	(g) Fiber	(g) Sug.	(g) Prot.	(mg) Sod.
Bob's Red Mill, Brownie Mix, Prepared									
1 brownie	180	0.5	0	0	27	2	17	2	180
Bob's Red Mill, Chocolate Cake Mix									
1/16 package, baked	170	0.5	0	0	24	2	12	2	85
Bob's Red Mill, Cinnamon Raisin Bread Mix									
1/17 of package, baked	190	1.5	0	0	29	2	1	2	230
Bob's Red Mill, Cornbread Mix									
1/16 package, baked	180	0.5	0	0	28	2	4	2	270
Bob's Red Mill, Pancake Mix, Prepared									
2 4″ pancakes	190	0.5	0	0	32	2	3	2	540
Bob's Red Mill, Pizza Crust Mix, Prepared									
1 slice	250	1	0	0	45	4	2	3	370
Bob's Red Mill, Vanilla Cake Mix, Prepared									
1/16th of package	190	0	0	0	29	0	16	0	180
Canyon Bakehouse, Cranberry Crunch Muffins									
1 muffin	380	18	2.5	30	52	2	19	4	250
Cause You're Special, Gluten-Free Famous Pizza Crust Mix (Small Size)									
1 crust	130	0.3	0.1	0	31	1	2	1	231
Cause You're Special, Gluten-Free Hearty Biscuit Mix (Small Size)									
2 biscuits	147	0.3	0.1	0	34	1	4	2	470
Cause You're Special, Gluten-Free Hearty Pancake and Waffle Mix, Dry									
1/4 cup	138	0.3	0.1	0	32	1	3	2	401
Cause You're Special, Gluten-Free Homestyle Pie Crust Mix									
1 slice	163	0.4	NA	0	37	1.3	1.5	3	301
Cause You're Special, Gluten-Free Homestyle Pie Crust Mix, Prepared 9" Crust									
1/8 of crust	82	0.2	0.1	0	19	1	1	1	150
Cause You're Special, Gluten-Free Sweet Corn Muffin Mix									
3 tbsp	127	0.4	0	0	29	1	10	2	314
Chatila's Bakery, Apple Pie (sweetened with Agave nector)									
1 slice	90	1	0	0	20	2	3	1	170
Chatila's Bakery, Blueberry Pie (sweetened with Agave nector)									
1 slice	90	1	0	0	20	3	4	1	150
Chatila's Bakery, Brownie (sweetened with Agave nector)									
2 brownies	110	6	1	35	12	3	4	3	15

Food Serving size	Cal.	(g) Total Fat	(g) Sat. Fat	(mg) Chol.	(g) Carb.	(g) Fiber	(g) Sug.	(g) Prot.	(mg) Sod.
Chatila's Bakery, Chocolate E'toile									
2.5 oz (75g)	110	5	2	20	27	2	0	1	0
Chatila's Bakery, Chocolate Swiss Roll									
85g	140	3.5	1.5	40	19	10	0	13	150
Chatila's Bakery, Chocolate with Chocolate Cream Donut									
1 donut	110	3.5	0.4	0	23	6	0	8	20
Chatila's Bakery, Chocolate with Vanilla Cream Donut									
1 donut	110	3.5	0.4	0	23	6	0	8	20
Chatila's Bakery, Cinnamon Roll (sweetened with Agave nectar)									
100g	220	9	2	30	30	2	4	6	200
Chatila's Bakery, Coconut Truffle									
125g	160	2.5	2	0	41	13	1	12	105
Chatila's Bakery, French Napoleon (sweetened with Agave nectar)									
70g	190	112	2.5	0	20	1	4	2	95
Chatila's Bakery, Gluten-Free Swiss Roll									
105g	120	0.5	0	35	30	2	1	8	95
Chatila's Bakery, Mini Éclair (2)									
30g	50	3.5	0.5	25	4	0	<1	1	15
Chatila's Bakery, New Generation Blueberry Muffin									
1 muffin	90	2	0	0	18	2	>1	7	10
Chatila's Bakery, New Generation Chocolate Chip Muffin									
1 muffin	90	2	0	0	14	3	>1	7	10
Chatila's Bakery, New Generation Double Chocolate Muffin									
1 muffin	80	2.5	0	0	12	4	>1	6	15
Chatila's Bakery, New Generation Lemon Poppy Muffin									
1 muffin	80	2.5	0	0	11	3	>1	6	15
Chatila's Bakery, New Generation Oat Bran Muffin									
1 muffin	90	2.5	0	0	12	3	>1	7	15
Chatila's Bakery, New Generation Peanut Chip Muffin									
1 muffin	90	2.5	0	0	15	3	>1	6	10
Chatila's Bakery, New Generation Pistachio Muffin									
1 muffin	80	2.5	0	0	11	3	>1	7	10
Chatila's Bakery, New Generation Pumpkin Muffin									
1 muffin	80	2.5	0	0	11	3	>1	7	15

Food Serving size	Cal.	(g) Total Fat	(g) Sat. Fat	(mg) Chol.	(g) Carb.	(g) Fiber	(g) Sug.	(g) Prot.	(mg) Sod.
Chatila's Bakery, Original Blueberry Muffin									
1 muffin	130	3	0	10	28	4	1	4	75
Chatila's Bakery, Original Corn Muffin									
1 muffin	140	2.5	0	25	32	3	0	4	220
Chatila's Bakery, Pumpkin Pie (sweetened with Agave nector)									
1 slice	130	6	1.5	35	18	3	3	3	200
Chatila's Bakery, Pumpkin Swiss Roll									
85g	130	3.5	1.5	40	19	7	0	12	130
Chatila's Bakery, Vanilla Swiss Roll									
110g	140	5	1	45	19	5	0	14	90
Chatila's Bakery, Vanilla with Chocolate Cream Donut									
1 serving	110	3	0.4	0	23	6	0	8	20
Chatila's Bakery, Vanilla with Vanilla Cream Donut									
1 serving	110	3	0.4	0	23	6	0	8	20
Chatila's Bakery, Whoopie Pie (sweetened with Agave nector)									
80g	80	0.5	0	10	15	1	3	3	105
Chebe, All-Purpose Dry Bread Mix									
21g	70	0	0	0	17	0	0	0	140
Chebe, Breadsticks Frozen Dough									
2 oz	167	6	1.5	17	25	0	<1	3	280
Chebe, Ciabatta Rolls Frozen Dough									
3 oz	250	9	2.5	26	37	0	<1	4	416
Chebe, Dry Focaccia Mix									
21g	70	0	0	0	17	0	0	0	150
Chebe, Garlic-Onion Dry Breadstick Mix, Gluten-Free									
21g	70	0	0	0	17	0	0	0	103
Chebe, Gluten-Free All-Purpose Bread Mix, Dry									
.75 oz	70	0	0	0	17	0	0	0	140
Chebe, Gluten-Free Cinnamon Roll Mix, Dry									
1.5 tbsp	70	0	0	0	18	0	3	0	110
Chebe, Gluten-Free Focaccia Bread Mix, Dry									
.75 oz	70	0	0	0	17	0	0	0	150
Chebe, Gluten-Free Frozen Pizza Crust									
2 slices	209	8	2	22	31	0	0	4	347

Food Serving size	Cal.	(g) Total Fat	(g) Sat. Fat	(mg) Chol.	(g) Carb.	(g) Fiber	(g) Sug.	(g) Prot.	(mg) Sod.
Chebe, Gluten-Free Garlic-Onion Breadstick Mix, Dry									
.75 oz	70	0	0	0	17	0	0	0	103
Chebe, Gluten-Free Original Cheese Bread Mix, Dry									
.75 oz	70	0	0	0	17	0	0	0	103
Chebe, Gluten-Free Pizza Crust Mix, Dry									
.75 oz	70	0	0	0	17	0	0	0	103
Chebe, Original Cheese Dry Bread Mix									
21g	70	0	0	0	17	0	0	0	103
Chebe, Original Cheese Rolls Frozen Dough									
2 oz	167	6	1.5	17	25	0	<1	3	280
Chebe, Pizza Crust Frozen Dough									
2 oz	167	6	1.5	17	25	0	<1	3	280
Chebe, Pizza Dry Crust Mix									
21g	70	0	0	0	17	0	0	0	103
Chebe, Tomato-Basil Breadsticks Frozen Dough									
2 oz	167	6	1.5	17	25	0	<1	3	280
Cherrybrook Kitchen, Chocolate Cake Mix									
1/8 of cake	190	0.5	0	0	47	2	25	1	220
Cherrybrook Kitchen, Chocolate Chip Pancake Mix									
1/8 cup	90	1.5	1	0	19	0	5	1	230
Cherrybrook Kitchen, Fudge Brownie Mix									
1 brownie	140	3	1.5	0	30	2	16	2	170
Cherrybrook Kitchen, Pancake Mix									
1 4" pancake	80	0	0	0	19	0	4	1	210
Cherrybrook Kitchen, Yellow Cake Mix									
1/4 cup dry mix	210	0	0	0	50	0	23	2	240
Cravings Place, Gluten-Free Crumble Coffeecake & Scone Mix									
42g	160	0.5	0	0	36	1	18	2	60
Cravings Place, Gluten-Free Grandma's Unsweetened Cornbread Mix									
22g	80	0	0	0	16	0	0	0	220
Cravings Place, Gluten-Free Pancake and Waffle Mix									
23g	70	0	0	0	17	1	0	0	300
Cravings Place, Gluten-Free Quick Bread and Muffin Mix									
29g	100	0.5	0	0	21	1	0	2	350

Food Serving size	Cal.	(g) Total Fat	(g) Sat. Fat	(mg) Chol.	(g) Carb.	(g) Fiber	(g) Sug.	(g) Prot.	(mg) Sod.
Ener-G, Bread Crumbs 1/4 cup	140	6	0.5	0	21	4	1	1	210
Ener-G, Brownies 1 piece	130	7	0	0	22	1	13	1	45
Ener-G, Corn Mix 1/4 cup	110	0.5	0	0	24	1	0	3	135
Ener-G, Focaccia Crust 1/2 crust	110	5	0	0	14	3	1	1	160
Ener-G, Plain Croutons 1 tbsp	25	1	0	0	3	0	0	0	25
Ener-G, Plain Doughnut Holes 1 doughnut hole	35	1.5	0.5	10	5	1	4	1	75
Ener-G, Plain Doughnuts 1 donut	90	3.5	1.5	25	14	3	10	4	210
Ener-G, Poundcake 1 piece	150	9	0.5	35	23	1	13	2	150
Ener-G, Rice Pizza Shells, 10" Crust 1/8 crust	70	3.5	0	0	9	2	1	0	105
Ener-G, Rice Pizza Shells, 6" Crust 1/4 crust	60	3	0	0	7	1	1	0	85
Ener-G, Yeast-Free Rice Pizza Shells, 10" Crust 1/8 crust	80	3	0	0	12	2	0	1	160
Ener-G, Yeast-Free Rice Pizza Shells, 6" Crust 1/4 crust	60	2.5	0	0	10	1	0	1	115
French Meadow, Chocolate Cupcakes 1 cupcake	220	8	4.5	20	35	1	27	2	240
French Meadow, Fudge Brownie 1 brownie	170	8	1	30	24	1	17	1	120
French Meadow, Gluten-Free Pizza Crust 1/3 pizza crust	130	3	0.5	10	23	1	1	1	220
French Meadow, Yellow Cupcakes 1 cupcake	230	9	5	20	35	0	28	2	230

Food Serving size	Cal.	(g) Total Fat	(g) Sat. Fat	(mg) Chol.	(g) Carb.	(g) Fiber	(g) Sug.	(g) Prot.	(mg) Sod.
Gilbert's Gourmet Goodies, Chocolate Brownie									
40g	180	10	4	30	21	<1	11	2	10
Gillian's Foods, Gluten-Free Plain Bread Crumbs									
1/4 cup	60	0	0	0	12	0	0	1	30
Gillian's Foods, Italian Gluten-Free Bread Crumbs									
1/4 cup	60	0.5	0	0	14	1	1	2	290
Gluten-Free Naturals, Pizzeria-Style Pizza Crust Mix, Prepared									
1/8 slice prepared	150	0	0	0	26	1	2	3	300
Gluten-Free Pantry, Chocolate Truffle Brownie Mix, Dry									
3 tbsp	150	2.5	1.5	0	31	2	23	1	70
Gluten-Free Pantry, Favorite Sandwich Bread Mix, Dry									
3 tbsp	110	0	0	0	24	0	5	3	150
Gluten-Free Pantry, French Bread and Pizza Mix									
3 tbsp	110	0	0	0	25	0	0	1	125
Gluten-Free Pantry, Old Fashioned Cake and Cookie Mix									
3 tbsp	130	0	0	0	32	0	14	1	90
Gluten-Free Pantry, Perfect Pie Crust Mix									
4 tbsp	130	0	0	0	29	1	0	2	150
Gluten-Free Pantry, Yankee Cornbread and Muffin Mix									
3 tbsp	130	0	0	0	30	1	0	3	115
Gluten-Free Naturals, Cornbread & Corn Muffin Mix, Prepared									
1/10 slice cornbread	150	0	0	0	20	<1	3	2	230
Gluten-Free Naturals, Homemade Brownie Mix, Prepared									
1 brownie	160	0	0	0	22	1	16	<1	100
Gluten-Free Naturals, Pancake Mix, Prepared									
3/4″ pancakes	210	0.5	0	0	29	2	2	4	370
Gluten-Free Naturals, Yellow Cake Mix, Prepared									
1/6 cake	310	0.5	0	0	44	1	27	3	350
Glutino, Bread & Pizza Mix, Dry									
3 tbsp	110	0	0	0	25	<1	0	1	125
Glutino, Brown Rice Pancake & Waffle Mix									
2.5 tbsp	130	1	0	5	29	0	4	3	280

Food Serving size	Cal.	(g) Total Fat	(g) Sat. Fat	(mg) Chol.	(g) Carb.	(g) Fiber	(g) Sug.	(g) Prot.	(mg) Sod.
Glutino, Chocolate Chip Cookie & Cake Mix									
2 tbsp	120	2	1	0	25	<1	14	1	80
Glutino, Chocolate Truffle Brownie Mix									
3 tbsp	130	2.5	1.5	0	31	1	23	1	70
Glutino, Decadent Chocolate Cake Mix									
3 tbsp	130	1	0.5	0	36	0	19	2	100
Glutino, Gluten-Free Bread Crumbs									
1/3 cup	110	0	0	0	25	0	3	3	135
Glutino, Gluten-Free Glazed Chocolate Donuts									
1 donut	180	8	3.5	20	25	2	11	3	180
Glutino, Gluten-Free Glazed Original Donuts									
1 donut	180	7	3	30	26	0	12	3	190
Glutino, Muffin & Scone Mix, Dry									
2.5 tbsp	100	0	0	0	24	0	7	1	190
Glutino, Old Fashioned Cake & Cookie Mix, Dry									
3 tbsp	130	0	0	0	32	0	14	1	90
Glutino, Perfect Pie Crust, Dry Mix									
4 tbsp	130	0	0	0	29	<1	0	2	150
Glutino, Premium Pizza Crusts									
1 crust	270	4.5	0	0	56	3	2	1	550
Glutino, Yankee Cornbread & Muffin Mix, Dry									
3 tbsp	130	0	0	0	30	0	12	3	320
Goldbaum's, Gluten-Free Cup Ice Cream Cones									
1 cone	14	0	0	0	4	0	0	0	7
Goldbaum's, Gluten-Free Sugar Cocoa Ice Cream Cones									
1 cone	45	0.42	0.18	0	10.2	0	3.2	0	29
Goldbaum's, Gluten-Free Sugar Ice Cream Cones									
1 cone	11	0	0	0	9	0	3	0	27
Hain Pure Foods, Gluten-Free Featherweight Baking Powder									
1/8 tsp	0	0	NA	NA	0	NA	NA	0	0
Hodgson Mill, Gluten-Free Apple Cinnamon Muffin Mix with Milled Flax Seed									
1/4 cup	120	2	0	0	26	3	5	3	215
Hodgson Mill, Gluten-Free Bread Mix									
1/4 cup dry	120	1	0	0	26	2	3	2	135

Food Serving size	Cal.	(g) Total Fat	(g) Sat. Fat	(mg) Chol.	(g) Carb.	(g) Fiber	(g) Sug.	(g) Prot.	(mg) Sod.
Hodgson Mill, Gluten-Free Brownie Mix									
28g	100	0.5	0	0	24	1.7	13	1	106
Hodgson Mill, Gluten-Free Chocolate Cake Mix									
43g	153	1	1	0	35	2.5	16	3	197
Hodgson Mill, Gluten-Free Multi Purpose Baking Mix, Dry									
1/4 cup	100	1	0	0	22	3	0	3	0
Hodgson Mill, Gluten-Free Pancake & Waffle Mix with Flaxseed, Dry									
1/3 cup	140	2	1	0	30	3	0	4	200
Hodgson Mill, Gluten-Free Pizza Crust Mix									
57g	192	1	0.5	0	45	1.7	1	3	228
Hodgson Mill, Gluten-Free Seasoned Coating Mix, Dry, 10 oz.									
4 tsp	45	0	0	0	10	<1	1	1	490
Hodgson Mill, Gluten-Free Sweet Yellow Cornbread Mix, 12 oz.									
3 tbsp	100	0	0	0	25	<1	4	1	300
Hodgson Mill, Gluten-Free Yellow Cake Mix									
43g	160	0	0	0	38	0	15	2	185
Homestead Gluten Free, Soft 'n Hearty "Easy Roll Mix"									
1/4 cup	140	0	0	0	33	1	6	1	200
I.M. Healthy, Corn Flake Crumbs									
2 tbsp	40	0	0	0	9	0	1	1	50
I.M. Healthy, Tortilla Crumbs									
2 tbsp	40	0	0	0	9	0	1	1	50
Ian's Natural Foods, AF Gluten-Free Italian Panko Breadcrumbs									
1/4 cup	70	0	0	0	15	1	0	1	310
Ian's Natural Foods, AF Gluten-Free Panko Breadcrumbs									
1/4 cup	70	0	0	0	16	1	0	1	135
Joan's GF Great Bakes, Corn Toaster Muffins									
1 muffin	220	8	4	15	36	2	15	2	160
Joan's GF Great Bakes, Double Chocolate Muffins									
1 muffin	280	14	2.5	30	37	2	22	3	260
King Arthur Flour, Gluten-Free Bread Mix, Prepared									
3 tbsp	160	0	0	0	26	1	2	1	180
King Arthur Flour, Gluten-Free Brownie Mix, Prepared									
3 tbsp	170	1	0.5	0	27	1	18	1	105

Food Serving size	Cal.	(g) Total Fat	(g) Sat. Fat	(mg) Chol.	(g) Carb.	(g) Fiber	(g) Sug.	(g) Prot.	(mg) Sod.
King Arthur Flour, Gluten-Free Chocolate Cake Mix 1/4 cup	280	2	1.5	0	37	2	22	1	300
King Arthur Flour, Gluten-Free Muffin Mix, Prepared 4 tbsp	210	0.5	0	0	33	3	17	1	360
King Arthur Flour, Gluten-Free Pancake Mix, Prepared 1/3 cup	280	0.5	0	0	41	1	4	2	560
King Arthur Flour, Gluten-Free Pizza Crust Mix, Prepared 4 tbsp	180	0	0	0	29	1	2	1	200
King Arthur Flour, Gluten-Free Yellow Cake Mix 1/4 cup	270	0	0	0	40	0	22	1	240
Kinnikinnick, Angel Food Cake Mix 45g	170	0	0	0	42	0	33	0	50
Kinnikinnick, Blueberry Muffins 1 muffin	190	7	2	10	32	3	18	1	320
Kinnikinnick, Bread Cubes, Dry 4.2 oz dry	60	1.5	0.2	15	10	1	2	1	150
Kinnikinnick, Carrot Muffins 1 muffin	170	6	1	15	27	3	13	2	300
Kinnikinnick, Chocolate Cake Mix 33g	120	0.5	0.4	0	28	2	16	1	250
Kinnikinnick, Chocolate Chip Muffins 1 muffin	170	9	2	20	28	2	15	1	170
Kinnikinnick, Chocolate Dipped Donuts 1 donut	220	6	3	0	41	2	19	2	200
Kinnikinnick, Chocolate Lovers Jumbo Muffin 1 muffin	460	26	4.5	80	50	2	24	4	350
Kinnikinnick, Cinnamon and Brown Sugar Homestyle Waffles 1 waffle	110	3.5	0.2	5	18	1	3	1	240
Kinnikinnick, Cinnamon Sugar Donuts 1 donut	170	4.5	2.5	5	30	1	11	2	230
Kinnikinnick, Crepe Mix 30g	100	0.5	0.2	20	24	2	5	2	220
Kinnikinnick, Fruit Cake 1 slice	90	3	1.5	15	21	1	12	1	35

Food Serving size	Cal.	(g) Total Fat	(g) Sat. Fat	(mg) Chol.	(g) Carb.	(g) Fiber	(g) Sug.	(g) Prot.	(mg) Sod.
Kinnikinnick, Graham Style Cracker Crumbs									
1/2 cup	50	3	1.5	0	13	0	4	0	70
Kinnikinnick, Harvest Crunch Jumbo Muffin									
1 muffin	490	29	3.5	85	53	2	19	6	400
Kinnikinnick, JB Brownie Squares									
1 piece	160	10	4	50	34	1	20	2	140
Kinnikinnick, Kinni-Kwik Bread & Bun Mix									
31g	110	1	0.4	20	24	1	3	3	240
Kinnikinnick, Lemon Poppy Seed Jumbo Muffin									
1 muffin	470	27	3.5	90	53	1	22	4	420
Kinnikinnick, Maple Glazed Donuts									
1 donut	220	6	3.5	0	41	1	20	2	190
Kinnikinnick, Original Homestyle Waffles									
1 waffle	110	3.5	0.4	10	19	1	3	1	210
Kinnikinnick, Pancake and Waffle Mix									
43g	160	1	0.3	20	34	1	7	3	490
Kinnikinnick, Panko Style Bread Crumbs									
30g	110	1	0.4	0	24	2	0	1	350
Kinnikinnick, Personal Size Pizza Crust									
1/2 crust	248	7	1	26	41	5	4	4	180
Kinnikinnick, Personal Size Thin Crusts									
1 crust	220	5	2.5	40	39	4	2	3	400
Kinnikinnick, Pie Crust									
24g slice	100	6	3	10	11	0	0	1	125
Kinnikinnick, Pumpkin Spice Donut									
1 donut	220	5	3.5	0	45	2	18	2	190
Kinnikinnick, Tapioca Rice Cinnamon Buns									
1 bun	180	6	0.5	60	41	6	15	4	340
Kinnikinnick, Vanilla Glazed Donuts									
1 donut	212	5	2.5	5	39	1	17	3	230
Kinnikinnick, White Cake Mix									
33g	120	0	0	0	29	1	16	1	320
La Tortilla Factory Smart & Delicious Wheat & Gluten-Free Softwraps									
1 wrap	180	5	0.5	0	30	3	0	2	320

Food Serving size	Cal.	(g) Total Fat	(g) Sat. Fat	(mg) Chol.	(g) Carb.	(g) Fiber	(g) Sug.	(g) Prot.	(mg) Sod.
Let's Do..., Gluten-Free Ice Cream Cones 1 cone	12	0	0	0	2	0	0	0	4
Lucini, Cinque e Cinque – Fiery Tuscan Chili 42g	160	3	0	0	24	5	5	9	25
Lucini, Cinque e Cinque – Rosemary 42g	160	3	0	0	24	5	5	9	25
Lucini, Cinque e Cinque – Traditional 42g	160	3	0	0	24	5	5	9	25
Maple Grove Farms, Gluten-Free All Purpose Baking Mix, Dry 1/4 cup	90	0	0	0	22	1	3	1	650
Maple Grove Farms, Gluten-Free Pancake & Waffle Mix, Prepared 1/4 cup	200	0	0	0	27	2	4	4	320
Mary's Gone Crackers, Caraway Crumbs 1/2 cup	160	3	0	0	28	3	0	3	190
Mary's Gone Crackers, Original Crumbs 1/2 cup	160	3	0	0	28	3	0	3	190
Mary's Gone Crackers, Savory Crumbs 1/2 cup	160	3	0	0	28	3	0	3	190
Nature's Path, Buckwheat Wildberry Frozen Waffles 2 waffles	190	7	1	0	33	1	5	2	330
Nature's Path, Chia Plus Frozen Waffles 2 waffles	210	7	1	0	34	2	5	2	370
Nature's Path, Homestyle Frozen Waffles 2 waffles	210	7	1	0	34	<1	4	1	450
Nature's Path, Mesa Sunrise Frozen Waffles 2 waffles	200	7	1	0	34	1	4	2	450
Pamela's Cornbread & Muffin Mix, Prepared 2″ x 2″ piece	140	0	0	0	38	1	0	1	200
Pamela's Gluten-Free Bread Mix, Prepared 1/16th loaf	170	1	0	0	28	3	9	1	280
Pamela's, Baking & Pancake Mix 2 4-inch pancakes	250	3.5	0.5	5	27	1.5	3	4	390
Pamela's, Chocolate Brownie Mix, Prepared 1 brownie	190	1.5	1	0	24	1	10	1	140

Food Serving size	Cal.	(g) Total Fat	(g) Sat. Fat	(mg) Chol.	(g) Carb.	(g) Fiber	(g) Sug.	(g) Prot.	(mg) Sod.
Pamela's, Chocolate Cake Mix, Prepared 1/12th of cake	260	1	0	0	41	4	22	2	670
Pamela's, Chocolate Fudge Cake 1 inch slice	320	13	4	50	51	3	32	3	480
Pamela's, Classic Vanilla Cake Mix, Prepared 1/12th of cake	240	1	0	0	42	4	20	0.5	490
Pamela's, Coffee Cake 1 inch slice	310	17	7	50	37	1	31	4	270
Pamela's, Gluten-Free Baking and Pancake Mix 4 lb (Dry Mix) 1/3 cup	160	3.5	0.5	5	27	1.5	3	4	390
Rudi's Gluten-Free Bakery, Pizza Crust 1/2 pizza shell	150	1.5	0	30	32	1	1	2	460
Schar, Bread Crumbs 3 tbsp	120	4	2	10	19	2	1	2	120
Schar, Gluten-Free Bread Crumbs 3 tbsp	120	4	2	10	19	2	1	2	120
Schar, Gluten-Free Classic White Bread Mix 3 tbsp	100	0.5	0	0	23	2	1	1	120
Schar, Gluten-Free Pizza Crusts (two per package) 1/3 of one crust	130	0.5	0.5	0	30	2	<1	2	270
Schar, Pizza Crusts 1/3 pizza crust	130	0.5	0.5	0	30	2	<1	2	270
Simply Organic Foods, Banana Bread Mix, Dry 2 tbsp dry mix	90	0	0	0	21	1	8	1	200
Simply Organic Foods, Carrot Cake Mix, Dry 1/4 cup dry mix	180	0	0	0	41	1	27	1	370
Simply Organic Foods, Chai Spice Scone Mix, Dry 3 tbsp dry mix	130	0.5	0	0	29	2	10	2	220
Simply Organic Foods, Cocoa Brownie Mix 2 tbsp	110	0.5	0	0	27	2	17	1	85
Simply Organic Foods, Cocoa Cayenne Cupcake Mix 2 tbsp	90	0	0	0	21	1	12	1	230
Simply Organic Foods, Devil's Food Cake Mix, Dry 1/4 cup dry mix	150	1	0	0	34	2	19	2	400

Food Serving size	Cal.	(g) Total Fat	(g) Sat. Fat	(mg) Chol.	(g) Carb.	(g) Fiber	(g) Sug.	(g) Prot.	(mg) Sod.
Simply Organic Foods, Golden Vanilla Cake Mix, Dry									
1/4 cup dry mix	170	0	0	0	40	1	23	1	240
Simply Organic Foods, Pancake & Waffle Mix, Dry									
1/3 cup dry mix	170	1	0	0	39	3	4	2	430
Simply Organic Foods, Pizza Crust Mix, Dry									
1/4 cup dry mix	130	0.5	0	0	28	1	0	1	125
The Really Great Food Company, Gluten-Free Angel Food Cake Mix									
1 slice	130	0	0	0	31	0	18	1	200
The Really Great Food Company, Gluten-Free Apple Spice Muffin Mix									
1/12th package	110	0	0	0	24	1	7	1	230
The Really Great Food Company, Gluten-Free Banana Bread Cake Mix									
1 slice	180	0	0	0	42	<1	19	1	340
The Really Great Food Company, Gluten-Free Biscuit Mix (Old Time Biscuit)									
1 biscuit	130	0	0	0	30	1	4	1	570
The Really Great Food Company, Gluten-Free Brownie Mix (Aunt Tootsie's)									
1 brownie	90	0	0	0	22	1	16	<1	70
The Really Great Food Company, Gluten-Free Chocolate Cake Mix									
1 slice	170	0.5	0	0	43	1	25	1	310
The Really Great Food Company, Gluten-Free Cinnamon Bread Mix									
1 slice	100	0	0	0	24	1	5	1	160
The Really Great Food Company, Gluten-Free Coffee Crumb Cake									
1 piece	120	0	0	0	30	0	16	1	380
The Really Great Food Company, Gluten-Free Cornbread Muffin Mix									
1/12th package	110	0	0	0	24	1	6	1	270
The Really Great Food Company, Gluten-Free Cupcake Mix (Chocolate)									
1 cupcake	180	2	1	0	42	3	23	2	290
The Really Great Food Company, Gluten-Free Devils Food Cake Mix									
1 slice	170	1	NA	0	41	3	23	2	280
The Really Great Food Company, Gluten-Free French Bread Mix									
1 slice	80	0	0	0	19	1	3	1	210
The Really Great Food Company, Gluten-Free French Bread/Pizza Crust									
32g	80	0	0	0	19	1	3	1	210
The Really Great Food Company, Gluten-Free Golden Cake Mix									
1 slice	180	0	0	0	44	0	23	1	410

Food Serving size	Cal.	(g) Total Fat	(g) Sat. Fat	(mg) Chol.	(g) Carb.	(g) Fiber	(g) Sug.	(g) Prot.	(mg) Sod.
The Really Great Food Company, Gluten-Free Homestyle Cornbread Mix									
1 slice	80	0	NA	0	20	1	7	1	220
The Really Great Food Company, Gluten-Free Irish Soda Bread Mix									
1 slice	100	0	0	0	25	1	14	1	330
The Really Great Food Company, Gluten-Free Lemon Poppy Cake Mix									
1 slice	180	1	NA	0	41	<1	22	1	340
The Really Great Food Company, Gluten-Free Maple Raisin Muffin Mix									
1/12th package	100	0	0	0	24	<1	9	1	200
The Really Great Food Company, Gluten-Free Orange Cake Mix									
1 slice	120	0	0	0	32	0	20	1	320
The Really Great Food Company, Gluten-Free Pancake Mix (Brown Rice Style)									
1 large pancake	140	1	NA	0	30	2	1	2	290
The Really Great Food Company, Gluten-Free Pancake Mix (Classic Pancake)									
1 large pancake	130	0	0	0	31	<1	4	1	390
The Really Great Food Company, Gluten-Free Pancake Mix (Jumbo Classic Size)									
1 large pancake	130	0	0	0	31	<1	4	1	390
The Really Great Food Company, Gluten-Free Pie Crust Mix									
1 slice	100	0	0	0	24	1	5	1	160
The Really Great Food Company, Gluten-Free Pineapple Cake Mix									
1 piece	120	0	0	0	31	0	17	1	300
The Really Great Food Company, Gluten-Free Pizza Crust Mix									
1 slice	100	0	0	0	23	0	2	2	310
The Really Great Food Company, Gluten-Free Pound Cake Mix									
1 slice	110	0	0	0	29	0	16	1	250
The Really Great Food Company, Gluten-Free Pumpkin Bread Cake Mix									
1 slice	170	0	NA	0	42	<1	19	1	360
The Really Great Food Company, Gluten-Free Pumpkin Spice Cake Mix									
1 slice	130	0	0	0	32	1	17	1	310
The Really Great Food Company, Gluten-Free Rye Style Bread Mix									
1 slice	110	0	0	0	25	1	3	1	210
The Really Great Food Company, Gluten-Free Vanilla Muffin Mix									
1/12th package	100	0	0	0	23	<1	6	1	240
The Really Great Food Company, Gluten-Free White Bread Mix (Original)									
1 slice	100	0	0	0	24	1	4	1	180

Food Serving size	Cal.	(g) Total Fat	(g) Sat. Fat	(mg) Chol.	(g) Carb.	(g) Fiber	(g) Sug.	(g) Prot.	(mg) Sod.
The Really Great Food Company, Gluten-Free White Cake Mix									
1/9th package	130	0	0	0	31	<1	18	<1	200
The Really Great Food Company, Gluten-Free Yellow Cake Mix									
1 slice	190	0	0	0	45	<1	24	1	200
Udi's Gluten Free, Blueberry Muffins									
1 muffin	260	10	2.5	75	39	1	19	3	270
Udi's Gluten Free, Blueberry Oat Muffin Tops									
1 muffin top	140	5	1.5	35	26	5	10	2	140
Udi's Gluten Free, Chocolate Chia Muffin Tops									
1 muffin top	150	8	3	40	23	6	11	3	180
Udi's Gluten Free, Cinnamon Rolls									
1 roll with 1/2 of icing	300	6	1	0	59	3	30	5	370
Udi's Gluten Free, Double Chocolate Muffins									
1 muffin	300	13	5	70	42	3	27	4	320
Udi's Gluten Free, Foods Pizza Crusts (2 package Frozen)									
1/2 of one crust	190	5	0	0	31	1	5	4	340
Udi's Gluten Free, Lemon Streusel Muffins									
1 muffin	310	13	4	75	46	1	23	3	340
Udi's Gluten Free, Margherita Pizza									
1/2 pizza	260	10	4	20	32	4	2	12	460
Van's, Wheat Free/Gluten-Free Apple Cinnamon Waffles									
2 waffles	230	7	0.5	0	39	1	5	2	390
Van's, Wheat Free/Gluten-Free Blueberry Waffles									
2 waffles	230	7	0.5	0	39	1	5	2	380
Van's, Wheat Free/Gluten-Free Buckwheat Waffles									
2 waffles	240	7	1	0	42	3	6	2	370
Van's, Wheat Free/Gluten-Free Flax Waffles									
2 waffles	230	7	1	0	37	2	4	3	370
Van's, Wheat Free/Gluten-Free Minis Waffles									
4 mini waffles	150	5	0.5	0	25	1	3	2	250
Van's, Wheat Free/Gluten-Free Totally Natural Waffles									
2 waffles	230	7	1	0	39	1	4	2	400

Food Serving size	Cal.	(g) Total Fat	(g) Sat. Fat	(mg) Chol.	(g) Carb.	(g) Fiber	(g) Sug.	(g) Prot.	(mg) Sod.
Breads									
Against the Grain, Gourmet Dairy-free Cinnamon Raisin Bagel									
1 bagel	196	10	3	39	26	1	3	1	246
Against the Grain, Gourmet Dairy-free Vermont Country Roll									
1 roll	208	11	3	41	27	1	2	2	259
Against the Grain, Gourmet Original Baguette									
1/3 baguette	250	14	3	54	27	0	0	5	332
Against the Grain, Gourmet Original Rolls									
1 roll	265	14	3	56	29	0	0	6	364
Against the Grain, Gourmet Pumpernickel Rolls									
1 roll	295	15	3	58	35	9	0	6	241
Against the Grain, Gourmet Rosemary Baguette									
1/3 baguette	250	14	3	54	27	0	0	5	332
Against the Grain, Gourmet Rosemary Rolls									
1 roll	265	14	3	56	29	0	0	6	364
Against the Grain, Gourmet Sesame Bagel									
1 bagel	250	13	3	51	28	0	0	5	328
Against the Grain, Gourmet Sun-dried Tomato and Basil Bagel									
1 bagel	241	13	3	52	27	0	0	5	293
Aleia's Gluten-Free Bakery, Cinnamon Raisin Bread									
1 slice	130	4	0	20	21	3	5	3	105
Aleia's Gluten-Free Bakery, Farmhouse White Bread									
1 slice	120	4	0	20	18	2	3	2	100
Bob's Red Mill, Hearty Whole Grain Bread									
1/16 of package, baked	190	3.5	0	0	23	4	3	4	170
Bob's Red Mill, Homemade Wonderful Bread									
1 slice prepared	150	0.5	0	0	22	3	2	2	180
Canyon Bakehouse, 7-Grain Bread									
1 slice	90	1	0	10	18	2	2	2	100
Canyon Bakehouse, Cinnamon Raisin Bread									
1 slice	90	1.5	0	5	19	2	5	2	85
Canyon Bakehouse, Colorado Caraway Bread									
1 slice	70	1.5	0	15	13	2	0	2	140

Food Serving size	Cal.	(g) Total Fat	(g) Sat. Fat	(mg) Chol.	(g) Carb.	(g) Fiber	(g) Sug.	(g) Prot.	(mg) Sod.
Canyon Bakehouse, Hamburger Buns									
1 bun	200	4	1	35	40	4	5	4	300
Canyon Bakehouse, Mountain White Bread									
1 slice	90	1	0	10	17	2	3	2	110
Canyon Bakehouse, Rosemary & Thyme Focaccia									
57g	140	4	0.5	15	26	3	2	3	250
Ener-G, Brown Rice Hamburger Buns									
1 bun	140	5	0	0	22	2	3	1	180
Ener-G, Brown Rice Loaf Bread									
1 slice	100	3	0	0	16	1	2	1	25
Ener-G, Corn Loaf Bread									
1 slice	40	2	0	0	7	3	1	0	50
Ener-G, Egg-Free Raisin Loaf Bread									
1 slice	100	3	0	0	17	1	4	1	125
Ener-G, English Muffins									
1 muffin	250	9	0.5	0	41	4	4	2	360
Ener-G, High Fiber Loaf Bread									
1 slice	80	4	0	0	14	5	2	1	150
Ener-G, Light Brown Rice Loaf Bread									
1 slice	50	2	0	0	7	1	1	0	75
Ener-G, Light Tapioca Loaf Bread									
1 slice	45	1.5	0	0	7	1	1	0	60
Ener-G, Light White Rice Flax Loaf Bread									
1 slice	50	2	0	7	7	1	1	1	60
Ener-G, Light White Rice Loaf Bread									
1 slice	50	2	0	0	8	1	1	0	40
Ener-G, Maninis Miracolo Pane Bread									
1 slice	90	3	0	5	15	4	2	2	190
Ener-G, Maninis Papas Pane Bread									
1 slice	100	4	0	5	14	2	2	2	230
Ener-G, Papas Loaf Bread									
1 slice	70	3	0	0	11	2	0	1	65
Ener-G, Rice Starch Loaf Bread									
1 slice	90	2	0	0	20	5	4	0	0

Food Serving size	Cal.	(g) Total Fat	(g) Sat. Fat	(mg) Chol.	(g) Carb.	(g) Fiber	(g) Sug.	(g) Prot.	(mg) Sod.
Ener-G, Seattle Brown Loaf Bread 1 slice	90	2.5	0	0	16	1	2	1	100
Ener-G, Seattle Hamburger Buns 1 bun	190	6	0	0	33	3	4	2	210
Ener-G, Seattle Hot Dog Buns 1 bun	190	6	0	0	33	3	4	2	210
Ener-G, Tapioca Dinner Rolls 1 roll	100	2.5	0	0	18	4	2	1	125
Ener-G, Tapioca Hamburger Buns 1 bun	120	3	0	0	21	4	3	1	150
Ener-G, Tapioca Hot Dog Buns 1 bun	120	3	0	0	21	4	3	1	150
Ener-G, Tapioca Loaf – Regular Sliced Bread 1 slice	100	4.5	0	0	15	3	1	1	125
Ener-G, Tapioca Loaf – Thin Sliced Bread 1 slice	80	3	0	0	11	2	1	1	95
Ener-G, White Rice Flax Loaf Bread 1 slice	100	4.5	0	0	14	2	2	2	110
Ener-G, White Rice Hamburger Buns 1 bun	180	7	0	0	29	2	3	2	200
Ener-G, White Rice Loaf Bread 1 slice	100	3.5	0	0	17	1	2	1	120
Ener-G, Yeast-Free Brown Rice Loaf Bread 1 slice	90	3	0	0	15	2	0	1	200
Ener-G, Yeast-Free Flax Meal Loaf Bread 1 slice	100	4.5	0	0	15	3	0	1	170
Ener-G, Yeast-Free White Rice Loaf Bread 1 slice	100	3.5	0	0	18	2	0	1	140
Everybody Eats, Baguette 2 oz	170	2.5	0	0	33	1	2	3	260
Everybody Eats, Deli Rolls 1 roll	210	3	0	0	42	2	3	4	320
Everybody Eats, Egg Challah (Dairy Free) 1″ slice	150	4	1	65	26	1	4	3	170

Food Serving size	Cal.	(g) Total Fat	(g) Sat. Fat	(mg) Chol.	(g) Carb.	(g) Fiber	(g) Sug.	(g) Prot.	(mg) Sod.
Everybody Eats, Multi-Grain High-Fiber Loaf									
1 slice	130	1.5	0	0	26	3.96	4	4.01	146.6
Everybody Eats, White Bread									
1 slice	140	3	1	10	25	1	4	2	130
Food for Life, Ezekiel 4:9 Sprouted Grain Taco Size Tortillas									
1 taco	150	3.5	0.5	0	NA	5	NA	6	140
Food for Life, Ezekiel 4:9 Sprouted Whole Grain Flourless Tortillas									
1 serving	150	3.5	0.1	NA	24	5	NA	6	140
Food for Life, Wheat & Gluten-Free Brown Rice Bread									
1 slice	110	2	0	0	21	2	3	2	120
Food for Life, Wheat and Gluten-Free Almond Rice Bread									
1 slice	120	2.5	0	0	22	2	3	2	5
Food for Life, Wheat Free and Gluten-Free Brown Rice Tortillas									
1 serving	130	2.5	NA	NA	24	2	NA	2	160
Food for Life, Wheat Free Sprouted Corn Tortillas									
2 tortillas	120	2	0	0	23	3	1	3	10
French Meadow, Cinnamon Raisin Bread									
1 slice	150	5	3	0	23	1	2	2	260
French Meadow, Gluten-Free Tortilla									
1 tortilla	120	1	0	0	24	1	0	1	300
French Meadow, Mulitgrain Bread									
1 slice	150	4.5	2	0	23	3	0	4	230
French Meadow, Sandwich Bread									
1 slice	130	4	2.5	0	20	1	0	2	310
GFL Foods, Gluten-Free Pita									
1 pita	163	2	0	0	37	0	NA	0	376
Glutino, Favorite Sandwich Bread									
3 tbsp	110	0	0	0	24	<1	5	3	160
Glutino, Genius by Glutino Multigrain Sandwich Bread									
1 slice	80	3.5	0	0	10	<1	1	2	110
Glutino, Genius by Glutino White Sandwich Bread									
1 slice	80	3.5	0	0	11	<1	<1	2	140
Glutino, Gluten-Free MultiGrain Bagel									
1/2 bagel	220	6	1	5	36	2	5	4	340

Food Serving size	Cal.	(g) Total Fat	(g) Sat. Fat	(mg) Chol.	(g) Carb.	(g) Fiber	(g) Sug.	(g) Prot.	(mg) Sod.
Glutino, Gluten-Free Premium Cinnamon & Raisin Bread									
1 slice	110	1.5	0	0	22	1	4	<1	170
Glutino, Gluten-Free Premium Cinnamon 'N Raisin Bagels									
1/2 bagel	200	4.5	0.5	10	39	1	12	3	310
Glutino, Gluten-Free Premium English Muffins									
1 muffin	190	2.5	0	0	38	1	5	4	410
Glutino, Gluten-Free Premium Fiber Bread									
1 slice	90	1.5	0	0	17	2	0	<1	160
Glutino, Gluten-Free Premium Flax Seed Bread									
1 slice	90	2.5	0	0	17	1	2	<1	210
Glutino, Gluten-Free Premium Plain Bagels									
1/2 bagel	200	6	1	5	36	1	5	3	330
Glutino, Gluten-Free Premium Poppy Seed Bagels									
1/2 bagel	190	5	0.5	10	33	1	6	3	330
Glutino, Gluten-Free Premium Sesame Bagels									
1/2 bagel	220	8	1.5	5	34	2	5	4	310
Joan's GF Great Bakes, Bagels									
1 bagel	270	4	0.5	0	53	2	2	5	460
Joan's GF Great Bakes, Bialys									
1 bun	240	3	0	0	48	2	0	5	480
Joan's GF Great Bakes, Corn Bread									
2 oz	190	8	4	35	27	1	8	2	220
Joan's GF Great Bakes, English Muffins									
1 muffin	200	5	0	0	35	2	1	4	550
Joan's GF Great Bakes, Italian Bread									
1/4 loaf	120	2	0	0	25	1	0	2	390
Joan's GF Great Bakes, Multi Grain English Muffins									
1 muffin	160	1.5	0	0	34	3	4	3	370
Kinnikinnick, Brown Sandwich Bread									
1 slice	70	2	0.3	15	14	2	2	2	160
Kinnikinnick, Candadi Yeast Free Multigrain Rice Bread									
1 slice	90	3.5	0.4	20	16	1	1	2	270
Kinnikinnick, Festive Bread									
1 slice	100	1.5	0.3	15	19	1	5	1	170

Food Serving size	Cal.	(g) Total Fat	(g) Sat. Fat	(mg) Chol.	(g) Carb.	(g) Fiber	(g) Sug.	(g) Prot.	(mg) Sod.
Kinnikinnick, Italian White Tapioca Rice Bread									
1 slice	90	2.5	0.3	20	20	1	4	2	190
Kinnikinnick, Many Wonder Multigrain Rice Bread									
1 slice	90	3.5	0.4	20	18	3	2	2	120
Kinnikinnick, Raisin Tapioca Rice Bread									
1 slice	100	2.5	0.3	20	23	2	7	2	135
Kinnikinnick, Robins Honey Brown Rice Bread									
1 slice	80	3	0.4	0	20	1	3	1	210
Kinnikinnick, Soft Dinner Rolls									
1 roll	100	3	0.5	0	17	3	0	2	135
Kinnikinnick, Soft Hamburger Buns									
1 bun	150	5	1	0	26	5	1	2	210
Kinnikinnick, Soft Hotdog Buns									
1 bun	180	5	1	0	30	6	1	3	250
Kinnikinnick, Soft Multigrain Bread									
2 slices	150	6	1	0	20	5	1	3	180
Kinnikinnick, Soft White Bread									
2 slices	140	4	1	0	24	5	1	2	200
Kinnikinnick, Sunflower Flax Rice Bread									
1 slice	90	4.5	0.4	0	16	2	2	2	280
Kinnikinnick, Tapioca Rice Bread									
1 slice	90	2.5	0.3	20	20	1	5	2	130
Kinnikinnick, Tapioca Rice Cinnamon Raisin Bagels									
1 bagel	220	6	2	25	51	5	19	4	340
Kinnikinnick, Tapioca Rice English Muffins									
1 English muffin	242	3.5	0.3	0	41	2	6	3	260
Kinnikinnick, Tapioca Rice Hot Cross Buns									
1 bun	171	3.5	0.5	15	35	4	16	2	290
Kinnikinnick, Tapioca Rice New York Style Plain Bagels									
1 bagel	210	7	2.5	35	46	3	9	4	430
Kinnikinnick, Tapioca Rice Sesame Bagels									
1 bagel	210	7	2.5	30	49	5	12	4	390
Kinnikinnick, White Sandwich Bread									
1 slice	70	2	0.2	15	15	2	2	1	150

Food Serving size	Cal.	(g) Total Fat	(g) Sat. Fat	(mg) Chol.	(g) Carb.	(g) Fiber	(g) Sug.	(g) Prot.	(mg) Sod.
Kinnikinnick, Yeast Free Tapioca Bread									
1 slice	80	2	0.3	15	17	2	3	1	170
Rudi's Gluten-Free Bakery, Cinnamon Raisin Bread									
1 slice	90	1.5	0	0	19	1	7	1	110
Rudi's Gluten-Free Bakery, Fiesta Tortillas									
1 tortilla	90	2.5	0	0	17	5	1	1	190
Rudi's Gluten-Free Bakery, Multigrain Bread									
1 slice	90	2	0	0	17	1	3	1	135
Rudi's Gluten-Free Bakery, Multigrain Hamburger Rolls									
1 bun	170	6	0	0	30	2	4	2	220
Rudi's Gluten-Free Bakery, Multigrain Hot Dog Rolls									
1 roll	130	4.5	0	0	23	2	3	1	160
Rudi's Gluten-Free Bakery, Original Bread									
1 slice	90	2	0	0	17	1	3	1	135
Rudi's Gluten-Free Bakery, Plain Tortillas									
1 tortilla	90	2.5	0	0	17	5	1	1	190
Rudi's Gluten-Free Bakery, Spinach Tortillas									
1 tortilla	90	2.5	0	0	17	5	1	1	180
Schar, Baguettes									
1/4 baguette	100	1	0	0	20	2.5	1	1	220
Schar, Ciabatta Parbaked Rolls									
1 roll	100	1	0	0	21	4	2	2	350
Schar, Classic Gluten-Free White Sandwich Bread									
1 slice	60	1	0.5	0	11	2	1	1	120
Schar, Classic White Bread									
1 slice	60	1	0.5	0	11	2	1	1	120
Schar, Classic White Bread Mix									
3 tbsp	100	0.5	0	0	23	2	1	1	120
Schar, Classic White Rolls									
1 roll	170	2	0	0	34	4	3	3	380
Schar, Crispbread									
4 slices	100	0.5	0	0	22	<1	<1	2	250
Schar, Deli-Style Bread									
1 slice	120	1.5	0	0	21	3	2	2	320

Food Serving size	Cal.	(g) Total Fat	(g) Sat. Fat	(mg) Chol.	(g) Carb.	(g) Fiber	(g) Sug.	(g) Prot.	(mg) Sod.
Schar, Gluten-Free Baguettes 1/4 baguette	100	1	0	0	20	2.5	1	1	220
Schar, Gluten-Free Ciabatta Parbaked Bread Rolls 1 roll	100	1	0	0	21	4	2	2	350
Schar, Gluten-Free Classic White Rolls 1 roll	170	2	0	0	34	4	3	3	380
Schar, Gluten-Free Italian Bread Sticks 7 breadsticks	130	2	1	0	26	0	<1	1	250
Schar, Gluten-Free Multigrain Sandwich Bread 1 slice	70	1	0.5	0	13	2	1	2	150
Schar, Gluten-Free Sub Sandwich Parbaked Rolls 1 roll	160	2	0	0	34	5	2	2	380
Schar, Hearty Grain Frozen Bread 1 slice	80	2	0.5	0	13	2	0	2	160
Schar, Hearty White Frozen Bread 1 slice	70	1.5	0.5	0	13	2	0	1	160
Schar, Italian Breadsticks 7 breadsticks	130	2	1	0	26	0	<1	1	250
Schar, Multigrain Bread 1 slice	70	1	0.5	0	13	2	1	2	150
Schar, Multigrain Ciabatta 1 roll	140	4	0	0	20	4	2	3	200
Schar, Sub Sandwich Rolls 1 roll	160	2	0	0	34	5	2	2	380
Udi's Gluten Free, Cinnamon Raisin Bread 2 slices	140	3	0	0	25	1	9	4	200
Udi's Gluten Free, Cinnamon Rolls 1 roll with 1/2 of icing	300	6	1	0	59	3	30	5	370
Udi's Gluten Free, Classic Hamburger Buns 1 bun	210	6	0.5	0	35	4	4	5	390
Udi's Gluten Free, Classic Hot Dog Buns 1 bun	170	4.5	0	0	29	4	4	4	330
Udi's Gluten Free, Millet-Chia Bread 2 slices	150	5	0	0	26	5	3	5	270

Food Serving size	Cal.	(g) Total Fat	(g) Sat. Fat	(mg) Chol.	(g) Carb.	(g) Fiber	(g) Sug.	(g) Prot.	(mg) Sod.
Udi's Gluten Free, Omega Flax & Fiber Bread 2 slices	150	6	0.5	0	23	6	3	5	260
Udi's Gluten Free, Soft & Chewy Cinnamon Raisin Bagels 1 bagel	320	10	1	0	51	3	11	7	530
Udi's Gluten Free, Soft & Chewy Plain Bagels 1 bagel	320	10	1	0	48	3	4	8	590
Udi's Gluten Free, Soft & Chewy Whole Grain Bagels 1 bagel	310	11	1	0	49	3	5	8	570
Udi's Gluten Free, White Sandwich Bread 2 slices	140	4	0	0	22	1	2	4	300
Udi's Gluten Free, Whole Grain Bread 2 slices	140	4	0	0	22	1	3	4	280
Udi's Gluten Free, Whole Grain Hamburger Buns 1 bun	190	6	0.5	0	34	6	4	6	370

Cereals

Food Serving size	Cal.	(g) Total Fat	(g) Sat. Fat	(mg) Chol.	(g) Carb.	(g) Fiber	(g) Sug.	(g) Prot.	(mg) Sod.
Amy's, Cream of Rice Hot Cereal Bowl 9 oz	170	1	0	0	39	2	8	2	220
Ancient Harvest, Original Quinoa Flakes 1/3 cup dry	131	2	0	0	23	2.4	2	4.3	2
Arrowhead Mills, Maple Buckwheat Flakes Cereal 1 cup with milk	210	1	0	0	35	1	5	4	190
Arrowhead Mills, Organic Rice and Shine Hot Cereal 1/4 cup	150	1	0	0	32	2	0	3	0
Arrowhead Mills, Organic Yellow Corn Grits Hot Cereal 1/4 cup	140	0.5	0	0	31	3	0	2	5
Arrowhead Mills, Rice Flakes Sweetened Cereal 1 cup with milk	230	1	0	0	40	1	8	3	190
Attune Erewhon, Cocoa Crispy Brown Rice Cereal 1 cup	200	1.5	0	0	44	1	11	3	190
Attune Erewhon, Corn Flakes Cereal 1 cup	130	0	0	0	30	1	0	3	60
Attune Erewhon, Crispy Brown Rice – GF Cereal 1 cup	110	0.5	0	0	25	0	<1	2	160

Food Serving size	Cal.	(g) Total Fat	(g) Sat. Fat	(mg) Chol.	(g) Carb.	(g) Fiber	(g) Sug.	(g) Prot.	(mg) Sod.
Attune Erewhon, Crispy Brown Rice – No Salt Added Cereal									
1 cup	110	0.5	0	0	25	0	<1	2	10
Attune Erewhon, Crispy Brown Rice with Mixed Berries Cereal									
1 cup	120	0.5	0	0	27	1	6	2	100
Attune Erewhon, Rice Twice Cereal									
3/4 cup	120	0	0	0	26	0	8	2	60
Attune Erewhon, Strawberry Crispy Cereal									
3/4 cup	120	0.5	0	0	28	1	6	2	125
Bakery on Main, Apple Raisin Walnut Granola									
3/4 cup	260	12	1	0	35	3	11	4	45
Bakery on Main, Cranberry Orange Cashew Granola									
3/4 cup	240	11	1	0	35	2	12	4	40
Bakery on Main, Extreme Fruit & Nut Granola									
3/4 cup	260	13	2	0	34	3	11	4	45
Bakery on Main, Nutty Cranberry Maple Granola									
3/4 cup	260	11	1	0	36	3	13	4	45
Bakery on Main, Rainforest Granola									
3/4 cup	250	12	1.5	0	34	2	9	4	45
Barbara's Bakery, Brown Rice Crisps Cereal									
1 cup	120	1	0	0	25	<1	1	2	95
Barbara's Bakery, Puffins Honey Rice Cereal									
3/4 cup	120	1	0	0	25	3	6	2	80
Barbara's Bakery, Puffins Multigrain Cereal									
3/4 cup	110	0	0	0	25	3	6	2	80
Birkett Mills, Pocono Cream of Buckwheat									
1/4 cup	140	0	0	0	36	0	0	0	0
Birkett Mills, Wolff's Cream of Buckwheat									
1/4 cup	140	0	0	0	36	0	0	0	0
Bob's Red Mill, Creamy Brown Rice Farina									
1/4 cup dry	150	1	0	0	32	2	0	3	5
Bob's Red Mill, Gluten-Free Muesli									
1/4 cup dry	110	3	0.5	0	19	2	5	3	0
Bob's Red Mill, Mighty Tasty Hot Cereal									
1/4 cup	150	1.5	0	0	31	4	0	4	5

Food Serving size	Cal.	(g) Total Fat	(g) Sat. Fat	(mg) Chol.	(g) Carb.	(g) Fiber	(g) Sug.	(g) Prot.	(mg) Sod.
Bob's Red Mill, Millet Grits/Meal									
1/4 cup dry	150	1.5	0	0	34	3	0	5	NA
Bob's Red Mill, Organic Brown Rice Farina									
1/4 cup	150	1	0	0	32	2	0	3	5
Bob's Red Mill, Organic Creamy Buckwheat									
1/4 cup	140	1	0	0	30	3	0	5	0
Bob's Red Mill, Quick Rolled Oats, Dry									
1/2 cup	180	3	0.5	0	29	5	1	7	0
Bob's Red Mill, Rolled Oats, Dry									
1/2 cup	160	2.5	0.5	0	27	4	1	7	0
Bob's Red Mill, Soy Grits (defatted)									
1/4 cup	130	1	0	0	14	7	4	19	0
Bob's Red Mill, Steel Cut Oats, Dry									
1/4 cup	140	2.5	0.5	0	27	4	0	6	0
Bob's Red Mill, Thick Rolled Oats									
1/2 cup dry	180	3	0	0	34	5	0	5	0
Bob's Red Mill, Whole Grain Teff									
1/4 cup	180	1	0	0	37	4	0	7	5
Chex, Apple Cinnamon Gluten-Free Cereal									
3/4 cup with 1/2 cup skim milk	170	2	0	0	26	<1	8	1	190
Chex, Chocolate Gluten-Free Cereal									
3/4 cup with 1/2 cup skim milk	170	2.5	0	0	26	1	8	2	210
Chex, Cinnamon Gluten-Free Cereal									
3/4 cup with 1/2 cup skim milk	160	2	0	0	25	1	8	1	180
Chex, Corn Chex Gluten-Free Cereal									
1 cup with 1/2 cup skim milk	160	0.5	0	0	26	2	3	2	240
Chex, Gluten Honey Nut Free Cereal									
3/4 cup with 1/2 cup skim milk	160	0.5	0	0	28	1	9	2	200
Chex, Rice Chex Gluten-Free Cereal									
1 cup with 1/2 cup skim milk	140	0	0	0	23	1	2	2	240
Eden Foods, Buckwheat, 100% Whole Grain, Organic, Uncooked									
1/4 cup	160	1	0	0	31	5	0	5	0
Enjoy Life Foods, Cinnamon Raisin Crunch Granola									
1/2 cup	170	1.5	0	0	35	2	11	3	10

Food Serving size	Cal.	(g) Total Fat	(g) Sat. Fat	(mg) Chol.	(g) Carb.	(g) Fiber	(g) Sug.	(g) Prot.	(mg) Sod.
Enjoy Life Foods, Crunchy Flax Cereal 3/4 cup	200	3	0	0	42	6	2	7	115
Enjoy Life Foods, Crunchy Rice Cereal 3/4 cup	210	1	0	0	46	2	5	4	110
Enjoy Life Foods, Double Chocolate Crunch Granola 1/2 cup	180	4	2	0	35	4	11	3	40
Enjoy Life Foods, Very Berry Crunch Granola 1/2 cup	170	1.5	0	0	35	2	11	3	10
Food for Life, Ezekiel 4:9 Sprouted Whole Grain Flourless Almond Cereal 1 serving	200	3	NA	NA	38	6	1	8	190
Food for Life, Ezekiel 4:9 Sprouted Whole Grain Flourless Golden Flax Cereal 1 serving	180	2.5	NA	NA	37	6	NA	NA	190
Food for Life, Ezekiel 4:9 Whole Grain Flourless Cereal Original 1 serving	190	1	NA	NA	40	6	NA	8	200
Food for Life, Whole Grain Flourless Cinnamon Raisin Cereal 1 serving	190	1	NA	NA	41	5	8	7	160
GlutenFreeda, Apple Almond Honey Gluten-Free Granola 1/4 cup	120	4	0	0	19	3	5	3	5
GlutenFreeda, Apple Cinnamon with Flax Instant Gluten-Free Oatmeal 50g	180	2.5	0.5	0	35	4	8	6	110
GlutenFreeda, Banana Maple with Flax Instant Gluten-Free Oatmeal 1 package	180	2.5	0.5	0	35	4	9	6	110
GlutenFreeda, Cranberry Cashew Honey Gluten-Free Granola 1/4 cup	120	4	0.5	0	19	2	6	3	0
GlutenFreeda, Maple Raisin with Flax Instant Gluten-Free Oatmeal 1 package	180	2.5	0	0	36	4	10	6	90
GlutenFreeda, Natural Instant Gluten-Free Oatmeal 1 package	190	3	0.5	0	34	5	1	8	0
GlutenFreeda, Raisin Almond Honey Gluten-Free Granola 1/4 cup	120	4	0	0	19	2	5	3	0
Glutino, Gluten-Free Apples & Cinnamon Rings Cereal 1/2 cup	120	1	0	0	26	1	4	1	120
Glutino, Gluten-Free Berry Sensible Beginnings Corn Rice Flakes Cereal 1 cup	120	0	0	0	27	1	9	2	125

Food Serving size	Cal.	(g) Total Fat	(g) Sat. Fat	(mg) Chol.	(g) Carb.	(g) Fiber	(g) Sug.	(g) Prot.	(mg) Sod.
Glutino, Gluten-Free Frosted Sensible Beginnings Corn Rice Flakes Cereal									
1 cup	120	0	0	0	28	1	10	2	120
Glutino, Gluten-Free Honey Nut Rings Cereal									
1/2 cup	120	1.5	0	0	26	1	4	1	120
Glutino, Gluten-Free Sensible Beginnings Corn Rice Flakes Cereal									
1 cup	120	0	0	0	27	1	8	2	130
Hodgson Mill, Gluten-Free Buckwheat Cereal with Milled Flaxseed									
1/4 cup	150	1	0	0	33	1	0	2	0
I.M. Healthy, Granola with Fruit									
1.12 oz	150	3.5	1	0	24	3	7	4	30
I.M. Healthy, Peanut/Nut Free Plain Granola									
1.12 oz	150	3.5	1	0	24	3	6	5	30
Kay's Naturals, Apple Cinnamon Cereal									
1.2 oz	120	1.5	0	0	19	4	3	12	150
Kay's Naturals, French Vanilla Cereal									
1.2 oz	120	1.5	0	0	18	4	3	12	140
Kay's Naturals, Honey Almond Cereal									
1.2 oz	120	1.5	0	0	18	4	3	12	140
Kinnikinnick, KinniKrisp Rice Cereal									
1 cup	100	0.4	0.1	0	22	0	1	2	80
Nature's Path, Amazon Frosted Flakes									
2/3 cup with skim milk	160	0	0	0	26	2	6	2	115
Nature's Path, Crispy Rice Cereal									
3/4 cup with 125ml fortified skim milk	150	15	0	0	24	2	2	2	160
Nature's Path, Fruit Juice Sweetened Corn Flakes									
3/4 cup with 125ml fortified skim milk	160	0.4	0	0	27	0	3	2	125
Nature's Path, Fruit Juice Sweetened Corn Flakes – ECO PAC									
3/4 cup	160	0.4	0	0	27	0	3	2	125
Nature's Path, Gorilla Munch Cereal									
3/4 cup with 125ml fortified milk	160	0	0	0	27	2	8	2	110
Nature's Path, Honey'd Corn Flakes									
3/4 cup with 125ml fortified skim milk	160	0	0	0	27	1	2	4	105

Food Serving size	Cal.	(g) Total Fat	(g) Sat. Fat	(mg) Chol.	(g) Carb.	(g) Fiber	(g) Sug.	(g) Prot.	(mg) Sod.
Nature's Path, Koala Crisp Cereal 3/4 cup with 125ml fortified skim milk									
	150	1	0	0	25	2	11	2	100
Nature's Path, Koala Crisp Cereal – ECO PAC 3/4 cup with 125ml fortified skim milk									
	150	1	0	0	25	2	11	2	100
Nature's Path, Leapin Lemurs Cereal 3/4 cup with 128ml fortified skim milk									
	160	1.5	0	0	25	2	8	2	115
Nature's Path, Mesa Sunrise Flakes 3/4 cup with 125ml fortified skim milk									
	160	1	0	0	24	3	4	3	125
Nature's Path, Mesa Sunrise Flakes – ECO PAC 3/4 cup with 125ml fortified skim milk									
	160	1	0	0	24	3	4	3	125
Nature's Path, Mesa Sunrise Flakes with Raisins – ECO PAC 1 cup	250	1	0	0	47	2	12	3	200
Nature's Path, Panda Puffs Cereal 3/4 cup with 125ml fortified skim milk									
	170	2.5	0	0	24	2	7	2	130
Nature's Path, Qi'a Superfood – Chia, Buckwheat & Hemp Cereal Apple Cinnamon 2 tbsp	130	6	0.5	0	15	4	3	6	0
Nature's Path, Qi'a Superfood – Chia, Buckwheat & Hemp Cereal Cranberry Vanilla 2 tbsp	140	6	0.5	0	14	4	3	6	0
Nature's Path, Qi'a Superfood – Chia, Buckwheat & Hemp Cereal Original Flavor 2 tbsp	140	7	0.5	0	13	4	0	6	0
Nature's Path, Sunrise Crunchy Maple Cereal 2/3 cup with 125ml fortified skim milk									
	150	1	0	0	25	3	7	2	130
Nature's Path, Sunrise Crunchy Vanilla Cereal 3/4 cup with 125ml fortified skim milk									
	150	1	0	0	25	3	7	2	130

Food Serving size	Cal.	(g) Total Fat	(g) Sat. Fat	(mg) Chol.	(g) Carb.	(g) Fiber	(g) Sug.	(g) Prot.	(mg) Sod.
Nature's Path, Whole O's Cereal 2/3 cup with 125ml fortified skim milk	160	15	0	0	25	3	4	2	115
Post Cereal, Cocoa Pebbles 3/4 cup with 1/2 cup fat free milk	160	1	1	0	25	0	10	1	170
Post Cereal, Fruity Pebbles 3/4 cup with 1/2 cup fat free milk	150	1	1	0	23	0	9	1	170
Post Cereal, Marshmallow Pebbles 3/4 cup with 1/2 cup fat free milk	150	0.5	0.5	0	24	0	10	1	180
Rice Krispies Gluten-Free with Brown Rice, Cereal 1 cup with 1/2 cup skim milk	150	0.5	0	0	25	<1	1	2	180
Udi's Gluten Free, Au Naturel Granola 1/4 cup	140	4.5	0.5	0	22	2	7	3	0
Udi's Gluten Free, Cranberry Granola 1/4 cup	140	5	0.5	0	21	2	8	3	0
Udi's Gluten Free, Gluten-Free Vanilla Granola 1/4 cup	140	6	0.5	0	21	2	7	4	0
Udi's Gluten Free, Original Granola 1/4 cup	140	6	1	0	21	2	7	3	0

Cereal Bars

Food Serving size	Cal.	(g) Total Fat	(g) Sat. Fat	(mg) Chol.	(g) Carb.	(g) Fiber	(g) Sug.	(g) Prot.	(mg) Sod.
Attune, Dark Chocolate Probiotic Bar 1 bar	80	6	3.5	0	11	3	6	1	0
Attune, Milk Chocolate Crisp Probiotic Bar 1 bar	90	6	3.5	0	12	3	8	1	20
Attune, Mint Chocolate Probiotic Bar 1 bar	90	6	3.5	0	12	3	8	1	15
Bakery on Main, Cranberry Maple Nut Granola Bar 1 bar	170	5	0.5	0	30	2	11	3	85
Bakery on Main, Extreme Trail Mix Granola Bar 1 bar	170	5	1	0	29	2	11	3	100

Food Serving size	Cal.	(g) Total Fat	(g) Sat. Fat	(mg) Chol.	(g) Carb.	(g) Fiber	(g) Sug.	(g) Prot.	(mg) Sod.
Bakery on Main, Peanut Butter Chocolate Granola Bar									
1 bar	170	6	1	0	29	2	11	3	140
Enjoy Life Foods, Caramel Apple Chewy Bars									
1 bar	120	2.5	0	0	24	3	7	2	60
Enjoy Life Foods, Cocoa Loco Chewy Bars									
1 bar	120	3.5	0.5	0	21	1	5	2	80
Enjoy Life Foods, Sunbutter Crunch Chewy Bars									
1 bar	140	4.5	0.5	0	23	3	4	3	100
Enjoy Life Foods, Very Berry Chewy Bars									
1 bar	120	2	0	0	24	2	7	1	70
Glutino, Gluten-Free Apple Breakfast Bars									
1 bar	130	2	0	0	28	3	11	2	5
Glutino, Gluten-Free Blueberry Breakfast Bars									
1 bar	130	2	0	0	27	3	11	2	0
Glutino, Gluten-Free Cherry Breakfast Bars									
1 bar	160	3	0	0	30	3	13	3	50
Glutino, Gluten-Free Chocolate & Peanuts Organic Bars									
1 bar	110	3	0.5	0	19	1	8	2	50
Glutino, Gluten-Free Strawberry Breakfast Bars									
1 bar	160	3	0	0	30	3	13	3	50
Nature's Path, Berry Crispy Rice Bars									
1 bar	110	3	0	0	21	1	7	1	70
Nature's Path, Chocolate Crispy Rice Bars									
1 bar	110	2.5	0.5	0	21	1	8	1	75
Nature's Path, Fruity Burst Crispy Rice Bars									
1 bar	110	2.5	0.5	0	21	1	8	1	65
Nature's Path, Peanut Butter Crispy Rice Bars									
1 bar	110	3	0	0	20	1	7	2	65
Nature's Path, Peanut Choco Drizzle Crispy Rice Bars									
1 bar	120	4.5	1	0	18	1	8	2	50
Post Cereal, Cocoa Pebbles Treats									
1 bar	90	2	1.5	0	18	0	9	1	110
Post Cereal, Fruity Pebbles Treats									
1 bar	90	2	1.5	0	18	0	9	1	100

Food Serving size	Cal.	(g) Total Fat	(g) Sat. Fat	(mg) Chol.	(g) Carb.	(g) Fiber	(g) Sug.	(g) Prot.	(mg) Sod.
Cookies									
1-2-3 Gluten Free, Cinnamon Thin Cookies									
1 serving	130	4.5	1.5	0	21	1	13	2	180
Aleia's Gluten-Free Bakery, Almond Horn									
1 cookie	120	7	0	0	14	1	11	3	5
Aleia's Gluten-Free Bakery, Chocolate Chip									
1 cookie	90	4	1.5	10	13	0	6	1	35
Aleia's Gluten-Free Bakery, Chocolate Coconut Macaroon									
1 cookie	30	1	0	0	6	2	2	1	0
Aleia's Gluten-Free Bakery, Coconut Macaroon									
1 cookie	30	1	0	0	6	2	2	1	0
Aleia's Gluten-Free Bakery, Ginger Snap									
1 cookie	60	2	1	10	11	0	5	1	30
Aleia's Gluten-Free Bakery, Oatmeal & Golden Raisin									
1 cookie	80	2.5	1.5	10	13	1	7	1	60
Aleia's Gluten-Free Bakery, Peanut Butter									
1 cookie	90	6	2	15	10	0	4	2	45
Aleia's Gluten-Free Bakery, Snickerdoodle									
1 cookie	80	3	1.5	15	13	0	6	1	40
Amy's, Gluten-Free Almond Shortbread Cookies									
1 cookie	90	7	2.5	10	6	1	3	2	30
Amy's, Gluten-Free Chocolate Chip Shortbread Cookies									
1 cookie	90	7	3	10	7	1	3	1	30
Amy's, Gluten-Free Classic Shortbread Cookies									
1 cookie	90	7	3	10	7	1	3	1	30
Andean Dream, Chocolate Chip Cookies									
2 cookies	140	7	3	0	20	<1	7	1	55
Andean Dream, Cocoa-Orange Cookies									
2 cookies	140	6	3	0	21	1	6	<1	65
Andean Dream, Coconut Cookies									
2 cookies	140	6	3	0	21	1	5	1	65
Andean Dream, Orange Essence Cookies									
2 cookies	140	6	3	0	21	1	5	<1	65

Food Serving size	Cal.	(g) Total Fat	(g) Sat. Fat	(mg) Chol.	(g) Carb.	(g) Fiber	(g) Sug.	(g) Prot.	(mg) Sod.
Andean Dream, Raisins & Spice Cookies									
2 cookies	140	6	3	0	21	<1	6	1	65
Annie's, Gluten-Free Cocoa & Vanilla Bunny Cookies									
27 cookies	120	3.5	1.5	0	22	1	9	2	90
Annie's, Gluten-Free Ginger Snap Bunny Cookies									
29 cookies	130	4	2	0	21	1	8	2	55
Annie's, Gluten-Free SnickerDoodle Bunny Cookies									
27 cookies	130	4	2	0	21	1	9	2	90
Barkat Gluten Free, Chocolate Cream Filled Wafers									
2 wafers	80	4	3	0	9	<1	5	0	9
Barkat Gluten Free, Lemon Cream Filled Wafers									
2 wafers	80	4	2.5	0	10	0	4	0	10
Betty Crocker, Dessert Mixes, Gluten-Free Chocolate Chip Cookie Mix									
2 tbsp	150	2	1	0	23	<1	13	1	125
Bob's Red Mill, Chocolate Chip Cookie Mix, Prepared									
2 cookies	260	2	1	0	41	2	24	2	180
Bob's Red Mill, Shortbread Cookie Mix, Prepared									
2 2-1/2" cookies	190	0	0	0	29	0.5	8	1	80
Chatila's Bakery, Chocolate Chocolate Chip Cookies									
1 cookie	50	0.5	0	15	9	2	0	2	20
Chatila's Bakery, Cream Horn									
2 cream horns, 35g	150	0	3.5	0	9	0	0	1	75
Chatila's Bakery, Dipped Macaroons									
1 cookie	130	8	7	0	20	4	1	3	40
Chatila's Bakery, Lemon Cookie									
1 cookie	45	0.5	0	20	10	2	0	3	40
Chatila's Bakery, Macaroon Cookie									
1 cookie	80	5	4.5	0	12	3	<1	2	30
Chatila's Bakery, Peanut Cookie									
1 cookie	60	3.5	0	15	8	2	0	2	30
Chatila's Bakery, Pistachio Cookie									
1 cookie	45	0	0	20	9	2	0	2	25
Chatila's Bakery, Vanilla Chip Cookie									
1 cookie	45	0.5	0	15	9	2	0	2	20

Food Serving size	Cal.	(g) Total Fat	(g) Sat. Fat	(mg) Chol.	(g) Carb.	(g) Fiber	(g) Sug.	(g) Prot.	(mg) Sod.
Chatila's Bakery, Vanilla Walnut Cookie									
1 cookie	45	0	0	15	10	1	0	1	20
Cherrybrook Kitchen, Chocolate Chip Cookie Mix									
1 cookie	90	1.5	1	0	19	0	9	1	105
Cherrybrook Kitchen, Sugar Cookie Mix									
1 cookie	70	0	0	0	18	0	7	1	60
Cravings Place, Gluten-Free Chocolate Chunk Cookie Mix									
19g	80	1.5	1	0	12	1	5	1	30
Cravings Place, Gluten-Free Peanut Butter Cookie Mix									
14g	50	0	0	0	10	0	3	1	15
Ener-G, Chocolate Chip Biscotti									
2 cookies	120	5	0.5	0	17	0	7	1	115
Ener-G, Cinnamon Cookies									
2 cookies	160	9	5	0	21	0	9	0	10
Ener-G, Communion Wafers									
1 wafer	0	0	0	0	<1	0	1	<1	0
Ener-G, Cranberry Biscotti									
2 cookies	110	4.5	0	0	17	0	8	1	110
Ener-G, Ginger Cookies									
1 cookie	50	1.5	0.5	0	9	0	4	0	30
Ener-G, Promo: Sunflower Cookies									
2 cookies	160	10	1.5	0	13	3	9	5	100
Ener-G, Raisin Biscotti									
2 cookies	130	5	0	0	20	1	9	1	125
Ener-G, Sunflower Cookies									
2 cookies	160	10	1.5	0	13	3	9	5	100
Ener-G, Vanilla Cookies									
1 cookie	90	4	0	10	11	0	5	1	45
Enjoy Life Foods, Chocolate Chip Soft Baked Cookies									
2 cookies	130	5	1	0	21	2	12	1	105
Enjoy Life Foods, Crunchy Chocolate Chip Cookies									
2 cookies	120	7	3.5	0	15	1	9	1	115
Enjoy Life Foods, Crunchy Double Chocolate Brownie									
2 cookies	110	6	3.5	0	14	1	8	1	95

Food Serving size	Cal.	(g) Total Fat	(g) Sat. Fat	(mg) Chol.	(g) Carb.	(g) Fiber	(g) Sug.	(g) Prot.	(mg) Sod.
Enjoy Life Foods, Double Chocolate Brownie									
2 cookies	120	4.5	1	0	20	2	12	1	105
Enjoy Life Foods, Gingerbread Spice Soft Baked Cookies									
2 cookies	120	4	0	0	19	2	10	1	120
Enjoy Life Foods, Happy Apple Soft Baked Cookies									
2 cookies	120	4	0	0	21	2	12	1	90
Enjoy Life Foods, Lively Lemon Soft Baked Cookies									
2 cookies	130	4.5	0	0	22	2	14	1	110
Enjoy Life Foods, No-Oats Oatmeal Soft Baked Cookies									
2 cookies	120	3.5	0	0	21	1	10	1	50
Enjoy Life Foods, Snickerdoodle Soft Baked Cookies									
2 cookies	130	4.5	0	0	21	2	14	1	110
Enjoy Life Foods, Sugar Crisp Cookies									
2 cookies	110	5	2.5	0	15	0	7	1	90
Enjoy Life Foods, Vanilla Honey Graham Cookies									
2 cookies	110	6	2.5	0	15	0	8	1	85
Everybody Eats, Chocolate Chip Cookies									
1 cookie	140	7	3.5	15	19	1	13	1	120
Get Fresh Bakehouse, Bill's Excellent Butterscotch Walnut Cookie									
43g	210	12	5	15	25	1	15	2	160
Get Fresh Bakehouse, Blondie Bar									
52g	270	17	8	35	31	1	21	2	60
Get Fresh Bakehouse, Brownie Bar									
54g	240	12	6	55	33	2	23	3	105
Get Fresh Bakehouse, Chocolate Chip Cookies									
42.5g	190	10	5	25	26	1	16	2	90
Get Fresh Bakehouse, Midnight 2x Chip Cookies									
49g	230	12	6	25	30	1	19	2	80
Get Fresh Bakehouse, Oatmeal Plus Cookies									
42.5g	180	7	4.5	25	27	1	17	2	105
Gilbert's Gourmet Goodies, Chewy Chocolate Chip Bite Sized Cookies									
4 cookies	140	6	4	20	20	<1	12	1	<5
Gilbert's Gourmet Goodies, Chewy Chocolate Chip Cookie Dough									
1 oz	130	5	3	15	19	0	11	1	5

Food Serving size	Cal.	(g) Total Fat	(g) Sat. Fat	(mg) Chol.	(g) Carb.	(g) Fiber	(g) Sug.	(g) Prot.	(mg) Sod.
Gilbert's Gourmet Goodies, Chewy Chocolate Chip Giant Cookie									
1/2 cookie	150	6	4	20	22	<1	13	1	<5
Gilbert's Gourmet Goodies, Double Chocolate Brownie Bite Size Cookies									
4 cookies	280	16	10	45	31	2	15	3	15
Gilbert's Gourmet Goodies, Double Chocolate Brownie Cookie Dough									
1 oz	140	8	5	25	15	1	7	2	10
Gilbert's Gourmet Goodies, Double Chocolate Brownie Giant Cookie									
1/2 cookie	170	9	6	30	19	1	8	2	10
Gilbert's Gourmet Goodies, Sensational Sugar Cookie Bite Size Cookies									
4 cookies	140	8	5	25	16	<1	8	1	<5
Gilbert's Gourmet Goodies, Sensational Sugar Cookie Dough									
1 oz	140	8	5	25	15	<1	7	1	5
Gilbert's Gourmet Goodies, Sensational Sugar Cookie Giant Cookie									
1/2 cookie	160	9	6	25	18	<1	9	2	5
Gilbert's Gourmet Goodies, Simply Chocolate Bite Size Cookies									
4 cookies	280	15	10	50	31	2	13	3	20
Gilbert's Gourmet Goodies, Simply Chocolate Giant Size Cookie									
1/2 cookie	170	9	6	30	19	1	8	2	10
Gilbert's Gourmet Goodies, Super Dooper Snickerdoodle Bite Size Cookies									
4 cookies	150	9	5	25	17	<1	9	1	10
Gilbert's Gourmet Goodies, Super Dooper Snickerdoodle Giant Cookie									
1/2 cookie	170	10	5	25	18	<1	10	1	10
Gluten-Free Naturals, Multi-Purpose Cookie Blend									
1/4 cup	110	1	0	0	22	<1	<1	4	0
Glutino, Gluten-Free Chocolate Chip Cookies									
4 cookies	130	5	2.5	5	20	<1	9	1	65
Glutino, Gluten-Free Chocolate Vanilla Crème Cookies									
2 cookies	140	6	2	0	20	<1	11	1	90
Glutino, Gluten-Free Lemon Flavored Wafer Cookies									
4 wafers	160	8	5	5	19	0	14	1	25
Glutino, Gluten-Free Milk Chocolate Coated Chocolate Wafer Cookies									
4 wafers	160	8	5	5	19	0	14	1	25
Glutino, Gluten-Free Vanilla Crème Cookies									
2 cookies	140	6	2	0	20	0	11	<1	60

Food Serving size	Cal.	(g) Total Fat	(g) Sat. Fat	(mg) Chol.	(g) Carb.	(g) Fiber	(g) Sug.	(g) Prot.	(mg) Sod.
Glutino, Gluten-Free Vanilla Flavored Wafer Cookies 4 wafers	160	8	5	5	19	0	14	1	25
Hodgson Mill, Gluten-Free Cookie Mix 2 cookies	101	0	0	0	24	1	8	1	100
Ian's Natural Foods, Animal Cookies 10 cookies	130	4	1	10	22	2	9	3	85
Ian's Natural Foods, Chocolate Chip Cookie Buttons 23 cookies	130	4.5	1.5	5	21	1	11	2	130
Ian's Natural Foods, Chocolate Covered Wafer Bites 5 wafer bites	160	9	4	0	19	0	11	<1	30
Ian's Natural Foods, Crunchy Cinnamon Cookie Buttons 23 cookies	120	5	0.4	0	22	1	9	1	80
Jo-sefs Gluten Free, Chocolate Cookie Squares 2 cookies	140	6	3	0	18	1	8	3	100
Jo-sefs Gluten Free, Chocolate O's Sandwich Cookies 3 cookies	160	8	4	0	21	1	11	3	110
Jo-sefs Gluten Free, Cinnamon Cookie Squares 2 cookies	140	7	3	0	18	1	8	2	70
Jo-sefs Gluten Free, Cinnamon O's Sandwich Cookies 3 cookies	160	8	4	0	21	1	11	2	75
Jo-sefs Gluten Free, Vanilla Cookie Squares 2 cookies	140	7	3	0	18	1	8	2	70
Jo-sefs Gluten Free, Vanilla O's Sandwich Cookies 3 cookies	160	8	4	0	21	1	11	2	75
Jovial Foods, Chocolate Chocolate Cream Cookies 2 cookies	160	7	2.5	15	20	1	9	2	75
Jovial Foods, Chocolate Vanilla Cream Cookies 2 cookies	160	7	2.5	15	21	1	10	2	75
Jovial Foods, Fig Fruit Filled Cookies 2 cookies	130	4	1.5	5	23	1	12	1	65
King Arthur Flour, Gluten-Free Cookie Mix, Prepared 2 tbsp	110	0	0	0	16	0	7	0	160
Kinnikinnick, Chocolate Cookie Crumbs, Dry Mix 4 oz	380	20	15	5	91	16	22	12	1570

Food Serving size	Cal.	(g) Total Fat	(g) Sat. Fat	(mg) Chol.	(g) Carb.	(g) Fiber	(g) Sug.	(g) Prot.	(mg) Sod.
Kinnikinnick, Chocolate KinniKritter Animal Cookies									
8 cookies	60	2.5	1	0	14	0	6	0	55
Kinnikinnick, Ginger Snaps Cookies									
1 cookie	40	1	0.5	0	7	0	2	0	50
Kinnikinnick, Gingerbread Cookie Mix									
30g	96	0.5	0.1	0	23	1	0	1	190
Kinnikinnick, Graham Style KinniKritter Animal Cookies									
8 cookies	60	3	1.5	0	13	1	4	0	75
Kinnikinnick, KinniKritter Animal Cookies									
8 cookies	90	1.5	1	0	17	1	2	1	25
Kinnikinnick, KinniToos Chocolate Vanilla Sandwich Cookies									
1 cookie	150	6	3	0	23	0	11	0	105
Kinnikinnick, KinniToos Fudge Sandwich Crème Cookies									
1 cookie	60	2.5	1	0	9	1	4	0	50
Kinnikinnick, KinniToos Vanilla Sandwich Crème Cookies									
1 cookie	150	6	3	0	24	0	12	0	55
Kinnikinnick, Montanas Chocolate Chip Cookies									
1 cookie	36	1.5	0.8	0	6	0	3	0	90
Kinnikinnick, Sugar Cookie Mix									
30g	102	0.3	0.1	0	25	1	6	2	95
Lucy's Gluten Free, Chocolate Chip Cookies									
3 cookies	130	5	2	0	20	2	12	2	170
Lucy's Gluten Free, Chocolate Cookies									
3 cookies	130	5	2	0	20	2	12	2	170
Lucy's Gluten Free, Cinnamon Thin Cookies									
3 cookies	130	4.5	1.5	0	21	1	13	2	180
Lucy's Gluten Free, Ginger Snap Cookies									
3 cookies	120	4.5	1	0	18	1	9	2	170
Lucy's Gluten Free, Maple Bliss Cookies									
3 cookies	120	4.5	1	0	18	1	9	2	170
Lucy's Gluten Free, Oatmeal Cookies									
3 cookies	120	4.5	1	0	18	1	9	2	170
Lucy's Gluten Free, Sugar Cookies									
3 cookies	130	4.5	1.5	0	21	1	13	2	180

Food Serving size	Cal.	(g) Total Fat	(g) Sat. Fat	(mg) Chol.	(g) Carb.	(g) Fiber	(g) Sug.	(g) Prot.	(mg) Sod.
Mary's Gone Crackers, "N" Oatmeal Raisin Cookies									
2 cookies	120	4	23	0	20	1.5	9	1	110
Mary's Gone Crackers, Chocolate Chip Cookies									
2 cookies	130	6	3	0	19	1.5	9	1	95
Mary's Gone Crackers, Double Chocolate Cookies									
2 cookies	130	6	3	0	19	1.5	9	1	100
Mary's Gone Crackers, Ginger Snaps Cookies									
3 cookies	140	5	3	0	23	1	9	1	120
Nana's Cookie Company, Gluten-Free Berry Vanilla Cookie Bars									
1 bar	130	4	0	0	22	1	7	1	135
Nana's Cookie Company, Gluten-Free Chocolate Cookie									
1/2 cookie	180	6	0	0	31	1	10	2	190
Nana's Cookie Company, Gluten-Free Chocolate Crunch Cookie									
1/2 cookie	180	6	0	0	31	1	10	2	190
Nana's Cookie Company, Gluten-Free Chocolate Mint									
1 bar	170	9	7	0	25	0.5	10	1	90
Nana's Cookie Company, Gluten-Free Chocolate Munch Cookie Bars									
1 bar	130	4.5	0	0	22	1	7	2	130
Nana's Cookie Company, Gluten-Free Chocolate Rush									
1 bar	170	9	7	0	25	0.5	10	1	90
Nana's Cookie Company, Gluten-Free Fudge Cookie Bites									
1 cookie	130	5	0	0	21	0.5	8	1	130
Nana's Cookie Company, Gluten-Free Ginger Cookie									
1/2 cookie	180	5	0	0	32	1	9	2	85
Nana's Cookie Company, Gluten-Free Ginger Spice Cookie Bites									
1 cookie	130	3.5	0	0	23	0.5	7	1	60
Nana's Cookie Company, Gluten-Free Lemon Cookie									
1/2 cookie	180	7	0	0	30	1	10	2	85
Nana's Cookie Company, Gluten-Free Lemon Dreams Cookie Bites									
1 cookie	130	4.5	0	0	20	0.5	8	1	140
Nana's Cookie Company, Gluten-Free Nana Banana Cookie Bars									
1 bar	130	4.5	0	0	23	0	7	1	130
Pamela's, Almond Anise Biscotti									
1 biscotti	120	6	2.5	10	18	1	5	1	150

Food Serving size	Cal.	(g) Total Fat	(g) Sat. Fat	(mg) Chol.	(g) Carb.	(g) Fiber	(g) Sug.	(g) Prot.	(mg) Sod.
Pamela's, Butter Shortbread									
1 cookie	110	7	4	15	13	0	3	0	70
Pamela's, Chocolate Chip Walnut Cookies									
1 cookie	120	7	1	10	13	0.5	6	1	80
Pamela's, Chocolate Chunk Cookies Mix									
1 cookie	150	3	2	0	16	0	6	1	120
Pamela's, Chocolate Chunk Pecan Shortbread Organic Cookies									
2 cookies	190	12	5	15	22	1	9	1	120
Pamela's, Chocolate Walnut Biscotti									
1 biscotti	120	6	2.5	10	18	1	6	1	140
Pamela's, Chunky Chocolate Chip Cookies									
1 cookie	120	6	1	10	14	0.5	7	1	80
Pamela's, Dark Chocolate-Chocolate Chunk Organic Cookies									
2 cookies	170	9	5	5	21	1.5	14	1	60
Pamela's, Espresso Chocolate Chunk Organic Cookies									
2 cookies	150	8	4	20	22	1	13	1	120
Pamela's, Ginger Cookies with Sliced Almonds									
1 cookie	110	5	0.5	0	15	0.5	5	1	60
Pamela's, Lemon Almond Biscotti									
1 biscotti	120	6	2.5	10	18	1	5	1	190
Pamela's, Lemon Shortbread									
1 cookie	120	6	4	15	15	0.5	5	0.5	50
Pamela's, Old Fashion Raisin Walnut Organic Cookies									
1 cookie	100	6	0.5	10	10	1	4	1	70
Pamela's, Peanut Butter Chocolate Chip Organic Cookies									
2 cookies	180	10	3	10	20	1	12	3	160
Pamela's, Peanut Butter Cookies									
1 cookie	100	5	1	15	11	0.5	7	3	120
Pamela's, Pecan Shortbread									
1 cookie	130	8	4	20	14	0.5	5	1	70
Pamela's, Shortbread Swirl									
1 cookie	120	7	4	15	14	0.5	5	1	70
Pamela's, Simplebites Chocolate Chip Mini Cookies									
4 cookies	130	6	2.5	10	18	0.5	10	1	120

Food Serving size	Cal.	(g) Total Fat	(g) Sat. Fat	(mg) Chol.	(g) Carb.	(g) Fiber	(g) Sug.	(g) Prot.	(mg) Sod.
Pamela's, Simplebites Extreme Chocolate Mini Cookies									
4 cookies	130	7	3	10	17	1.5	11	1	150
Pamela's, Simplebites Ginger Mini Snapz									
4 cookies	115	4	2	5	20	0.5	12	1	170
Pamela's, Spicy Ginger Cookies with Crystallized Ginger Organic Cookies									
2 cookies	150	6	2.5	5	23	1	12	1	120
Schar, Chocolate O's									
3 cookies	150	7	4	<5	19	1	9	2	120
Schar, Chocolate Sandwich Cremes									
2 cookies	130	6	3	0	16	0	8	2	100
Schar, Cocoa Wafers									
4 cookies	160	9	5	0	18	0	6	1	20
Schar, Gluten-Free Chocolate Hazelnut Bars									
1 bar	200	12	6	<5	21	<1	14	2	30
Schar, Gluten-Free Chocolate O's Chocolate Flavored Cookies									
3 cookies	150	7	4	<5	19	1	9	2	120
Schar, Gluten-Free Chocolate Sandwich Cremes Cookies									
2 cookies	130	6	3	0	16	0	8	2	100
Schar, Gluten-Free Chocolate-Dipped Cookies									
3 cookies	150	7	3.5	0	21	1	6	1	60
Schar, Gluten-Free Hazelnut Wafers									
1 package	260	13	6	0	34	2	17	2	20
Schar, Gluten-Free Ladyfingers									
3 cookies	110	2	0.5	40	22	1	10	2	40
Schar, Gluten-Free Shortbread Cookies									
4 cookies	130	5	2.5	10	20	0	5	1	56
Schar, Gluten-Free Vanilla Sandwich Cremes Cookies									
2 cookies	130	0	3	0	16	0	9	2	100
Schar, Gluten-Free Vanilla Wafers									
4 cookies	160	0	5	0	20	0	10	1	20
Schar, Hazelnut Wafers									
1 package	260	13	6	0	34	2	17	2	20
Schar, Ladyfingers									
3 cookies	110	2	0.5	40	22	1	10	2	40

Food Serving size	Cal.	(g) Total Fat	(g) Sat. Fat	(mg) Chol.	(g) Carb.	(g) Fiber	(g) Sug.	(g) Prot.	(mg) Sod.
Schar, Shortbread Cookies									
4 cookies	130	5	2.5	10	20	0	5	1	56
Schar, Vanilla Sandwich Cremes									
2 cookies	130	6	3	0	16	0	9	2	100
Schar, Vanilla Wafers									
4 cookies	160	8	5	0	20	0	10	1	20
Simply Organic Foods, Spice Cookie Mix									
2 tbsp dry mix	100	0	0	0	23	1	12	1	190
The Really Great Food Company, Gluten-Free Chocolate Crinkle Cookie Mix									
3 cookies	60	0.5	NA	0	14	1	8	1	115
The Really Great Food Company, Gluten-Free Versatile Cookie Mix									
13g	45	0	0	0	11	0	2	0	80
The Really Great Food Company, Mi-Del Ginger Snaps									
5 cookies	140	6	0	0	21	1	12	2	85
Udi's Gluten Free, Chocolate Chip Cookies									
2 cookies	210	10	6	30	30	1	16	2	120
Udi's Gluten Free, Dark Chocolate Brownie Bites									
2 brownies	180	8	5	35	26	1	16	2	100
Udi's Gluten Free, Oatmeal Raisin Cookies									
2 cookies	200	8	4.5	35	30	2	15	3	130
Udi's Gluten Free, Snickerdoodle Cookies									
2 cookies	200	8	4.5	35	32	1	16	1	140

Crackers

Food Serving size	Cal.	(g) Total Fat	(g) Sat. Fat	(mg) Chol.	(g) Carb.	(g) Fiber	(g) Sug.	(g) Prot.	(mg) Sod.
Blue Diamond, Natural Almond Nut-Thins, Almond Flavor, Nut & Rice Cracker Snacks									
16 crackers	130	2.5	0	0	23	<1	0	3	115
Blue Diamond, Natural Almond Nut-Thins, Cheddar Cheese Flavor, Nut & Rice Cracker Snacks									
16 crackers	130	4	0.5	0	22	<1	0	3	250
Blue Diamond, Natural Almond Nut-Thins, Country Ranch Flavor, Nut & Rice Cracker Snacks									
16 crackers	130	3.5	0	0	22	<1	1	3	220
Blue Diamond, Natural Almond Nut-Thins, Hazelnut Flavor, Nut & Rice Cracker Snacks									
16 crackers	130	3	0	0	23	<1	0	2	115

Food Serving size	Cal.	(g) Total Fat	(g) Sat. Fat	(mg) Chol.	(g) Carb.	(g) Fiber	(g) Sug.	(g) Prot.	(mg) Sod.
Blue Diamond, Natural Almond Nut-Thins, Hint of Sea Salt Flavor, Nut & Rice Cracker Snacks									
17 crackers	130	2.5	0	0	24	1	0	3	80
Blue Diamond, Natural Almond Nut-Thins, Pecan Flavor, Nut & Rice Cracker Snacks									
16 crackers	130	3.5	0	0	23	<1	0	2	130
Blue Diamond, Natural Almond Nut-Thins, Pepper Jack Cheese Flavor, Nut & Rice Cracker Snacks									
16 crackers	130	3.5	0	0	22	<1	1	3	210
Blue Diamond, Natural Almond Nut-Thins, Smokehouse Flavor, Nut & Rice Cracker Snacks									
16 crackers	130	3	0	0	23	<1	0	3	160
Crunchmaster, 7 Ancient Grains, Cracked Pepper & Herb Gluten-Free Crackers									
14 crackers	130	2.5	0	0	24	1	0	2	55
Crunchmaster, 7 Ancient Grains, Hint of Sea Salt Gluten-Free Crackers									
15 crackers	130	2.5	0	0	24	1	0	2	80
Crunchmaster, Gluten-Free Multigrain, Roasted Vegetable Crackers									
15 crackers	120	3	0	0	23	3	2	2	90
Crunchmaster, Gluten-Free Multigrain, Sea Salt Crackers									
16 crackers	120	3	0	0	23	3	2	2	135
Crunchmaster, Gluten-Free Multigrain, White Cheddar Crackers									
15 crackers	120	3	0	0	23	3	2	2	125
Crunchmaster, Gluten-Free Multiseed, Original Crackers									
15 crackers	140	5	0.5	0	20	2	0	3	110
Crunchmaster, Gluten-Free Multiseed, Roasted Garlic Crackers									
14 crackers	140	5	0.5	0	20	2	1	3	150
Crunchmaster, Gluten-Free Multiseed, Rosemary and Olive Oil Crackers									
14 crackers	140	5	0.5	0	20	2	1	3	90
Crunchmaster, Gluten-Free Multiseed, Toasted Onion Crackers									
14 crackers	140	5	0.5	0	20	2	1	3	95
Crunchmaster, Multi-Grain Cracker Crisps									
30 crackers	140	5	0.5	0	20	2	0	3	110

Food Serving size	Cal.	(g) Total Fat	(g) Sat. Fat	(mg) Chol.	(g) Carb.	(g) Fiber	(g) Sug.	(g) Prot.	(mg) Sod.
Crunchmaster, Multi-Grain Crackers, Roasted Vegetable									
15 crackers	120	3	0	0	23	3	2	2	90
Crunchmaster, Multi-Grain Crackers, Sea Salt									
16 crackers	120	3	0	0	23	3	2	2	135
Crunchmaster, Multi-Grain Crackers, White Cheddar									
15 crackers	120	3	0	0	23	3	2	2	125
Crunchmaster, Multi-Seed Crackers, Original									
15 crackers	140	5	0.5	0	20	2	0	3	110
Crunchmaster, Multi-Seed Crackers, Roasted Garlic									
14 crackers	140	5	0.5	0	20	2	1	3	150
Crunchmaster, Multi-Seed Crackers, Rosemary & Olive Oil									
14 crackers	140	5	0.5	0	20	2	1	3	90
Crunchmaster, Multi-Seed Crackers, Toasted Onion									
14 crackers	140	5	0.5	0	20	2	1	3	95
Eden Foods, Brown Rice Crackers									
8 crackers	120	2	0	0	22	2	<1	3	230
Eden Foods, Nori Maki Rice Crackers, Hand Wrapped									
15 crackers	110	0	0	0	24	2	0	3	160
Edward & Sons, Brown Rice Snaps, Black Sesame Crackers (with organic brown rice)									
8 crackers	60	2	0	0	11	1	0	2	70
Edward & Sons, Brown Rice Snaps, Onion Garlic Crackers									
9 crackers	50	1	0.5	0	10	<1	0	1	50
Edward & Sons, Brown Rice Snaps, Tamari Seaweed Crackers									
9 crackers	60	0	0	0	12	<1	0	1	120
Edward & Sons, Brown Rice Snaps, Tamari Sesame Crackers									
9 crackers	60	0.5	0	0	13	<1	0	1	120
Edward & Sons, Brown Rice Snaps, Toasted Onion Crackers (with organic brown rice)									
8 crackers	60	1	0	0	12	<1	<1	1	30
Edward & Sons, Brown Rice Snaps, Unsalted Plain Crackers (with organic brown rice)									
8 crackers	60	1	0	0	12	<1	<1	1	0

Food Serving size	Cal.	(g) Total Fat	(g) Sat. Fat	(mg) Chol.	(g) Carb.	(g) Fiber	(g) Sug.	(g) Prot.	(mg) Sod.
Edward & Sons, Brown Rice Snaps, Unsalted Sesame Crackers									
9 crackers	60	1	0	0	12	<1	0	1	0
Edward & Sons, Brown Rice Snaps, Vegetable Crackers (with organic brown rice)									
8 crackers	60	1.5	0	0	12	<1	<1	1	40
Edward & Sons, Exotic Rice Toast, Jasmine Rice & Spring Onion Crackers									
7 crackers	60	1	0	0	13	0	<1	1	140
Edward & Sons, Exotic Rice Toast, Purple Rice & Black Sesame Crackers									
7 crackers	60	1	0	0	12	0	<1	1	35
Edward & Sons, Exotic Rice Toast, Thai Red Rice & Flaxseeds Crackers									
7 crackers	60	1	0	0	13	<1	<1	1	35
Edward & Sons, Rice Snax, Bar-B-Que Rice Snax									
30g	110	1.5	0	0	22	1	1	2	170
Edward & Sons, Rice Snax, Lightly Salted Rice Snax									
30g	120	1.5	0	0	23	1	0	2	120
Edward & Sons, Rice Snax, Onion Garlic Rice Snax									
30g	130	1.5	0	0	23	1	0	2	150
Edward & Sons, Rice Snax, Salt & Vinegar Rice Snax									
30g	110	1.5	0	0	22	1	0	2	170
Ener-G, Cinnamon Crackers									
10 crackers	100	4	0	0	18	1	7	0	75
Ener-G, Cinnamon Crackers Pieces									
1 cup	240	9	0.5	0	42	2	17	1	35
Ener-G, Communion Wafers in Jar									
1 wafer	0	0	0	0	<1	0	<1	<1	0
Ener-G, Flax Crackers									
10 crackers	90	4.5	1	0	11	3	1	2	140
Ener-G, Gourmet Crackers									
3 crackers	160	7	3	0	24	0	1	1	320
Ener-G, Seattle Crackers									
13 crackers	100	5	0	0	10	1	2	1	230
Food Should Taste Good, Sea Salt Brown Rice Crackers									
About 10 crackers	130	5	0	0	19	1	3	3	100

Food Serving size	Cal.	(g) Total Fat	(g) Sat. Fat	(mg) Chol.	(g) Carb.	(g) Fiber	(g) Sug.	(g) Prot.	(mg) Sod.
Glutino, Gluten-Free Cheddar Crackers 8 crackers	140	5	2.5	10	21	<1	<1	2	180
Glutino, Gluten-Free Multigrain Crackers 8 crackers	140	4.5	2.5	5	22	<1	1	<1	260
Glutino, Gluten-Free Original Crackers 8 crackers	140	5	2	5	22	<1	1	<1	260
Glutino, Gluten-Free Table Crackers 3 crackers	160	7	3	0	24	0	0	<1	270
Glutino, Gluten-Free Vegetable Crackers 8 crackers	130	4.5	2	5	22	<1	1	<1	260
Kinnikinnick, S'moreables Graham Style Crackers 1 cookie	60	2	0.5	0	9	0	2	0	60
Mary's Gone Crackers, Black Pepper Crackers 13 crackers	140	5	0.5	0	21	3	0	3	180
Mary's Gone Crackers, Caraway Crackers 13 crackers	140	5	0.5	0	21	3	0	3	190
Mary's Gone Crackers, Herb Crackers 13 crackers	140	5	0.5	0	21	3	0	3	180
Mary's Gone Crackers, Onion Crackers 13 crackers	140	5	0.5	0	21	3	0	3	190
Mary's Gone Crackers, Original Seed Crackers 13 crackers	140	5	0.5	0	21	3	0	3	190
Quaker Oats, Quaker Rice Cakes, Apple Cinnamon 1 cake	50	0	0	NA	11	NA	3	1	0
Quaker Oats, Quaker Rice Cakes, Butter Popped Corn 1 cake	35	0	0	NA	8	NA	0	1	45
Quaker Oats, Quaker Rice Cakes, Caramel Corn 1 cake	50	0	0	NA	11	NA	3	1	30
Quaker Oats, Quaker Rice Cakes, Chocolate Crunch 1 cake	60	1	0	NA	11	NA	3	1	30
Quaker Oats, Quaker Rice Cakes, Lightly Salted 1 cake	35	0	0	0	7	NA	NA	1	15
Quaker Oats, Quaker Rice Cakes, Salt Free 1 cake	35	0	0	0	7	NA	NA	1	0

Food Serving size	Cal.	(g) Total Fat	(g) Sat. Fat	(mg) Chol.	(g) Carb.	(g) Fiber	(g) Sug.	(g) Prot.	(mg) Sod.
Quaker Oats, Quaker Rice Cakes, White Cheddar									
1 cake	45	0.5	0	NA	8	NA	1	NA	105
RW Garcia, Onion & Chive 5-Seed Crackers									
1 oz, about 16 crackers	140	7	1	0	18	2	0	2	50
RW Garcia, Rosemary & Garlic 5-Seed Crackers									
1 oz, about 16 crackers	140	7	1	0	18	2	0	2	50
RW Garcia, Tellicherry Cracked Pepper 5-Seed Crackers									
1 oz, about 16 crackers	140	7	1	0	18	2	0	2	50
San-J, Tamari Black Sesame Brown Rice Crackers									
5 crackers	140	6	1	0	17	2	0	4	170
San-J, Tamari Brown Rice Crackers									
6 crackers	120	0.5	0	0	26	<1	0	3	220
San-J, Tamari Brown Sesame Brown Rice Crackers									
5 crackers	140	6	1	0	17	1	0	4	160
San-J, Teriyaki Sesame Brown Rice Crackers									
5 crackers	130	5	1	6	18	<1	<1	4	140
Schar Gluten Free, Cheese Bites									
33 pieces	140	5	3	<5	20	1	2	2	270
Schar Gluten Free, Crispibread									
4 slices	100	0.5	0	0	22	<1	<1	2	250
Schar Gluten Free, Table Crackers									
5 crackers	130	3	2	10	24	<1	1	1	300
Schar, Cheese Bites Crackers									
33 pieces	140	5	3	<5	20	1	2	2	270
Schar, Snack Crackers									
8 crackers	240	11	5	0	29	2	1.5	5	330
Schar, Table Crackers									
5 crackers	130	3	2	10	24	<1	1	1	300
The Kitchen Table Baker's, Aged Parmesan Crisps									
3 crackers	80	6	3.5	15	<1	0	0	7	150
The Kitchen Table Baker's, Aged Parmesan Mini Crisps									
15 crisps	80	6	3.5	15	<1	0	0	7	150
The Kitchen Table Baker's, Everything Parmesan Crisps									
3 crackers	80	6	3.5	15	2	1	0	7	150

Food Serving size	Cal.	(g) Total Fat	(g) Sat. Fat	(mg) Chol.	(g) Carb.	(g) Fiber	(g) Sug.	(g) Prot.	(mg) Sod.
The Kitchen Table Baker's, Flax Seed Parmesan Crisps									
3 crackers	80	6	3.5	15	<2	1	0	6	150
The Kitchen Table Baker's, Garlic Parmesan Crisps									
3 crackers	80	6	3.5	15	2	1	0	6	150
The Kitchen Table Baker's, Italian Herb Parmesan Crisps									
3 crackers	80	6	3.5	15	2	0	0	6	150
The Kitchen Table Baker's, Jalapeno Parmesan Crisps									
3 crackers	80	6	3.5	15	2	1	0	6	150
The Kitchen Table Baker's, Rosemary Parmesan Crisps									
3 crackers	80	6	3.5	15	<1	1	0	7	150
The Kitchen Table Baker's, Sesame Parmesan Crisps									
3 crackers	80	6	3.5	15	2	1	0	6	150
The Really Great Food Company, Communion Wafers									
1 wafer	0	0	0	0	<1	0	<1	<1	0
The Really Great Food Company, Mi-Del Animal Crackers									
10 cookies	130	4	1	10	23	2	9	2	85
Wellaby's Gluten Free, Classic Cheese Crackers									
1 cup	122	4.5	2.5	15	18	<1	0	4	320
Wellaby's Gluten Free, Feta, Oregano & Olive Oil Crackers									
8 crackers	130	4.5	2.5	15	19	1	1	4	130
Wellaby's Gluten Free, Parmesan and Sun Dried Tomato Crackers									
8 crackers	130	4.5	2.5	15	19	1	1	4	130
Wellaby's Gluten Free, Parmesan Cheese Ups Crackers									
1 cup	122	4.5	2.5	15	18	<1	0	4	320
Wellaby's Gluten Free, Rosemary and Onion Crackers									
8 crackers	130	4.5	2.5	15	19	1	1	4	130
Wellaby's Gluten Free, Smoked Cheese Ups Crackers									
1 cup	122	4.5	2.5	15	18	<1	0	4	320

Flours & Baking Ingredients

Food Serving size	Cal.	(g) Total Fat	(g) Sat. Fat	(mg) Chol.	(g) Carb.	(g) Fiber	(g) Sug.	(g) Prot.	(mg) Sod.
Arrowhead Mills, Organic Blue Corn Meal									
1/3 cup	130	1.5	0	0	25	5	0	3	0
Arrowhead Mills, Organic Brown Rice Flour									
1/3 cup	130	1	0	0	27	2	0	3	0

Food Serving size	Cal.	(g) Total Fat	(g) Sat. Fat	(mg) Chol.	(g) Carb.	(g) Fiber	(g) Sug.	(g) Prot.	(mg) Sod.
Arrowhead Mills, Organic Buckwheat Flour									
1/3 cup	115	1.5	0	0	20	6	<1	5	0
Arrowhead Mills, Organic Millet Flour									
1/3 cup	130	1.5	0	0	26	3	0	4	0
Arrowhead Mills, Organic Soy Flour									
1/4 cup	100	4.5	1	0	9	4	0	7	0
Arrowhead Mills, Organic White Rice Flour									
1/3 cup	120	0	0	0	28	<1	0	2	0
Arrowhead Mills, Organic Yellow Corn Meal									
1/3 cup	120	1	0	0	27	3	0	3	0
Better Batter, Gluten-Free Flour (2.5-lb bag)									
1/4 cup	100	0	0	0	22	1	0	1	15
Better Batter, Gluten-Free Flour (20-oz bag)									
1/4 cup	100	0	0	0	22	1	0	1	15
Better Batter, Gluten-Free Flour (5-lb bag)									
1/4 cup	100	0	0	0	22	1	0	1	15
Birkett Mills, Pocono Buckwheat Flour									
1/4 cup	100	1	NA	NA	22	3	NA	4	0
Bob's Red Mill, All Purpose Baking Flour									
1/4 cup	100	1	0	0	22	3	1	3	0
Bob's Red Mill, Almond Meal/Flour									
1/4 cup	160	14	1	0	6	3	1	6	10
Bob's Red Mill, Arrowroot Starch									
1/4 cup	110	0	0	0	28	1	0	0	10
Bob's Red Mill, Baking Powder									
1 tsp	5	0	0	0	1	0	0	0	590
Bob's Red Mill, Baking Soda									
1/4 tsp	0	0	0	0	0	0	0	0	270
Bob's Red Mill, Black Bean Flour									
1/4 cup	120	0	0	0	22	5	1	8	0
Bob's Red Mill, Brown Rice Flour									
1/4 cup	140	1	0	0	31	2	0	3	5
Bob's Red Mill, Corn Flour									
1/4 cup	110	1	0	0	22	4	0	2	2

Food Serving size	Cal.	(g) Total Fat	(g) Sat. Fat	(mg) Chol.	(g) Carb.	(g) Fiber	(g) Sug.	(g) Prot.	(mg) Sod.
Bob's Red Mill, Corn Starch									
1 tbsp	30	0	0	0	7	0	0	0	0
Bob's Red Mill, Fava Bean Flour									
1/4 cup	110	0.5	0	0	19	8	1	9	0
Bob's Red Mill, Garbanzo Bean Flour									
1/4 cup dry	110	2	0	0	18	5	3	6	5
Bob's Red Mill, Garbanzo Fava Flour									
1/4 cup	110	1.5	0	0	18	6	3	6	5
Bob's Red Mill, Gluten-Free Active Dry Yeast									
1 tbsp	20	0.5	0	0	5	2	0	0	0
Bob's Red Mill, Golden Masa Harina									
1/4 cup	100	1	0	0	21	2	0	3	0
Bob's Red Mill, Green Pea Flour									
1-1/2 tbsp	50	0	0	0	9	4	1	4	2
Bob's Red Mill, Guar Gum									
1 tbsp	20	0	0	0	6	6	0	0	2
Bob's Red Mill, Hazelnut Flour/Meal									
1/4 cup	180	17	1	0	5	3	1	4	0
Bob's Red Mill, Medium Cornmeal									
1/4 cup	110	1	0	0	23	5	0	2	10
Bob's Red Mill, Millet Flour									
1/4 cup dry	110	1	0	0	22	4	0	3	2
Bob's Red Mill, Oat Bran									
1/3 cup	150	3	0.5	0	27	6	0	5	0
Bob's Red Mill, Oat Flour									
1/3 cup	160	3	0.5	0	25	4	0	7	0
Bob's Red Mill, Organic Amaranth Flour									
1/4 cup dry	110	2	0.5	0	20	3	0	4	6
Bob's Red Mill, Organic Brown Rice Flour									
1/4 cup	140	1	0	0	31	1	0	3	5
Bob's Red Mill, Organic Coconut Flour									
2 tbsp	60	1.5	1	0	10	6	0	2	0
Bob's Red Mill, Organic Quinoa Flour									
1/4 cup dry	120	2	0	0	21	4	0	4	8

Food Serving size	Cal.	(g) Total Fat	(g) Sat. Fat	(mg) Chol.	(g) Carb.	(g) Fiber	(g) Sug.	(g) Prot.	(mg) Sod.
Bob's Red Mill, Organic White Rice Flour									
1/4 cup	150	0.5	0	0	32	1	0	2	0
Bob's Red Mill, Potato Flour									
3 tbsp	120	0.5	0	0	27	2	0	3	10
Bob's Red Mill, Potato Starch, Dry									
1 tbsp	40	0	0	0	10	0	0	0	0
Bob's Red Mill, Sorghum Flour									
1/4 cup	120	1	0	0	25	3	0	4	0
Bob's Red Mill, Sweet White Rice Flour									
1/4 cup	180	0.5	0	0	40	1	1	3	0
Bob's Red Mill, Tapioca Flour									
1/4 cup	100	0	0	0	26	0	0	0	0
Bob's Red Mill, Teff Flour									
1/4 cup	113	1	0	0	22	4	0	4	5
Bob's Red Mill, White Rice Flour									
1/4 cup	150	0.5	0	0	32	1	0	2	0
Bob's Red Mill, Xanthan Gum									
1 tbsp	30	0	0	0	7	7	0	0	10
Eden Foods, Kuzu Root Starch, Organic									
1 tbsp	30	0	NA	0	8	NA	0	0	0
Eden Foods, Short Grain Brown Rice Flour (100% Whole Grain, Organic)									
1/4 cup	150	1.5	0	0	35	3	1	3	0
Ener-G, Baking Powder									
1 tsp	5	0	0	0	1	0	0	0	0
Ener-G, Baking Soda									
1 tsp	0	0	0	0	0	0	0	0	0
Ener-G, Brown Rice Flour									
1/4 cup	150	1	0	0	31	2	0	3	0
Ener-G, Potato Flour									
1/4 cup	150	0	0	0	34	3	0	3	15
Ener-G, Potato Starch Flour									
1/4 cup	160	0	0	0	41	0	0	0	0
Ener-G, Sweet Rice Flour									
1/4 cup	120	0	0	0	28	0	0	2	5

Food Serving size	Cal.	(g) Total Fat	(g) Sat. Fat	(mg) Chol.	(g) Carb.	(g) Fiber	(g) Sug.	(g) Prot.	(mg) Sod.
Ener-G, Tapioca Flour									
1/2 cup	170	0	0	0	42	0	0	0	0
Ener-G, White Rice Flour									
1/4 cup	150	0.5	0	0	32	<1	0	2	0
Ener-G, Xanthan Gum									
2 tbsp	80	0	0	0	20	20	0	0	420
Enjoy Life Foods, Mega Chunks Chocolate for Baking									
1 tbsp	75	5	3	0	9	1	7	1	0
Enjoy Life Foods, Mini Chips Chocolate for Baking									
1-1/3 tbsp	75	5	3	0	9	1	7	1	0
Gluten-Free Pantry, Gluten-Free All Purpose Flour									
1 oz	100	0	0	0	23	0	0	1	115
Gluten-Free Naturals, All Purpose Flour									
1/3 cup	110	0	0	0	27	2	<1	1	20
Gluten-Free Naturals, Multi-Grain Bread Flour									
1/4 cup	100	0	0	0	23	2	<1	1	20
Gluten-Free Naturals, Sandwich Bread Flour									
1/3 cup	110	0	0	0	27	2	<1	1	20
Glutino, All-Purpose Gluten-Free Baking Flour Mix, Dry									
1 oz	90	0	0	0	26	<1	0	1	115
Hodgson Mill, Gluten-Free All Purpose Flour									
1/4 cup	110	0	0	0	24	1	0	1	0
Hodgson Mill, Gluten-Free Xanthan Gum									
.32 oz	30	0	0	0	7	7	0	0	200
King Arthur Flour, Gluten-Free Multi-Purpose Flour									
3 tbsp	110	0	0	0	24	0	0	2	0
Kinnikinnick, All Purpose Flour Blend									
30g	100	0.2	0	0	25	1	0	1	15
Let's Do...Organic, Organic Cornstarch									
1 tbsp	30	0	0	0	7	0	0	1	0
Lundberg Family Farms, Eco-Farmed Brown Rice Flour, Dry									
1/4 cup	110	1.5	0	0	22	2	1	2	0

Food Serving size	Cal.	(g) Total Fat	(g) Sat. Fat	(mg) Chol.	(g) Carb.	(g) Fiber	(g) Sug.	(g) Prot.	(mg) Sod.
Lundberg Family Farms, Organic Brown Rice Flour, Dry									
1/4 cup	110	1.5	0	0	22	2	1	2	0
The Really Great Food Company, Gluten-Free All Purpose Flour Mix									
30g	100	0	0	0	24	<1	0	2	0

Pasta & Pasta Products

Food Serving size	Cal.	Total Fat	Sat. Fat	Chol.	Carb.	Fiber	Sug.	Prot.	Sod.
Ancient Harvest Quinoa, Gluten-Free Linguine Pasta									
2 oz dry	205	1	0	0	46	4	1	4	4
Ancient Harvest Quinoa, Gluten-Free Pasta Elbows									
2 oz dry	205	1	0	0	46	4	<1	4	4
Ancient Harvest Quinoa, Gluten-Free Pasta Shells									
2 oz dry	205	1	0	0	46	4	<1	4	4
Ancient Harvest Quinoa, Gluten-Free Spaghetti Pasta									
2 oz dry	205	1	0	0	46	4	<1	4	4
Ancient Harvest, Garden Pagodas									
2 oz dry	205	1	0	0	46	4	<1	4	4
Ancient Harvest, Macaroni & Cheese, Prepared									
2 oz, about 1 cup	243	2	0.5	3	50	4	1	5	409
Andean Dream, Quinoa Fusilli									
2 oz	207	1	0	0	42	3	3	6	0
Andean Dream, Quinoa Macaroni									
2 oz	207	1	0	0	42	3	3	6	0
Andean Dream, Quinoa Shells									
2 oz	207	1	0	0	42	3	3	6	0
Andean Dream, Quinoa Spaghetti									
2 oz	207	1	0	0	42	3	3	6	0
Annie Chun's, Chinese Chow Mein Noodle Express									
1/2 tray	160	4	0.5	0	27	1	3	5	510
Annie Chun's, Chow Mein Noodles									
2 oz	200	1	0	0	39	3	1	8	350
Annie Chun's, Maifun Brown Rice Noodles									
2 oz	200	1	0.5	0	44	4	1	4	10
Annie Chun's, Maifun Rice Noodles									
2 oz	190	0	0	0	43	1	0	4	0

Food Serving size	Cal.	(g) Total Fat	(g) Sat. Fat	(mg) Chol.	(g) Carb.	(g) Fiber	(g) Sug.	(g) Prot.	(mg) Sod.
Annie Chun's, Organic Buckwheat Soba FreshPak Noodles									
(2 servings for package)									
1 serving	250	1	0	0	52	2	1	8	460
Annie Chun's, Organic Chow Mein FreshPak Noodles									
(2 servings for package)									
1 serving	250	0.5	0	0	53	2	0	7	460
Annie Chun's, Organic Japanese-Style Udon FreshPak Noodles									
(2 servings for package)									
1 serving	240	0.5	0	0	51	2	0	6	470
Annie Chun's, Pad Thai Brown Rice Noodles									
2 oz	200	1	0.5	0	44	4	1	4	10
Annie Chun's, Pad Thai Rice Noodles									
2 oz	190	0	0	0	43	1	0	4	0
Annie Chun's, Soba Noodles									
2 oz	200	1	0	0	39	3	1	8	390
Annie Chun's, Spicy Szechuan Noodle Express									
1/2 tray	170	3	0	0	29	1	4	4	470
Annie Chun's, Teriyaki Noodle Express									
1/2 tray	160	2	0	0	31	1	5	5	510
Annie Chun's, Thai Curry Noodle Express									
1/2 tray	180	7	1	0	29	2	3	4	500
Annie Chun's, Thai Peanut Noodle Express									
1/2 tray	200	7	1	0	29	1	5	6	300
Barkat Gluten-Free, Alphabet Shapes Pasta									
100g, 17.6 package	370	1	0	0	86	4	0	3	20
Barkat Gluten-Free, Animal Shapes Pasta									
100g, 17.6 package	370	1	0	0	86	4	0	3	20
Barkat Gluten-Free, Pasta Spirals, Dry									
1 cup	196	0.6	0	0	40	2	2	4.5	0
Barkat Gluten-Free, Spaghetti Pasta									
100g, 17.6 package	370	1	0	0	86	4	0	3	0
DeBoles, Rice Angel Hair Pasta									
1/4 package	210	0.5	0	0	46*	<1	0	4	15
DeBoles, Rice Angel Hair Pasta, Plus Golden Flax									
1/4 package	210	1.5	0	0	44	1	0	4	10

Food Serving size	Cal.	(g) Total Fat	(g) Sat. Fat	(mg) Chol.	(g) Carb.	(g) Fiber	(g) Sug.	(g) Prot.	(mg) Sod.
DeBoles, Rice Elbow Style Pasta & Cheese, Prepared									
1/4 package	260	1.5	1	5	19	0	0	3	100
DeBoles, Rice Fettuccini Pasta									
1/4 package	210	0.5	0	0	46	<1	0	4	15
DeBoles, Rice Lasagna Pasta									
1/4 package	260	0.5	0	0	56	1	0	5	15
DeBoles, Rice Penne Pasta									
1/4 package	210	0.5	0	0	46	<1	0	4	15
DeBoles, Rice Shells Pasta & Cheddar, Prepared									
1/4 package	260	1.5	1	5	19	0	0	3	100
DeBoles, Rice Spaghetti Style Pasta									
1/4 package	210	0.5	0	0	46	<1	0	4	15
DeBoles, Rice Spirals Pasta									
1/4 package	210	0.5	0	0	46	<1	0	4	15
DeBoles, Rice Spirals Pasta, Plus Golden Flax									
1/4 package	210	1.5	0	0	44	1	0	4	10
DeBoles, Wheat Free Corn Elbow Style Pasta									
1/6 package	200	2	0	0	43	5	0	4	15
DeBoles, Wheat Free Corn Spaghetti Style Pasta									
1/4 package	200	2	0	0	43	5	0	4	15
DeBoles, Whole Grain Penne Pasta									
1/4 package	200	1.5	0	0	46	3	0	5	0
DeBoles, Whole Grain Spaghetti Style Pasta									
1/4 package	200	1.5	0	0	46	3	0	5	0
Eden Foods, Bifun (Rice) Pasta, Japanese									
2 oz	200	0.5	0	0	44	0	0	5	5
Eden Foods, Kuzu Pasta									
2 oz	200	0	0	0	48	2	0	0	0
Eden Foods, Mung Bean Pasta (Harusame)									
2 oz	190	0	0	NA	47	0	0	0	5
Ener-G, White Rice Lasagna									
56g	180	0	0	0	42	2	0	4	0
Ener-G, White Rice Macaroni									
56g	180	0	0	0	43	3	0	4	0

Food Serving size	Cal.	(g) Total Fat	(g) Sat. Fat	(mg) Chol.	(g) Carb.	(g) Fiber	(g) Sug.	(g) Prot.	(mg) Sod.
Ener-G, White Rice Small Shells									
56g	180	0	0	0	42	2	0	4	0
Ener-G, White Rice Spaghetti									
56g	180	0	0	0	42	2	0	4	0
Ener-G, White Rice Vermicelli									
56g	180	0	0	0	41	2	0	4	0
Food for Life, Ezekiel 4:9 Sprouted Grain Fettuccine Pasta									
1 serving	210	2	0.1	NA	39	7	NA	9	10
Food for Life, Ezekiel 4:9 Sprouted Grain Linguine Pasta									
2 oz	210	2	0.5	0	39	7	NA	9	10
Food for Life, Ezekiel 4:9 Sprouted Grain Penne Pasta									
1 serving	210	2	0.1	NA	39	7	NA	9	10
Food for Life, Ezekiel 4:9 Sprouted Grain Spaghetti Pasta									
1 serving	210	2	0.1	NA	39	7	NA	9	10
Gillian's Foods, Gluten-Free Brown Rice Penne Pasta									
1 cup	200	0	0	0	45	1	<1	5	1
Gillian's Foods, Gluten-Free Brown Rice Spaghetti Pasta									
1 cup	200	0	0	0	45	1	<1	5	1
Hodgson Mill, Gluten-Free Brown Rice Angel Hair Pasta with Golden Milled Flax Seed, Dry									
2 oz	209	1	0	0	44	2	0	5	0
Hodgson Mill, Gluten-Free Brown Rice Elbows with Golden Milled Flax Seed, Dry									
2 oz	209	1	0	0	44	2	0	5	0
Hodgson Mill, Gluten-Free Brown Rice Lasagna with Golden Milled Flax Seed, Dry									
2 oz	209	1	0	0	44	2	0	5	0
Hodgson Mill, Gluten-Free Brown Rice Linguine with Golden Milled Flax Seed, Dry									
2 oz	209	1	0	0	44	2	0	5	0
Hodgson Mill, Gluten-Free Brown Rice Penne with Golden Milled Flax Seed, Dry									
2 oz	209	1	0	0	44	2	0	5	0
Hodgson Mill, Gluten-Free Brown Rice Spaghetti with Golden Milled Flax Seed, Dry									
2 oz	209	1	0	0	44	2	0	5	0
Jovial Foods, Brown Rice Pasta									
(including Spaghetti, Capellini, Penne Rigate, Fusilli, and Caserecce)									
2 oz	210	2	0	0	43	2	0	5	0

Food Serving size	Cal.	(g) Total Fat	(g) Sat. Fat	(mg) Chol.	(g) Carb.	(g) Fiber	(g) Sug.	(g) Prot.	(mg) Sod.
Lundberg Family Farms, Butternut Squash Risotto, Cooked									
1/2 cup	140	1	0	0	31	1	1	4	500
Lundberg Family Farms, Creamy Parmesan Risotto, Cooked									
1/2 cup	140	1.5	0.5	5	27	1	1	5	490
Lundberg Family Farms, Elbow Pasta, Dry									
55g	190	3	0.5	0	40	4	1	4	0
Lundberg Family Farms, Garlic Primavera Risotto, Cooked									
1/2 cup	140	1	0	0	29	1	1	4	520
Lundberg Family Farms, Italian Herb Risotto, Cooked									
1/2 cup	140	1	0	0	28	1	1	4	530
Lundberg Family Farms, Organic Alfredo Risotto									
40g	140	1	0.5	0	29	1	1	5	400
Lundberg Family Farms, Organic Florentine Risotto, Cooked									
1/2 cup	140	0	0	0	31	1	2	3	410
Lundberg Family Farms, Organic Porcini Mushroom Risotto, Cooked									
1/2 cup	143	1	0.5	0	31	1	1	4	535
Lundberg Family Farms, Organic Tuscan Risotto, Cooked									
1/2 cup	140	0	0	0	31	1	2	3	735
Lundberg Family Farms, Penne Pasta, Dry									
55g	190	3	0.5	0	40	4	1	4	0
Lundberg Family Farms, Rotini Pasta, Dry									
55g	190	3	0.5	0	40	4	1	4	0
Lundberg Family Farms, Spaghetti Pasta, Dry									
55g	190	3	0.5	0	40	4	1	4	0
Pastariso, Gluten-Free Potato Spaghetti Pasta									
2 oz	191	0.8	0	0	42	5	3	4	0
Pastariso, Organic Brown Rice Gluten-Free Pasta (including Elbows, Lasagna, Penne, Spaghetti, Linguine, Fettucine)									
2 oz	190	0.6	0	0	42	3	3	4	5
Schar, Anellini Pasta									
1/3 cup	190	1.5	0.5	0	40	1	0	5	30
Schar, Fusilli Pasta									
1/2 cup	190	1.5	0.5	0	40	<1	0	5	30
Schar, Gluten-Free Anellini Pasta									
1/3 cup	190	1.5	0.5	0	40	1	0	5	30

Food Serving size	Cal.	(g) Total Fat	(g) Sat. Fat	(mg) Chol.	(g) Carb.	(g) Fiber	(g) Sug.	(g) Prot.	(mg) Sod.
Schar, Gluten-Free Fusilli Pasta									
1/2 cup	190	1.5	0.5	0	40	<1	0	5	30
Schar, Gluten-Free Multigrain Penne Rigate Pasta									
1/2 cup	190	1	0.5	0	42	1	0	4	15
Schar, Gluten-Free Penne Pasta									
1/2 cup	190	1.5	0.5	0	40	<1	0	5	30
Schar, Gluten-Free Spaghetti Pasta									
2 oz	200	1.5	0	0	42	1	0	5	10
Schar, Multigrain Penne Rigate									
1/2 cup	190	1	0.5	0	42	1	0	4	15
Schar, Penne Pasta									
1/2 cup	190	1.5	0.5	0	40	<1	0	5	30
Schar, Spaghetti Pasta									
2 oz	200	1.5	0	0	42	1	0	5	30
Schar, Tagliatelle Gluten-Free Pasta									
1/2 cup	180	1	0.5	0	43	1	0	3	10
Schar, Tagliatelle Pasta									
1/2 cup	180	1	0.5	0	43	1	0	3	10
Thai Kitchen, Stir-Fry Rice Noodles									
2 oz	210	1	0	0	46	0	0	4	20
Thai Kitchen, Thin Rice Noodles									
2 oz	180	1	0	0	40	1	0	3	0
The Really Great Food Company, Tinkyada Rice Pasta – Vegetable Spirals									
2 oz	210	1	0	0	45	2	0	5	10
The Really Great Food Company, Tinkyada Rice Pasta									
(including Spaghetti, Penne, Elbows, Shells, Fusilli, Fettuccini, Lasagna)									
2 oz	210	2	0.5	0	43	2	0	4	15
Tinkyada Gluten Free, Brown Rice Lasagne Pasta									
56g	210	2	0.5	0	43	2	NA	4	15
Tinkyada Gluten Free, Brown Rice Little Dreams Pasta									
2 oz	210	2	0.5	0	43	2	0	4	15
Tinkyada Gluten Free, Brown Rice Pasta Shells, Dry									
2 oz	210	2	0.5	0	43	2	0	4	15
Tinkyada Gluten Free, Spinach & Brown Rice Spaghetti Style Pasta									
2 oz	210	2	0.5	0	43	2	0	4	15

Food Serving size	Cal.	(g) Total Fat	(g) Sat. Fat	(mg) Chol.	(g) Carb.	(g) Fiber	(g) Sug.	(g) Prot.	(mg) Sod.
Tinkyada Organic, Gluten-Free Brown Rice Elbow Pasta, Dry									
2 oz	200	1.5	0	0	44	1	0	4	25
Tinkyada Organic, Gluten-Free Brown Rice Penne Pasta, Dry									
2 oz	210	2	1	0	43	2	0	4	15
Tinkyada Organic, Gluten-Free Brown Rice Spaghetti Style Pasta									
2 oz	200	1.5	0	0	44	1	0	4	25

Rice / Grains

Food Serving size	Cal.	(g) Total Fat	(g) Sat. Fat	(mg) Chol.	(g) Carb.	(g) Fiber	(g) Sug.	(g) Prot.	(mg) Sod.
Ancient Harvest, Inca Red Original Quinoa, Dry									
1/4 cup	180	3	0	0	33	6	3	6	2
Ancient Harvest, Traditional Original Quinoa, Dry									
1/4 cup	172	2.8	0	0	31	3	3	6	1
Annie Chun's, Black Pearl Sticky Rice									
1 tray	270	2	NA	NA	57	2	NA	6	5
Annie Chun's, Multi-Grain Sticky Rice									
1 tray	270	2	NA	NA	57	3	NA	6	5
Annie Chun's, Sprouted Brown Sticky Rice									
1 tray	270	1	NA	NA	59	3	NA	6	0
Annie Chun's, White Sticky Rice									
1 tray	300	0	NA	NA	67	NA	NA	6	0
Arrowhead Mills, Amaranth									
1/4 cup	180	3	1	0	31	7	1	7	10
Arrowhead Mills, Brown Basmati Rice									
1/4 cup	140	1.5	0	0	31	2	1	3	0
Arrowhead Mills, Buckwheat Groats									
1/4 cup	150	1	0	0	31	4	1	5	0
Arrowhead Mills, Hulled Millet									
1/4 cup	150	1.5	0	0	33	1	0	4	0
Arrowhead Mills, Long Grain Brown Rice									
1/4 cup	160	1	0	0	32	1	0	3	0
Arrowhead Mills, Quinoa									
1/3 cup	160	2.5	0	0	30	3	0	6	10
Birkett Mills, Pocono Kasha									
1/4 cup	170	1	0	0	35	2	0	6	10

Food Serving size	Cal.	(g) Total Fat	(g) Sat. Fat	(mg) Chol.	(g) Carb.	(g) Fiber	(g) Sug.	(g) Prot.	(mg) Sod.
Birkett Mills, Pocono Whole Buckwheat Groats									
1/4 cup	150	1	0	0	32	2	0	5	10
Birkett Mills, Wolff's Kasha									
1/4 cup	170	1	0	0	35	2	0	6	10
Birkett Mills, Wolff's Whole Buckwheat Groats									
1/4 cup	150	1	0	0	32	2	0	5	10
Bob's Red Mill, Corn Grits/Polenta, Dry									
1/4 cup	130	0	0	0	27	2	0	3	0
Bob's Red Mill, Hulled Millet, Prepared									
1/8 cup	140	1	0	0	18	4	0	3	0
Bob's Red Mill, Organic Amaranth Grain									
1/4 cup	190	3.5	1	0	34	7	1	8	10
Bob's Red Mill, Organic Buckwheat Groats									
1/4 cup	150	1.5	0	0	32	5	1	6	0
Bob's Red Mill, Rice Bran, Dry									
2 tbsp	60	2.5	0.5	0	8	3	0	2	0
Eden Foods, Millet, 100% Whole Grain, Organic, Uncooked									
1/4 cup	160	2	0	0	30	4	0	5	5
Eden Foods, Quinoa, 100% Whole Grain, Organic									
1/4 cup	170	2.5	0	0	31	4	1	5	0
Eden Foods, Red Quinoa, 100% Whole Grain, Organic, Uncooked									
1/4 cup	170	2	0	0	32	5	2	6	5
Eden Foods, Short Grain Brown Rice, 100% Whole Grain, Organic									
1/4 cup	150	1.5	0	0	35	3	1	3	0
Eden Foods, Sprouted Brown Rice Mochi									
1 square	110	1	0.2	0	25	1	0	2	0
Eden Foods, Sweet Brown Rice Mochi, 100% Whole Grain									
1 square	110	1	0	0	25	1	0	2	0
Eden Foods, Wild Rice, 100% Whole Grain									
1/4 cup	160	0.5	0	0	35	3	0	6	15
Ener-G, Rice Bran									
1/2 cup	220	14	2.5	0	34	19	3	10	5
Ener-G, Rice Mix									
1/2 cup	130	0	0	0	28	<1	0	2	85

Food Serving size	Cal.	(g) Total Fat	(g) Sat. Fat	(mg) Chol.	(g) Carb.	(g) Fiber	(g) Sug.	(g) Prot.	(mg) Sod.
Frieda's, Organic Polenta Basil and Garlic Rice									
1/4 package	90	0	0	0	19	0	0	2	300
Frieda's, Organic Polenta Green Chile and Cilantro Rice									
1/4 package	90	0	0	0	18	0	0	2	300
Frieda's, Organic Polenta Mushroom and Onion Rice									
1/4 package	90	0	0	0	19	1	0	2	300
Frieda's, Organic Polenta Sun Dried Tomato and Garlic Rice									
1/4 package	90	0	0	0	19	1	0	2	310
Frieda's, Organic Polenta Traditional Flavor Rice									
2-1/2 slices	70	NA	NA	NA	15	1	1	2	310
Lotus Foods, Bhutanese Red Rice									
1/3 cup	200	0	0	0	48	3	0	4	0
Lotus Foods, Cambodian Mekong Flower Rice									
1/3 cup dry	190	0	0	0	45	1	0	4	0
Lotus Foods, Forbidden Rice									
1/3 cup	200	2	0	0	43	3	1	6	0
Lotus Foods, Indonesian Volcano Rice									
1/3 cup	200	0	0	0	44	1	0	6	0
Lotus Foods, Kalijira Rice									
1/4 cup	150	0	NA	0	42	0	0	5	0
Lotus Foods, Madagascar Pink Rice									
1/3 cup	200	1.5	0.5	0	44	2	0	4	0
Lotus Foods, Organic Brown Jasmine Rice									
1/3 cup	230	1	0	0	47	1	1	5	0
Lotus Foods, Organic Carnaroli Rice									
1/3 cup	240	0	0	0	53	2	0	5	0
Lotus Foods, Organic Forbidden Rice									
1/3 cup	200	2	0	0	43	3	1	6	0
Lotus Foods, Organic Jade Pearl Rice									
1/3 cup	210	0	0	0	43	0	0	4	0
Lotus Foods, Organic Jasmine Rice									
1/3 cup	210	1.5	0.5	0	45	2	0	5	0
Lundberg Family Farms, Christmas Rice									
1/4 cup	170	1.5	0	0	37	3	1	4	0

Food Serving size	Cal.	(g) Total Fat	(g) Sat. Fat	(mg) Chol.	(g) Carb.	(g) Fiber	(g) Sug.	(g) Prot.	(mg) Sod.
Lundberg Family Farms, Eco-Farmed Brown Sweet Rice									
1/4 cup	180	1.5	0	0	40	2	0	4	0
Lundberg Family Farms, Eco-Farmed California Brown Basmati Rice, Dry									
1/4 cup	150	1.5	0	0	33	2	1	4	0
Lundberg Family Farms, Eco-Farmed California White Basmati Rice, Dry									
1/4 cup	160	0.5	0	0	36	0	0	3	0
Lundberg Family Farms, Eco-Farmed California White Jasmine Rice, Dry									
1/4 cup	160	0.5	0	0	36	0	0	3	0
Lundberg Family Farms, Eco-Farmed Long Grain Brown Rice, Dry									
1/4 cup	150	2	0	0	35	3	0	3	0
Lundberg Family Farms, Eco-Farmed Short Grain Brown Rice, Dry									
1/4 cup	150	1.5	0	0	35	3	0	3	0
Lundberg Family Farms, Eco-Farmed White Arborio Rice, Dry									
1/4 cup	160	1	0	0	35	1	0	5	0
Lundberg Family Farms, Lundberg Black Japonica									
45g	150	1.5	0	0	33	3	0	4	0
Lundberg Family Farms, Lundberg Black Japonica Rice									
1/4 cup	150	1.5	0	0	33	3	0	4	0
Lundberg Family Farms, Lundberg Countrywild Brown Rice									
210g	280	25	0	0	65	6	0	6	0
Lundberg Family Farms, Lundberg Jubilee Rice									
1/4 cup	170	1.5	0	0	35	3	0	3	0
Lundberg Family Farms, Lundberg Wehani Rice									
45g	150	1.5	0	0	35	2	0	3	0
Lundberg Family Farms, Lundberg Wild Blend Rice									
45g	160	1	0	0	34	3	1	4	0
Lundberg Family Farms, Mediterranean Curry Brown Rice Couscous									
45g	150	1.5	0	0	34	3	1	3	460
Lundberg Family Farms, Olde World Pilaf									
1/4 cup	153	1.5	0	0	33	4.5	1	5	0
Lundberg Family Farms, Organic Brown Sweet Rice									
45g	150	1	0	0	35	2	0	3	0
Lundberg Family Farms, Organic Brown Sweet Rice, Dry									
1/4 cup	150	1	0	0	35	2	0	3	0

Food Serving size	Cal.	(g) Total Fat	(g) Sat. Fat	(mg) Chol.	(g) Carb.	(g) Fiber	(g) Sug.	(g) Prot.	(mg) Sod.
Lundberg Family Farms, Organic California Brown Basmati Rice, Dry									
1/4 cup	150	1.5	0	0	33	2	1	4	0
Lundberg Family Farms, Organic California Brown Jasmine Rice, Dry									
1/4 cup	150	1.5	0	0	33	2	1	4	0
Lundberg Family Farms, Organic California White Basmati Rice									
45g	160	0.5	0	0	34	1	0	3	0
Lundberg Family Farms, Organic California White Jasmine Rice, Dry									
1/4 cup	160	0.5	0	0	36	1	0	3	0
Lundberg Family Farms, Organic California White Sushi Rice									
45g	150	0	0	0	35	1	0	4	0
Lundberg Family Farms, Organic California White Sushi Rice, Dry									
1/4 cup	150	0	0	0	35	1	0	4	5
Lundberg Family Farms, Organic Golden Rose Brown Rice, Dry									
1/4 cup	160	1	0	0	34	1	0	3	0
Lundberg Family Farms, Organic Long Grain Brown Rice									
45g	150	1.5	0	0	35	3	0	3	0
Lundberg Family Farms, Organic Long Grain Brown Rice, Dry									
1/4 cup	150	1.5	0	0	35	3	0	3	0
Lundberg Family Farms, Organic Long Grain White Rice, Dry									
1/4 cup	160	0	0	0	36	0	0	4	0
Lundberg Family Farms, Organic Quick Wild Rice, Dry									
1/4 cup	150	0.5	0	NA	33	2	1	6	0
Lundberg Family Farms, Organic Short Grain Brown Rice, Dry									
1/4 cup	150	1.5	0	0	35	3	1	3	0
Lundberg Family Farms, Organic White Arborio Rice									
1/4 cup	160	1	0	0	43	1	0	6	0
Lundberg Family Farms, Organic Wild Blend									
1/4 cup	150	1.5	0	0	35	3	0	4	0
Lundberg Family Farms, Organic Wild Rice, Dry									
.25 cup	150	1	0	0	33	2	1	6	0
Lundberg Family Farms, Roasted Garlic & Olive Oil Brown Rice Couscous, Dry									
45g	150	1.5	0	0	34	2	1	3	340

Food Serving size	Cal.	(g) Total Fat	(g) Sat. Fat	(mg) Chol.	(g) Carb.	(g) Fiber	(g) Sug.	(g) Prot.	(mg) Sod.
Lundberg Family Farms, Roasted Organic Plain Original Brown Rice Couscous, Dry									
45g	150	1.5	0	0	35	3	1	3	0
Lundberg Family Farms, Savory Herb Brown Rice Couscous									
45g	150	1.5	0	0	34	2	1	3	300
Tasty Bite, Basmati Rice									
1/2 pack	170	2	0	0	37	1	0	3	0
Tasty Bite, Brown Rice									
1/2 pack	240	3	0	0	48	2	0	5	0
Tasty Bite, Garlic Brown Rice									
1/2 pack	220	5	0.5	0	39	2	1	5	420
Tasty Bite, Ginger Lentil Rice									
1/2 pack	190	3.5	1.5	0	35	3	2	5	380
Tasty Bite, Jasmine Rice									
1/2 pack	210	4	0	0	39	<1	0	3	0
Thai Kitchen, Green Chili & Garlic Jasmine Rice									
3 tbsp	210	2	1.5	0	43	1	3	4	510
Thai Kitchen, Jasmine Rice									
2 tbsp	160	0	0	0	36	1	0	3	0
Thai Kitchen, Lemongrass & Ginger Jasmine Rice									
66g	250	3.5	0.5	0	50	1	3	4	840
Thai Kitchen, Roasted Red Chili Paste									
1 tbsp	50	3	0	5	4	0	2	2	130
Thai Kitchen, Spicy Thai Chili Jasmine Rice									
66g	250	0	0	0	47	1	3	5	250
Thai Kitchen, Sweet Chili & Onion Jasmine Rice									
3 tbsp	210	1.5	1.5	0	43	2	2	4	470
Thai Kitchen, Thai Yellow Curry Jasmine Rice									
2 tbsp	170	0	0	0	38	1	2	3	370
The Really Great Food Company, Gluten-Free Brown Rice Bread Mix									
1 slice, prepared	100	0	0	0	22	<1	4	<1	180

Vegetables

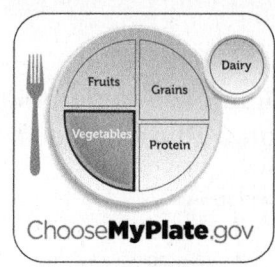

ChooseMyPlate.gov

Why Eat Vegetables?

The main reason to include vegetables in your diet is that they are gluten-free. In addition, eating a diet rich in vegetables and fruits as part of an overall healthy diet may reduce risk for heart disease, including heart attack and stroke. Most vegetables are naturally low in fat and calories, and none have cholesterol, although added sauces or seasonings may add fat, calories, cholesterol, and gluten. Vegetables are important sources of many nutrients, including potassium, dietary fiber, folate (folic acid), vitamin A, and vitamin C. Diets rich in potassium may help to maintain healthy blood pressure. Vitamin A keeps eyes and skin healthy and helps to protect against infections. Vitamin C helps heal cuts and wounds, keeps teeth and gums healthy, and aids in iron absorption.

Daily Goal

Two and a half cups for an adult on a 2,000 calorie diet.
One-cup equivalents:

1 cup cooked vegetable	3" tomato
2 cups raw vegetables	1 cup cooked dry peas or beans
2 medium carrots	1 cup starchy vegetable

Gluten-Free Shopping Tips

- Choose vegetables rich in color—red, orange, or dark green
- Buy fresh vegetables in season
- Purchase locally grown vegetables when possible
- Stock up on frozen or canned vegetables for fast preparation
- Remember that over a quarter of your plate should be vegetables
- Avoid vegetables that are in sauces or fried
- Season with fresh herbs and spices

Gluten-Free Shopping List Essentials

Tomatoes	Cauliflower	Squash
Peppers	Green Beans	Fresh Herbs & Spices
Carrots	Spinach	
Broccoli	Sweet Potatoes/Yams	

Approved Vegetables and Those to Avoid on a Gluten-Free Diet

Gluten-Free

- Fresh, frozen, and canned vegetables
- Vegetable juices

May Contain Gluten

- Vegetables with sauces
- French-fried potatoes (especially where gluten-containing foods may be cooked in the same oil)
- Scalloped potatoes (containing wheat flour)
- Deep-fried, battered vegetables

Caution

Canned vegetables can be high in sodium. Look for salt-free canned vegetables, or rinse canned vegetables before using. Frozen vegetables may have added sauces that contain gluten and add calories, fat, and salt. Choose frozen vegetables without sauces and seasonings.

Food Serving size	Cal.	(g) Total Fat	(g) Sat. Fat	(mg) Chol.	(g) Carb.	(g) Fiber	(g) Sug.	(g) Prot.	(mg) Sod.

Potatoes

Betty Crocker, Potato Bud Gluten Free Mashed Potatoes

.33 cup	80	0	0	0	18	1	0	0	20

Dr. Praeger's Sensible Foods, Potato Littles

2 pieces	60	3	0	15	7	<1	0	1	115

Dr. Praeger's Sensible Foods, Sweet Potato Littles

2 pieces	60	2	0	0	9	<1	2	<1	85

Dr. Praeger's Sensible Foods, Sweet Potato Pancakes

1 pancake	80	2	0	0	12	3	6	2	140

Edward & Sons, Organic Home Style Mashed Potatoes

1/2 cup prepared	150	0	0	0	20	2	1	2	190

Edward & Sons, Organic Roasted Garlic Mashed Potatoes

1/2 cup prepared	150	0	0	0	20	2	1	2	190

Ener-G, Potato Mix

1/4 cup	160	0	0	0	40	<1	0	0	130

Ian's Natural Foods, Allergy Friendly Sweet Potato Fries

About 15 pieces	180	2	0	0	37	3	14	3	50

Ian's Natural Foods, Alphatots

14 fries	140	7	3	5	18	3	1	2	290

Idahoan, Baby Reds Flavored Mashed Potatoes

1/2 cup	110	3	1	0	21	2	2	2	400

Idahoan, Baby Reds with Roasted Garlic and Parmesan Flavored Mashed Potatoes

1/2 cup	110	2	1	0	21	2	1	3	560

Idahoan, Butter & Herb Flavored Mashed Potatoes

1/2 cup	110	3	1	0	20	1	2	2	520

Idahoan, Buttery Homestyle Flavored Mashed Potatoes

1/2 cup	110	3	1	0	20	1	2	2	450

Idahoan, Four Cheese Flavored Mashed Potatoes

1/2 cup	110	2.5	1	0	20	1	2	2	590

Idahoan, Golden Selects Flavored Mashed Potatoes

1/2 cup	110	3	1	0	21	2	2	2	400

Idahoan, Honest Earth All Natural Creamy Mash

1/2 cup	180	1	0	0	17	2	1	2	270

Food Serving size	Cal.	(g) Total Fat	(g) Sat. Fat	(mg) Chol.	(g) Carb.	(g) Fiber	(g) Sug.	(g) Prot.	(mg) Sod.
Idahoan, Italian Romano White Cheese Flavored Mashed Potatoes									
1/2 cup	110	2.5	1	0	20	1	2	2	560
Idahoan, Original Mashed Potatoes									
1/2 cup	180	0	0	0	17	1	1	2	15
Idahoan, Roasted Garlic Flavored Mashed Potatoes									
1/2 cup	110	3	1	0	20	1	2	2	590
Idahoan, Southwest Flavored Mashed Potatoes									
1/2 cup	110	3	1	0	20	1	2	2	500
Tasty Bite, Bombay Potatoes									
1/2 pack	130	4	0.5	0	19	4	3	5	530

Spices / Seasonings / Herbs

Food Serving size	Cal.	(g) Total Fat	(g) Sat. Fat	(mg) Chol.	(g) Carb.	(g) Fiber	(g) Sug.	(g) Prot.	(mg) Sod.
Eden Foods, Black & Tan Gomasio (Sesame Salt), Organic									
1 tsp	20	1.5	0	0	<1	0	0	<1	80
Eden Foods, Black Gomasio (Sesame Salt), Organic									
1 tsp	20	1.5	0	0	<1	0	0	<1	80
Eden Foods, Dulse Flakes, Sea Vegetable, Organic, Wild, Hand Harvested, Raw									
1 tsp	3	0	0	0	0	0	0	0	15
Eden Foods, Dulse Whole Leaf, Sea Vegetable, Organic, Wild, Hand Harvested									
1/4 cup	10	0	0	0	2	1	0	<1	60
Eden Foods, Eden Shake (Sesame and Sea Vegetable Seasoning) (Furikake)									
1/2 tsp	5	0	0	0	1	1	0	0	25
Eden Foods, Garlic Gomasio (Sesame Salt), Organic									
1 tsp	15	1.5	0	0	<1	0	0	<1	80
Eden Foods, Gomasio (Sesame Salt), Organic									
1 tsp	15	1.5	0	0	<1	0	0	<1	80
Eden Foods, Sea Salt, French									
1/4 tsp	0	0	NA	NA	0	NA	NA	NA	392
Eden Foods, Sea Salt, Portuguese									
1/4 tsp	0	0	0	0	0	0	0	0	408
Eden Foods, Seaweed Gomasio (Sesame Salt), Organic									
1 tsp	15	1.5	0	0	<1	0	0	<1	80
Eden Foods, Shiso Leaf Powder (Pickled Beefsteak Leaf)									
1 tsp	0	0	0	0	0	0	0	0	200

Food Serving size	Cal.	(g) Total Fat	(g) Sat. Fat	(mg) Chol.	(g) Carb.	(g) Fiber	(g) Sug.	(g) Prot.	(mg) Sod.
Eden Foods, Wasabi Powder									
1 tsp	10	0	0	0	1	0.5	0	0	0
Eden Foods, Yansen (Dandelion Root Concentrate)									
1/4 tsp	5	0	0	0	1	0	<1	0	0
Simply Organic Foods, Black Bean Seasoning Mix									
2 tsp	15	0	0	0	3	0	0	0	260
Simply Organic Foods, Citrus 'n Herb Seasoning									
1/4 tsp	5	0	0	0	0	0	0	0	0
Simply Organic Foods, Dirty Rice Seasoning Mix									
2 tsp	20	0	0	0	4	1	0	1	410
Simply Organic Foods, Fajita Seasoning									
2 tsp	20	0	0	0	5	1	0	0	270
Simply Organic Foods, Gumbo Base Seasoning Mix									
1 tbsp	25	0	0	0	6	1	0	1	410
Simply Organic Foods, Jambalaya Seasoning Mix									
2 tsp	15	0	0	0	3	1	0	1	460
Simply Organic Foods, Mild Chili Seasoning Mix									
2 tsp	15	0	0	0	3	1	1	0	280
Simply Organic Foods, Orange Ginger Seasoning									
1/4 tsp	5	0	0	0	<1	0	0	0	60
Simply Organic Foods, Red Bean Seasoning Mix									
2 tsp	15	0	0	0	3	1	0	0	250
Simply Organic Foods, Roasted Chicken Gravy Seasoning Mix									
2 tsp	20	0	0	0	4	0	0	0	290
Simply Organic Foods, Roasted Turkey Gravy Seasoning Mix									
2 tsp	20	0	0	0	4	0	0	0	290
Simply Organic Foods, Salsa Verde Seasoning									
1/2 tsp	5	0	0	0	1	0	0	0	80
Simply Organic Foods, Seafood Seasoning									
1/4 tsp	0	0	0	0	0	0	0	0	40
Simply Organic Foods, Sloppy Joe Seasoning Mix									
1 tsp	15	0	0	0	3	0	1	0	300
Simply Organic Foods, Spicy Chili Seasoning Mix									
2 tsp	15	0	0	0	3	1	0	1	210

Food Serving size	Cal.	(g) Total Fat	(g) Sat. Fat	(mg) Chol.	(g) Carb.	(g) Fiber	(g) Sug.	(g) Prot.	(mg) Sod.
Simply Organic Foods, Spicy Steak Seasoning									
1/4 tsp	0	0	0	0	0	0	0	0	35
Simply Organic Foods, Spicy Taco									
2 tsp	25	0.5	0	0	5	1	1	1	330
Simply Organic Foods, Steak Seasoning									
1/4 tsp	0	0	0	0	0	0	0	0	85
Simply Organic Foods, Sweet Basil Pesto									
2 tsp	10	0	0	0	2	0	0	0	200
Simply Organic Foods, Vegetable Seasoning									
1/4 tsp	0	0	0	0	0	0	0	0	40
Simply Organic Foods, Vegetarian Chili Seasoning Mix									
2 tsp	15	0	0	0	3	1	0	1	210

Vegetable Products (Including Canned Items)

Food Serving size	Cal.	(g) Total Fat	(g) Sat. Fat	(mg) Chol.	(g) Carb.	(g) Fiber	(g) Sug.	(g) Prot.	(mg) Sod.
505 Southwestern, Chunky Organic Medium Salsa									
2 tbsp	10	0	NA	NA	2	NA	1	0	120
505 Southwestern, Salsa									
2 tbsp	14	0	NA	NA	2	NA	1	0	120
Amy's, Black Bean & Corn Salsa									
2 tbsp	15	0	0	0	3	<1	1	1	170
Amy's, Medium Salsa									
2 tbsp	10	0	0	0	2	0	1	0	190
Amy's, Mild Salsa									
2 tbsp	10	0	0	0	2	0	1	0	190
Amy's, Organic Light in Sodium, Spicy Chili									
1 cup	280	9	1	0	35	7	5	15	340
Bhuja, Crunchy Seasoned Peas									
.88 oz	119	5	1	0	14	3	1	5	109
Boar's Head, Sauerkraut									
2 tbsp	5	0	0	0	1	<1	0	0	180
Boar's Head, Sweet Vidalia Onions in Sauce									
1 tbsp	10	0	0	0	2	0	2	0	15
Campbell's, Healthy Request, Tomato Juice									
8 oz	50	0	0	0	10	2	7	2	480

Food Serving size	Cal.	(g) Total Fat	(g) Sat. Fat	(mg) Chol.	(g) Carb.	(g) Fiber	(g) Sug.	(g) Prot.	(mg) Sod.
Campbell's, Low Sodium Tomato Juice 8 fl oz	50	0	0	0	10	2	7	2	140
Campbell's, Tomato Juice 6 oz	50	0	0	0	10	2	7	2	660
Dr. Praeger's Sensible Foods, Broccoli Littles 2 pieces	40	2.5	0	0	4	<1	0	1	100
Dr. Praeger's Sensible Foods, Spinach Littles 2 pieces	45	3	0	0	5	<1	0	1	100
Eden Foods, Agar, Agar Flakes, Sea Vegetable, Wild, Hand Harvested 1 tbsp	0	0	0	0	1	1	0	0	10
Eden Foods, Arame, Sea Vegetable, Wild, Hand Harvested 1/2 cup	30	0	0	0	7	7	0	1	120
Eden Foods, Crushed Tomatoes with Basil, Organic 1/4 cup	20	0	0	0	3	1	2	1	0
Eden Foods, Crushed Tomatoes with Onions and Garlic, Organic 1/4 cup	20	0	0	0	3	1	2	1	0
Eden Foods, Crushed Tomatoes with Roasted Onion, Organic 1/4 cup	20	0	0	0	3	1	2	1	0
Eden Foods, Crushed Tomatoes with Sweet Basil, Organic 1/4 cup	20	0	0	0	3	1	2	1	0
Eden Foods, Crushed Tomatoes, Organic 1/4 cup	20	0	0	0	3	1	2	1	0
Eden Foods, Daikon Radish, Shredded and Dried 2 tbsp	45	0	0	0	9	3	6	1	20
Eden Foods, Diced Tomatoes with Basil, Organic 1/2 cup	30	0	0	0	6	2	4	1	5
Eden Foods, Diced Tomatoes with Green Chiles, Organic 1/2 cup	30	0	0	0	5	2	3	2	35
Eden Foods, Diced Tomatoes with Roasted Onion, Organic 1/2 cup	30	0	0	0	6	2	4	1	5
Eden Foods, Diced Tomatoes, Organic 1/2 cup	30	0	0	0	6	2	4	1	5
Eden Foods, Hiziki, Sea Vegetable, Wild, Hand Harvested 1 tsp	0	0	0	0	0	1	0	0	15

Food Serving size	Cal.	(g) Total Fat	(g) Sat. Fat	(mg) Chol.	(g) Carb.	(g) Fiber	(g) Sug.	(g) Prot.	(mg) Sod.
Eden Foods, Instant Wakame Flakes, Sea Vegetable, Cultivated									
1 tsp	0	0	0	0	0	0	0	0	90
Eden Foods, Kombu, Sea Vegetable, Wild, Hand Harvested									
1/2 of 7" piece	10	0	0	0	2	1	0	0	90
Eden Foods, Lotus Root									
About 5 slices	35	0	0	0	8	2	1	1	25
Eden Foods, Maitake Mushrooms, Dried									
About 10 pieces	35	0	0	0	7	4	0	2	0
Eden Foods, Mekabu Wakame, Sea Vegetable, Wild, Hand Harvested									
1 tsp	0	0	0	0	0	0	0	0	35
Eden Foods, Nori Krinkles, Sea Vegetables, Cultivated, Toasted									
1/2 cup	10	0	0	0	1	1	0	1	5
Eden Foods, Nori, Sea Vegetable, Cultivated, Raw									
1 sheet	10	0	0	0	0	1	0	1	5
Eden Foods, Pickled Daikon Radish									
2 whole pieces	5	0	NA	NA	1	NA	0	0	250
Eden Foods, Sauerkraut, Organic									
1/4 cup	5	0	NA	0	2	1	0	0	150
Eden Foods, Shiitake Mushrooms, Dried Sliced									
About 6 slices	35	0	0	0	7	5	2	2	0
Eden Foods, Shiitake Mushrooms, Whole Dried									
3 mushrooms	35	0	0	0	7	5	2	2	0
Eden Foods, Sushi Nori, Sea Vegetable, Cultivated									
1 toasted sheet	10	0	0	0	0	1	0	1	5
Eden Foods, Wakame, Sea Vegetable, Cultivated, Hand Harvested, Raw									
1/2 cup	25	0	0	0	4	4	0	2	660
Eden Foods, Whole Roma Tomatoes with Sweet Basil, Organic									
1/2 cup	30	0	0	0	4	1	2	1	10
Frieda's, Dried Red Tomatoes, Chopped									
1 serving	72	0	0	0	16	3	7	4	265
Frieda's, Fresh Mild Salsa									
2 tbsp	10	0	0	0	4	0	1	0	75
Frieda's, Fresh Hot Salsa									
2 tbsp	10	0	0	0	1	0	1	0	75

Food Serving size	Cal.	(g) Total Fat	(g) Sat. Fat	(mg) Chol.	(g) Carb.	(g) Fiber	(g) Sug.	(g) Prot.	(mg) Sod.
Frito-Lay, Tostitos, All Natural Hot Chunky Salsa									
2 tbsp	10	0	0	0	2	<1	2	0	250
Frito-Lay, Tostitos, All Natural Medium Chunky Salsa									
2 tbsp	10	0	0	0	2	<1	2	0	250
Frito-Lay, Tostitos, All Natural Mild Chunky Salsa									
2 tbsp	10	0	0	0	2	<1	2	0	250
Frito-Lay, Tostitos, Creamy Spinach Dip									
2 tbsp	50	4	0	<5mg	2	<1	<1	1	200
Frito-Lay, Tostitos, Restaurant Style Salsa									
2 tbsp	15	0	0	0	3	<1	1	<1	210
Ian's Natural Foods, Allergy Friendly Onion Rings									
5 rings	130	6	0	0	18	1	2	2	115
Jovial Foods, Organic Tomatoes (including diced, whole peeled, and crushed)									
1/2 cup	30	0	0	0	6	1	4	1	30
Lucini, Hearty Artichoke Tomato Sauce									
1/2 cup	50	1.5	0	0	7	3	<1	2	230
Lucini, Rustic Tomato Basil Sauce									
1/2 cup	80	5	0.5	0	8	2	6	2	490
Lucini, Rustic Tomato Basil Sauce Pouch									
1/2 cup	70	4.5	0.5	0	8	1	6	1	380
Lucini, Spicy Tuscan Tomato Sauce									
1/2 cup	80	4.5	1	0	8	2	5	2	480
Lucini, Spicy Tuscan Tomato Sauce Pouch									
1/2 cup	70	4	0.5	0	7	1	5	1	480
Lucini, Tuscan Harvest Plum Tomatoes, Diced Peeled 100% Organic									
1/2 cup	19	0	0	0	4	3	4	1	80
Lucini, Tuscan Harvest Plum Tomatoes, Whole Peeled 100% Organic									
1/2 cup	19	0	0	0	4	3	4	1	80
Mariani Premium Fruit, Sun-Dried Tomatoes, Tomato Halves									
1 tbsp	15	0	0	0	3	1	2	0	10
Mariani Premium Fruit, Sun-Dried Tomatoes, Tomatoes Julienne									
1 tbsp	15	0	0	0	3	1	2	0	10
Mezzetta Roasted Red Bell Peppers									
1.5 tbsp	5	0	0	0	1	0	1	0	110

Food Serving size	Cal.	(g) Total Fat	(g) Sat. Fat	(mg) Chol.	(g) Carb.	(g) Fiber	(g) Sug.	(g) Prot.	(mg) Sod.
Mezzetta Sandwich Spreads									
1 tbsp	40	4	0.5	0	1	0	0	0	150
Mezzetta Sun Ripened Tomatoes									
1 tomato	30	2	0	0	3	1	2	1	40
Mezzetta Sundried Tomato Sandwich Spread									
1 tbsp	25	2	0	0	1	0	1	0	65
Mezzetta, Artichoke Hearts									
2 pieces	20	2	NA	NA	2	NA	NA	NA	NA
Mezzetta, Banana Peppers, Sweet									
3 peppers	10	0	0	0	1	0	0	0	320
Mezzetta, Capers, Drained									
1 tbsp	2	0.07	0.02	0	0.42	0.3	0.04	0.2	255
Mezzetta, Cherry Peppers									
3 pieces	15	0	0	0	2	1	1	1	340
Mezzetta, Chicago Style Giardiniera									
1 serving	90	10	1	0	1	NA	NA	0	310
Mezzetta, Chimichurri Sandwich Spread									
1 tbsp	40	4	0.5	0	1	0	0	0	150
Mezzetta, Giardiniera									
5 pieces	5	0	0	0	0	1	0	0	410
Mezzetta, Grape Leaves									
1 grape leaf	5	0	0	0	1	NA	NA	0	100
Mezzetta, Green Chili Peppers									
2 tbsp	10	0	0	0	2	0	0	0	180
Mezzetta, Habanero Peppers									
1 serving	10	0	0	0	2	1	NA	0	310
Mezzetta, Hot Chili Peppers									
5 pieces	10	0	0	0	1	0	1	0	330
Mezzetta, Jalapeno Peppers, Deli-Sliced, Hot									
1/4 cup	5	0	0	0	1	0	0	0	380
Mezzetta, Jalapeno Sandwich Spread									
1 tbsp	40	3.5	NA	NA	1	NA	NA	1	NA
Mezzetta, Onions									
8 onions	5	0	0	0	1	0	1	0	300

Food Serving size	Cal.	(g) Total Fat	(g) Sat. Fat	(mg) Chol.	(g) Carb.	(g) Fiber	(g) Sug.	(g) Prot.	(mg) Sod.
Mezzetta, Peperoncini 3 peppers	10	0	0	0	1	0	0	0	390
Native Forest, Artichoke Hearts, Marinated 1 oz	20	2	0	0	0	1	0	0	30
Native Forest, Artichoke Hearts, Quartered 4 oz	35	0	0	0	6	4	1	2	390
Native Forest, Artichoke Hearts, Whole 4 oz	35	0	0	0	6	4	1	2	390
Native Forest, Green Asparagus Cuts & Tips 1/2 cup	30	0	0	0	3	1	0	3	260
Native Forest, Green Asparagus Spears 1/2 cup	30	0	0	0	3	1	0	3	260
Native Forest, Organic Bamboo Shoots 1/2 cup	15	0	0	0	3	1	2	1	5
Native Forest, Organic Cut Baby Corn 1/2 cup	25	0	0	0	4	2	1	2	280
Native Forest, Organic Hearts of Palm 1 oz	15	0	0	0	2	1	0	1	120
Native Forest, Organic Mushrooms Pieces & Stems 1/2 cup	20	0	0	0	3	1	1	2	390
Nestlé, Libby's, 100% Pure Pumpkin 1/2 cup	40	0.5	0	0	9	5	4	2	5
Nestlé, Libby's, Easy Pumpkin Pie Mix 1/3 cup	90	0.5	0	0	20	3	17	1	120
Newman's Own, Black Bean and Corn Salsa 2 tbsp	20	0	0	0	5	2	1	1	140
Newman's Own, Farmer's Garden Salsa 2 tbsp	15	0	0	0	4	0	2	1	220
Newman's Own, Hot Salsa 2 tbsp	10	0	0	0	2	<1	1	0	150
Newman's Own, Mango Salsa 2 tbsp	20	0	0	0	5	0	3	0	180
Newman's Own, Medium Salsa 2 tbsp	10	0	0	0	2	<1	1	0	105

Food Serving size	Cal.	(g) Total Fat	(g) Sat. Fat	(mg) Chol.	(g) Carb.	(g) Fiber	(g) Sug.	(g) Prot.	(mg) Sod.
Newman's Own, Mild Salsa 2 tbsp	10	0	0	0	2	<1	1	0	65
Newman's Own, Peach Chunky Salsa 2 tbsp	25	0	0	0	6	<1	5	0	90
Newman's Own, Pineapple Salsa 2 tbsp	15	0	0	0	3	<1	3	0	90
Newman's Own, Roasted Garlic Chunky Salsa 2 tbsp	10	0	0	0	2	<1	1	1	150
Newman's Own, Tequila Lime Salsa 2 tbsp	15	0	0	0	3	0	2	0	170
Pace, Salsas, Chunky Salsa, Hot 2 tbsp	10	0	NA	0	3	1	2	0	230
Pace, Salsas, Chunky Salsa, Medium 2 tbsp	10	0	NA	0	3	1	2	0	230
Pace, Salsas, Chunky Salsa, Mild 2 tbsp	10	0	0	0	3	0	2	0	220
Pace, Salsas, Chunky Salsa, Mild, Medium, Hot 2 tbsp	10	0	0	0	3	1	2	0	230
Pace, Salsas, Pico de Gallo 2 tbsp	10	0	0	0	3	NA	2	0	150
Pace, Salsas, Pineapple Mango Chipotle Salsa 2 tbsp	20	0	0	0	4	NA	4	0	130
Pace, Salsas, Restaurant Style, Medium 2 tbsp	10	0	0	0	2	0	NA	0	130
Pace, Salsas, Salsa Verde 2 tbsp	15	0.5	NA	0	2	0	2	0	230
Sabra, Babaganoush Vegetarian Side 2 tbsp	80	8	0.5	5	2	0	1	0	135
Sabra, Caponata Vegetarian Side 2 tbsp	25	2	0	0	2	0	0	0	90
Sabra, Chunky Pico De Gallo Salsa 2 tbsp	10	0	0	0	2	0	1	0	200
Sabra, Classic Guacamole 2 tbsp	50	4.5	0.5	0	3	2	0	1	160

Food Serving size	Cal.	(g) Total Fat	(g) Sat. Fat	(mg) Chol.	(g) Carb.	(g) Fiber	(g) Sug.	(g) Prot.	(mg) Sod.
Sabra, Classic Salsa 2 tbsp	10	0	0	0	2	0	1	0	160
Sabra, Classic Tahini Vegetarian Side 2 tbsp	80	8	1	0	2	1	0	2	150
Sabra, Cucumber & Dill Greek Yogurt Style Vegetable Dip 2 tbsp	35	2.5	1.5	10	2	0	1	2	95
Sabra, Grilled Eggplant Vegetarian Side 2 tbsp	40	3.5	0	0	2	1	1	1	110
Sabra, Homestyle Salsa 2 tbsp	10	0	0	0	2	0	1	0	170
Sabra, Moroccan Matbuch Vegetarian Side 2 tbsp	30	0.5	0	0	2	0	1	1	180
Sabra, Onion Veggie Dip 2 tbsp	35	1.5	0.5	5	2	0	1	3	150
Sabra, Roasted Garlic Veggie Dip 2 tbsp	40	1.5	1	5	3	0	1	3	150
Sabra, Southwestern Style Salsa 2 tbsp	15	0	0	0	3	1	2	0	110
Sabra, Spanish Eggplant Vegetarian Side 2 tbsp	80	7	1	0	5	1	2	1	410
Sabra, Spicy Guacamole 2 tbsp	45	4	0.5	0	3	2	0	1	130
Sabra, Spinach & Artichoke Veggie Dip 2 tbsp	30	1.5	0.5	5	2	0	1	3	160
Sabra, Turkish Salad Vegetarian Side 2 tbsp	35	2	0	0	3	1	1	1	260
Simply Organic Foods, French Onion Dip 1/2 tsp	5	0	0	0	1	0	0	0	125
Simply Organic Foods, Salsa Mix 1/2 tsp	5	0	0	0	1	0	0	0	60
Squash, Summer, All Varieties, Raw 1 large (323g)	52	1	0	0	11	3.6	7	4	6
Squash, Summer, Crookneck and Straightneck, Raw 1 cup, sliced (127g)	24	0	0	0	5	1.3	4	1	3

Food Serving size	Cal.	(g) Total Fat	(g) Sat. Fat	(mg) Chol.	(g) Carb.	(g) Fiber	(g) Sug.	(g) Prot.	(mg) Sod.
Squash, Summer, Scallop, Raw 1 cup, slices (130g)	23	0	0	0	5	NA	NA	2	1
Squash, Summer, Zucchini, Including Skin, Raw 1 cup, sliced (113g)	19	0	0	0	4	1.1	3	1	9
Squash, Winter, Acorn, Raw 1 squash (4 inch dia) (431g)	172	0	0	0	45	6.5	NA	3	13
Squash, Winter, All Varieties, Raw 1 cup, cubes (116g)	39	0	0	0	10	1.7	3	1	5
Squash, Winter, Butternut, Raw 1 cup, cubes (140g)	63	0	0	0	16	2.8	3	1	6
Squash, Winter, Hubbard, Raw 1 cup, cubes (116g)	46	1	0	0	10	NA	NA	2	8
Squash, Winter, Spaghetti, Raw 1 cup, cubes (101g)	31	1	0	0	7	NA	NA	1	17
Squash, Zucchini, Baby, Raw 1 medium (11g)	2	0	0	0	0	0.1	NA	0	0
Tasty Bite, Agra Peas & Greens 1/2 pack	150	8	2	3	13	4	3	6	460
Tasty Bite, Aloo Palak 1/2 pack	100	3	0	0	13	3	3	3	400
Thumann's, Cole Slaw 1/4 lb	210	20	3	10	7	2	5	1	420
Thumann's, Sauerkraut 2 tsp	5	0	0	0	1	0	0	0	160
Thumann's, Sweet Roasted Peppers 1 oz	15	0	0	0	5	1	4	1	250
V8 Vegetable Juice, Essential Antioxidants V8 8 fl oz	60	0	0	0	12	2	7	2	480
V8 Vegetable Juice, High Fiber V8 8 fl oz	60	0	0	0	13	5	8	2	480
V8 Vegetable Juice, Low Sodium Spicy Hot V8 8 fl oz	50	0	0	0	11	2	8	2	140
V8 Vegetable Juice, Low Sodium V8 8 fl oz	50	0	0	0	10	2	7	2	140

Food Serving size	Cal.	(g) Total Fat	(g) Sat. Fat	(mg) Chol.	(g) Carb.	(g) Fiber	(g) Sug.	(g) Prot.	(mg) Sod.
V8 Vegetable Juice, Spicy Hot V8 8 fl oz	50	0	0	0	10	2	8	2	480
V8, 100% Vegetable Juice 8 fl oz	50	0	0	0	10	2	7	2	420
Wholly Avocado, Chunky Dip 2 tbsp	60	6	1	0	3	2	0	1	0
Wholly Guacamole, Classic Dip 2 tbsp	60	5	1	0	3	2	0	1	90
Wholly Salsa, Avocado Verde Dip 2 tbsp	25	1.5	0	0	2	1	1	0	135
Wholly Salsa, Guacamole & Spicy Pico Dip 2 tbsp	35	2.5	0	0	2	1	0	0	115
Wholly Salsa, Hot Dip 2 tbsp	10	0	0	0	2	0	1	0	160
Wholly Salsa, Medium Dip 2 tbsp	10	0	0	0	2	0	1	0	160
Wholly Salsa, Mild Dip 2 tbsp	10	0	0	0	2	0	1	0	160
Wholly Salsa, Pineapple Dip 2 tbsp	15	0	0	0	4	0	3	0	25
Wholly Salsa, Red Pepper Mango Dip 2 tbsp	25	0	0	0	6	0	5	0	25
Wholly Salsa, Roasted Tomato Dip 2 tbsp	10	0	0	0	3	0	2	0	120

Vegetables

Food Serving size	Cal.	Total Fat	Sat. Fat	Chol.	Carb.	Fiber	Sug.	Prot.	Sod.
Artichokes (Globe or French), Cooked, Boiled, Drained, with Salt .5 cup, hearts (84g)	45	0	0	0	10	7.2	1	2	50
Artichokes (Globe or French), Cooked, Boiled, Drained, Without Salt .5 cup, hearts (84g)	45	0	0	0	10	7.2	1	2	50
Artichokes (Globe or French), Frozen, Cooked, Boiled, Drained, Without Salt 1 package (9 oz), yields (240g)	108	1	0	0	22	11	2	7	127
Artichokes (Globe or French), Raw 1 artichoke, large (162g)	76	0	0	0	17	8.7	2	5	152

Food Serving size	Cal.	(g) Total Fat	(g) Sat. Fat	(mg) Chol.	(g) Carb.	(g) Fiber	(g) Sug.	(g) Prot.	(mg) Sod.
Arugula, Raw .5 cup (10g)	3	0	0	0	0	0.2	0	0	3
Asparagus, Cooked, Boiled, Drained 4 spears (1/2" base) (60g)	13	0	0	0	2	1.2	1	1	8
Asparagus, Cooked, Boiled, Drained, with Salt 4 spears (1/2" base) (60g)	13	0	0	0	2	1.2	1	1	144
Asparagus, Frozen, Cooked, Boiled, Drained, Without Salt 1 package (10 oz) yields (293g)	53	1	0	0	6	4.7	1	9	9
Asparagus, Raw 1 spear, small (5" long or less) (12g)	2	0	0	0	0	0.3	0	0	0
Avocados, Raw, All Commercial Varieties 1 cup, pureed (230g)	368	34	5	0	20	15.4	2	5	16
Avocados, Raw, California 1 fruit, without skin and seed (136g)	227	21	3	0	12	9.2	0	3	11
Avocados, Raw, Florida 1 fruit, without skin and seeds (304g)	365	31	6	0	24	17	7	7	6
Basil, Fresh 5 leaves (2.5g)	1	0	0	0	0	0	0	0	0
Broccoli, Cooked, Boiled, Drained, Without Salt 1 stalk, medium (7-1/2" – 8" long) (180g)	63	1	0	0	13	5.9	3	4	74
Broccoli, Flower Clusters, Raw 1 floweret (11g)	3	0	0	0	1	NA	NA	0	3
Garlic, Raw 1 tsp (2.8g)	4	0	0	0	1	0.1	0	0	0
Ginger Root, Raw .25 cup, slices (1" dia) (24g)	19	0	0	0	4	0.5	0	0	3
Lemon Grass (Citronella), Raw 1 tbsp (4.8g)	5	0	0	0	1	NA	NA	0	0
Lentils, Mature Seeds, Cooked, Boiled, Without Salt 1 tbsp (12.3g)	14	0	0	0	2	1	0	1	0

Food Serving size	Cal.	(g) Total Fat	(g) Sat. Fat	(mg) Chol.	(g) Carb.	(g) Fiber	(g) Sug.	(g) Prot.	(mg) Sod.
Lentils, Pink, Raw 1 cup (192g)	662	4	1	0	114	20.7	NA	48	13
Lentils, Raw 1 tbsp (12g)	42	0	0	0	7	3.7	0	3	1
Lentils, Sprouted, Raw 1 cup (77g)	82	0	0	0	17	NA	NA	7	8
Lettuce, Butterhead (Including Boston and Bibb Types), Raw 1 head (5″ dia) (163g)	21	0	0	0	4	1.8	2	2	8
Lettuce, Cos and Romaine, Raw 1 leaf, inner (6g)	1	0	0	0	0	0.1	0	0	0
Lettuce, Green Leaf, Raw 1 head (360g)	54	1	0	0	10	4.7	3	5	101
Lettuce, Iceberg (Including Crisphead Types), Raw 1 cup, chopped (1/2″ pieces, loosely packed) (57g)	8	0	0	0	2	0.7	1	1	6
Lettuce, Red Leaf, Raw 1 leaf, inner (2.6g)	0	0	NA	NA	0	0	0	0	1
Lima Beans, Immature Seeds, Cooked, Boiled, Drained, with Salt 1 cup (170g)	209	1	0	0	40	9	3	12	430
Lima Beans, Immature Seeds, Frozen, Baby, Cooked, Boiled, Drained, with Salt 1 package (10 oz) yields (311g)	327	1	0	0	60	18.7	4	21	824
Lima Beans, Immature Seeds, Frozen, Fordhook, Cooked, Boiled, Drained, with Salt 1 package (10 oz) yields (311g)	320	1	0	0	60	18	4	19	899
Lima Beans, Large, Mature Seeds, Cooked, Boiled, with Salt 1 cup (188g)	216	1	0	0	39	13.2	5	15	447
Lima Beans, Large, Mature Seeds, Raw 1 tbsp (11.1g)	38	0	0	0	7	2.1	1	2	2
Lima Beans, Thin Seeded (Baby), Mature Seeds, Cooked, Boiled, with Salt 1 cup (182g)	229	1	0	0	42	14	NA	15	435
Lima Beans, Thin Seeded (Baby), Mature Seeds, Cooked, Boiled, Without Salt 1 cup (182g)	229	1	0	0	42	14	NA	15	5

Food Serving size	Cal.	(g) Total Fat	(g) Sat. Fat	(mg) Chol.	(g) Carb.	(g) Fiber	(g) Sug.	(g) Prot.	(mg) Sod.
Lima Beans, Thin Seeded (Baby), Mature Seeds, Raw									
1 cup (202g)	677	2	0	0	127	41.6	17	42	26
Lotus Root, Cooked, Boiled, Drained, with Salt									
10 slices (2-1/2″ dia) (89g)	59	0	0	0	14	2.8	NA	1	250
Lotus Root, Cooked, Boiled, Drained, Without Salt									
10 slices (2-1/2″ dia) (89g)	59	0	0	0	14	2.8	0	1	40
Lotus Root, Raw									
1 root (9-1/2″ long) (115g)	85	0	0	0	20	5.6	NA	3	46
Malabar Spinach, Cooked									
1 bunch (17g)	4	0	NA	0	0	0.4	NA	1	9
Mountain Yam, Hawaii, Cooked, Steamed, Without Salt									
1 cup, cubes (145g)	119	0	0	0	29	NA	NA	3	17
Mountain Yam, Hawaii, Raw									
1 yam (420g)	281	0	0	0	69	NA	NA	6	55
Mushrooms, Brown, Italian or Crimini, Raw									
1 cup, sliced (72g)	16	0	0	0	3	0.4	1	2	4
Mushrooms, Chanterelle, Raw									
1 piece (5.4g)	2	0	NA	NA	0	0.2	0	0	0
Mushrooms, Enoki, Raw									
1 medium (3g)	1	0	0	0	0	0.1	0	0	0
Mushrooms, Maitake, Raw									
1 piece, whole (1.1g)	0	0	0	0	0	0	0	0	0
Mushrooms, Morel, Raw									
1 piece (12.9g)	4	0	0	NA	1	0.4	0	0	3
Mushrooms, Oyster, Raw									
1 small (15g)	5	0	0	0	1	0.3	0	0	3
Mushrooms, Portobello, Raw									
1 piece, whole (84g)	18	0	0	0	3	1.1	2	2	8
Mushrooms, Shiitake, Cooked, Without Salt									
4 mushrooms (72g)	40	0	0	0	10	1.5	3	1	3
Mushrooms, Shiitake, Raw									
1 piece, whole (19g)	6	0	NA	NA	1	0.5	0	0	2
Mushrooms, White, Cooked, Boiled, Drained, Without Salt									
1 tbsp (9.8g)	3	0	0	0	1	0.2	0	0	0

Food Serving size	Cal.	(g) Total Fat	(g) Sat. Fat	(mg) Chol.	(g) Carb.	(g) Fiber	(g) Sug.	(g) Prot.	(mg) Sod.
Mushrooms, White, Raw									
1 cup, whole (96g)	21	0	0	0	3	1	2	3	5
Mustard Greens, Cooked, Boiled, Drained, Without Salt									
1 cup, chopped (140g)	21	0	0	0	3	2.8	0	3	22
Mustard Greens, Raw									
1 cup, chopped (56g)	15	0	0	0	3	1.8	1	2	14
Mustard Spinach (Tendergreen), Raw									
1 cup, chopped (150g)	33	0	0	0	6	4.2	NA	3	32
New Zealand Spinach, Cooked, Boiled, Drained, Without Salt									
1 cup, chopped (180g)	22	0	0	0	4	NA	NA	2	193
New Zealand Spinach, Raw									
1 cup, chopped (56g)	8	0	0	0	1	NA	NA	1	73
Okra, Cooked, Boiled, Drained, Without Salt									
8 pods (3″ long) (85g)	19	0	0	0	4	2.1	2	2	5
Okra, Raw									
8 pods (3″ long) (95g)	29	0	0	0	7	3	1	2	8
Onions, Raw									
1 cup, sliced (115g)	46	0	0	0	11	2	5	1	5
Onions, Spring or Scallions (Including Tops and Bulb), Raw									
1 tbsp, chopped (6g)	2	0	0	0	0	0.2	0	0	1
Onions, Sweet, Raw									
1 NLEA serving (148g)	47	0	NA	0	11	1.3	7	1	12
Onions, Young Green, Tops Only									
1 stalk (12g)	3	0	0	0	1	0.2	1	0	2
Parsley, Raw									
1 tbsp (3.8g)	1	0	0	0	0	0.1	0	0	2
Parsnips, Cooked, Boiled, Drained, Without Salt									
1 parsnip (9″ long) (160g)	114	0	0	0	27	5.8	8	2	16
Parsnips, Raw									
1 cup, slices (133g)	100	0	0	0	24	6.5	6	2	13
Peas, Edible-podded, Raw									
1 cup, whole (63g)	26	0	0	0	5	1.6	3	2	3
Peas, Green, Raw									
1 cup (145g)	117	1	0	0	21	7.4	8	8	7

Food Serving size	Cal.	(g) Total Fat	(g) Sat. Fat	(mg) Chol.	(g) Carb.	(g) Fiber	(g) Sug.	(g) Prot.	(mg) Sod.
Peas, Mature Seeds, Sprouted, Raw 1 cup (120g)	149	1	0	0	33	NA	NA	11	24
Peppers, Hot Chili, Red, Raw .5 cup, chopped or diced (75g)	30	0	0	0	7	1.1	4	1	7
Peppers, Hungarian, Raw 1 pepper (27g)	8	0	0	0	2	NA	NA	0	0
Peppers, Jalapeno, Raw 1 pepper (14g)	4	0	0	0	1	0.4	1	0	0
Peppers, Sweet, Green, Raw 1 cup, sliced (92g)	18	0	0	0	4	1.6	2	1	3
Peppers, Sweet, Yellow, Raw 10 strips (52g)	14	0	0	0	3	0.5	NA	1	1
Potato, Baked, Flesh and Skin, Without Salt 1 potato, medium (173g)	161	0	0	0	37	3.8	2	4	17
Potato, Flesh and Skin, Raw 1 potato, medium (2-1/4" to 3-1/4" dia) (213g)	164	0	0	0	37	4.7	2	4	13
Potatoes, Baked, Flesh, Without Salt 1 potato (2-1/3" x 4-3/4") (156g)	145	0	0	0	34	2.3	3	3	8
Potatoes, Baked, Skin, Without Salt 1 skin (58g)	115	0	0	0	27	4.6	1	2	12
Potatoes, Boiled, Cooked in Skin, Flesh, Without Salt 1 potato (2-1/2" dia, sphere) (136g)	118	0	0	0	27	2.4	1	3	5
Potatoes, Boiled, Cooked in Skin, Without Salt 1 skin (34g)	27	0	0	0	6	1.1	NA	1	5
Potatoes, Boiled, Cooked Without Skin, Flesh, Without Salt 1 medium (2-1/4" to 3-1/4" dia.) (167g)	144	0	0	0	33	3	1	3	8
Potatoes, Raw, Skin 1 skin (38g)	22	0	0	0	5	1	NA	1	4
Potatoes, Red, Flesh and Skin, Baked 1 potato, medium (2-1/4" to 3-1/4" dia.) (173g)	154	0	0	0	34	3.1	2	4	21

Food Serving size	Cal.	(g) Total Fat	(g) Sat. Fat	(mg) Chol.	(g) Carb.	(g) Fiber	(g) Sug.	(g) Prot.	(mg) Sod.
Potatoes, Red, Flesh and Skin, Raw 1 potato, medium (2-1/4″ to 3-1/4″ dia) (213g)	149	0	0	0	34	3.6	3	4	38
Potatoes, Russet, Flesh and Skin, Baked 1 potato, medium (2-1/4″ to 3-1/4″ dia.) (173g)	168	0	0	0	37	4	2	5	24
Potatoes, Russet, Flesh and Skin, Raw 1 potato, medium (2-1/4″ to 3-1/4″ dia) (213g)	168	0	0	0	38	2.8	1	5	11
Potatoes, White, Flesh and Skin, Baked 1 potato, medium (2-1/4″ to 3-1/4″ dia) (138g)	130	0	0	0	29	2.9	2	3	10
Potatoes, White, Flesh and Skin, Raw 1 potato, medium (2-1/4″ to 3-1/4″ dia) (213g)	147	0	0	0	33	5.1	2	4	34
Pumpkin, Raw 1 cup (1″ cubes) (116g)	30	0	0	0	8	0.6	2	1	1
Purslane, Cooked, Boiled, Drained, Without Salt 1 squash (431g)	78	1	NA	0	15	NA	NA	6	190
Purslane, Raw 1 plant (3g)	0	0	NA	0	0	NA	NA	0	1
Quinoa, Cooked 1 cup (185g)	222	4	NA	0	39	5.2	NA	8	13
Quinoa, Uncooked 1 cup (170g)	626	10	1	0	109	11.9	NA	24	9
Radicchio, Raw 1 leaf (8g)	2	0	0	0	0	0.1	0	0	2
Radish Seeds, Sprouted, Raw 1 cup (38g)	16	1	0	0	1	NA	NA	1	2
Radishes, Oriental, Cooked, Boiled, Drained, Without Salt 1 cup, sliced (147g)	25	0	0	0	5	2.4	3	1	19
Radishes, Oriental, Raw 1 radish (7″ long) (338g)	61	0	0	0	14	5.4	8	2	71
Radishes, Raw 1 large (1″ to 1-1/4″ dia) (9g)	1	0	0	0	0	0.1	0	0	4

Food Serving size	Cal.	(g) Total Fat	(g) Sat. Fat	(mg) Chol.	(g) Carb.	(g) Fiber	(g) Sug.	(g) Prot.	(mg) Sod.
Radishes, White Icicle, Raw 1 radish (7″ long) (17g)	2	0	0	0	0	0.2	NA	0	3
Rhubarb, Raw 1 stalk (51g)	11	0	0	0	2	0.9	1	0	2
Roselle, Raw 1 cup, without refuse (57g)	28	0	NA	0	6	NA	NA	1	3
Rutabagas, Cooked, Boiled, Drained, Without Salt 1 cup, mashed (240g)	94	1	0	0	21	4.3	14	3	48
Rutabagas, Raw 1 large (772g)	278	2	0	0	63	19.3	43	9	154
Salsify (Vegetable Oyster), Raw 1 cup, slices (133g)	109	0	NA	0	25	4.4	NA	4	27
Salsify, Cooked, Boiled, Drained, Without Salt 1 cup, sliced (135g)	92	0	0	0	21	4.2	4	4	22
Shallots, Raw 1 tbsp, chopped (10g)	7	0	0	0	2	NA	NA	0	1
Spinach, Cooked, Boiled, Drained, Without Salt 1 cup (180g)	41	0	0	0	7	4.3	1	5	126
Spinach, Raw 1 bunch (340g)	78	1	0	0	12	7.5	1	10	269
Succotash (Corn and Limas), Cooked, Boiled, Drained, Without Salt 1 cup (192g)	221	2	0	0	47	8.6	NA	10	33
Succotash (Corn and Limas), Frozen, Cooked, Boiled, Drained, Without Salt 1 cup (170g)	158	2	0	0	34	7	4	7	77
Tapioca, Pearl, Dry 1 cup (152g)	544	0	0	0	135	1.4	5	0	2
Taro Leaves, Cooked, Steamed, Without Salt 1 cup (145g)	35	1	0	0	6	2.9	NA	4	3
Taro Leaves, Raw 1 leaf (11″ x 6-1/2″) (10g)	4	0	0	0	1	0.4	0	0	0
Taro Shoots, Cooked, Without Salt 1 cup, slices (140g)	20	0	0	0	4	NA	NA	1	3
Taro Shoots, Raw 1 shoot (83g)	9	0	0	0	2	NA	NA	1	1

Food Serving size	Cal.	(g) Total Fat	(g) Sat. Fat	(mg) Chol.	(g) Carb.	(g) Fiber	(g) Sug.	(g) Prot.	(mg) Sod.
Taro, Cooked, Without Salt 1 cup, sliced (132g)	187	0	0	0	46	6.7	1	1	20
Taro, Leaves, Cooked, Steamed, with Salt 1 cup (145g)	35	1	0	0	6	2.9	NA	4	345
Taro, Raw 1 cup, sliced (104g)	116	0	0	0	28	4.3	0	2	11
Taro, Tahitian, Cooked, Without Salt 1 cup, slices (137g)	60	1	0	0	9	NA	NA	6	74
Taro, Tahitian, Raw 1 cup, slices (125g)	55	1	0	0	9	NA	NA	3	63
Tomatoes, Green, Raw 1 large (182g)	42	0	0	0	9	2	7	2	24
Tomatoes, Orange, Raw 1 tomato (111g)	18	0	0	0	4	1	NA	1	47
Tomatoes, Red, Ripe, Cooked 2 medium (246g)	44	0	0	0	10	1.7	6	2	27
Tomatoes, Red, Ripe, Raw 1 cup, chopped or sliced (180g)	32	0	0	0	7	2.2	5	2	9
Tomatoes, Sun-dried 1 piece (2g)	5	0	0	0	1	0.2	1	0	42
Tomatoes, Yellow, Raw 1 tomato (212g)	32	1	0	0	6	1.5	NA	2	49
Turnip Greens and Turnips, Frozen, Cooked, Boiled, Drained, Without Salt 1 cup (163g)	57	1	0	0	8	5.1	2	5	31
Turnip Greens, Cooked, Boiled, Drained, Without Salt 1 cup, chopped (144g)	29	0	0	0	6	5	1	2	42
Turnip Greens, Frozen, Cooked, Boiled, Drained, Without Salt 1 package (10 oz) yields (220g)	64	1	0	0	11	7.5	2	7	33
Turnip Greens, Raw 1 cup, chopped (55g)	18	0	0	0	4	1.8	0	1	22
Turnips, Cooked, Boiled, Drained, Without Salt 1 cup, mashed (230g)	51	0	0	0	12	4.6	7	2	37
Turnips, Raw 1 large (183g)	51	0	0	0	12	3.3	7	2	123

Food Serving size	Cal.	(g) Total Fat	(g) Sat. Fat	(mg) Chol.	(g) Carb.	(g) Fiber	(g) Sug.	(g) Prot.	(mg) Sod.
Water Chestnuts, Chinese (Matai), Raw 4 water chestnuts (36g)	35	0	0	0	9	1.1	2	1	5
Watercress, Raw 1 sprig (2.5g)	0	0	0	0	0	0	0	0	1
Waxgourd (Chinese Preserving Melon), Cooked, Boiled, Drained, Without Salt 1 cup, cubes (175g)	25	0	0	0	5	1.8	2	1	187
Waxgourd (Chinese Preserving Melon), Raw 1 waxgourd (5700g)	741	11	1	0	171	165.3	NA	23	6327
Yam, Cooked, Boiled, Drained or Baked, Without Salt .5 cup, cubes (68g)	79	0	0	0	19	2.7	0	1	5
Yam, Raw 1 cup, cubes (150g)	177	0	0	0	42	6.2	1	2	14
Yambean (Jicama), Raw 1 cup (130g)	49	0	0	0	11	6.4	2	1	5
Yardlong Bean, Cooked, Boiled, Drained, Without Salt 1 pod (14g)	7	0	0	0	1	NA	NA	0	1
Yardlong Bean, Raw 1 pod (12g)	6	0	0	0	1	NA	NA	0	0
Yardlong Beans, Mature Seeds, Cooked, Boiled, Without Salt 1 cup (171g)	202	1	0	0	36	6.5	NA	14	9
Yardlong Beans, Mature Seeds, Raw 1 cup (167g)	579	2	1	0	103	18.4	NA	41	28

Fruits

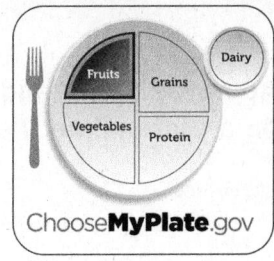

ChooseMyPlate.gov

Why Eat Fruits?

All fruits are gluten-free. Additionally, fruits provide nutrients vital for health and maintenance of your body. Most fruits are naturally low in fat, sodium, and calories. None
have cholesterol. Fruits are sources of many essential nutrients that are under-con-
sumed, including potassium, dietary fiber, vitamin C, and folate (folic acid). Diets rich
in potassium may help to maintain healthy blood pressure. Dietary fiber from fruits,
as part of an overall healthy diet, helps reduce blood cholesterol levels and may lower
risk of heart disease. Vitamin C is important for growth and repair of all body tissues,
helps heal cuts and wounds, and keeps teeth and gums healthy.

Daily Goal

Two cups for an adult on a 2,000 calorie diet.
One-cup equivalents:
  2.5" whole fruit
  1 cup chopped or sliced fruit
  ½ cup dried fruit
  8 oz. fruit juice (100%)
  32 seedless grapes
  8 large strawberries

Gluten-Free Shopping Tips

- Eat a variety of fruits
- Choose fresh, in-season fruits
- Buy locally grown fruits when available
- Buy fruits that are frozen and canned in water or 100% juice
- Refrigerate or freeze cut-up fruit to store for use later
- Stay away from dates and fruits with sauces

Gluten-Free Shopping List Essentials

Apples
Bananas
Berries
Melon
Grapes
Oranges
Grapefruits

Approved Fruits and Those to Avoid on a Gluten-Free Diet

Gluten-Free

Fresh, frozen, and canned fruits and juices

May Contain Gluten

- Dates may be dusted with flour containing gluten
- Fruits with sauces

Caution

Fruit juice can add calories and sugar and eliminate fiber and nutrients. Eat the whole fruit for all the nutrients. Make sure that fruit drinks are 100% fruit and not sugar water with a little fruit juice. When purchasing frozen or canned fruit, be aware of any added sugar and calories.

Food Serving size	Cal.	(g) Total Fat	(g) Sat. Fat	(mg) Chol.	(g) Carb.	(g) Fiber	(g) Sug.	(g) Prot.	(mg) Sod.
Fruit Juices									
AriZona Fruit Flavored Juice Drinks, Mucho Mango 8 fl oz	120	0	0	0	27	0	25	0	10
AriZona Fruit Flavored Juice Drinks, Orangeade 8 fl oz	120	0	0	0	27	0	26	0	20
AriZona Fruit Flavored Juice Drinks, Watermelon 8 fl oz	100	0	0	0	25	0	24	0	10
Diet V8 Splash, Juice Drink, Diet Berry Blend 8 fl oz	10	0	0	0	3	0	2	0	30
Diet V8 Splash, Juice Drink, Diet Tropical Blend 8 fl oz	10	0	0	0	3	0	2	0	30
Eden Foods, Apple Cider Vinegar, Organic – Raw, Unpasteurized 1 tbsp	0	0	0	0	0	0	0	0	0
Eden Foods, Apple Juice, Organic 8 oz	90	0	0	0	24	0	12	0	0
Eden Foods, Cherry Juice Concentrate, Organic 2 tbsp	110	0	0	0	26	0	21	1	20
Eden Foods, Concord Grape Juice, Organic 8 oz	150	0	NA	NA	37	<1	32	<1	35
Eden Foods, Montmorency Tart Cherry Juice, Organic 8 oz	140	0	0	0	33	0	25	1	30
Hansen's Natural, Aguas Frescas Juice, Jamaica 8 fl oz	70	0	NA	NA	18	NA	18	0	0
Hansen's Natural, Aguas Frescas Juice, Mango 8 fl oz	80	0	NA	NA	21	NA	21	0	10
Hansen's Natural, Aguas Frescas Juice, Melon 8 fl oz	80	0	NA	NA	20	NA	20	0	1
Hansen's Natural, Aguas Frescas Juice, Pina 8 fl oz	80	0	NA	NA	19	NA	19	0	0
Hansen's Natural, Aguas Frescas Juice, Tamarindo 8 fl oz	90	0	NA	NA	23	NA	22	0	75
Hansen's Natural, Hansen's Organic Junior Juice, Apple 1 package (125mL)	60	0	NA	NA	15	NA	15	NA	10

Food Serving size	Cal.	(g) Total Fat	(g) Sat. Fat	(mg) Chol.	(g) Carb.	(g) Fiber	(g) Sug.	(g) Prot.	(mg) Sod.
Hansen's Natural, Hansen's Organic Junior Juice, Berry Medley									
1 package (125mL)	60	0	NA	NA	15	NA	15	NA	10
Hansen's Natural, Junior Juice, Apple									
1 package (125mL)	60	0	NA	NA	15	NA	14	NA	5
Hansen's Natural, Junior Juice, Apple Grape									
1 package (125mL)	60	0	NA	NA	16	NA	16	NA	5
Hansen's Natural, Junior Juice, Fruit Punch									
1 package (125mL)	60	0	NA	NA	15	NA	14	NA	5
Hansen's Natural, Junior Juice, Island Splash									
8 fl oz	110	0	NA	NA	29	NA	29	0	5
Hansen's Natural, Junior Juice, Mixed Fruit									
1 package (125mL)	60	0	NA	NA	15	NA	14	NA	5
Hansen's Natural, Kids Junior Juice, Coconut Water Twist, Orange Creamsicle									
1 box	70	0	0	NA	17	NA	17	0	50
Hansen's Natural, Kids Junior Juice, Coconut Water Twist, Pineapple									
1 box	70	0	0	NA	17	NA	17	0	50
Hansen's Natural, Kids Junior Juice, Coconut Water Twist, Tropical Punch									
1 box	70	0	0	NA	17	NA	17	0	60
Hansen's Natural, Kids Junior Juice, Coconut Water Twist, Very Berry									
1 box	70	0	0	NA	17	NA	17	0	50
Nature Factor, Organic Coconut Water									
1 can	80	0	NA	NA	16	NA	9	0	50
Nestlé, Juicy Juice, Apple									
8 fl oz	110	0	0	0	28	0	26	0	20
Nestlé, Juicy Juice, Apple Raspberry									
8 fl oz	120	0	0	0	30	0	28	0	20
Nestlé, Juicy Juice, Berry									
8 fl oz	120	0	0	0	29	0	27	0	20
Nestlé, Juicy Juice, Cherry									
8 fl oz	120	0	0	0	29	0	27	0	20
Nestlé, Juicy Juice, Grape									
8 fl oz	120	0	0	0	29	0	28	0	20
Nestlé, Juicy Juice, Kiwi Strawberry									
8 fl oz	120	0	0	0	29	0	24	0	20

Food Serving size	Cal.	(g) Total Fat	(g) Sat. Fat	(mg) Chol.	(g) Carb.	(g) Fiber	(g) Sug.	(g) Prot.	(mg) Sod.
Nestlé, Juicy Juice, Mango 8 fl oz	120	0	0	0	29	0	27	0	20
Nestlé, Juicy Juice, Orange Tangerine 8 fl oz	130	0	0	0	32	0	31	0	25
Nestlé, Juicy Juice, Punch 8 fl oz	120	0	0	0	28	0	26	0	20
Nestlé, Juicy Juice, Strawberry Banana 8 fl oz	120	0	0	0	29	0	27	0	20
Nestlé, Juicy Juice, Tropical 8 fl oz	120	0	0	0	29	0	27	0	20
Nestlé, Juicy Juice, White Grape 8 fl oz	150	0	0	0	38	0	34	0	25
Passion-fruit Juice, Purple, Raw 1 fl oz (30.9g)	16	0	0	0	4	0.1	4	0	2
V8 Splash, Juice Drink, Berry Blend 8 fl oz	70	0	0	0	18	0	18	0	50
V8 Splash, Juice Drink, Cherry Pomegranate 8 fl oz	70	0	0	0	18	0	18	0	50
V8 Splash, Juice Drink, Fruit Medley 8 fl oz	70	0	0	0	18	0	18	0	50
V8 Splash, Juice Drink, Mango Peach 8 fl oz	80	0	0	0	20	0	18	0	40
V8 Splash, Juice Drink, Strawberry Kiwi 8 fl oz	70	0	0	0	18	0	16	0	50
V8 Splash, Juice Drink, Tropical Blend 8 fl oz	70	0	0	0	18	0	16	0	50
V8 Splash, Smoothies, Strawberry Banana 8 fl oz	90	0	0	0	20	0	18	3	70
V8 Splash, Smoothies, Tropical Colada 8 fl oz	100	0	0	0	21	1	18	3	50
V8 Splash, Smoothies, Wild Berry 8 fl oz	120	0	0	0	29	2	21	1	90
V8 V-Fusion Juice, Açaí Mixed Berry 8 fl oz	110	0	0	0	27	0	24	0	90

Food Serving size	Cal.	(g) Total Fat	(g) Sat. Fat	(mg) Chol.	(g) Carb.	(g) Fiber	(g) Sug.	(g) Prot.	(mg) Sod.
V8 V-Fusion Juice, Concord Grape Raspberry 8 fl oz	140	0	0	0	35	0	31	0	125
V8 V-Fusion Juice, Cranberry Blackberry 8 fl oz	100	0	0	0	26	0	21	0	90
V8 V-Fusion Juice, Goji Raspberry 1 cup	110	0	0	0	27	0	24	0	120
V8 V-Fusion Juice, Light Açaí Mixed Berry 8 fl oz	50	0	0	0	12	0	11	0	70
V8 V-Fusion Juice, Light Concord Grape Raspberry 8 fl oz	70	0	0	0	17	0	14	0	50
V8 V-Fusion Juice, Light Cranberry Blackberry 8 fl oz	50	0	0	0	12	0	10	0	70
V8 V-Fusion Juice, Light Peach Mango 8 fl oz	50	0	0	0	12	0	10	0	60
V8 V-Fusion Juice, Light Pomegranate Blueberry 8 fl oz	50	0	0	0	13	0	10	0	115
V8 V-Fusion Juice, Light Strawberry Banana 8 fl oz	50	0	0	0	12	0	10	0	60
V8 V-Fusion Juice, Peach Mango 8 fl oz	120	0	0	0	28	0	26	1	70
V8 V-Fusion Juice, Pineapple Mango with Green Tea 8 fl oz	50	0	0	0	13	0	10	0	60
V8 V-Fusion Juice, Pomegranate Blueberry 8 fl oz	100	0	0	0	25	0	23	0	60
V8 V-Fusion Juice, Pomegranate with Green Tea 8 fl oz	50	0	0	0	13	0	10	0	60
V8 V-Fusion Juice, Raspberry Green Tea 8 fl oz	50	0	0	0	13	0	10	0	60
V8 V-Fusion Juice, Strawberry Banana 8 fl oz	120	0	0	0	28	2	25	1	70
V8 V-Fusion Juice, Tropical Orange 8 fl oz	120	0	0	0	28	0	25	1	80
V8 V-Fusion Smoothies, Mango 8 fl oz	130	0	0	0	32	2	21	1	90

Food Serving size	Cal.	(g) Total Fat	(g) Sat. Fat	(mg) Chol.	(g) Carb.	(g) Fiber	(g) Sug.	(g) Prot.	(mg) Sod.
V8 V-Fusion Smoothies, Strawberry Banana 8 fl oz	130	0	0	0	32	2	22	1	90
V8 V-Fusion Smoothies, Wild Berry 8 fl oz	120	0	0	0	29	2	21	1	90
V8 V-Fusion Sparkling Juice, Black Cherry Pomegranate 1 can	50	0	0	0	14	0	12	0	80
V8 V-Fusion Sparkling Juice, Tangerine Raspberry 1 can	60	0	0	0	14	0	13	0	80
V8 V-Fusion, Energy, Peach Mango + Energy 1 can	50	0	0	0	13	0	10	0	40
V8 V-Fusion, Energy, Pomegranate Blueberry + Energy 1 can	50	0	0	0	13	0	10	0	90
Welch's, 100% Black Cherry Concord Grape Juice 8 fl oz	170	0	0	NA	42	NA	41	0	20
Welch's, 100% Grape Juice 8 fl oz	140	0	0	NA	38	3	36	1	15
Welch's, 100% Grape Juice with Calcium 8 fl oz	140	0	0	NA	38	NA	36	1	15
Welch's, 100% Grape Juice with Fiber 8 fl oz	150	0	0	NA	41	NA	36	1	15
Welch's, 100% White Grape Cherry Juice 8 fl oz	140	0	0	NA	35	NA	33	0	15
Welch's, 100% White Grape Juice 8 fl oz	160	0	0	NA	39	NA	38	0	20
Welch's, 100% White Grape Peach Juice 8 fl oz	160	0	0	NA	39	NA	37	0	15
Welch's, Chillers Juice Drink, Fruit Punch 8 fl oz	130	0	0	NA	31	NA	30	0	20
Welch's, Chillers Juice Drink, Grape Flavor 8 fl oz	140	0	0	NA	34	NA	33	NA	35
Welch's, Chillers Juice Drink, Mango Passion Fruit Flavor 8 fl oz	130	0	0	NA	31	NA	30	0	45
Welch's, Chillers Juice Drink, Strawberry Kiwi Flavor 8 fl oz	120	0	0	NA	29	NA	28	0	25

Food Serving size	Cal.	(g) Total Fat	(g) Sat. Fat	(mg) Chol.	(g) Carb.	(g) Fiber	(g) Sug.	(g) Prot.	(mg) Sod.
Welch's, Essentials Juice Cocktail Blend, Concord Grape									
8 fl oz	150	0	0	NA	37	NA	NA	0	20
Welch's, Essentials Juice Cocktail Blend, Concord Grape-Cranberry									
8 fl oz	150	0	0	NA	37	NA	NA	0	20
Welch's, Essentials Juice Cocktail Blend, Orange Pineapple Apple									
8 fl oz	140	0	0	NA	35	NA	34	0	20
Welch's, Essentials Juice Cocktail Blend, White Grape Peach Mango									
8 fl oz	150	0	0	NA	37	NA	NA	0	20
Welch's, Frozen 100% Purple Grape Juice Concentrate									
60ml	140	0	0	NA	38	NA	36	1	15
Welch's, Frozen 100% White Grape Cranberry Juice Concentrate									
60ml	160	0	0	NA	41	NA	39	0	0
Welch's, Frozen 100% White Grape Juice Concentrate									
60ml	160	0	0	NA	41	NA	39	0	0
Welch's, Frozen 100% White Grape Peach Juice Concentrate									
60ml	160	0	0	NA	41	NA	39	0	0
Welch's, Frozen 100% White Grape Pear Juice Concentrate									
60ml	160	0	0	NA	41	NA	39	0	0
Welch's, Frozen 100% White Grape Raspberry Juice Concentrate									
60ml	160	0	0	NA	41	NA	39	0	0
Welch's, Frozen Apple Grape Cherry Cocktail Concentrate									
60ml	150	0	0	NA	38	NA	37	0	40
Welch's, Frozen Apple Grape Raspberry Cocktail Concentrate									
60ml	150	0	0	NA	38	NA	37	0	40
Welch's, Frozen Berry Sunsplash Cocktail Concentrate									
60ml	150	0	0	NA	38	NA	37	0	40
Welch's, Frozen Cranberry Cocktail Concentrate									
60ml	150	0	0	NA	38	NA	37	0	40
Welch's, Frozen Fruit Harvest Punch Cocktail Concentrate									
60ml	150	0	0	NA	38	NA	37	0	40
Welch's, Frozen Grape Apple Cocktail Concentrate									
60ml	150	0	0	NA	38	NA	37	0	40
Welch's, Frozen Harvest Blend Cocktail Concentrate									
60ml	150	0	0	NA	38	NA	37	0	40

Food Serving size	Cal.	(g) Total Fat	(g) Sat. Fat	(mg) Chol.	(g) Carb.	(g) Fiber	(g) Sug.	(g) Prot.	(mg) Sod.
Welch's, Frozen Light Cranberry Cocktail Concentrate									
60ml	150	0	0	NA	38	NA	37	0	40
Welch's, Frozen Light Purple Grape Juice Cocktail Concentrate									
60ml	150	0	0	NA	38	NA	37	0	40
Welch's, Frozen Orange Pineapple Apple Juice Cocktail Concentrate									
60ml	150	0	0	NA	38	NA	37	0	40
Welch's, Frozen Purple Grape Juice Cocktail Concentrate									
60ml	150	0	0	NA	38	NA	37	0	40
Welch's, Frozen White Grape Juice Cocktail Concentrate									
60ml	150	0	0	NA	38	NA	NA	0	40
Welch's, Healthy Start 100% Grape Juice									
8 fl oz	140	0	0	NA	38	NA	36	1	15
Welch's, Light, Concord Grape Flavor									
8 fl oz	45	0	0	NA	12	NA	11	0	75
Welch's, Light, White Grape Flavor									
8 fl oz	45	0	0	NA	12	NA	11	0	75
Welch's, Pourable 100% Apple Juice Concentrate									
60ml	160	0	0	NA	41	NA	39	0	0
Welch's, Pourable 100% Fruit Fantastic Juice Concentrate									
60ml	160	0	0	NA	41	NA	39	0	0
Welch's, Pourable 100% Grape Juice Concentrate									
60ml	160	0	0	NA	41	NA	39	0	0
Welch's, Pourable 100% Tropical Orange Passion Juice Concentrate									
60ml	160	0	0	NA	41	NA	39	0	0
Welch's, Red 100% Grape Juice									
8 fl oz	170	0	0	NA	44	NA	42	0	20
Welch's, Refrigerated Juice Cocktails, Berry Pineapple Passion Fruit									
8 fl oz	140	0	0	NA	34	NA	33	0	5
Welch's, Refrigerated Juice Cocktails, Concord Grape									
8 fl oz	140	0	0	NA	34	NA	33	0	20
Welch's, Refrigerated Juice Cocktails, Guava Pineapple									
8 fl oz	140	0	0	NA	35	NA	35	0	5
Welch's, Refrigerated Juice Cocktails, Mango Twist									
8 fl oz	150	0	0	NA	38	NA	37	0	5

Food Serving size	Cal.	(g) Total Fat	(g) Sat. Fat	(mg) Chol.	(g) Carb.	(g) Fiber	(g) Sug.	(g) Prot.	(mg) Sod.
Welch's, Refrigerated Juice Cocktails, Mountain Berry 8 fl oz	140	0	0	NA	34	NA	33	0	5
Welch's, Refrigerated Juice Cocktails, Orange Pineapple Apple 8 fl oz	140	0	0	NA	35	NA	34	0	20
Welch's, Refrigerated Juice Cocktails, Passion Fruit 8 fl oz	150	0	0	NA	38	NA	37	0	5
Welch's, Refrigerated Juice Cocktails, Strawberry Breeze 8 fl oz	130	0	0	NA	33	NA	32	0	5
Welch's, Refrigerated Juice Cocktails, Strawberry Peach 8 fl oz	140	0	0	NA	34	NA	33	0	20
Welch's, Refrigerated Juice Cocktails, Tropical Cherry 8 fl oz	140	0	0	NA	36	NA	35	0	5
Welch's, Refrigerated Juice Cocktails, White Grape Peach 8 fl oz	150	0	0	NA	36	NA	35	0	5
Welch's, Sparkling Juice Cocktails, Blueberry Grape 8 fl oz	150	0	0	NA	38	NA	37	0	45
Welch's, Sparkling Juice Cocktails, Cranberry 8 fl oz	160	0	0	NA	40	NA	38	0	45
Welch's, Sparkling Juice Cocktails, Cranberry (Walmart) 8 fl oz	160	0	0	NA	40	NA	38	0	45
Welch's, Sparkling Juice Cocktails, Lemonade Flavor 8 fl oz	140	0	0	NA	36	NA	35	0	45
Welch's, Sparkling Juice Cocktails, Mango Passion Fruit Flavor 8 fl oz	130	0	0	NA	32	NA	31	0	45
Welch's, Sparkling Juice Cocktails, Raspberry Limeade Flavor 8 fl oz	140	0	0	NA	34	NA	33	0	45
Welch's, Sparkling Juice Cocktails, Red Grape 8 fl oz	160	0	0	NA	40	NA	38	0	45
Welch's, Sparkling Juice Cocktails, Red Grape (Holiday) 8 fl oz	160	0	0	NA	45	NA	38	0	45
Welch's, Sparkling Juice Cocktails, Red Grape (Target) 8 fl oz	160	0	0	NA	45	NA	38	0	45
Welch's, Sparkling Juice Cocktails, Red Grape (Walmart) 8 fl oz	160	0	0	NA	45	NA	38	0	45

Food Serving size	Cal.	(g) Total Fat	(g) Sat. Fat	(mg) Chol.	(g) Carb.	(g) Fiber	(g) Sug.	(g) Prot.	(mg) Sod.
Welch's, Sparkling Juice Cocktails, Strawberry Lemonade Flavor									
8 fl oz	140	0	0	NA	36	NA	35	0	45
Welch's, Sparkling Juice Cocktails, White Grape									
8 fl oz	160	0	0	NA	40	NA	38	0	45
Welch's, Sparkling Juice Cocktails, White Grape (Holiday)									
8 fl oz	160	0	0	NA	45	NA	38	0	45
Welch's, Sparkling Juice Cocktails, White Grape (Target)									
8 fl oz	160	0	0	NA	45	NA	38	0	45
Welch's, Sparkling Juice Cocktails, White Grape (Walmart)									
8 fl oz	160	0	0	NA	45	NA	38	0	45

Fruits

Food Serving size	Cal.	(g) Total Fat	(g) Sat. Fat	(mg) Chol.	(g) Carb.	(g) Fiber	(g) Sug.	(g) Prot.	(mg) Sod.
Apples, Raw, with Skin									
1 cup, slices (109g)	57	0	0	0	15	2.6	11	0	1
Apples, Raw, Without Skin									
1 large (3-1/4″ dia) (216g)	104	0	0	0	28	2.8	22	1	0
Apples, Raw, Without Skin, Cooked, Boiled									
1 cup, slices (171g)	91	1	0	0	23	4.1	19	0	2
Apples, Raw, Without Skin, Cooked, Microwave									
1 cup, slices (170g)	95	1	0	0	24	4.8	20	0	2
Apricots, Raw									
1 cup, sliced (165g)	79	1	0	0	18	3.3	15	2	2
Bananas, Raw									
1 cup, sliced (150g)	134	0	0	0	34	3.9	18	2	2
Blackberries, Raw									
1 cup (144g)	62	1	0	0	14	7.6	7	2	1
Blueberries, Raw									
50 berries (68g)	39	0	0	0	10	1.6	7	1	1
Carambola (Starfruit), Raw									
1 cup, sliced (108g)	33	0	0	0	7	3	4	1	2
Carissa (Natal-plum), Raw									
1 fruit, without skin and seeds (20g)	12	0	NA	0	3	NA	NA	0	1
Chayote, Fruit, Raw									
1 chayote (5-3/4″) (203g)	39	0	0	0	9	3.5	3	2	4

Food Serving size	Cal.	(g) Total Fat	(g) Sat. Fat	(mg) Chol.	(g) Carb.	(g) Fiber	(g) Sug.	(g) Prot.	(mg) Sod.
Cherimoya, Raw 1 cup, pieces (160g)	120	1	0	0	28	4.8	21	3	11
Cherries, Sour, Red, Raw 1 cup, with pits yields (103g)	52	0	0	0	13	1.6	9	1	3
Cherries, Sweet, Raw 1 cup, without pits (154g)	97	0	0	0	25	3.2	20	2	0
Clementines, Raw 1 fruit (74g)	35	0	NA	NA	9	1.3	7	1	1
Crabapples, Raw 1 cup, slices (110g)	84	0	0	0	22	NA	NA	0	1
Cranberries, Raw 1 cup, whole (100g)	46	0	0	0	12	4.6	4	0	2
Currants, European Black, Raw 1 cup (112g)	71	0	0	0	17	NA	NA	2	2
Currants, Red and White, Raw 1 cup (112g)	63	0	0	0	15	4.8	8	2	1
Dates, Deglet Noor 1 date, pitted (7.1g)	20	0	0	0	5	0.6	4	0	0
Dates, Medjool 1 date, pitted (24g)	66	0	NA	NA	18	1.6	16	0	0
Eden Foods, Apple Butter, Organic 1 tbsp	20	0	0	NA	4	1	4	0	0
Eden Foods, Apple Cherry Butter, Organic 1 tbsp	25	0	0	NA	6	<1	5	0	0
Eden Foods, Apple Cherry Sauce, Organic 1/2 cup	70	0	0	0	17	3	12	0	10
Eden Foods, Apple Cinnamon Sauce, Organic 1/2 cup	60	0	0	0	14	2	12	0	10
Eden Foods, Apple Sauce, Organic 1/2 cup	60	0	0	NA	13	2	10	0	10
Eden Foods, Apple Strawberry Sauce, Organic 1/2 cup	60	0	0	NA	13	2	10	0	10
Eden Foods, Cherry Butter, Montmorency Tart, Organic 1 tbsp	35	0	NA	NA	9	1	8	0	0

Food Serving size	Cal.	(g) Total Fat	(g) Sat. Fat	(mg) Chol.	(g) Carb.	(g) Fiber	(g) Sug.	(g) Prot.	(mg) Sod.
Eden Foods, Plum Balls									
3g	10	0	0	0	1	0	0	0	1
Eden Foods, Thompson Raisins, Organic									
1/4 cup	130	0	0	0	32	1.5	24	1	0
Eden Foods, Umeboshi Plums									
1 tsp	0	0	NA	0	0	0	0	0	520
Eden Foods, Wild Berry Mix, Organic									
3 tbsp	150	8	1	0	13	4	1	5	10
Elderberries, Raw									
1 cup (145g)	106	1	0	0	27	10.2	NA	1	9
Figs, Raw									
1 medium (2-1/4″ dia) (50g)	37	0	0	0	10	1.5	8	0	1
Gooseberries, Raw									
1 cup (150g)	66	1	0	0	15	6.5	NA	1	2
Grapefruit, Raw, Pink and Red and White, All Areas									
.5 large (approx 4-1/2″ dia) (166g)	53	0	0	0	13	1.8	12	1	0
Grapefruit, Raw, Pink and Red, All Areas									
.5 fruit (3-3/4″ dia) (123g)	52	0	0	0	13	2	8	1	0
Grapefruit, Raw, Pink and Red, California and Arizona									
.5 fruit (3-3/4″ dia) (123g)	46	0	0	0	12	NA	NA	1	1
Grapefruit, Raw, Pink and Red, Florida									
.5 fruit (3-3/4″ dia) (123g)	37	0	0	0	9	1.4	NA	1	0
Grapefruit, Raw, White, All Areas									
.5 fruit (3-3/4″ dia) (118g)	39	0	0	0	10	1.3	9	1	0
Grapefruit, Raw, White, California									
.5 fruit (3-3/4″ dia) (118g)	44	0	0	0	11	NA	NA	1	0
Grapefruit, Raw, White, Florida									
.5 fruit (3-3/4″ dia) (118g)	38	0	0	0	10	NA	NA	1	0
Grapes, American Type (Slip Skin), Raw									
1 grape (2.4g)	2	0	0	0	0	0	0	0	0
Grapes, Muscadine, Raw									
1 grape (6g)	3	0	NA	NA	1	0.2	NA	0	0

Food Serving size	Cal.	(g) Total Fat	(g) Sat. Fat	(mg) Chol.	(g) Carb.	(g) Fiber	(g) Sug.	(g) Prot.	(mg) Sod.
Grapes, Red or Green (European Type, Such as Thompson Seedless), Raw									
10 grapes (49g)	34	0	0	0	9	0.4	8	0	1
Guavas, Common, Raw									
1 fruit, without refuse (55g)	37	1	0	0	8	3	5	1	1
Guavas, Strawberry, Raw									
1 fruit, without refuse (6g)	4	0	0	0	1	0.3	NA	0	2
Jackfruit, Raw									
1 cup, 1" pieces (151g)	143	1	0	0	35	2.3	29	3	3
Java-plum (Jambolan), Raw									
3 fruit (9g)	5	0	NA	0	1	NA	NA	0	1
Kiwifruit, Gold, Raw									
1 fruit (86g)	52	0	0	NA	12	1.7	9	1	3
Kiwifruit, Green, Raw									
1 fruit (2" dia) (69g)	42	0	0	0	10	2.1	6	1	2
Kumquats, Raw									
1 fruit, without refuse (19g)	13	0	0	0	3	1.2	2	0	2
Lemon Peel, Raw									
1 tsp (2g)	1	0	0	0	0	0.2	0	0	0
Lemons, Raw, Without Peel									
1 fruit (2-1/8" dia) (58g)	17	0	0	0	5	1.6	1	1	1
Let's Do...Organic, Organic Coconut Flakes									
3 tbsp	110	10	9	0	4	2	<1	1	5
Let's Do...Organic, Organic Creamed Coconut									
1 tbsp	190	18	16	0	7	5	2	2	10
Let's Do...Organic, Organic Reduced Fat Shredded Coconut									
4 tbsp	70	6	5	0	4	2	0	1	0
Let's Do...Organic, Organic Shredded Coconut									
3 tbsp	110	10	9	0	4	2	<1	1	5
Litchis, Raw									
1 fruit, without refuse (9.6g)	6	0	0	0	2	0.1	1	0	0
Longans, Raw									
1 fruit, without refuse (3.2g)	2	0	NA	0	0	0	NA	0	0
Loquats, Raw									
1 large (20g)	9	0	0	0	2	0.3	NA	0	0

Food Serving size	Cal.	(g) Total Fat	(g) Sat. Fat	(mg) Chol.	(g) Carb.	(g) Fiber	(g) Sug.	(g) Prot.	(mg) Sod.
Mammy-apple (Mamey), Raw									
1 fruit, without refuse (846g)	431	4	1	0	106	25.4	NA	4	127
Mangos, Raw									
1 fruit, without refuse (336g)	202	1	0	0	50	5.4	46	3	3
Mariani Premium Fruit, Berries 'N Apples									
1/3 cup	130	0	0	0	32	2	26	0	30
Mariani Premium Fruit, Berries 'N Cherries									
1/3 cup	140	0	0	0	33	2	28	1	10
Mariani Premium Fruit, Berry Defense									
1/4 cup	130	0	0	0	31	3	25	1	0
Mariani Premium Fruit, Berry Thrive									
1/4 cup	130	0.5	0	0	32	2	27	0	5
Mariani Premium Fruit, Cherries									
1/4 cup	140	0	0	0	33	1	27	1	0
Mariani Premium Fruit, Cherry Pie Cherries									
1/4 cup	130	0	0	0	31	2	27	1	15
Mariani Premium Fruit, Chopped Dates									
1/3 cup	130	0	0	0	33	3	26	0	0
Mariani Premium Fruit, Cranberries									
1/3 cup	130	0	0	0	32	2	27	0	30
Mariani Premium Fruit, Cranberries (Snack Box)									
1 box	140	0	NA	NA	35	2	29	0	30
Mariani Premium Fruit, Orchard Fruit, California Apricots									
1/4 cup	110	0	0	0	25	4	20	1	15
Mariani Premium Fruit, Orchard Fruit, Mediterranean Apricots									
1/4 cup	110	0	0	0	25	2	15	1	10
Mariani Premium Fruit, Orchard Fruit, Mixed Fruit									
1/4 cup	110	0	0	0	25	4	17	1	20
Mariani Premium Fruit, Orchard Fruit, Plum Support with Glucosamine									
1/4 cup	110	0	0	0	25	3	17	1	5
Mariani Premium Fruit, Orchard Fruit, Sliced Apples									
1/3 cup	100	0	0	0	25	3	13	1	130
Mariani Premium Fruit, Orchard Fruit, Ultimate Apricots									
1/4 cup	100	0	0	0	24	2	13	1	15

Food Serving size	Cal.	(g) Total Fat	(g) Sat. Fat	(mg) Chol.	(g) Carb.	(g) Fiber	(g) Sug.	(g) Prot.	(mg) Sod.
Mariani Premium Fruit, Pitted Dates 6-7 Dates	120	0	0	0	30	3	25	1	0
Mariani Premium Fruit, Raisins 1/4 cup	120	0	0	0	32	1	24	1	0
Mariani Premium Fruit, Strawberries 1/4 cup	140	0	0	0	32	2	28	0	15
Mariani Premium Fruit, Tropical Fruit, Banana Chips 1/3 cup	160	9	7	0	19	4	5	0	0
Mariani Premium Fruit, Tropical Fruit, Island Fruits 1/4 cup	140	0	0	0	34	1	30	0	120
Mariani Premium Fruit, Tropical Fruit, Mango 5 slices	140	0	0	0	36	1	28	0	15
Mariani Premium Fruit, Tropical Fruit, Philippine Mango 6 slices	130	0	0	0	32	1	27	1	60
Mariani Premium Fruit, Tropical Fruit, Tropical Medley 1/3 cup	130	0	0	0	31	3	22	1	40
Mariani Premium Fruit, Tropical Fruit, Tropical Pineapple 1/3 cup	140	0	0	0	35	1	31	0	85
Mariani Premium Fruit, Wild Blueberries 1/4 cup	140	0	0	0	35	2	30	0	0
Mariani Premium Fruit, Yogurt Coated, Cranberry Crunch 1 bag	160	2	NA	NA	34	2	28	1	25
Mariani Premium Fruit, Yogurt Coated, Vanilla Raisins 2 tbsp	150	7	6	0	19	1	17	2	25
Mariani Premium Fruit, Yogurt Coated, Vanilla Raisins (Snack Box) 1 box	210	10	9	NA	28	1	24	2	35
Mariani Premium Tropical Fruit, Pineapple Tango 1/3 cup	130	0	0	0	33	2	25	0	110
Melon, Cantaloupe, Raw 1 cup, cubes (160g)	54	0	0	0	13	1.4	13	1	26
Melon, Casaba, Raw 1 melon (1640g)	459	2	0	0	108	14.8	93	18	148
Melon, Honeydew, Raw 1 cup, diced (approx 20 pieces per cup) (170g)	61	0	0	0	15	1.4	14	1	31

Food Serving size	Cal.	(g) Total Fat	(g) Sat. Fat	(mg) Chol.	(g) Carb.	(g) Fiber	(g) Sug.	(g) Prot.	(mg) Sod.
Mulberries, Raw 10 fruit (15g)	6	0	0	0	1	0.3	1	0	2
Native Forest, Organic Mango Chunks 1/2 cup	70	0	0	0	19	2	17	0	0
Native Forest, Organic Mangosteen 1/2 cup	90	0	0	0	23	<1	22	0	10
Native Forest, Organic Papaya Chunks 1/2 cup	60	0	0	0	14	1	11	<1	0
Native Forest, Organic Pineapple Chunks 1/2 cup	60	0	0	0	15	1	13	0	10
Native Forest, Organic Pineapple Crushed 1/2 cup	60	0	0	0	15	1	13	0	10
Native Forest, Organic Pineapple Slices 1/2 cup	60	0	0	0	15	1	13	0	10
Native Forest, Organic Rambutan 1/2 cup	100	0	0	0	24	<1	23	0	10
Native Forest, Organic Sliced Asian Pears 1/2 cup	45	0	0	0	11	2	8	0	5
Native Forest, Organic Sliced Peaches 1/2 cup	50	0	0	0	14	2	12	<1	5
Native Forest, Organic Tropical Fruit Salad 1/2 cup	70	0	0	0	16	1	14	<1	0
Nectarines, Raw 1 small (2-1/3″ dia) (129g)	57	0	0	0	14	2.2	10	1	0
Ocean Spray, Gluten Free Fruit Shapes Assorted Fruit 1 pouch	80	0	0	0	19	NA	12	0	25
Ocean Spray, Gluten Free Fruit Shapes Berries and Cherries 1 pouch	80	0	0	0	19	NA	12	0	25
Oheloberries, Raw 10 fruit (11g)	3	0	NA	0	1	NA	NA	0	0
Orange Peel, raw 1 tsp (2g)	2	0	0	0	1	0.2	NA	0	0
Orange, Raw, California, Valencia 1 fruit (2-5/8″ dia) (121g)	59	0	0	0	14	3	NA	1	0

Food Serving size	Cal.	(g) Total Fat	(g) Sat. Fat	(mg) Chol.	(g) Carb.	(g) Fiber	(g) Sug.	(g) Prot.	(mg) Sod.
Oranges, Raw, All Commercial Varieties 1 large (3-1/16″ dia) (184g)	86	0	0	0	22	4.4	17	2	0
Oranges, Raw, Florida 1 fruit (2-5/8″ dia) (141g)	65	0	0	0	16	3.4	13	1	0
Oranges, Raw, Navels 1 fruit (2-7/8″ dia) (140g)	69	0	0	0	18	3.1	12	1	1
Oranges, Raw, with Peel 1 fruit, without seeds (159g)	100	0	0	0	25	7.2	NA	2	3
Papayas, Raw 1 cup, mashed (230g)	99	1	0	0	25	3.9	18	1	18
Passion-fruit (Granadilla), Purple, Raw 1 fruit, without refuse (18g)	17	0	0	0	4	1.9	2	0	5
Peaches, Raw 1 small (2-1/2″ dia) (130g)	51	0	0	0	12	2	11	1	0
Pears, Asian, Raw 1 fruit, 3-3/8″ high x 3″ diameter (275g)	116	1	0	0	29	9.9	19	1	0
Pears, Raw 1 medium (178g)	103	0	0	0	28	5.5	17	1	2
Persimmons, Japanese, Raw 1 fruit (2-1/2″ dia) (168g)	118	0	0	0	31	6	21	1	2
Persimmons, Native, Raw 1 fruit, without refuse (25g)	32	0	NA	0	8	NA	NA	0	0
Pineapple, Raw, All Varieties 1 fruit (905g)	453	1	0	0	119	12.7	89	5	9
Pineapple, Raw, Extra Sweet Variety 1 slice (4-2/3″ dia x 3/4″ thick) (166g)	85	0	NA	NA	22	2.3	17	1	2
Pineapple, Raw, Traditional Variety 1 slice (4-2/3″ dia x 3/4″ thick) (175g)	79	0	NA	NA	21	NA	15	1	2
Plantains, Raw 1 medium (179g)	218	1	0	0	57	4.1	27	2	7

Food Serving size	Cal.	(g) Total Fat	(g) Sat. Fat	(mg) Chol.	(g) Carb.	(g) Fiber	(g) Sug.	(g) Prot.	(mg) Sod.
Plums, Raw 1 fruit (2-1/8″ dia) (66g)	30	0	0	0	8	0.9	7	0	0
Pomegranates, Raw .5 cup, arils (seed/juice sacs) (87g)	72	1	0	0	16	3.5	12	1	3
Prickly Pears, Raw 1 fruit, without refuse (103g)	42	1	0	0	10	3.7	NA	1	5
Prunes, Dehydrated (Low-moisture), Uncooked 1 cup (132g)	447	1	0	0	118	NA	NA	5	7
Pummelo, Raw 1 fruit, without refuse (609g)	231	0	NA	0	59	6.1	NA	5	6
Quinces, Raw 1 fruit, without refuse (92g)	52	0	0	0	14	1.7	NA	0	4
Raisins, Golden, Seedless 1 cup (not packed) (145g)	438	1	0	0	115	5.8	86	5	17
Raisins, Seeded 1 cup (not packed) (145g)	429	1	0	0	114	9.9	NA	4	41
Raisins, Seedless 1 cup (not packed) (145g)	434	1	0	0	115	5.4	86	4	16
Raspberries, Raw 1 pint, as purchased, yields (312g)	162	2	0	0	37	20.3	14	4	3
Strawberries, Raw 1 cup, pureed (232g)	74	1	0	0	18	4.6	11	2	2
Tamarinds, Raw 1 fruit (3″ x 1″) (2g)	5	0	0	0	1	0.1	1	0	1
Tangerines (Mandarin Oranges), Raw 1 small (2-1/4″ dia) (76g)	40	0	0	0	10	1.4	8	1	2
Tomatillos, Raw .5 cup, chopped or diced (66g)	21	1	0	0	4	1.3	3	1	1
Watermelon, Raw 1 cup, diced (152g)	46	0	0	0	11	0.6	9	1	2

Dairy

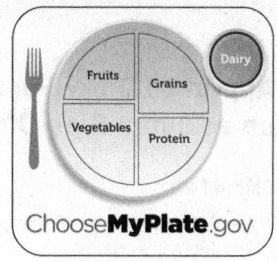

ChooseMyPlate.gov

Why Eat Dairy?

Basic dairy products are gluten-free, and consuming dairy products provides health benefits — especially improved bone health. Intake of dairy products is also associated with a reduced risk of cardiovascular disease and type 2 diabetes, and with lower blood pressure in adults. Foods in the Dairy Group provide nutrients that are vital for health and maintenance of your body. These nutrients include calcium, potassium, vitamin D, and protein. Calcium is used for building bones and teeth and in maintaining bone mass. Diets rich in potassium may help to maintain healthy blood pressure. Vitamin D functions in the body to maintain proper levels of calcium and phosphorous, thereby helping to build and maintain bones.

Daily Goal

Three cups for an adult on a 2,000 calorie diet.
One-cup equivalents:

1 cup milk	⅓ cup shredded cheese
1 cup yogurt	2 oz processed cheese
1½ oz hard cheese	2 cups cottage cheese

Gluten-Free Shopping Tips

- Choose low-fat or fat-free dairy products
- If you don't or can't consume milk, choose lactose-free products or milk alternatives
- Look for good sources of calcium—10% DV or higher
- Use fat-free or low-fat yogurt as a snack or to make dips or smoothies
- Check flavored yogurt, cheese sauces and spreads, malted milk, and ice creams for gluten ingredients

Gluten-Free Shopping List Essentials

Milk, low-fat or fat-free
Yogurt, low-fat or fat-free
Cottage Cheese, low-fat or fat-free
Soy Milk, calcium fortified
Cheese, reduced-fat
Lactose-free milk, if needed

Approved Dairy Foods and Those to Avoid on a Gluten-Free Diet

Gluten-Free

- Milk, cream, buttermilk
- Most ice cream
- Plain regular and frozen yogurt
- Cheese, cream cheese, processed cheese, processed cheese foods, and cottage cheese

May Contain Gluten

- Malted milk
- Flavored ice cream
- Flavored regular and frozen yogurt
- Cheese sauces, cheese spreads, and seasoned (flavored) shredded cheese made with ingredients to avoid (see page xi)
- Non-dairy beverages (nut, potato, soy, and rice) made with barley malt extract, barley-malt flavoring, or oats

Caution

The fat in dairy products is highly saturated, so the lower the fat content, the better. Move from whole milk to reduced-fat, to low-fat, to skim or fat-free gradually to let your taste buds adjust.

Food Serving size	Cal.	(g) Total Fat	(g) Sat. Fat	(mg) Chol.	(g) Carb.	(g) Fiber	(g) Sug.	(g) Prot.	(mg) Sod.
Cheeses									
Applegate Farms, American Cheese									
1 oz	90	7	6	20	1	0	1	6	350
Applegate Farms, American Cheese									
1 slice	80	7	5	25	1	0	0	5	270
Applegate Farms, Cheddar Cheese									
1 oz	110	9	5	30	0	0	0	7	180
Applegate Farms, Cheddar Cheese									
1 slice	70	6	4	20	0	0	0	5	120
Applegate Farms, Emmentaler Swiss Cheese									
1 oz	110	8	5	25	0	0	0	9	45
Applegate Farms, Emmentaler Swiss Cheese									
1 slice	80	6	4	15	0	0	0	5	35
Applegate Farms, Extra Sharp Aged Cheddar Cheese									
1 slice	110	9	5	30	0	0	0	7	180
Applegate Farms, Havarti Cheese									
1 slice	180	15	11	37	0	0	0	7	225
Applegate Farms, Monterey Jack Cheese									
1 slice	70	5	3.5	20	0	0	0	5	110
Applegate Farms, Muenster Cheese									
1 slice	70	6	4	20	0	0	0	5	140
Applegate Farms, Organic American Cheese									
1 slice	80	7	5	25	1	0	0	5	270
Applegate Farms, Organic Mild Cheddar Cheese									
1 slice	80	6	4	20	0	0	0	5	130
Applegate Farms, Organic Monterey Jack Cheese									
1 slice	80	6	4	20	0	0	0	5	130
Applegate Farms, Organic Muenster Cheese									
1 slice	85	6	4	20	0	0	0	5	130
Applegate Farms, Organic Provolone Cheese									
1 slice	70	5	3	15	0	0	0	5	160
Applegate Farms, Provolone Cheese									
1 oz	70	5	2.5	15	0	0	0	5	160

Food Serving size	Cal.	(g) Total Fat	(g) Sat. Fat	(mg) Chol.	(g) Carb.	(g) Fiber	(g) Sug.	(g) Prot.	(mg) Sod.
Applegate Farms, Provolone Cheese									
1 slice	70	5	2.5	15	0	0	0	5	160
Applegate Farms, Yogurt Cheese									
1 slice	80	6	4	15	<1	0	0	5	105
Boar's Head, 25% Lower Sodium / 25% Lower Fat American Cheese (Yellow & White)									
1 oz	90	6	4.5	20	2	0	0	7	300
Boar's Head, 3 Pepper Colby Jack Cheese									
1 oz	100	8	5	25	1	0	0	6	170
Boar's Head, 42% Lower Sodium Provolone Cheese									
1 oz	100	7	4.5	20	1	0	0	7	140
Boar's Head, All Natural Muenster Cheese									
1 oz	100	8	5	25	0	0	0	6	190
Boar's Head, American Cheese (Yellow & White)									
1 oz	110	9	6	25	1	0	0	6	350
Boar's Head, Asiago Cheese									
1 oz	100	9	6	25	1	0	0	6	220
Boar's Head, Baby Swiss Cheese									
1 oz	110	9	6	25	<1	0	0	7	135
Boar's Head, Chipotle Gouda Cheese									
1 oz	100	8	5	20	<1	0	0	6	240
Boar's Head, Colby Jack Cheese									
1 oz	110	9	6	25	0	0	0	6	180
Boar's Head, Cream Havarti Cheese									
1 oz	110	10	7	35	0	0	0	6	210
Boar's Head, Double Gloucester Cheddar Cheese									
1 oz	110	10	6	35	0	0	0	7	200
Boar's Head, Edam Cheese									
1 oz	90	7	5	20	NA	NA	NA	7	280
Boar's Head, Gold Label Premium Imported Swiss Cheese									
1 oz	110	8	5	20	<1	0	0	8	70
Boar's Head, Gouda Cheese									
1 oz	110	9	5	30	0	NA	NA	6	280

Food Serving size	Cal.	(g) Total Fat	(g) Sat. Fat	(mg) Chol.	(g) Carb.	(g) Fiber	(g) Sug.	(g) Prot.	(mg) Sod.
Boar's Head, Horseradish Cheddar Cheese									
1 oz	110	9	6	30	2	0	0	6	190
Boar's Head, Lacey Swiss Cheese									
1 oz	90	6	4	15	0	0	0	9	35
Boar's Head, Longhorn Colby Cheese									
1 oz	110	9	5	30	<1	0	0	7	170
Boar's Head, Low Sodium Muenster Cheese									
1 oz	100	8	5	20	0	0	0	6	75
Boar's Head, Monterey Jack Cheese									
1 oz	100	9	5	25	0	0	0	6	180
Boar's Head, Monterey Jack Cheese with Jalapeno									
1 oz	100	9	5	25	0	0	0	6	180
Boar's Head, Mortadella									
2 oz	160	14	5	30	0	0	0	9	560
Boar's Head, Mortadella with Pistachio Nuts									
2 oz	170	14	5	30	2	0	0	10	560
Boar's Head, Natural Gouda Cheese									
1 oz	100	8	5	20	1	0	0	6	240
Boar's Head, Natural Swiss Cheese									
1 oz	110	8	5	20	0	0	0	8	65
Boar's Head, No Salt Added Natural Swiss Cheese									
1 oz	110	8	5	25	1	0	0	8	10
Boar's Head, Picante Sharp Provolone Cheese									
1 oz	100	8	5	25	1	0	0	7	250
Boar's Head, Sharp American Cheese (White)									
1 oz	110	9	6	20	1	0	1	6	350
Boar's Head, Sharp Cheddar Cheese (White)									
1 oz	110	9	5	30	<1	0	0	7	190
Boar's Head, Sharp Cheddar Cheese (Yellow)									
1 oz	110	9	5	30	<1	0	0	7	190
Boar's Head, Vermont Cheddar Cheese (White)									
1 oz	110	10	6	30	0	0	0	7	180
Boar's Head, Vermont Cheddar Cheese (Yellow)									
1 oz	110	10	6	30	0	0	0	7	180

Food Serving size	Cal.	(g) Total Fat	(g) Sat. Fat	(mg) Chol.	(g) Carb.	(g) Fiber	(g) Sug.	(g) Prot.	(mg) Sod.
Boar's Head, Whole Milk Low Moisture Mozzarella Cheese									
1 oz	90	7	4.5	20	1	0	0	6	150
Galaxy Nutritional Foods, Rice Cheese Mozzarella Flavor									
1 slice	40	2.5	0	0	<1	0	0	3	220
Galaxy Nutritional Foods, Rice Mozzarella Flavor Cheese Block									
1 oz	70	4	0.5	0	2	0	0	6	220
Galaxy Nutritional Foods, Rice Shreds									
1/3 cup	70	4	1	0	3	0	0	6	370
Galaxy Nutritional Foods, Rice-Based Grated Parmesan Flavor Topping									
2 tsp	15	0.5	0	0	0	0	0	2	75
Galaxy Nutritional Foods, Vegan American Flavor Cheese (Soy Vegan Slices)									
1 slice	40	2	0	0	5	0	0	1	120
Galaxy Nutritional Foods, Vegan Cheddar Flavor (Soy Vegan Block)									
1 oz	60	3	0.5	0	6	0	0	1	290
Galaxy Nutritional Foods, Vegan Cream Cheese Alternative									
2 tbsp	90	9	4.5	0	1	0	0	1	120
Galaxy Nutritional Foods, Vegan Grated Parmesan Flavor Topping									
2 tsp	15	0	0	0	1	<1	0	2	55
Galaxy Nutritional Foods, Vegan Mozzarella Style Shreds									
1/4 cup	90	6	0	0	7	0	0	1	190
Galaxy Nutritional Foods, Veggie Cream Cheese Soy Cheese Alternative									
2 tbsp	90	9	4.5	0	1	0	0	1	120
Galaxy Nutritional Foods, Veggie Grated Parmesan Flavor Topping									
2 tsp	15	0.5	0	0	0	0	0	2	95
Galaxy Nutritional Foods, Veggie Shreds Mozzarella Soy-Based Shreds									
1/3 cup	70	4.5	0.5	<5	<1	0	0	6	260
Galaxy Nutritional Foods, Veggie Slices Cheddar Flavor (Soy-Based)									
1 slice	40	2.5	0	0	<1	0	0	3	220
Galaxy Nutritional Foods, Veggie Soy-Based Block Mozzarella Flavor									
1 oz	70	4	0	0	2	0	0	6	290
Lifeway Foods, Farmer Cheese									
2 tbsp	40	1.5	1	6	4	NA	4	3	10
Lifeway Foods, Farmer Cheese Fat Free									
2 tbsp	20	0	0	<5	NA	NA	2	2	2

Food Serving size	Cal.	(g) Total Fat	(g) Sat. Fat	(mg) Chol.	(g) Carb.	(g) Fiber	(g) Sug.	(g) Prot.	(mg) Sod.
Lifeway Foods, Farmer Cheese Lite									
2 tbsp	25	1	0.5	<5	2	NA	1	3	10
Lifeway Foods, Organic Farmer Cheese									
2 tbsp	40	1.5	1	6	4	0	4	3	10
Lifeway Foods, White Cheese									
1 oz	50	3	0	11	2	NA	1	3	11
Lisanetti Foods, SoySation, 3-Cheese Blend Shreds									
1 oz	60	3	0	0	2	1	0	7	190
Lisanetti Foods, SoySation, Cheddar Style Chunks									
1 oz	60	3	0	0	2	1	0	7	190
Lisanetti Foods, SoySation, Cheddar Style Shreds									
1 oz	63	3	0	0	2	1	0	7	190
Lisanetti Foods, SoySation, Cheddar Style Slices									
1 slice	40	2.5	0	0	1	0	0	4	180
Lisanetti Foods, SoySation, Mozzarella Style Chunks									
1 oz	60	3	0	0	2	1	0	7	190
Lisanetti Foods, SoySation, Mozzarella Style Shreds									
1 oz	63	3	0	0	2	1	0	7	190
Lisanetti Foods, SoySation, Parmesan Style Shreds									
1 oz	60	3	0	0	2	1	0	7	290
Lisanetti Foods, SoySation, RiceCheeze, Cheddar Style Chunks									
1 oz	60	3	0	0	2	1	0	6	190
Lisanetti Foods, SoySation, RiceCheeze, Mozzarella Style Chunks									
1 oz	60	3	0	0	2	1	0	6	190
Lisanetti Foods, SoySation, RiceCheeze, Pepper Jack Chunks									
1 oz	60	3	0	0	2	1	0	6	190
Lisanetti Foods, SoySation, RiceCheeze, Snack Sticks American Style Snack Sticks									
1 stick	60	3	0	0	2	1	0	6	190
Lisanetti Foods, SoySation, RiceCheeze, Snack Sticks Mozzarella Style Snack Sticks									
1 stick	60	3	0	0	2	1	0	6	190
Lisanetti Foods, SoySation, Swiss Style Slices									
1 slice	40	2.5	0	0	1	0	0	4	180

Food Serving size	Cal.	(g) Total Fat	(g) Sat. Fat	(mg) Chol.	(g) Carb.	(g) Fiber	(g) Sug.	(g) Prot.	(mg) Sod.
Lisanetti Foods, SoySation, Vegan Cheeze Shreds, Cheddar Style									
1 oz	70	5	0.5	0	3	2	0	2	130
Lisanetti Foods, SoySation, Vegan Cheeze Shreds, Mozzarella Style									
1 oz	70	5	0.5	0	4	2	0	2	120
Lisanetti Foods, The Original Almond, Cheddar Style Chunks									
1 oz	50	1	0	0	3	1	0	7	190
Lisanetti Foods, The Original Almond, Cheddar Style Shred									
1 oz	63	3	0	0	2	1	0	7	190
Lisanetti Foods, The Original Almond, Garlic-Herb Style Chunks									
1 oz	50	1	0	0	3	1	0	7	190
Lisanetti Foods, The Original Almond, Jalapeno Jack Style Chunks									
1 oz	50	1	0	0	3	1	0	7	190
Lisanetti Foods, The Original Almond, Mozzarella Style Chunks									
1 oz	50	1	0	0	3	1	0	7	190
Lisanetti Foods, The Original Almond, Mozzarella Style Shred									
1 oz	63	3	0	0	2	1	0	7	190
Thumann's, American Cheese									
1 oz	100	9	5	25	1	0	0	6	430
Thumann's, Baby Swiss Cheese									
1 oz	100	8	5	25	0	0	0	7	110
Thumann's, Cream Cheese									
1 oz	100	9	6	30	2	0	1	2	100
Thumann's, Hot Pepper Jack Cheese									
1 oz	100	8	5	25	1	0	<1	5	470
Thumann's, Mozzarella Cheese – Low Moisture									
1 oz	90	7	4	25	1	0	1	6	290
Thumann's, Muenster Cheese									
1 oz	110	9	6	30	0	0	0	7	180
Thumann's, Provolone Cheese									
1 oz	100	8	5	25	1	0	0	7	250
Thumann's, Sharp Cheddar Cheese – Yellow									
1 oz	110	9	6	25	0	0	0	7	180
Thumann's, Swiss Cheese – Domestic									
1 oz	100	8	5	25	1	0	0	8	60

Food Serving size	Cal.	(g) Total Fat	(g) Sat. Fat	(mg) Chol.	(g) Carb.	(g) Fiber	(g) Sug.	(g) Prot.	(mg) Sod.
Thumann's, Swiss Lace Cheese – Lower Sodium									
1 oz	100	8	5	25	0	0	0	7	35

Dairy

Food Serving size	Cal.	Total Fat	Sat. Fat	Chol.	Carb.	Fiber	Sug.	Prot.	Sod.
Milk, Chocolate, Fluid, Commercial, Low Fat, with Added Vitamins A and D									
1 quart (1000g)	630	10	6	30	104	5	99	32	610
Milk, Chocolate, Fluid, Commercial, Reduced Fat, with Added Calcium									
1 fl oz (31.2g)	24	1	0	2	4	0.2	3	1	21
Milk, Chocolate, Fluid, Commercial, Reduced Fat, with Added Vitamins A and D									
1 fl oz (31.2g)	24	1	0	2	4	0.2	3	1	21
Milk, Chocolate, Fluid, Commercial, Whole, with Added Vitamins A and D									
1 fl oz (31.2g)	26	1	1	4	3	0.2	3	1	19
Milk, Condensed, Evaporated, Non-fat, with Added Vitamins A and D									
1 fl oz (31.9g)	25	0	0	1	4	0	4	2	37
Milk, Condensed, Evaporated, with Added Vitamin D, No Added Vitamin A									
1 fl oz (31.5g)	42	2	1	9	3	0	3	2	33
Milk, Condensed, Evaporated, with Vitamin A									
.5 cup (126g)	169	10	6	37	13	0	NA	9	134
Milk, Condensed, Evaporated, Without Added Vitamins A and D									
1 fl oz (31.5g)	43	2	1	9	3	0	3	2	33
Milk, Dry, Non-fat, Calcium Reduced									
.25 lb (113g)	400	0	0	2	59	0	NA	40	2576
Milk, Dry, Whole, with Added Vitamin D									
.25 cup (32g)	159	9	5	31	12	0	12	8	119
Milk, Dry, Whole, Without Added Vitamin D									
.25 cup (32g)	159	9	5	31	12	0	12	8	119
Milk, Fluid, Non-fat, Calcium Fortified (Fat Free or Skim)									
1 fl oz (30.9g)	11	0	0	1	1	0	0	1	16
Milk, Low Fat, Fluid, 1% Milk Fat, Protein Fortified, with Added Vitamins A and D									
1 quart (984g)	472	12	7	39	54	0	NA	39	571
Milk, Low Fat, Fluid, 1% Milk Fat, with Added Vitamins A and D									
1 fl oz (30.5g)	13	0	0	2	2	0	2	1	13
Milk, Low Sodium, Fluid, Whole									
1 fl oz (30.5g)	19	1	1	4	1	0	1	1	1

Food Serving size	Cal.	(g) Total Fat	(g) Sat. Fat	(mg) Chol.	(g) Carb.	(g) Fiber	(g) Sug.	(g) Prot.	(mg) Sod.
Milk, Non-fat, Fluid, Protein Fortified, with Added Vitamins A and D (Fat Free or Skim)									
1 quart (984g)	403	2	2	20	55	0	NA	39	581
Milk, Non-fat, Fluid, with Added Vitamins A and D (Fat Free or Skim)									
1 fl oz (30.6g)	10	0	0	1	2	0	2	1	13
Milk, Non-fat, Fluid, Without Added Vitamins A and D (Fat Free or Skim)									
1 quart (980g)	333	1	0	20	49	0	50	33	412
Milk, Producer, Fluid, 3.7% Milk Fat									
1 quart (976g)	625	36	22	137	45	0	NA	32	478
Milk, Reduced Fat, Fluid, 2% Milk Fat, Protein Fortified, with Added Vitamins A and D									
1 quart (984g)	551	19	12	79	54	0	52	39	581
Milk, Reduced Fat, Fluid, 2% Milk Fat, with Added Vitamins A and D									
1 fl oz (30.5g)	15	1	0	2	1	0	2	1	14
Milk, Whole, 3.25% Milk Fat, with Added Vitamin D									
1 tbsp (15g)	9	0	0	2	1	0	1	0	6
Milk, Whole, 3.25% Milk Fat, Without Added Vitamins A and D									
1 tbsp (15g)	9	0	0	2	1	0	1	0	6
Smart Balance, Omega-3 Grade A Natural Large Eggs (All natural eggs are gluten free; egg substitutes may not be)									
1 egg	70	4	1	185	0	NA	NA	6	70

Dairy Alternatives (Soy Milk & Yogurts, Coconut Milk, Almond Milk, etc.)

Food Serving size	Cal.	Total Fat	Sat. Fat	Chol.	Carb.	Fiber	Sug.	Prot.	Sod.
8th Continent, Complete Vanilla Soymilk									
8 fl oz	80	2.5	0	0	8	3	6	6	95
8th Continent, Fat Free Original Soymilk									
8 fl oz	60	0	0	0	8	0	7	6	100
8th Continent, Fat Free Vanilla Soymilk									
8 fl oz	70	0	0	0	11	0	10	6	100
8th Continent, Light Chocolate Soymilk									
8 fl oz	90	1.5	0	0	12	<1	11	7	120
8th Continent, Light Original Soymilk									
8 fl oz	50	2	0	0	2	0	2	6	115
8th Continent, Light Vanilla Soymilk									
8 fl oz	60	2	0	0	5	0	5	6	110

Food Serving size	Cal.	(g) Total Fat	(g) Sat. Fat	(mg) Chol.	(g) Carb.	(g) Fiber	(g) Sug.	(g) Prot.	(mg) Sod.
8th Continent, Original Soymilk 8 fl oz	80	2.5	0	0	7	0	7	8	95
8th Continent, Vanilla Soymilk 8 fl oz	100	2.5	0	0	11	0	11	8	85
Blue Diamond, Almond Breeze, Chocolate Flavored Almond Milk 1 cup	120	3	0	0	22	1	20	1	150
Blue Diamond, Almond Breeze, Refrigerated Almond Milk, Original 1 cup	60	2.5	0	0	18	1	7	1	150
Blue Diamond, Almond Breeze, Refrigerated Almond Milk, Original (Unsweetened) 8 fl oz	40	3	0	0	2	1	0	1	180
Blue Diamond, Almond Breeze, Shelf Stable, Chocolate Almond Milk 1 cup	120	3	0	0	22	1	20	1	150
Blue Diamond, Almond Breeze, Shelf Stable, Chocolate Almond Milk (Unsweetened) 1 cup	45	3.5	0	0	3	1	0	2	180
Blue Diamond, Almond Breeze, Shelf Stable, Original Almond Milk 1 cup	60	2.5	0	0	8	1	7	1	150
Blue Diamond, Almond Breeze, Shelf Stable, Original Almond Milk (Unsweetened) 1 cup	40	3.5	0	0	2	1	0	1	180
Blue Diamond, Almond Breeze, Shelf Stable, Vanilla Almond Milk 1 cup	90	2.5	0	0	16	1	15	1	150
Blue Diamond, Almond Breeze, Shelf Stable, Vanilla Almond Milk (Unsweetened) 1 cup	40	3.5	0	0	2	1	0	1	180
Blue Diamond, Almond Breeze, Vanilla Flavored Almond Milk 1 cup	90	2.5	0	0	16	1	7	1	150
Blue Diamond, Almond Breeze, Vanilla Almond Milk (Unsweetened) 1 cup	40	3.5	0	0	2	1	7	1	180
Blue Diamond, Refrigerated, Almond Coconut, Original Almondmilk Coconutmilk Blend 1 cup	60	3	1	0	7	1	6	1	125
Blue Diamond, Refrigerated, Almond Coconut, Original Almondmilk Coconutmilk Blend (Unsweetened) 1 cup	45	3.5	1	0	1	1	0	1	125

Food Serving size	Cal.	(g) Total Fat	(g) Sat. Fat	(mg) Chol.	(g) Carb.	(g) Fiber	(g) Sug.	(g) Prot.	(mg) Sod.
Blue Diamond, Shelf Stable, Almond Coconut, Vanilla Almondmilk Coconutmilk Blend									
1 cup	70	3	1	0	10	1	9	1	130
Blue Diamond, Shelf Stable, Almond Coconut, Vanilla Almondmilk Coconutmilk Blend (Unsweetened)									
1 cup	45	3.5	1	0	2	1	0	1	130
Chocolate Dream, Dairy Free, Dark Chocolate – Raspberry Chocolate Bar									
3.2 oz, 1/2 bar	240	15	9	0	24	1	22	2	15
Chocolate Dream, Dairy Free, Dark Chocolate – Rice Crunch Chocolate Bar									
3.2 oz, 1/2 bar	240	14	8	0	25	1	23	3	15
Chocolate Dream, Dairy Free, Dark Chocolate Dream – Almond Chocolate Bar									
3.2 oz, 1/2 bar	250	17	8	0	21	1	19	3	15
Chocolate Dream, Dairy Free, Dark Chocolate Dream – Pure Dark Chocolate Bar									
3.2 oz, 1/2 bar	240	14	8	0	25	1	23	3	15
Chocolate Dream, Dairy Free, Semi Sweet Baking Chips Chocolate Bar									
2 tbsp	70	4	2.5	0	9	1	8	0.5	1
Chocolate Dream, Dairy Free, Sweet Chocolate – Creamy Sweet Chocolate Bar									
3.2 oz, 1/2 bar	230	13	8	0	25	1	20	2	10
Earth Balance, Chocolate Soymilk									
1 cup	130	3	0.5	0	21	2	19	5	100
Earth Balance, Organic Soy Nog									
1/2 cup	80	1.5	0	0	12	1	11	3	75
Earth Balance, Original Soymilk									
1/2 cup	90	4	0.5	0	8	1	7	7	120
Earth Balance, Unsweetened Soymilk									
1 cup	80	4	0.5	0	3	1	2	7	85
Earth Balance, Vanilla Soymilk									
1 cup	90	3.5	0.5	0	9	1	8	6	95
Eden Foods, EdenBlend, Organic Rice and Soymilk									
8 fl oz	120	3	0.5	0	18	<1	8	7	90
Eden Foods, Unsweetened Edensoy, Organic Soymilk									
8 fl oz	120	6	1	0	5	<1	2	12	5
Ener-G, Egg Replacer									
1-1/2 tsp	15	0	0	0	4	0	0	0	5

Food Serving size	Cal.	(g) Total Fat	(g) Sat. Fat	(mg) Chol.	(g) Carb.	(g) Fiber	(g) Sug.	(g) Prot.	(mg) Sod.
Good Karma, Organic, Chocolate Whole Grain Ricemilk									
1 cup 8 fl oz	120	2.5	0	0	25	3	18	1	180
Good Karma, Organic, Original Whole Grain Ricemilk									
1 cup 8 fl oz	100	3	0	0	19	3	9	1	150
Good Karma, Organic, Rice Divine, Banana Fudge Non-Dairy Frozen Dessert									
1/2 cup	150	6	0	0	25	1	16	0	85
Good Karma, Organic, Rice Divine, Carrot Cake Non-Dairy Frozen Dessert									
1/2 cup	160	7	1	0	25	1	15	0	105
Good Karma, Organic, Rice Divine, Chocolate Chip Non-Dairy Frozen Dessert									
1/2 cup	170	9	3	0	23	2	13	0	60
Good Karma, Organic, Rice Divine, Chocolate Chocolate Bars Non-Dairy Frozen Dessert									
1 bar	200	13	7	0	22	1	12	0	55
Good Karma, Organic, Rice Divine, Chocolate Peanut Butter Fudge Non-Dairy Frozen Dessert									
1/2 cup	200	10	1	0	27	2	16	1	120
Good Karma, Organic, Rice Divine, Coconut Mango Non-Dairy Frozen Dessert									
1/2 cup	150	6	1	0	23	1	14	0	75
Good Karma, Organic, Rice Divine, Key Lime Pie Non-Dairy Frozen Dessert									
1/2 cup	140	6	0	0	23	1	13	0	55
Good Karma, Organic, Rice Divine, Mint Chocolate Swirl Non-Dairy Frozen Dessert									
1/2 cup	150	6	0.5	0	24	1	15	0	80
Good Karma, Organic, Rice Divine, Mudd Pie Non-Dairy Frozen Dessert									
1/2 cup	170	8	1	0	26	2	15	1	85
Good Karma, Organic, Rice Divine, Very Cherry Non-Dairy Frozen Dessert									
1/2 cup	160	6	0	0	26	1	17	0	55
Good Karma, Organic, Rice Divine, Very Vanilla Bars Non-Dairy Frozen Dessert									
1 bar	200	13	7	0	21	1	13	0	55
Good Karma, Organic, Rice Divine, Very Vanilla Non-Dairy Frozen Dessert									
1/2 cup	150	7	0.5	0	22	1	12	0	75
Good Karma, Organic, Vanilla Whole Grain Ricemilk									
1 cup 8 fl oz	120	3	0	0	26	3	13	1	150
Good Karma, Original Flax Milk									
1 cup 8 fl oz	60	2.5	0	0	11	0	11	0	80

Food Serving size	Cal.	(g) Total Fat	(g) Sat. Fat	(mg) Chol.	(g) Carb.	(g) Fiber	(g) Sug.	(g) Prot.	(mg) Sod.
Good Karma, Unsweetened Flax Milk									
1 cup 8 fl oz	25	2.5	0	0	1	0	0	0	80
Good Karma, Vanilla Flax Milk									
1 cup 8 fl oz	60	2.5	0	0	11	0	11	0	80
Living Harvest, Chocolate Fudge Ice Cream Bar									
1 bar	100	4	3	0	18	2	8	1	60
Living Harvest, Chocolate Fudge Tempt Non-Dairy Frozen Dessert									
1/2 cup	200	11	1.5	0	26	2	16	1	85
Living Harvest, Chocolate Tempt Hempmilk									
1 cup	170	6	0.5	0	23	1	22	2	135
Living Harvest, Coconut Lime Tempt Non-Dairy Frozen Dessert									
1/2 cup	150	7	1.5	0	22	1	11	0	75
Living Harvest, Coffee Biscotti Tempt Non-Dairy Frozen Dessert									
1/2 cup	140	7	1	0	24	1	8	0	75
Living Harvest, Coffee with Cream Swirls Ice Cream Bar									
1 bar	100	4	3	0	18	1	8	0	65
Living Harvest, High Protein Hemp Protein Powder									
4 tbsp	135	3	NA	NA	5	4	1	22	NA
Living Harvest, Mint Chip Tempt Non-Dairy Frozen Dessert									
1/2 cup	170	9	3	0	21	1	10	0	70
Living Harvest, Organic Hemp Oil Ice Cream Bar									
1 tbsp	130	14	1.5	0	0	NA	NA	0	0
Living Harvest, Original Hemp Protein Powder									
4 tbsp	120	4	NA	NA	7	9	1	13	NA
Living Harvest, Original Tempt Hempmilk									
1 cup	100	6	0.5	0	9	0	6	2	110
Living Harvest, Unsweetened Original Tempt Hempmilk									
1 cup	70	6	0.5	0	1	0	0	2	125
Living Harvest, Unsweetened Vanilla Tempt Hempmilk									
1 cup	70	6	0.5	0	1	0	0	2	135
Living Harvest, Vanilla Bean Tempt Non-Dairy Frozen Dessert									
1/2 cup	140	7	0.5	0	20	1	9	0	75
Living Harvest, Vanilla Spice Hemp Protein Powder									
4 tbsp	120	3	NA	NA	13	7	7	10	NA

Food Serving size	Cal.	(g) Total Fat	(g) Sat. Fat	(mg) Chol.	(g) Carb.	(g) Fiber	(g) Sug.	(g) Prot.	(mg) Sod.
Living Harvest, Vanilla Tempt Hempmilk 1 cup	120	6	0.5	0	13	0	9	2	135
Living Harvest, Vanilla with Blueberry Pomegranate Swirls Ice Cream Bar 1 bar	100	3.5	2.5	0	18	1	9	0	60
Living Harvest, Vanilla with Fudge Swirls Ice Cream Bar 1 bar	100	3.5	2.5	0	19	1	10	0	65
Native Forest, Organic Coconut Milk 1/4 cup	100	10	9	0	3	0	1	<1	25
Native Forest, Organic Light Coconut Milk 1/4 cup	45	4	3.5	0	2	0	<1	<1	15
Nestlé, Coffee-Mate, Belgian Chocolate Toffee Liquid 1 tbsp	35	1.5	0	0	6	0	6	0	5
Nestlé, Coffee-Mate, Café Latte Liquid 1 tbsp	25	1.5	0	0	3	0	3	0	0
Nestlé, Coffee-Mate, Café Mocha Liquid 1 tbsp	35	1.5	0	0	5	0	5	0	0
Nestlé, Coffee-Mate, Caramel Macchiato Liquid 1 tbsp	35	1.5	0	0	5	0	5	0	0
Nestlé, Coffee-Mate, Chocolate Raspberry Liquid 1 tbsp	35	1.5	0	0	5	0	5	0	30
Nestlé, Coffee-Mate, Cinnamon Vanilla Liquid 1 tbsp	35	1.5	0	0	5	0	5	0	30
Nestlé, Coffee-Mate, Coconut Crème Liquid 1 tbsp	35	1.5	0	0	5	0	5	0	0
Nestlé, Coffee-Mate, French Vanilla Fat Free Liquid 1 tbsp	25	0	0	0	5	0	5	0	25
Nestlé, Coffee-Mate, French Vanilla Fat Free Powder 4 tsp	50	0	0	0	11	0	6	0	15
Nestlé, Coffee-Mate, French Vanilla Liquid 1 tbsp	35	1.5	0	0	5	0	5	0	30
Nestlé, Coffee-Mate, French Vanilla Powder 4 tsp	60	2.5	2	0	9	0	7	0	15
Nestlé, Coffee-Mate, French Vanilla Sugar Free Liquid 1 tbsp	15	1	0	0	2	0	0	0	0

Food Serving size	Cal.	(g) Total Fat	(g) Sat. Fat	(mg) Chol.	(g) Carb.	(g) Fiber	(g) Sug.	(g) Prot.	(mg) Sod.
Nestlé, Coffee-Mate, French Vanilla Sugar Free Powder									
1 tbsp	30	2.5	2	0	2	0	0	0	15
Nestlé, Coffee-Mate, Hazelnut Fat Free Liquid									
1 tbsp	25	0	0	0	5	0	5	0	0
Nestlé, Coffee-Mate, Hazelnut Liquid									
1 tbsp	35	1.5	0	0	5	0	5	0	30
Nestlé, Coffee-Mate, Hazelnut Powder									
4 tsp	60	3	2.5	0	9	0	7	0	15
Nestlé, Coffee-Mate, Hazelnut Sugar Free Liquid									
1 tbsp	15	1	0	0	2	0	0	0	5
Nestlé, Coffee-Mate, Hazelnut Sugar Free Powder									
1 tbsp	30	2.5	2	0	2	0	0	0	15
Nestlé, Coffee-Mate, Irish Crème Liquid									
1 tbsp	35	1.5	0	0	5	0	5	0	30
Nestlé, Coffee-Mate, Italian Sweet Crème Liquid									
1 tbsp	35	1.5	0	0	5	0	5	0	15
Nestlé, Coffee-Mate, Natural Bliss, Caramel Liquid									
1 tbsp	35	1.5	1	10	5	0	5	0	5
Nestlé, Coffee-Mate, Natural Bliss, Sweet Cream Liquid									
1 tbsp	35	1.5	0	10	5	0	5	0	5
Nestlé, Coffee-Mate, Natural Bliss, Vanilla Liquid									
1 tbsp	35	1.5	1	10	5	0	5	0	5
Nestlé, Coffee-Mate, Original Fat Free Liquid									
1 tbsp	10	0	0	0	1	0	1	0	0
Nestlé, Coffee-Mate, Original Fat Free Powder									
2 tsp	10	0	0	0	2	0	0	0	0
Nestlé, Coffee-Mate, Original Liquid									
1 tbsp	15	1	0	0	1	0	1	0	0
Nestlé, Coffee-Mate, Original Lite Powder									
1 tbsp	10	0	0	0	2	0	0	0	0
Nestlé, Coffee-Mate, Original Low Fat Liquid									
1 tbsp	10	0.5	0	0	1	0	1	0	5
Nestlé, Coffee-Mate, Original Powder									
1 tsp	10	0.5	0.5	0	1	0	0	0	0

Food Serving size	Cal.	(g) Total Fat	(g) Sat. Fat	(mg) Chol.	(g) Carb.	(g) Fiber	(g) Sug.	(g) Prot.	(mg) Sod.
Nestlé, Coffee-Mate, Vanilla Caramel Liquid									
1 tbsp	35	1.5	0	0	5	0	5	0	30
Nestlé, Coffee-Mate, Vanilla Caramel Powder									
4 tsp	60	3	2.5	0	9	0	7	0	15
Nestlé, Coffee-Mate, Vanilla Caramel Sugar Free Powder									
1 tbsp	30	2.5	2	0	2	0	0	0	15
Nestlé, Coffee-Mate, Vanilla Nut Liquid									
1 tbsp	35	1.5	0	0	5	0	5	0	30
Pacific Natural Foods, Hazelnut Chocolate Beverage									
8 fl oz	120	5	0.5	0	19	1	15	2	140
Pacific Natural Foods, Hazelnut Original Beverage									
8 fl oz	110	3.5	0	0	19	1	14	2	120
Pacific Natural Foods, Hemp Chocolate Beverage									
8 fl oz	190	5	1	0	35	2	23	3	150
Pacific Natural Foods, Hemp Original Beverage									
8 fl oz	140	5	0.5	0	20	1	14	3	130
Pacific Natural Foods, Hemp Vanilla Beverage									
8 fl oz	160	5	0.5	0	24	1	16	3	135
Pacific Natural Foods, Low Fat Plain Rice Beverage									
1 cup	130	2	0	0	27	0	14	1	60
Pacific Natural Foods, Low Fat Vanilla Rice Beverage									
1 cup	130	2	0	0	27	0	14	1	75
Pacific Natural Foods, Organic Almond Chocolate Beverage									
8 fl oz	100	3	0	0	19	1	16	1	140
Pacific Natural Foods, Organic Almond Original Beverage									
8 fl oz	60	2.5	0	0	8	0	6	1	140
Pacific Natural Foods, Organic Almond Vanilla Beverage									
8 fl oz	70	2.5	0	0	11	0	9	1	140
Pacific Natural Foods, Organic Unsweetened Almond Original Beverage									
8 fl oz	35	2.5	0	0	2	0	0	1	180
Pacific Natural Foods, Organic Unsweetened Almond Vanilla Beverage									
8 fl oz	40	2.5	0	0	3	0	0	1	180
Pacific Natural Foods, Organic Unsweetened Original Soy Beverage									
8 fl oz	90	4.5	0.5	0	4	2	2	9	15

Food Serving size	Cal.	(g) Total Fat	(g) Sat. Fat	(mg) Chol.	(g) Carb.	(g) Fiber	(g) Sug.	(g) Prot.	(mg) Sod.
Pacific Natural Foods, Select Soy – Low Fat Plain Soy Beverage									
8 fl oz	70	2.5	0	0	9	1	6	5	115
Pacific Natural Foods, Select Soy – Low Fat Vanilla Soy Beverage									
8 fl oz	80	2.5	0	0	11	1	9	5	115
Pacific Natural Foods, Ultra Soy – Plain Soy Beverage									
8 fl oz	120	4	0.5	0	11	1	8	10	150
Pacific Natural Foods, Ultra Soy – Vanilla Soy Beverage									
8 fl oz	130	4	0.5	0	14	1	10	10	150
Rice Dream, Cocoa Marble Fudge Non-Dairy Frozen Dessert									
1/2 cup	170	6	0.5	0	31	1	17	<1	90
Rice Dream, Enriched Refrigerated Non-Dairy Original Rice Drink									
1 cup, 8 fl oz	120	2.5	0	0	23	0	10	1	80
Rice Dream, Enriched Refrigerated Non-Dairy Vanilla Rice Drink									
1 cup, 8 fl oz	130	2.5	0	0	26	0	12	1	80
Rice Dream, Neapolitan Frozen Non-Dairy Dessert									
1/2 cup	160	6	0.5	0	26	>1	13	0	80
Rice Dream, Original Unsweetened Enriched Refrigerated Non-Dairy Rice Drink									
1 cup, 8 fl oz	90	2.5	0	0	15	0	<1	<1	130
Rice Dream, Shelf Stable, Classic Carob Rice Drink									
1 cup, 8 fl oz	150	2.5	0	0	30	<1	26	1	80
Rice Dream, Shelf Stable, Classic Original Rice Drink									
1 cup, 8 fl oz	120	2.5	0	0	24	0	11	1	100
Rice Dream, Shelf Stable, Classic Vanilla Rice Drink									
1 cup, 8 fl oz	130	2.5	0	0	27	0	12	1	105
Rice Dream, Shelf Stable, Enriched Chocolate Rice Drink									
1 cup, 8 fl oz	160	3	0	0	34	<1	28	2	90
Rice Dream, Shelf Stable, Enriched Original Rice Drink									
1 cup, 8 fl oz	120	2.5	0	0	23	0	10	1	100
Rice Dream, Shelf Stable, Enriched Vanilla Rice Drink									
1 cup, 8 fl oz	130	2.5	0	0	26	0	12	1	105
Rice Dream, Shelf Stable, Horchata Rice Drink									
1 cup, 8 fl oz	160	2.5	0	0	32	0	18	1	5
Rice Dream, Shelf Stable, Unsweetened Organic Original Enriched Rice Drink									
1 cup, 8 fl oz	70	2.5	0	0	11	0	>1	>1	125

Food Serving size	Cal.	(g) Total Fat	(g) Sat. Fat	(mg) Chol.	(g) Carb.	(g) Fiber	(g) Sug.	(g) Prot.	(mg) Sod.
Rice Dream, Strawberry Non-Dairy Frozen Dessert									
1/2 cup	170	6	0.5	0	30	0	16	0	85
Rice Dream, Vanilla Non-Dairy Frozen Dessert									
1/2 cup	160	6	0.5	0	26	0	14	0	85
So Delicious, Blueberry Cultured Coconut Milk Greek Yogurt									
1 container	130	4.5	3.5	0	25	8	11	2	130
So Delicious, Blueberry Cultured Coconut Milk Yogurt									
4 oz	100	3	3	0	18	3	13	0	60
So Delicious, Butter Pecan Frozen Dessert, Almond Based, Pint									
1/2 cup serving	160	8	1	0	25	5	7	2	100
So Delicious, Cherry Amaretto Frozen Dessert, Almond Based, Pint									
1/2 cup serving	130	4	0	0	27	5	6	1	65
So Delicious, Cherry Amaretto Frozen, Coconut Based Dessert									
1/2 cup	130	6	5	0	22	6	10	1	10
So Delicious, Chocolate Coconut Milk Beverage									
1 cup	100	5	4	0	12	1	10	1	160
So Delicious, Chocolate Coconut Milk Yogurt									
1 container	170	7	5	0	27	3	23	1	35
So Delicious, Chocolate Cultured Coconut Milk Greek Yogurt									
1 container	140	6	4.5	0	25	8	11	2	115
So Delicious, Chocolate Cultured Coconut Milk Yogurt									
1 container	170	7	5	0	27	3	23	1	35
So Delicious, Chocolate Frozen Dessert, Almond Based, Pint									
1/2 cup serving	120	2.5	0	0	28	5	9	2	75
So Delicious, Chocolate Frozen, Coconut Based Dessert									
1/2 cup	150	9	8	0	20	6	12	1	5
So Delicious, Chocolate Peanut Butter Frozen, Soy Based Dessert									
1/2 cup	140	4.5	1	0	23	2	13	2	60
So Delicious, Chocolate Peanut Butter Swirl Frozen, Coconut Based Dessert									
1/2 cup	210	13	9	0	21	6	12	3	40
So Delicious, Chocolate Velvet Frozen, Soy Based Dessert									
1/2 cup	130	3.5	0.5	0	23	1	14	2	50
So Delicious, Coconut Almond Chip Frozen, Coconut Based Dessert									
1/2 cup	180	12	8	0	20	6	12	5	5

Food Serving size	Cal.	(g) Total Fat	(g) Sat. Fat	(mg) Chol.	(g) Carb.	(g) Fiber	(g) Sug.	(g) Prot.	(mg) Sod.
So Delicious, Coconut Frozen, Coconut Based Dessert									
1/2 cup	170	10	9	0	19	6	11	1	5
So Delicious, Cookie Dough Frozen, Coconut Based Dessert									
1/2 cup	190	9	8	0	24	5	15	1	30
So Delicious, Creamy Fudge Frozen Bar, Soy Based Dessert									
1 bar	90	2	0	0	18	2	12	1	30
So Delicious, Creamy Vanilla Frozen, Soy Based Dessert									
1/2 cup	130	3	0	0	24	3	13	1	55
So Delicious, Fruit Sweetened Almond Pecan Frozen, Soy Based Dessert									
1/2 cup	139	4.5	0.5	0	24	3	12	2	175
So Delicious, Fruit Sweetened Awesome Chocolate Frozen, Soy Based Dessert									
1/2 cup	130	1.5	0	0	24	2	12	2	130
So Delicious, Fruit Sweetened Chocolate Almond Frozen, Soy Based Dessert									
1/2 cup	160	4.5	0.5	0	23	3	11	3	165
So Delicious, Fruit Sweetened Chocolate Peanut Butter Frozen, Soy Based Dessert									
1/2 cup	150	3.5	0.5	0	24	3	11	3	155
So Delicious, Fruit Sweetened Green Tea Frozen, Soy Based Dessert									
1/2 cup	110	1.5	0	0	24	2	9	2	130
So Delicious, Fruit Sweetened Vanilla Frozen, Soy Based Dessert									
1/2 cup	130	1.5	0	0	24	2	9	2	130
So Delicious, Fudge Minis Bar (Organic) Frozen, Coconut Based Dessert									
1 bar	70	3.5	3	0	10	3	6	1	0
So Delicious, German Chocolate Frozen, Coconut Based Dessert									
1/2 cup	180	12	9	0	22	6	14	1	15
So Delicious, Green Tea Frozen, Coconut Based Dessert									
1/2 cup	130	7	6	0	19	6	12	1	5
So Delicious, Hibiscus Sorbet Frozen, Coconut Based Dessert									
1/2 cup	100	0	0	0	26	3	23	0	160
So Delicious, Mint Chip Frozen Dessert, Almond Based, Pint									
1/2 cup serving	160	7	2	0	27	5	9	1	70
So Delicious, Mint Chip Frozen, Coconut Based Dessert									
1/2 cup	170	9	8	0	20	6	13	1	5
So Delicious, Mint Marble Fudge Frozen, Soy Based Dessert									
1/2 cup	140	3	0.5	0	27	2	17	1	55

Food Serving size	Cal.	(g) Total Fat	(g) Sat. Fat	(mg) Chol.	(g) Carb.	(g) Fiber	(g) Sug.	(g) Prot.	(mg) Sod.
So Delicious, Mocha Almond Fudge Bar Mini Novelty, Multipack									
1 bar	150	7	3	0	19	3	10	1	50
So Delicious, Mocha Almond Fudge Frozen Dessert, Almond Based, Pint									
1/2 cup serving	160	7	0.5	0	28	5	10	2	110
So Delicious, Mocha Almond Fudge Frozen, Coconut Based Dessert									
1/2 cup	180	9	6	0	21	5	14	2	30
So Delicious, Mocha Fudge Frozen, Soy Based Dessert									
1/2 cup	130	3	0	0	26	3	15	2	85
So Delicious, Neapolitan Frozen, Soy Based Dessert									
1/2 cup	120	3.5	0.5	0	23	2	13	2	55
So Delicious, No Sugar Added, Butter Pecan Frozen, Coconut Based Dessert									
1/2 cup	140	13	7	0	17	10	1	1	65
So Delicious, No Sugar Added, Chocolate Frozen, Coconut Based Dessert									
1/2 cup	100	8	7	0	18	10	1	1	70
So Delicious, No Sugar Added, Mint Chip Frozen, Coconut Based Dessert									
1/2 cup	120	11	9	0	18	10	1	1	65
So Delicious, No Sugar Added, Toasted Almond Chip Frozen, Coconut Based Dessert									
1/2 cup	140	12	9	0	18	10	1	2	80
So Delicious, No Sugar Added, Vanilla Bean Frozen, Coconut Based Dessert									
1/2 cup	100	8	7	0	18	10	1	1	70
So Delicious, Original Coconut Milk Beverage									
1 cup	80	5	5	0	7	0	6	1	15
So Delicious, Passionate Mango, Cultured Coconut Milk Yogurt									
1 container	130	6	6	0	20	2	16	1	10
So Delicious, Passionate Mango, Frozen Coconut Based Dessert									
1/2 cup	150	7	6	0	19	5	13	1	10
So Delicious, Pina Colada, Cultured Coconut Milk Yogurt									
1 container	140	6	5	0	20	2	20	1	10
So Delicious, Plain Cultured, Coconut Milk Greek Yogurt									
1 container	130	5	4.5	0	22	9	7	2	130
So Delicious, Plain Cultured, Coconut Milk Yogurt									
4 oz	80	4.5	4	0	12	3	8	0	5
So Delicious, Pomegranate Chip Frozen, Coconut Based Dessert									
1/2 cup	130	7	6	0	20	6	13	1	10

Food Serving size	Cal.	(g) Total Fat	(g) Sat. Fat	(mg) Chol.	(g) Carb.	(g) Fiber	(g) Sug.	(g) Prot.	(mg) Sod.
So Delicious, Purely Decadent, Chocolate Obsession, Frozen Soy Based Dessert									
1/2 cup	210	7	3	0	27	5	20	2	30
So Delicious, Purely Decadent, Cookie Dough, Frozen Soy Based Dessert									
1/2 cup	230	8	3.5	0	36	5	27	1	75
So Delicious, Purely Decadent, Mocha Almond Fudge, Frozen Soy Based Dessert									
1/2 cup	200	8	1	0	25	5	19	3	40
So Delicious, Purely Decadent, Peanut Butter Zig Zag, Frozen Soy Based Dessert									
1/2 cup	230	12	3	0	24	5	16	3	45
So Delicious, Purely Decadent, Pomegranate Chip, Frozen Soy Based Dessert									
1/2 cup	200	7	3	0	29	5	24	1	35
So Delicious, Purely Decadent, Praline Pecan, Frozen Soy Based Dessert									
1/2 cup	210	10	1	0	33	5	15	2	20
So Delicious, Purely Decadent, Turtle Trails, Frozen Soy Based Dessert									
1/2 cup	200	7	1	0	28	4	22	1	80
So Delicious, Raspberry Minis Sorbet Bar Frozen, Coconut Based Dessert									
1 cup	70	2	0	0	8	0	8	5	95
So Delicious, Raspberry, Cultured Coconut Milk Greek Yogurt									
1 container	130	4.5	3.5	0	25	8	11	2	140
So Delicious, Raspberry, Cultured Coconut Milk Yogurt									
1 container	140	6	6	0	24	2	20	1	5
So Delicious, Shelf Stable, Chocolate Coconut Milk Beverage									
1 cup	100	5	4	0	12	1	10	1	160
So Delicious, Shelf Stable, Original, Coconut Milk Beverage									
1 cup	80	5	5	0	7	0	6	1	15
So Delicious, Shelf Stable, Original, Sugar Free Coconut Milk Beverage									
1 cup	80	5	5	0	7	0	6	1	15
So Delicious, Shelf Stable, Unsweetened Coconut Milk Beverage									
1 cup	50	5	5	0	1	0	0	1	15
So Delicious, Shelf Stable, Vanilla Almond Plus Beverage									
1 cup	70	2	0	0	8	0	8	5	95
So Delicious, Shelf Stable, Vanilla Coconut Milk Beverage									
1 cup	90	5	5	0	9	0	7	1	15
So Delicious, Shelf Stable, Vanilla, Sugar Free Coconut Milk Beverage									
1 cup	50	4.5	4	0	2	1	0	0	65

Food Serving size	Cal.	(g) Total Fat	(g) Sat. Fat	(mg) Chol.	(g) Carb.	(g) Fiber	(g) Sug.	(g) Prot.	(mg) Sod.
So Delicious, Strawberry Banana, Cultured Coconut Milk Yogurt									
1 container	150	6	5	0	25	2	21	1	5
So Delicious, Strawberry, Cultured Coconut Milk Greek Yogurt									
1 container	130	4.5	3.5	0	25	8	11	2	115
So Delicious, Strawberry, Cultured Coconut Milk Yogurt									
1 container	130	6	5	0	21	2	18	1	5
So Delicious, Turtle Trails, Frozen, Coconut Based Dessert									
1/2 cup	160	8	6	0	26	5	19	1	40
So Delicious, Unsweetened Coconut Milk Beverage									
1 cup	50	5	5	0	1	0	0	1	15
So Delicious, Vanilla Bar Mini Novelty, Multipack									
1 bar	140	7	3	0	18	3	8	1	40
So Delicious, Vanilla Bean Frozen, Coconut Based Dessert									
1/2 cup	150	8	7	0	19	6	12	1	5
So Delicious, Vanilla Coconut Milk Beverage									
1 cup	90	5	5	0	9	0	7	1	15
So Delicious, Vanilla Cultured Coconut Milk Greek Yogurt									
1 container	140	4.5	3.5	0	27	8	12	2	115
So Delicious, Vanilla Cultured Coconut Milk Yogurt									
4 oz	90	4	3.5	0	15	1	12	0	0
So Delicious, Vanilla Frozen Dessert, Almond Based, Pint									
1/2 cup serving	130	4.5	0	0	26	5	7	1	75
Soy Dream, Butter Pecan, Non-Dairy Frozen Dessert									
1/2 cup	190	11	2	0	23	1	14	1	140
Soy Dream, Classic Non-Dairy Original Soy Beverage									
1 cup, 8 fl oz	130	4	0.5	0	16	2	9	7	150
Soy Dream, Enriched Refrigerated Non-Dairy Original Soy Beverage									
1 cup, 8 fl oz	100	3.5	0.5	0	9	2	5	8	140
Soy Dream, Enriched Refrigerated Non-Dairy Vanilla Soy Beverage									
1 cup, 8 fl oz	120	3.5	0.5	0	14	2	10	8	130
Soy Dream, French Vanilla, Non-Dairy Frozen Dessert									
1/2 cup	170	9	1.5	0	21	<1	13	1	150
Soy Dream, Shelf Stable, Non-Dairy Classic Vanilla Soy Beverage									
1 cup, 8 fl oz	140	4	0.5	0	18	2	10	7	135

Food Serving size	Cal.	(g) Total Fat	(g) Sat. Fat	(mg) Chol.	(g) Carb.	(g) Fiber	(g) Sug.	(g) Prot.	(mg) Sod.
Soy Dream, Shelf Stable, Non-Dairy Enriched Chocolate Soy Beverage									
1 cup, 8 fl oz	150	4	0.5	0	21	3	15	7	125
Soy Dream, Shelf Stable, Non-Dairy Enriched Original Soy Beverage									
1 cup, 8 fl oz	100	4	0.5	0	8	2	4	7	135
Soy Dream, Shelf Stable, Non-Dairy Enriched Vanilla Soy Beverage									
1 cup, 8 fl oz	120	4	0.5	0	14	2	10	7	135
Soy Dream, Vanilla Fudge Swirl, Non-Dairy Frozen Dessert									
1/2 cup	170	9	1.5	0	23	1	16	<1	150
Soy Dream, Vanilla, Non-Dairy Frozen Dessert									
1/2 cup	170	9	1.5	0	21	1	13	<1	150
Stonyfield Organic, O'Soy, Fruit on the Bottom, Blueberry Soy Yogurt									
6 oz, 1 container	170	3	0	0	29	2	26	7	30
Stonyfield Organic, O'Soy, Fruit on the Bottom, Peach Soy Yogurt									
6 oz, 1 container	170	3	0	0	30	2	28	7	45
Stonyfield Organic, O'Soy, Fruit on the Bottom, Raspberry Soy Yogurt									
6 oz, 1 container	170	2.5	0	0	29	2	27	7	75
Stonyfield Organic, O'Soy, Fruit on the Bottom, Strawberry Soy Yogurt									
6 oz, 1 container	170	3	0	0	29	2	26	7	55
Stonyfield Organic, O'Soy, Smooth and Creamy, Chocolate Soy Yogurt									
6 oz, 1 container	160	3	1	0	25	2	22	8	35
Stonyfield Organic, O'Soy, Smooth and Creamy, Peach & Strawberry Soy Yogurt									
4 oz, 1 container	100	2	0	0	15	1	13	5	25
Stonyfield Organic, O'Soy, Smooth and Creamy, Vanilla Soy Yogurt									
6 oz, 1 container	150	3	0	0	24	1	21	7	40
Thai Kitchen, Coconut Milk									
1/3 cup	140	14	12	0	3	0	1	1	20
Thai Kitchen, Lite Coconut Milk									
1/3 cup	40	4.5	4	0	1	0	0	0	5
Thai Kitchen, Organic Lite Coconut Milk									
.33 cup	50	5	4	0	1	0	0	0	5
ZenSoy Soy Milk – Cappuccino									
1 cup	150	3.5	1	NA	22	1	17	7	150
ZenSoy Soy Milk – Chocolate									
8 oz	170	4	1	0	27	2	23	7	160

Food Serving size	Cal.	(g) Total Fat	(g) Sat. Fat	(mg) Chol.	(g) Carb.	(g) Fiber	(g) Sug.	(g) Prot.	(mg) Sod.
ZenSoy Soy Milk – Plain									
8 oz	90	3.5	1	0	9	1	6	7	80
ZenSoy Soy Milk – Vanilla									
1 cup	110	3.5	1	NA	14	1	12	7	80
ZenSoy, Soy on the Go – Cappuccino Soy Milk									
8.25 oz	150	3.5	1	0	22	1	17	7	160
ZenSoy, Soy on the Go – Chocolate Soy Milk									
8.25 oz	170	4	1	0	27	2	23	7	160
ZenSoy, Soy on the Go – Vanilla Soy Milk									
8.25 oz	110	3.5	1	0	14	1	12	7	80
ZenSoy, Zen Pudding – Chocolate									
1 container	110	1	0	0	23	1	18	3	75
ZenSoy, Zen Pudding – Chocolate/Vanilla Swirl									
1 container	110	1	0	0	22	1	17	3	70
ZenSoy, Zen Pudding – Vanilla									
1 container	100	1	0	0	20	<1	14	2	60

Dairy Based Desserts (Puddings, Frozen Yogurts, Ice Cream)

Food Serving size	Cal.	(g) Total Fat	(g) Sat. Fat	(mg) Chol.	(g) Carb.	(g) Fiber	(g) Sug.	(g) Prot.	(mg) Sod.
Chatila's Bakery, Mini Chocolate Cheesecake									
85g	110	2.5	1	20	7	1	3	9	280
Chatila's Bakery, Mini Plain Cheesecake									
80g	100	3	1.5	20	6	0	3	8	300
Chatila's Bakery, Mini Strawberry Cheesecake									
85g	100	2	1	20	6	0	3	7	290
Chatila's Bakery, New York Chocolate Cheesecake (8 slices)									
115g	140	3	1.5	30	9	1	4	11	390
Chatila's Bakery, New York Plain Cheesecake (8 slices)									
115g	140	3	1.5	30	8	0	4	11	400
Chatila's Bakery, New York Strawberry Cheesecake (8 slices)									
115g	140	2.5	1.5	30	8	0	4	11	390
Kozy Shack, Banana Cream Pudding									
1/2 cup	150	4	2	20	24	0	19	4	160
Kozy Shack, Butterscotch Pudding									
4 oz	120	2	1	10	23	0	19	3	135

Food Serving size	Cal.	(g) Total Fat	(g) Sat. Fat	(mg) Chol.	(g) Carb.	(g) Fiber	(g) Sug.	(g) Prot.	(mg) Sod.
Kozy Shack, Chocolate Hazelnut Pudding									
4 oz	110	2	1	10	21	1	16	4	140
Kozy Shack, Chocolate Pudding									
1/2 cup	140	2.5	1.5	10	27	1	22	4	160
Kozy Shack, Chocolate Rice Pudding									
1/2 cup	160	4	2	15	27	0	18	5	140
Kozy Shack, Cinnamon Raisin Rice Pudding									
1/2 cup	150	2.5	1	15	28	0	18	4	140
Kozy Shack, Crème Caramel Flan									
1 cup	140	3	1.5	35	27	0	27	4	90
Kozy Shack, European Style Rice Pudding									
1/2 cup	140	2.5	1	20	24	0	16	4	150
Kozy Shack, Original Rice Pudding									
1/2 cup	130	2.5	1	15	24	0	16	4	150
Kozy Shack, Pumpkin Pudding									
1/2 cup	130	4.5	2.5	20	20	1	15	4	130
Kozy Shack, Tapioca Pudding									
1/2 cup	140	2	1	10	26	0	19	4	160
Let's Do...Organic, Organic Tapioca Granules									
1 tbsp	35	0	0	0	9	0	0	0	0
Let's Do...Organic, Organic Tapioca Pearls									
1 tbsp	35	0	0	0	9	0	0	0	0
Let's Do...Organic, Organic Tapioca Starch									
1 tbsp	35	0	0	0	9	0	0	0	0
Lifeway Foods, Greek Style Fro-Yo, Blood Orange Swirl									
1/2 cup	110	1	1	10	19	NA	17	6	25
Lifeway Foods, Greek Style Fro-Yo, Chocolate Swirl									
1/2 cup	110	1	0.5	10	19	NA	16	6	30
Lifeway Foods, Greek Style Fro-Yo, Honey Swirl									
1/2 cup	110	1	0	10	19	NA	17	6	25
Lifeway Foods, Sweet Kiss, Dessert Cheese Spread, Apple									
1 oz	50	1.5	0.5	<5	6	NA	6	3	10
Lifeway Foods, Sweet Kiss, Dessert Cheese Spread, Chocolate Chip									
2 tbsp	100	6.5	4.5	8	8	NA	7	1	50

Food Serving size	Cal.	(g) Total Fat	(g) Sat. Fat	(mg) Chol.	(g) Carb.	(g) Fiber	(g) Sug.	(g) Prot.	(mg) Sod.
Lifeway Foods, Sweet Kiss, Dessert Cheese Spread, Peach									
1 oz	50	1.5	0.5	<5	6	NA	6	3	10
Lifeway Foods, Sweet Kiss, Dessert Cheese Spread, Plain									
1 oz	50	2	0.5	<5	5	NA	5	3	10
Lifeway Foods, Sweet Kiss, Dessert Cheese Spread, Raisins									
1 oz	45	1	0.5	<5	6	NA	6	3	10
Lifeway Foods, Tart and Tangy, Chocolate Frozen Kefir									
1/2 cup	90	1	0	5	18	NA	16	4	65
Lifeway Foods, Tart and Tangy, Dulce de Leche Frozen Kefir									
1/2 cup	90	1	0.5	5	18	NA	16	4	75
Lifeway Foods, Tart and Tangy, Mango Frozen Kefir									
1/2 cup	90	1	0	5	18	0	16	4	55
Lifeway Foods, Tart and Tangy, Original Frozen Kefir									
1/2 cup	90	1	0.5	5	18	0	16	4	60
Lifeway Foods, Tart and Tangy, Pomegranate Frozen Kefir									
1/2 cup	90	1	0	5	18	0	16	4	60
Lifeway Foods, Tart and Tangy, Pumpkin Frozen Kefir									
1/2 cup	90	1	0.5	5	18	NA	16	4	60
Lifeway Foods, Tart and Tangy, Strawberry Frozen Kefir									
1/2 cup	90	1	0	5	18	0	16	4	55
Pamela's, Agave Sweetened New York Cheesecake									
1 slice	350	22	14	110	31	0.5	15	6	340
Pamela's, Hazelnut Cheesecake with Chocolate Crust									
1 slice	370	25	15	120	31	0.5	26	6	330
Pamela's, New York Cheesecake									
1 slice	370	25	15	120	31	0.5	26	6	330
Pamela's, White Chocolate Raspberry Cheesecake									
1 slice	360	23	14	110	32	0.5	25	6	310
Pamela's, Zesty Lemon Cheesecake									
1 slice	360	23	14	110	32	0.5	25	6	310
Stonyfield Organic, After Dark Chocolate Frozen Yogurt Bar									
1 bar	170	8	1	0	21	1	18	3	35
Stonyfield Organic, After Dark Chocolate Ice Cream									
16 oz, 1/2 cup	240	16	10	60	22	1	20	3	35

Food Serving size	Cal.	(g) Total Fat	(g) Sat. Fat	(mg) Chol.	(g) Carb.	(g) Fiber	(g) Sug.	(g) Prot.	(mg) Sod.
Stonyfield Organic, After Dark Chocolate Nonfat Frozen Yogurt									
16 oz, 1/2 cup	100	0	0	1	21	1	18	4	55
Stonyfield Organic, Crème Caramel Ice Cream									
16 oz, 1/2 cup	260	14	9	55	28	0	28	3	85
Stonyfield Organic, Gotta Have Java Nonfat Frozen Yogurt									
16 oz, 1/2 cup	100	0	0	1	21	0	18	4	65
Stonyfield Organic, Gotta Have Vanilla Frozen Yogurt Bar									
1 bar	170	8	1	0	20	1	18	4	40
Stonyfield Organic, Gotta Have Vanilla Ice Cream									
16 oz, 1/2 cup	250	16	10	60	21	0	20	3	45
Stonyfield Organic, Gotta Have Vanilla Nonfat Frozen Yogurt									
32 oz, 1/2 cup	100	0	0	<5	20	0	19	4	65
Stonyfield Organic, Low Fat Cookies 'n Cream Frozen Yogurt									
16 oz, 1/2 cup	130	2	1	1	25	0	20	4	110
Stonyfield Organic, Low Fat Crème Caramel Frozen Yogurt									
16 oz, 1/2 cup	130	2	1	5	26	0	25	4	95
Stonyfield Organic, Low Fat Minty Chocolate Chip Frozen Yogurt									
16 oz, 1/2 cup	140	3	2	1	25	1	21	4	50
Stonyfield Organic, Organic Nonfat Greek Frozen Yogurt, Blueberry									
16 oz, 1/2 cup	100	0	0	5	21	0	19	6	65
Stonyfield Organic, Organic Nonfat Greek Frozen Yogurt, Chocolate									
16 oz, 1/2 cup	100	0	0	5	19	1	16	6	55
Stonyfield Organic, Organic Nonfat Greek Frozen Yogurt, Honey									
16 oz, 1/2 cup	110	0	0	5	22	0	20	6	60
Stonyfield Organic, Organic Nonfat Greek Frozen Yogurt, Peach Mango									
16 oz, 1/2 cup	110	0	0	<5	21	0	20	6	60
Stonyfield Organic, Organic Nonfat Greek Frozen Yogurt, Super Fruits									
16 oz, 1/2 cup	110	0	0	<5	21	0	20	6	60
Stonyfield Organic, Organic Nonfat Greek Frozen Yogurt, Vanilla									
16 oz, 1/2 cup	100	0	0	5	19	0	17	6	65
Stonyfield Organic, Vanilla Fudge Swirl, Nonfat Frozen Yogurt									
16 oz, 1/2 cup	120	0	0	1	25	0	23	4	65

Food Serving size	Cal.	(g) Total Fat	(g) Sat. Fat	(mg) Chol.	(g) Carb.	(g) Fiber	(g) Sug.	(g) Prot.	(mg) Sod.
Milk									
Lifeway Foods, BioKefir – Black Cherry									
1 bottle	60	0	0	0	10	NA	10	5	50
Lifeway Foods, BioKefir – Blackberry									
1 bottle	60	0	0	0	10	NA	10	5	50
Lifeway Foods, BioKefir – Pomegranate / Blueberry									
1 bottle	60	0	0	0	10	NA	10	5	50
Lifeway Foods, BioKefir – Vanilla									
1 bottle	60	0	0	0	10	2	9	5	50
Lifeway Foods, Frozen ProBugs, Goo-Berry Pie									
1 tube	70	0.5	0	5	13	NA	12	3	45
Lifeway Foods, Frozen ProBugs, Orange Creamy Crawler									
1 tube	70	0.5	0	5	13	NA	12	3	45
Lifeway Foods, Frozen ProBugs, Strawnana Split									
1 tube	70	0.5	0	5	13	NA	12	4	45
Lifeway Foods, Greek Style Kefir									
1 cup	210	14	9	55	12	NA	12	8	120
Lifeway Foods, Greek Style Low Carb Kefir									
1 cup	210	14	9	55	12	NA	12	8	120
Lifeway Foods, Helios Nutrition, Organic Nonfat – Coconut Kefir									
1 cup	160	0	0	5	29	2	27	11	125
Lifeway Foods, Helios Nutrition, Organic Nonfat – Original Kefir									
1 cup	100	0	0	5	14	2	12	12	120
Lifeway Foods, Helios Nutrition, Organic Nonfat – Passion Fruit Kefir									
1 cup	120	0	0	15	23	0	23	8	85
Lifeway Foods, Helios Nutrition, Organic Nonfat – Plain Kefir									
1 cup	80	0	0	18	10	0	10	9	90
Lifeway Foods, Helios Nutrition, Organic Nonfat – Pomegranate/Acai Kefir									
1 cup	120	0	0	15	23	0	23	8	85
Lifeway Foods, Helios Nutrition, Organic Nonfat – Pomegranate/Blueberry Kefir									
1 cup	160	0	0	5	29	2	27	11	125
Lifeway Foods, Helios Nutrition, Organic Nonfat – Raspberry Kefir									
1 cup	160	0	0	5	29	2	27	11	125

Food Serving size	Cal.	(g) Total Fat	(g) Sat. Fat	(mg) Chol.	(g) Carb.	(g) Fiber	(g) Sug.	(g) Prot.	(mg) Sod.
Lifeway Foods, Helios Nutrition, Organic Nonfat – Strawberry Kefir									
1 cup	160	0	0	5	29	2	27	11	125
Lifeway Foods, Helios Nutrition, Organic Nonfat – Vanilla Kefir									
1 cup	160	0	0	5	29	2	27	11	125
Lifeway Foods, Lassi Mango									
1 cup	160	2	1.5	10	25	3	21	11	125
Lifeway Foods, Lassi Strawberry									
1 cup	160	2	1.5	10	25	3	21	11	125
Lifeway Foods, Low Fat Blueberry Kefir									
1 cup	140	2	1.5	10	20	NA	20	11	125
Lifeway Foods, Low Fat Cappuccino Kefir									
1 cup	140	2	1.5	10	20	NA ·	20	11	125
Lifeway Foods, Low Fat Cherry Kefir									
1 cup	140	2	1.5	10	20	NA	20	11	125
Lifeway Foods, Low Fat Chocolate Truffle Kefir									
1 cup	160	2	1.5	10	25	NA	21	11	125
Lifeway Foods, Low Fat Low Carb Plain Kefir									
1 cup	110	2	1.5	10	12	NA	12	11	125
Lifeway Foods, Low Fat Madagascar Vanilla Kefir									
1 cup	140	2	1.5	10	20	NA	20	11	125
Lifeway Foods, Low Fat Mango Kefir									
1 cup	140	2	1.5	10	20	NA	20	11	125
Lifeway Foods, Low Fat Peach Kefir									
1 cup	140	2	1.5	10	20	NA	20	11	125
Lifeway Foods, Low Fat Plain Kefir									
1 cup	110	2	1.5	10	12	NA	12	11	125
Lifeway Foods, Low Fat Pomegranate Kefir									
1 cup	140	2	1.5	10	20	NA	20	11	125
Lifeway Foods, Low Fat Raspberry Kefir									
1 cup	140	2	1.5	10	20	NA	20	11	125
Lifeway Foods, Low Fat Strawberry Kefir									
1 cup	140	2	1.5	10	20	NA	20	11	125
Lifeway Foods, Low Fat Strawberry-Banana Kefir									
1 cup	140	2	1.5	10	20	NA	20	11	125

Food Serving size	Cal.	(g) Total Fat	(g) Sat. Fat	(mg) Chol.	(g) Carb.	(g) Fiber	(g) Sug.	(g) Prot.	(mg) Sod.
Lifeway Foods, Non Fat Blueberry Kefir									
1 cup	150	0	0	5	27	NA	27	11	125
Lifeway Foods, Non Fat Low Carb Plain Kefir									
1 cup	90	0	0	5	12	NA	12	11	120
Lifeway Foods, Non Fat Plain Kefir									
1 cup	90	12	0	5	12	NA	12	11	120
Lifeway Foods, Non Fat Raspberry Kefir									
1 cup	150	0	0	5	27	NA	27	11	125
Lifeway Foods, Non Fat Strawberry Kefir									
1 cup	150	0	0	5	27	NA	27	11	125
Lifeway Foods, Non Fat Strawberry-Banana Kefir									
1 cup	150	0	0	5	27	NA	27	11	125
Lifeway Foods, Nonfat Greek Style Strawberry Kefir									
1 cup	150	0	0	5	27	NA	27	11	125
Lifeway Foods, Organic Green Kefir – Kiwi Passion Fruit									
1 cup	170	2	0	NA	25	4	21	12	137
Lifeway Foods, Organic Green Kefir – Pomegranate Acai Blueberry									
1 cup	170	2	0	NA	25	4	21	12	137
Lifeway Foods, Organic Low Fat Blueberry Kefir									
1 cup	140	2	1.5	10	20	NA	20	11	125
Lifeway Foods, Organic Low Fat Low Carb Plain Kefir									
1 cup	110	2	1.5	10	12	NA	12	11	125
Lifeway Foods, Organic Low Fat Peach Kefir									
1 cup	140	2	1.5	10	20	NA	20	11	125
Lifeway Foods, Organic Low Fat Plain Kefir									
1 cup	110	2	1.5	10	12	NA	12	11	125
Lifeway Foods, Organic Low Fat Pomegranate / Acai Kefir									
1 cup	140	2	1.5	10	20	NA	20	11	125
Lifeway Foods, Organic Low Fat Raspberry Kefir									
1 cup	140	2	1.5	10	20	NA	20	11	125
Lifeway Foods, Organic Low Fat Strawberries n' Cream Kefir									
1 cup	140	2	1.5	10	20	NA	20	11	125
Lifeway Foods, Organic Whole Milk Plain Kefir									
1 cup	160	8	5	30	12	NA	12	10	125

Food Serving size	Cal.	(g) Total Fat	(g) Sat. Fat	(mg) Chol.	(g) Carb.	(g) Fiber	(g) Sug.	(g) Prot.	(mg) Sod.
Lifeway Foods, Organic Whole Milk Strawberries n' Cream Kefir									
1 cup	190	8	5	30	20	NA	20	10	125
Lifeway Foods, Organic Whole Milk Wildberries Kefir									
1 cup	190	8	5	30	20	NA	20	10	125
Lifeway Foods, Original Kefir									
1 cup	150	8	5	30	12	0	12	8	125
Lifeway Foods, Original Low Carb Kefir									
1 cup	150	8	5	30	12	0	12	8	125
Lifeway Foods, ProBugs – Goo-Berry Pie									
1 unit	100	4	2	15	10	NA	10	7	60
Lifeway Foods, ProBugs – Orange Creamy Crawler									
1 unit	100	4	2	15	10	NA	10	7	60
Lifeway Foods, ProBugs – Strawnana Split									
1 unit	100	4	2	15	10	NA	10	7	60
Lifeway Foods, ProBugs – Sublime Slime Lime									
1 unit	100	4	2	15	10	NA	10	7	60
Lifeway Foods, Slim 6, Mixed Berry Low Carb Kefir									
1 cup	110	2	1.5	10	8	2	6	14	125
Lifeway Foods, Slim 6, Plain Low Carb Kefir									
1 cup	110	2	1.5	10	8	2	6	14	125
Lifeway Foods, Traditional Bazarny Kefir									
1 cup	164	9	6	35	12	NA	12	8	125
Lifeway Foods, Traditional Krestiansky Kefir									
1 cup	164	9	6	35	12	NA	12	8	125
Lifeway Foods, Traditional Ryazhenka Kefir									
1 cup	164	9	6	35	12	NA	12	8	125
Lifeway Foods, Traditional Weijski Kefir									
1 cup	164	9	6	35	12	NA	12	8	125
Nestlé, Carnation, Evaporated Milk									
2 tbsp	40	2	1.5	10	3	NA	3	2	30
Nestlé, Carnation, Fat Free Evaporated Milk									
2 tbsp	25	0	0	0	4	NA	4	2	40
Nestlé, Carnation, Instant Nonfat Dry Milk									
1/3 cup	80	0	0	<5	12	NA	12	8	125

Food Serving size	Cal.	(g) Total Fat	(g) Sat. Fat	(mg) Chol.	(g) Carb.	(g) Fiber	(g) Sug.	(g) Prot.	(mg) Sod.
Nestlé, Carnation, Low Fat Evaporated Milk									
2 tbsp	25	0.5	0	5	3	NA	3	2	35
Nestlé, Carnation, Sweetened Condensed Milk									
2 tbsp	100	2	1	10	17	NA	17	2	30
Nestlé, Nesquik, Banana Strawberry Lowfat Milk									
8 fl oz	170	3	2	15	29	0	28	8	130
Nestlé, Nesquik, Chocolate Fat Free Milk									
8 fl oz	150	0	0	<5	29	<1	28	8	160
Nestlé, Nesquik, Chocolate Lowfat Milk									
8 fl oz	150	2.5	1.5	15	25	<1	24	8	160
Nestlé, Nesquik, Double Chocolate Lowfat Milk									
8 fl oz	180	3	2	10	30	1	29	8	180
Nestlé, Nesquik, No Sugar Added, Chocolate Lowfat Milk									
8 fl oz	100	2	1.5	10	13	<1	12	8	140
Nestlé, Nesquik, Strawberry Lowfat Milk									
8 fl oz	180	2.5	1.5	15	31	0	30	8	130
Nestlé, Nesquik, Vanilla Lowfat Milk									
8 fl oz	170	3	1.5	10	30	0	29	8	130
Smart Balance, Fat Free Milk and Calcium									
1 cup	100	0	0	5	15	NA	15	11	150
Smart Balance, Fat Free Milk and Omega-3s									
1 cup	110	1	0	5	14	NA	14	10	150
Smart Balance, HeartRight, Fat Free Milk and Omega-3s									
1 cup	110	1	0	5	14	NA	14	10	150
Smart Balance, Lactose-Free Fat Free Milk and Omega-3s									
1 cup	110	1	0	5	14	NA	14	10	140
Smart Balance, Low Fat Milk and Omega-3s									
1 cup	130	3	1.5	15	15	NA	15	11	170
Stonyfield Organic, 1 % Milk Fat Organic Lowfat Milk, Half Gallon Size									
1 cup	110	3	2	15	12	0	12	8	125
Stonyfield Organic, 2 % Milk Fat Organic Reduced Fat Milk, Half Gallon Size									
1 cup	130	5	3	20	12	0	11	8	120
Stonyfield Organic, 2% Milk Fat, Organic Omega-3 Milk									
1 cup	130	5	3	20	12	0	11	8	120

Food Serving size	Cal.	(g) Total Fat	(g) Sat. Fat	(mg) Chol.	(g) Carb.	(g) Fiber	(g) Sug.	(g) Prot.	(mg) Sod.
Stonyfield Organic, Fat Free Organic Milk, Half Gallon Size									
1 cup	90	0	0	5	12	0	12	8	125
Stonyfield Organic, Half & Half Milk									
2 tbsp	40	4	2	10	1	0	1	1	10
Stonyfield Organic, Whole Milk Organic Milk, Half Gallon Size									
1 cup	150	8	5	30	12	0	11	8	120
Stonyfield Organic, Whole Milk Organic Omega-3 Milk									
1 cup	150	8	5	30	12	0	11	8	120

Yogurt

Food Serving size	Cal.	(g) Total Fat	(g) Sat. Fat	(mg) Chol.	(g) Carb.	(g) Fiber	(g) Sug.	(g) Prot.	(mg) Sod.
Brown Cow Farms, Chocolate on the Bottom									
1 container, 6 oz	190	6	4	20	28	0	26	5	80
Brown Cow Farms, Cream Top Fruit on the Bottom, Strawberry									
1 container, 6 oz	180	6	3.5	20	28	<1	26	5	75
Brown Cow Farms, Cream Top Fruit on the Bottom, Raspberry									
1 container, 6 oz	170	6	3.5	20	26	<1	25	5	75
Brown Cow Farms, Cream Top Smooth and Creamy, Plain									
1 container, 32 oz	170	10	6	35	12	0	12	8	125
Brown Cow Farms, Cream Top Smooth and Creamy, Vanilla									
1 container, 32 oz	210	9	6	35	25	0	24	7	115
Brown Cow Farms, Cream Top Yogurts, Coffee									
1 container, 6 oz	160	7	4	25	19	0	18	6	85
Brown Cow Farms, Cream Top Yogurts, Maple									
1 container, 6 oz	170	7	4	25	22	0	21	5	85
Brown Cow Farms, Cream Top Yogurts, Plain									
1 container, 6 oz	130	7	4.5	30	9	0	9	6	95
Brown Cow Farms, Cream Top Yogurts, Vanilla									
1 container, 6 oz	160	7	4	25	19	0	18	6	85
Brown Cow Farms, Fruit on the Bottom, Apricot Mango									
1 container, 6 oz	170	6	3.5	20	23	0	20	5	80
Brown Cow Farms, Fruit on the Bottom, Blueberry									
1 container, 6 oz	180	6	3.5	20	28	<1	25	5	75
Brown Cow Farms, Fruit on the Bottom, Cherry-Vanilla									
1 container, 6 oz	180	6	3.5	20	28	0	27	5	75

Food Serving size	Cal.	(g) Total Fat	(g) Sat. Fat	(mg) Chol.	(g) Carb.	(g) Fiber	(g) Sug.	(g) Prot.	(mg) Sod.
Brown Cow Farms, Fruit on the Bottom, Non Fat Greek, Blueberry									
5.3 oz	130	0	0	0	18	0	17	13	60
Brown Cow Farms, Fruit on the Bottom, Non Fat Greek, Strawberry									
5.3 oz	130	0	0	0	18	0	17	13	65
Brown Cow Farms, Fruit on the Bottom, Non Fat Yogurt, Strawberry									
1 container, 6 oz	130	0	0	0	25	0	23	6	95
Brown Cow Farms, Low Fat Fruit on the Bottom, Black Cherry									
1 container, 6 oz	150	2	1	5	27	0	25	6	100
Brown Cow Farms, Low Fat Fruit on the Bottom, Blueberry									
1 container, 6 oz	150	2	1	5	26	0	24	6	100
Brown Cow Farms, Low Fat Fruit on the Bottom, Boysenberry									
1 container, 6 oz	150	2	1	5	27	0	25	6	100
Brown Cow Farms, Low Fat Fruit on the Bottom, Lemon Twist									
1 container, 6 oz	150	2	1	5	27	0	25	6	105
Brown Cow Farms, Low Fat Fruit on the Bottom, Peach									
1 container, 6 oz	180	6	3.5	20	27	<1	26	5	75
Brown Cow Farms, Low Fat Fruit on the Bottom, Strawberry									
1 container, 6 oz	150	2	1	5	26	0	25	6	100
Brown Cow Farms, Low Fat Fruit on the Bottom, Vanilla Bean									
1 container, 6 oz	150	2	1	5	26	0	25	6	100
Brown Cow Farms, Low Fat Smooth and Creamy, Plain									
1 container, 32 oz	130	3	2	10	15	0	15	10	160
Brown Cow Farms, Low Fat Smooth and Creamy, Vanilla									
1 container, 32 oz	200	3	2	10	32	0	32	10	150
Brown Cow Farms, Non Fat Greek Yogurt, Bluberry, 4-pack									
1 container, 4 oz	100	0	0	0	13	0	13	10	45
Brown Cow Farms, Non Fat Greek Yogurt, Strawberry, 4-pack									
1 container, 4 oz	100	0	0	0	14	0	13	10	50
Brown Cow Farms, Smooth and Creamy, Blueberry									
1 container, 32 oz	210	9	6	35	26	0	25	7	160
Brown Cow Farms, Smooth and Creamy, Low Fat Yogurt, Peach									
1 container, 6 oz	150	2	1.5	10	26	0	25	7	120
Brown Cow Farms, Smooth and Creamy, Maple									
1 container, 32 oz	230	9	5	35	29	0	28	7	115

Food Serving size	Cal.	(g) Total Fat	(g) Sat. Fat	(mg) Chol.	(g) Carb.	(g) Fiber	(g) Sug.	(g) Prot.	(mg) Sod.
Brown Cow Farms, Smooth and Creamy, Non Fat Greek Yogurt, Plain									
1 container, 5.3 oz	80	0	0	0	6	0	6	15	60
Brown Cow Farms, Smooth and Creamy, Non Fat Greek Yogurt, Vanilla									
5.3 oz	110	0	0	0	12	0	12	14	55
Brown Cow Farms, Smooth and Creamy, Non Fat Greek, Plain									
16 oz	130	0	0	0	9	0	9	23	95
Brown Cow Farms, Smooth and Creamy, Non Fat Yogurt, Blueberry									
1 container, 6 oz	140	0	0	0	26	0	26	7	125
Brown Cow Farms, Smooth and Creamy, Non Fat Yogurt, Lemon									
1 container, 32 oz	180	0	0	0	36	0	35	9	140
Brown Cow Farms, Smooth and Creamy, Non Fat Yogurt, Plain									
1 container, 32 oz	110	0	0	0	16	0	15	10	160
Brown Cow Farms, Smooth and Creamy, Non Fat Yogurt, Vanilla									
1 container, 32 oz	180	0	0	0	34	0	33	9	140
Brown Cow Farms, Smooth and Creamy, Non Fat Yogurt, Vanilla									
1 container, 6 oz	130	0	0	0	25	0	25	7	105
Fage, Total 0%, Blueberry Acai Yogurt									
1 container	120	0	0	0	18	0	16	13	45
Fage, Total 0%, Cherry Pomegranate Yogurt									
1 container	130	0	0	0	19	0	16	13	50
Fage, Total 0%, Cherry Yogurt									
1 container	120	0	0	0	17	0	16	13	50
Fage, Total 0%, Family Size, Plain Yogurt									
1 cup, 8 oz	130	0	0	0	9	0	9	23	85
Fage, Total 0%, Mango Guanabana Yogurt									
1 container	120	0	0	0	18	0	17	13	45
Fage, Total 0%, Peach Yogurt									
1 container	120	0	0	0	17	0	16	13	45
Fage, Total 0%, Raspberry Yogurt									
1 container	120	0	0	0	18	0	16	13	45
Fage, Total 0%, Single Size Plain Yogurt									
1 container	100	0	0	0	7	0	7	18	65
Fage, Total 0%, Strawberry Goji Yogurt									
1 container	120	0	0	0	17	0	16	13	50

Food Serving size	Cal.	(g) Total Fat	(g) Sat. Fat	(mg) Chol.	(g) Carb.	(g) Fiber	(g) Sug.	(g) Prot.	(mg) Sod.
Fage, Total 0%, Strawberry Yogurt									
1 container	120	0	0	0	17	0	16	13	45
Fage, Total 2%, Blueberry Yogurt									
1 container	140	2.5	1.5	5	18	0	16	12	40
Fage, Total 2%, Cherry Yogurt									
1 container	140	2.5	1.5	5	17	0	16	12	40
Fage, Total 2%, Family Size, Plain Yogurt									
1 cup, 8 oz	170	4.5	3	15	9	0	9	23	75
Fage, Total 2%, Honey Yogurt									
1 container	190	2.5	1.5	5	29	0	29	12	40
Fage, Total 2%, Peach Yogurt									
1 container	140	2.5	1.5	5	17	0	16	12	40
Fage, Total 2%, Single Size, Plain Yogurt									
1 container	150	4	3	10	8	0	8	20	65
Fage, Total 2%, Strawberry Yogurt									
1 container	140	2.5	1.5	5	17	0	16	12	40
Fage, Total Classic, Blueberry Yogurt									
1 container	170	6	4.5	15	18	0	16	11	45
Fage, Total Classic, Cherry Yogurt									
1 container	170	6	4.5	15	17	0	16	11	45
Fage, Total Classic, Family Size, Plain Yogurt									
1 cup, 8 oz	220	11	8	30	9	0	9	20	80
Fage, Total Classic, Honey Yogurt									
1 container	210	6	4.5	15	29	0	29	11	45
Fage, Total Classic, Peach Yogurt									
1 container	170	6	4.5	15	17	0	16	11	45
Fage, Total Classic, Single Size, Plain Yogurt									
1 container	190	10	7	25	8	0	8	18	70
Fage, Total Classic, Strawberry Yogurt									
1 container	170	6	4.5	15	17	0	16	11	45
Noosa Finest Yoghurt, Blueberry									
4 oz	130	6	4	15	14	1	9	9	50
Noosa Finest Yoghurt, Honey									
4 oz	140	6	5	15	16	1	10	9	50

Food Serving size	Cal.	(g) Total Fat	(g) Sat. Fat	(mg) Chol.	(g) Carb.	(g) Fiber	(g) Sug.	(g) Prot.	(mg) Sod.
Noosa Finest Yoghurt, Mango									
4 oz	130	6	4	15	14	1	9	9	50
Noosa Finest Yoghurt, Peach									
4 oz	130	6	4	15	14	1	9	9	50
Noosa Finest Yoghurt, Raspberry									
4 oz	130	6	4	15	14	1	9	9	50
Noosa Finest Yoghurt, Strawberry Rhubarb									
4 oz	130	6	4	15	14	1	9	9	50
Stonyfield Organic, 0% Fat, Strawberry Fruit on the Bottom Yogurt									
6 oz, 1 container	110	0	0	<5	22	<1	21	6	125
Stonyfield Organic, Acai Fruit on the Bottom Yogurt									
6 oz, 1 container	120	0	0	0	22	<1	22	6	130
Stonyfield Organic, Activia, Blueberry Yogurt									
4 oz, 1 container	90	1	0.5	5	16	0	15	5	85
Stonyfield Organic, Activia, Peach Yogurt									
4 oz, 1 container	90	1	0.5	5	15	0	14	5	75
Stonyfield Organic, Activia, Strawberry Yogurt									
4 oz, 1 container	90	1	0.5	5	16	0	15	5	75
Stonyfield Organic, Activia, Vanilla Yogurt									
4 oz, 1 container	90	1	0.5	5	15	0	14	5	70
Stonyfield Organic, Blueberry Fruit on the Bottom Yogurt									
6 oz, 1 container	120	0	0	<5	22	<1	20	6	100
Stonyfield Organic, Chocolate Underground									
6 oz, 1 container	140	0	0	<5	29	<1	27	7	110
Stonyfield Organic, Fat Free, Smooth and Creamy, Black Cherry Yogurt									
6 oz, 1 container	100	0	0	<5	18	0	17	7	120
Stonyfield Organic, Fat Free, Smooth and Creamy, French Vanilla Yogurt									
6 oz, 1 container	100	0	0	<5	17	0	17	7	115
Stonyfield Organic, Fat Free, Smooth and Creamy, Key Lime Yogurt									
6 oz, 1 container	100	0	0	<5	17	0	16	7	125
Stonyfield Organic, Fat Free, Smooth and Creamy, Lemon Yogurt									
6 oz, 1 container	100	0	0	<5	18	0	17	7	120
Stonyfield Organic, Fat Free, Smooth and Creamy, Peach Yogurt									
6 oz, 1 container	100	0	0	<5	18	0	17	7	115

Food Serving size	Cal.	(g) Total Fat	(g) Sat. Fat	(mg) Chol.	(g) Carb.	(g) Fiber	(g) Sug.	(g) Prot.	(mg) Sod.
Stonyfield Organic, Fat Free, Smooth and Creamy, Plain Yogurt 6 oz, 1 container	80	0	0	<5	11	0	11	8	120
Stonyfield Organic, Fat Free, Smooth and Creamy, Pomegranate Berry Yogurt 6 oz, 1 container	100	0	0	<5	17	0	16	7	120
Stonyfield Organic, Fat Free, Smooth and Creamy, Strawberry Yogurt 6 oz, 1 container	100	0	0	<5	18	0	17	7	120
Stonyfield Organic, French Vanilla, Smooth and Creamy Yogurt 32 oz, 1 cup	130	0	0	<5	23	0	22	10	150
Stonyfield Organic, Fruit on the Bottom, Peach Yogurt 6 oz, 1 container	130	1.5	1	5	22	0	22	6	110
Stonyfield Organic, Fruit on the Bottom, Pomegranate Raspberry Yogurt 6 oz, 1 container	120	0	0	0	22	<1	22	6	130
Stonyfield Organic, Fruit on the Bottom, Strawberries & Cream 6 oz, 1 container	150	6	3.5	20	20	<1	19	5	105
Stonyfield Organic, Low Fat, Banilla Yogurt 32 oz, 1 cup	200	2.5	1.5	10	35	0	34	9	135
Stonyfield Organic, Low Fat, Blueberry Fruit on the Bottom Yogurt 6 oz, 1 container	120	1.5	1	5	21	<1	20	6	90
Stonyfield Organic, Low Fat, Blueberry Yogurt 32 oz, 1 cup	180	2	1.5	10	30	0	30	9	170
Stonyfield Organic, Low Fat, French Vanilla Yogurt 32 oz, 1 cup	170	2	1.5	10	29	0	28	9	140
Stonyfield Organic, Low Fat, Plain Yogurt 32 oz, 1 cup	120	2	1.5	10	15	0	14	10	150
Stonyfield Organic, Low Fat, Smooth and Creamy, Cherry Vanilla Yogurt 6 oz, 1 container	130	1.5	1	5	23	0	21	7	110
Stonyfield Organic, Low Fat, Smooth and Creamy, French Vanilla Yogurt 6 oz, 1 container	130	1.5	1	5	22	0	21	7	105
Stonyfield Organic, Low Fat, Smooth and Creamy, Mango Honey Yogurt 6 oz, 1 container	130	1.5	1	5	23	0	23	7	110
Stonyfield Organic, Low Fat, Smooth and Creamy, Plain Yogurt 6 oz, 1 container	90	1.5	1	5	11	0	11	7	110
Stonyfield Organic, Low Fat, Smooth and Creamy, Raspberry Yogurt 6 oz, 1 container	130	1.5	1	5	23	0	22	7	110

Food Serving size	Cal.	(g) Total Fat	(g) Sat. Fat	(mg) Chol.	(g) Carb.	(g) Fiber	(g) Sug.	(g) Prot.	(mg) Sod.
Stonyfield Organic, Low Fat, Smooth and Creamy, Strawberry Pomegranate Yogurt 6 oz, 1 container	130	1.5	1	5	23	0	22	7	110
Stonyfield Organic, Low Fat, Smooth and Creamy Strawberry Yogurt 32 oz, 1 cup	200	2.5	1.5	10	35	0	34	9	135
Stonyfield Organic, Low Fat, Strawberry, Fruit on the Bottom Yogurt 6 oz, 1 container	120	1.5	1	5	21	<1	20	6	120
Stonyfield Organic, Oikos, Fruit on the Bottom, Organic Greek Yogurt, Blueberry 5.3 oz, 1 container	120	0	0	0	16	0	15	13	70
Stonyfield Organic, Oikos, Fruit on the Bottom, Organic Greek Yogurt, Honey 5.3 oz, 1 container	120	0	0	0	18	0	17	13	50
Stonyfield Organic, Oikos, Fruit on the Bottom, Organic Greek Yogurt, Peach Mango 5.3 oz, 1 container	130	0	0	0	19	0	19	13	60
Stonyfield Organic, Oikos, Fruit on the Bottom, Organic Greek Yogurt, Strawberry 5.3 oz, 1 container	110	0	0	0	16	0	16	13	80
Stonyfield Organic, Oikos, Fruit on the Bottom, Organic Greek Yogurt, Superfruits 5.3 oz, 1 container	130	0	0	0	18	0	16	13	80
Stonyfield Organic, Oikos, Organic Greek, Nonfat Caramel Yogurt 4 oz, 1 container	110	0	0	0	17	0	16	10	60
Stonyfield Organic, Oikos, Organic Greek, Nonfat Chocolate Yogurt 4 oz, 1 container	100	0	0	0	17	<1	16	10	40
Stonyfield Organic, Oikos, Organic Greek, Nonfat, Fruit on the Bottom, Blueberry Yogurt 4 oz, 1 container	90	0	0	0	12	0	11	10	40
Stonyfield Organic, Oikos, Organic Greek, Nonfat, Fruit on the Bottom, Strawberry Yogurt 4 oz, 1 container	90	0	0	0	12	0	12	10	60
Stonyfield Organic, Oikos, Organic Greek, Nonfat, Honey Yogurt 4 oz, 1 container	90	0	0	0	13	0	13	10	40
Stonyfield Organic, Oikos, Organic Greek, Smooth and Creamy, Honey Fig Yogurt 5.3 oz, 1 container	110	0	0	0	14	0	14	14	65

Food Serving size	Cal.	(g) Total Fat	(g) Sat. Fat	(mg) Chol.	(g) Carb.	(g) Fiber	(g) Sug.	(g) Prot.	(mg) Sod.
Stonyfield Organic, Oikos, Organic Greek, Smooth and Creamy, Nonfat, Plain Yogurt									
4 oz, 1 container	70	0	0	0	5	0	5	12	45
Stonyfield Organic, Oikos, Organic Greek, Smooth and Creamy, Nonfat, Vanilla Yogurt									
4 oz, 1 container	80	0	0	0	9	0	8	11	45
Stonyfield Organic, Oikos, Organic Greek, Smooth and Creamy, Plain Yogurt									
16 oz, 1 cup	130	0	0	0	9	0	9	23	95
Stonyfield Organic, Oikos, Organic Greek, Smooth and Creamy, Plain Yogurt									
5.3 oz, 1 container	80	0	0	0	6	0	6	15	60
Stonyfield Organic, Oikos, Organic Greek, Smooth and Creamy, Vanilla Yogurt									
16 oz, 1 cup	160	0	0	0	18	0	17	22	90
Stonyfield Organic, Oikos, Organic Greek, Smooth and Creamy, Vanilla Yogurt									
5.3 oz, 1 container	110	0	0	0	12	0	11	15	60
Stonyfield Organic, Smooth and Creamy, French Vanilla Whole-Milk Yogurt									
6 oz, 1 container	170	6	4	25	22	0	22	6	90
Stonyfield Organic, Smooth and Creamy, French Vanilla Yogurt									
32 oz, 1 cup	230	8	5	30	30	0	29	8	125
Stonyfield Organic, Smooth and Creamy, French Vanilla Yogurt									
4 oz, 1 container	70	0	0	<5	11	0	11	5	75
Stonyfield Organic, Smooth and Creamy, Peach Yogurt									
4 oz, 1 container	70	0	0	<5	12	0	12	5	75
Stonyfield Organic, Smooth and Creamy, Plain Whole-Milk Yogurt									
32 oz, 1 cup	170	9	6	35	12	0	12	8	130
Stonyfield Organic, Smooth and Creamy, Plain Yogurt									
32 oz, 1 cup	110	0	0	<5	15	0	15	10	160
Stonyfield Organic, Smooth and Creamy, Raspberry Yogurt									
4 oz, 1 container	70	0	0	<5	12	0	12	5	80
Stonyfield Organic, Smooth and Creamy, Strawberry Yogurt									
4 oz, 1 container	70	0	0	<5	12	0	12	5	80
Stonyfield Organic, Smoothies, Peach									
10 oz, 1 bottle	230	3	2	10	41	<1	40	10	140
Stonyfield Organic, Smoothies, Peach									
6 oz, 1 bottle	140	2	1	5	24	0	24	6	85

Food Serving size	Cal.	(g) Total Fat	(g) Sat. Fat	(mg) Chol.	(g) Carb.	(g) Fiber	(g) Sug.	(g) Prot.	(mg) Sod.
Stonyfield Organic, Smoothies, Raspberry									
10 oz, 1 bottle	230	3	2	10	40	<1	39	10	150
Stonyfield Organic, Smoothies, Strawberry									
10 oz, 1 bottle	230	3	2	10	39	<1	38	10	150
Stonyfield Organic, Smoothies, Strawberry									
6 oz, 1 bottle	140	2	1	5	23	0	23	6	90
Stonyfield Organic, Smoothies, Strawberry Banana									
10 oz, 1 bottle	230	3	2	10	40	<1	38	10	150
Stonyfield Organic, Smoothies, Strawberry Banana									
6 oz, 1 bottle	140	2	1	5	24	0	23	6	90
Stonyfield Organic, Smoothies, Vanilla									
10 oz, 1 bottle	240	3	2	10	40	<1	37	10	140
Stonyfield Organic, Smoothies, Wild Berry									
10 oz, 1 bottle	230	3	2	10	39	<1	38	10	150
Stonyfield Organic, Smoothies, Wild Berry									
6 oz, 1 bottle	140	2	1	5	23	0	23	6	90
Yoplait Kids, Cars Vroom Vroom Vanilla									
85g container	70	1	0.5	<5	13	NA	9	3	45
Yoplait Kids, Dora the Explorer Strawberry									
85g container	70	1	0.5	<5	13	0	9	3	45
Yoplait Kids, Mickey Mouse Clubhouse Strawberry Banana Adventure									
85g container	70	1	0.5	<5	13	0	9	3	45
Yoplait, Go-Gurt, Banana Split									
1 tube	70	0.5	0	<5	13	0	10	2	30
Yoplait, Go-Gurt, Berry Blue Blast									
1 tube	70	0.5	0	<5	13	0	10	2	30
Yoplait, Go-Gurt, Burstin' Melon Berry									
1 tube	70	0.5	0	<5	13	0	10	2	30
Yoplait, Go-Gurt, Chill Out Cherry									
1 tube	70	0.5	0	<5	13	0	10	2	30
Yoplait, Go-Gurt, Cool Cotton Candy									
1 tube	70	0.5	0	<5	13	0	10	2	30
Yoplait, Go-Gurt, Phineas & Ferb Perry Berry									
1 tube	70	0.5	0	<5	13	0	10	2	30

Food Serving size	Cal.	(g) Total Fat	(g) Sat. Fat	(mg) Chol.	(g) Carb.	(g) Fiber	(g) Sug.	(g) Prot.	(mg) Sod.
Yoplait, Go-Gurt, Phineas & Ferb Summer Punch									
1 tube	70	0.5	0	<5	13	0	10	2	30
Yoplait, Go-Gurt, SpongeBob Sponge Berry									
1 tube	70	0.5	0	<5	13	0	10	2	30
Yoplait, Go-Gurt, SpongeBob Strawberry Riptide									
1 tube	70	0.5	0	<5	13	0	10	2	30
Yoplait, Go-Gurt, Strawberry Banana Burst									
1 tube	70	0.5	0	<5	13	0	10	2	30
Yoplait, Go-Gurt, Strawberry Kiwi Kick									
1 tube	70	0.5	0	<5	13	0	10	2	30
Yoplait, Go-Gurt, Strawberry Milkshake									
1 tube	70	0.5	0	<5	13	0	10	2	30
Yoplait, Go-Gurt, Strawberry Splash									
1 tube	70	0.5	0	<5	13	0	10	2	30
Yoplait, Go-Gurt, Victorious Poppin' Punch									
1 tube	70	0.5	0	<5	13	0	10	2	30
Yoplait, Go-Gurt, Victorious Smashin' Berry									
1 tube	70	0.5	0	<5	13	0	10	2	30
Yoplait, Go-Gurt, Watermelon Meltdown									
1 tube	70	0.5	0	<5	13	0	10	2	30
Yoplait, Greek 100, Black Cherry Yogurt									
5.3 oz, 1 container	100	0	0	<5	14	NA	9	10	45
Yoplait, Greek 100, Key Lime Yogurt									
5.3 oz, 1 container	100	0	0	<5	10	NA	7	13	55
Yoplait, Greek 100, Mixed Berry Yogurt									
5.3 oz, 1 container	100	0	0	<5	14	NA	9	10	45
Yoplait, Greek 100, Peach Yogurt									
5.3 oz, 1 container	100	0	0	<5	14	NA	9	10	45
Yoplait, Greek 100, Strawberry Yogurt									
5.3 oz, 1 container	100	0	0	<5	14	NA	9	10	45
Yoplait, Greek 100, Vanilla Yogurt									
5.3 oz, 1 container	100	0	0	<5	14	NA	9	10	45
Yoplait, Greek, Blueberry Yogurt									
4 oz, 1 container	160	0	0	10	26	NA	20	12	100

Food Serving size	Cal.	(g) Total Fat	(g) Sat. Fat	(mg) Chol.	(g) Carb.	(g) Fiber	(g) Sug.	(g) Prot.	(mg) Sod.
Yoplait, Greek, Blueberry Yogurt with Granola									
1 container	230	2.5	0	5	39	1	23	12	140
Yoplait, Greek, Cherry Pomegranate Yogurt									
4 oz, 1 container	110	0	0	5	16	NA	13	8	65
Yoplait, Greek, Coconut Yogurt									
4 oz, 1 container	110	0	0	5	19	NA	14	8	60
Yoplait, Greek, Honey Vanilla Yogurt									
4 oz, 1 container	150	0	0	10	22	NA	18	14	120
Yoplait, Greek, Key Lime Yogurt									
4 oz, 1 container	160	0	0	10	25	NA	20	14	100
Yoplait, Greek, Peach Yogurt									
4 oz, 1 container	160	0	0	10	25	NA	20	14	100
Yoplait, Greek, Peach Yogurt with Granola									
1 container	230	2.5	0	5	39	1	23	12	140
Yoplait, Greek, Plain Yogurt									
4 oz, 1 container	120	0	0	15	12	NA	9	17	115
Yoplait, Greek, Strawberry Yogurt									
4 oz, 1 container	160	0	0	10	25	NA	20	14	100
Yoplait, Greek, Strawberry Yogurt with Granola									
1 container	230	2.5	0	5	39	1	23	12	140
Yoplait, Lactose Free, Cherry									
1 container	170	1.5	1	10	33	NA	26	5	85
Yoplait, Lactose Free, Peach									
1 container	170	1.5	1	10	33	NA	26	5	85
Yoplait, Lactose Free, Strawberry									
1 container	170	1.5	1	10	33	NA	26	5	85
Yoplait, Lactose Free, Vanilla									
1 container	170	1.5	1	10	33	NA	26	5	85
Yoplait, Large Size, Creamy Harvest Peach Yogurt									
8 oz	210	1.5	1	10	42	0	33	7	100
Yoplait, Large Size, Creamy Strawberry Banana Yogurt									
8 oz	210	1.5	1	10	42	0	33	7	100
Yoplait, Large Size, Creamy Strawberry Yogurt									
8 oz	210	1.5	1	10	42	0	33	7	100

Food Serving size	Cal.	(g) Total Fat	(g) Sat. Fat	(mg) Chol.	(g) Carb.	(g) Fiber	(g) Sug.	(g) Prot.	(mg) Sod.
Yoplait, Large Size, Creamy Vanilla Yogurt									
8 oz	210	1.5	1	10	42	NA	33	7	100
Yoplait, Light Apple Turnover Yogurt									
1 container	90	0	0	<5	16	NA	10	5	80
Yoplait, Light Apricot Mango Yogurt									
1 container	90	0	0	<5	16	NA	10	5	80
Yoplait, Light Banana Cream Pie Yogurt									
1 container	90	0	0	<5	16	NA	10	5	80
Yoplait, Light Black Forrest Cake Yogurt									
1 container	90	0	0	<5	16	NA	10	5	80
Yoplait, Light Blackberry Yogurt									
1 container	90	0	0	<5	16	NA	10	5	80
Yoplait, Light Blueberry Patch Yogurt									
1 container	90	0	0	<5	16	NA	10	5	80
Yoplait, Light Blueberry with Granola Yogurt									
1 container	190	2.5	0	<5	35	1	19	5	105
Yoplait, Light Blueberry Yogurt with Fiber									
1 container, 113g	50	0	0	<5	13	5	4	3	55
Yoplait, Light Boston Cream Pie Yogurt									
1 container	90	0	0	<5	16	NA	10	5	80
Yoplait, Light Cherry with Granola Yogurt									
1 container	190	2.5	0	<5	35	1	19	5	105
Yoplait, Light Harvest Peach Yogurt									
1 container	90	0	0	<5	16	NA	10	5	80
Yoplait, Light Key Lime Pie Yogurt									
1 container	90	0	0	<5	16	NA	10	5	80
Yoplait, Light Key Lime Pie Yogurt with Fiber									
1 container, 113g	50	0	0	<5	13	5	4	3	55
Yoplait, Light Lemon Cream Pie Yogurt									
1 container	90	0	0	<5	16	NA	10	5	80
Yoplait, Light Orange Crème Yogurt									
1 container	90	0	0	<5	16	NA	10	5	80
Yoplait, Light Peach with Granola Yogurt									
1 container	190	2.5	0	<5	35	1	19	5	105

Food Serving size	Cal.	(g) Total Fat	(g) Sat. Fat	(mg) Chol.	(g) Carb.	(g) Fiber	(g) Sug.	(g) Prot.	(mg) Sod.
Yoplait, Light Pineapple Upside Down Cake Yogurt									
1 container	90	0	0	<5	16	NA	10	5	80
Yoplait, Light Raspberry Cheesecake Yogurt									
1 container	90	0	0	<5	16	NA	10	5	80
Yoplait, Light Raspberry Lemonade Yogurt									
1 container	90	0	0	<5	16	NA	10	5	80
Yoplait, Light Red Raspberry Yogurt									
1 container	90	0	0	<5	16	NA	10	5	80
Yoplait, Light Red Velvet Cake Yogurt									
1 container	90	0	0	<5	16	NA	10	5	80
Yoplait, Light Strawberry 'n Bananas Yogurt									
1 container	90	0	0	<5	16	NA	10	5	80
Yoplait, Light Strawberry Orange Sunrise Yogurt									
1 container	90	0	0	<5	16	NA	10	5	80
Yoplait, Light Strawberry Shortcake Yogurt									
1 container	90	0	0	<5	16	NA	10	5	80
Yoplait, Light Strawberry with Granola Yogurt									
1 container	190	2.5	0	<5	35	1	19	5	105
Yoplait, Light Strawberry Yogurt									
1 container	90	0	0	<5	16	NA	10	5	80
Yoplait, Light Strawberry Yogurt with Fiber									
1 container, 113g	50	0	0	<5	13	5	4	3	55
Yoplait, Light Thick & Creamy Blueberry Pie Yogurt									
1 container	100	0	0	<5	21	NA	14	5	90
Yoplait, Light Thick & Creamy Cherry Cobbler Yogurt									
1 container	100	0	0	<5	21	NA	14	5	90
Yoplait, Light Thick & Creamy Cinnamon Roll Yogurt									
1 container	100	0	0	<5	21	NA	14	5	90
Yoplait, Light Thick & Creamy French Vanilla Yogurt									
1 container	100	0	0	<5	21	NA	14	5	90
Yoplait, Light Thick & Creamy Key Lime Pie Yogurt									
1 container	100	0	0	<5	21	NA	14	5	90
Yoplait, Light Thick & Creamy Lemon Meringue Yogurt									
1 container	100	0	0	<5	21	NA	14	5	90

Food Serving size	Cal.	(g) Total Fat	(g) Sat. Fat	(mg) Chol.	(g) Carb.	(g) Fiber	(g) Sug.	(g) Prot.	(mg) Sod.
Yoplait, Light Thick & Creamy Strawberry Yogurt									
1 container	100	0	0	<5	21	NA	14	5	90
Yoplait, Light Triple Berry Torte Yogurt									
1 container	90	0	0	<5	16	NA	10	5	80
Yoplait, Light Vanilla Cherry Yogurt									
1 container	90	0	0	<5	16	NA	10	5	80
Yoplait, Light Vanilla Yogurt with Fiber									
1 container, 113g	50	0	0	<5	13	5	4	3	55
Yoplait, Light Very Cherry Yogurt									
1 container	90	0	0	<5	16	NA	10	5	80
Yoplait, Light Very Vanilla Yogurt									
1 container	90	0	0	<5	16	NA	10	5	80
Yoplait, Light White Chocolate Strawberry Yogurt									
1 container	90	0	0	<5	16	NA	10	5	80
Yoplait, Original Blackberry Harvest Yogurt									
1 container	170	1.5	1	10	33	NA	26	5	85
Yoplait, Original Blackberry Pomegranate Yogurt									
1 container	170	1.5	1	10	33	NA	26	5	85
Yoplait, Original Boston Cream Pie Yogurt									
1 container	170	1.5	1	10	33	NA	26	5	85
Yoplait, Original Cherry Orchard Yogurt									
1 container	170	1.5	1	10	33	NA	26	5	85
Yoplait, Original Cherry Pomegranate Yogurt									
1 container	170	1.5	1	10	33	NA	26	5	85
Yoplait, Original French Vanilla Yogurt									
1 container	170	1.5	1	10	33	NA	26	5	85
Yoplait, Original Harvest Peach Yogurt									
1 container	170	1.5	1	10	33	NA	26	5	85
Yoplait, Original Key Lime Pie Yogurt									
1 container	170	1.5	1	10	33	NA	26	5	85
Yoplait, Original Lemon Burst Yogurt									
1 container	170	1.5	1	10	33	NA	26	5	85
Yoplait, Original Mango Yogurt									
1 container	170	1.5	1	10	33	NA	26	5	85

Food Serving size	Cal.	(g) Total Fat	(g) Sat. Fat	(mg) Chol.	(g) Carb.	(g) Fiber	(g) Sug.	(g) Prot.	(mg) Sod.
Yoplait, Original Mixed Berry Yogurt									
1 container	170	1.5	1	10	33	NA	26	5	85
Yoplait, Original Mountain Blueberry Yogurt									
1 container	170	1.5	1	10	33	NA	26	5	85
Yoplait, Original Orange Crème Yogurt									
1 container	170	1.5	1	10	33	NA	26	5	85
Yoplait, Original Pina Colada Yogurt									
1 container	170	2	1.5	10	33	NA	27	5	80
Yoplait, Original Pineapple Yogurt									
1 container	170	1.5	1	10	33	NA	26	5	85
Yoplait, Original Red Raspberry Yogurt									
1 container	170	1.5	1	10	33	NA	26	5	85
Yoplait, Original Strawberry Banana Yogurt									
1 container	170	1.5	1	10	33	NA	26	5	85
Yoplait, Original Strawberry Cheesecake Yogurt									
1 container	170	1.5	1	10	33	NA	26	5	85
Yoplait, Original Strawberry Kiwi Yogurt									
1 container	170	1.5	1	10	33	NA	26	5	85
Yoplait, Original Strawberry Lemonade Yogurt									
1 container	170	1.5	1	10	33	NA	26	5	85
Yoplait, Original Strawberry Mango Yogurt									
1 container	170	1.5	1	10	33	NA	26	5	85
Yoplait, Original Strawberry Yogurt									
1 container	170	1.5	1	10	33	NA	26	5	85
Yoplait, Original, Thick and Creamy, Blackberry Harvest Yogurt									
1 container	180	2.5	1.5	15	31	NA	28	7	110
Yoplait, Original, Thick and Creamy, Key Lime Pie Yogurt									
1 container	180	2.5	1.5	15	31	NA	28	7	110
Yoplait, Original, Thick and Creamy, Strawberry Banana Yogurt									
1 container	180	2.5	1.5	15	31	NA	28	7	110
Yoplait, Original, Thick and Creamy, Strawberry Yogurt									
1 container	180	2.5	1.5	15	31	NA	28	7	110
Yoplait, Original, Thick and Creamy, Vanilla Yogurt									
1 container	180	2.5	1.5	15	31	NA	28	7	110

Food Serving size	Cal.	(g) Total Fat	(g) Sat. Fat	(mg) Chol.	(g) Carb.	(g) Fiber	(g) Sug.	(g) Prot.	(mg) Sod.
Yoplait, Simplait, Blackberry 1 container	200	7	4.5	30	28	NA	24	7	100
Yoplait, Simplait, Peach 1 container	200	7	4.5	30	28	NA	24	7	100
Yoplait, Simplait, Strawberry 1 container	200	7	4.5	30	28	NA	24	7	100
Yoplait, Simplait, Vanilla 1 container	200	7	4.5	30	28	NA	24	7	100
Yoplait, Simply Go-Gurt, Mixed Berry 1 tube	70	0.5	0	<5	13	0	10	2	30
Yoplait, Simply Go-Gurt, Strawberry 1 tube	70	0.5	0	<5	13	0	10	2	30
Yoplait, Splitz, Birthday Cake 92g container	100	1	1	<5	18	NA	13	3	60
Yoplait, Splitz, Rainbow Sherbert 92g container	90	1	0.5	<5	17	NA	12	3	60
Yoplait, Splitz, Strawberry Banana Split 92g container	90	1	0.5	<5	17	NA	12	3	60
Yoplait, Splitz, Strawberry Sundae 92g container	90	1	0.5	<5	17	NA	12	3	60
Yoplait, Trix, Cotton Candy 113g container	100	0.5	0.5	<5	20	NA	14	3	50
Yoplait, Trix, Raspberry Rainbow 113g container	100	0.5	0.5	<5	20	NA	14	3	50
Yoplait, Trix, Strawberry Banana Bash 113g container	100	0.5	0.5	<5	20	NA	14	3	50
Yoplait, Trix, Strawberry Punch 113g container	100	0.5	0.5	<5	20	NA	14	3	50
Yoplait, Trix, Triple Cherry 113g container	100	0.5	0.5	<5	20	NA	14	3	50
Yoplait, Whips!, Cherry Cheesecake 1 container	140	2.5	2	10	25	NA	21	5	75
Yoplait, Whips!, Chocolate Mousse 1 container	160	4	2.5	15	25	NA	22	5	105

Food Serving size	Cal.	(g) Total Fat	(g) Sat. Fat	(mg) Chol.	(g) Carb.	(g) Fiber	(g) Sug.	(g) Prot.	(mg) Sod.
Yoplait, Whips!, Chocolate Raspberry									
1 container	160	4	2.5	15	25	NA	22	5	105
Yoplait, Whips!, Key Lime Pie									
1 container	140	2.5	2	10	25	NA	21	5	75
Yoplait, Whips!, Lemon Burst									
1 container	140	2.5	2	10	25	NA	21	5	75
Yoplait, Whips!, Orange Crème									
1 container	140	2.5	2	10	25	NA	21	5	75
Yoplait, Whips!, Peaches 'n Cream									
1 container	140	2.5	2	10	25	NA	21	5	75
Yoplait, Whips!, Raspberry Mousse									
1 container	140	2.5	2	10	25	NA	21	5	75
Yoplait, Whips!, Strawberry Mist									
1 container	140	2.5	2	10	25	NA	21	5	75
Yoplait, Whips!, Vanilla Crème									
1 container	160	4	2.5	15	25	NA	22	5	105

Protein Foods

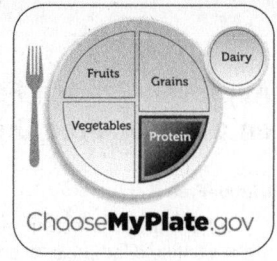

ChooseMyPlate.gov

Why Eat Protein?

Protein-rich foods such as meat, poultry, fish, eggs, nuts, and seeds are gluten-free. They provide nutrients that are vital for health and maintenance of your body. These include protein, B vitamins (niacin, thiamin, riboflavin, and B6), vitamin E, iron, zinc, and magnesium. Proteins function as building blocks for bones, muscles, cartilage, skin, and blood. B vitamins help the body release energy, play a vital role in the function of the nervous system, aid in the formation of red blood cells, and help build tissues. Iron is used to carry oxygen in the blood. Seafood contains a range of nutrients, notably the omega-3 fatty acids, EPA and DHA. Eating about 8 ounces per week of a variety of seafood contributes to the prevention of heart disease.

Daily Goal

Five and a half ounces for an adult on a 2,000 calorie diet.
Eight ounces of fish per week.
One ounce equivalents:
  1 ounce lean meat, poultry, or fish
  1 egg
  ½ ounce of seeds
  1 tsp peanut butter
  ¼ cup cooked, dried beans or peas
  ¼ cup tofu/roasted soybeans

Gluten-Free Shopping Tips

- Choose low-fat or lean cuts of plain, fresh meat
- Avoid meats that are marinated, seasoned, or contain fillers
- Vary your meals with more fish, beans, peas, nuts, and seeds
- Select fish rich in omega-3 fats: salmon, trout, or herring
- Trim visible fat and skin from meat before cooking
- Meat substitutes (vegetarian) often contain wheat ingredients
- Avoid baked beans that are thickened with wheat flour

Gluten-Free Shopping List Essentials

Lean beef	Fish	Beans
Chicken	Eggs	Nuts
Turkey	Almonds	

Approved Protein Foods and Those to Avoid on a Gluten-Free Diet

Gluten-Free

- Plain (fresh or frozen) meat, fish, or poultry
- Lentils, dried peas, dried beans (e.g., black, chickpeas or garbanzo, navy, pinto, soy, white), and plain tofu
- Plain nuts and seeds (chia, flax, sesame, pumpkin, sunflower), nut and seed butters (e.g., almond, peanut, sesame)
- Fresh, liquid, dried, or powdered eggs

May Contain Gluten

- Deli or luncheon meat (e.g., bologna, salami), hot dogs, frankfurters, sausages, pâtés, meat and sandwich spreads, frozen patties (meat, chicken, or fish), meat loaf, ham (ready to cook), dried meats (beef jerky), seasoned fish in pouches, imitation fish products (e.g., surimi), meat substitutes, and meat product extenders/fillers
- Frozen or fresh turkey with bread stuffing
- Frozen chicken breasts containing chicken broth (made with ingredients to avoid)
- Meat, poultry, or fish breaded with ingredients to avoid
- Flavored egg products (liquid or frozen). Baked beans and flavored tofu, tempeh, and miso
- Seasoned or dry roasted nuts and seasoned pumpkin or sunflower seeds

Caution

Cross-contamination of gluten can occur on grills, in pans, and in fryers that have previously been used to cook breaded or battered items. Make sure that cooking equipment is thoroughly cleaned before using for gluten-free cooking.

Choosing proteins that are high in saturated fat and cholesterol may increase your risk for coronary heart disease. These include fatty cuts of beef, pork, and lamb; regular (75% to 85% lean) ground beef; regular sausages, hot dogs, and bacon; some luncheon meats, such as regular bologna and salami; and some poultry, such as duck.

Food Serving size	Cal.	(g) Total Fat	(g) Sat. Fat	(mg) Chol.	(g) Carb.	(g) Fiber	(g) Sug.	(g) Prot.	(mg) Sod.
Beans, Peas & Legumes									
Amy's, Organic Black Bean Chili									
1 cup	200	3	0	0	31	13	3	13	680
Amy's, Organic Light in Sodium, Medium Chili									
1 cup	280	9	1	0	35	7	5	15	340
Amy's, Organic Light in Sodium, Refried Black Beans									
1/2 cup	140	3	0	0	21	6	1	8	220
Amy's, Organic Light in Sodium, Traditional Refried Beans									
1/2 cup	140	3	0	0	22	6	1	7	190
Amy's, Organic, Medium Chili									
1 cup	280	9	1	0	35	7	5	15	680
Amy's, Organic, Medium Chili with Vegetables									
1 cup	230	6	0.5	0	34	9	6	10	590
Amy's, Organic, Refried Beans with Green Chiles									
1/2 cup	130	3	0	0	20	6	1	7	440
Amy's, Organic, Refried Black Beans									
1/2 cup	140	3	0	0	21	6	1	8	440
Amy's, Organic, Spicy Chili									
1 cup	280	9	1	0	35	7	5	15	680
Amy's, Organic, Traditional Refried Beans									
1/2 cup	140	3	0	0	22	6	1	7	390
Amy's, Organic, Vegetarian Baked Beans									
1/2 cup	140	0.5	0	0	28	6	9	7	480
Amy's, Southwestern Black Bean Chili									
1 cup	240	4	0.5	0	40	10	5	12	680
Arrowhead Mills, Adzuki Beans									
1/4 cup	130	0	0	0	26	5	1	8	0
Arrowhead Mills, Anasazi Beans									
1/4 cup	140	1	0	0	26	6	2	7	10
Arrowhead Mills, Chickpeas (Garbanzos)									
1/4 cup	160	2.5	0	0	27	8	5	9	10
Arrowhead Mills, Green Lentils									
1/4 cup	150	1	0	0	27	7	1	10	5

Food Serving size	Cal.	(g) Total Fat	(g) Sat. Fat	(mg) Chol.	(g) Carb.	(g) Fiber	(g) Sug.	(g) Prot.	(mg) Sod.
Arrowhead Mills, Green Split Peas 1/4 cup	160	1	0	0	24	4	1	12	10
Arrowhead Mills, Pinto Beans 1/4 cup	150	0	0	0	27	10	2	9	0
Arrowhead Mills, Red Lentils 1/4 cup	170	1	0	0	28	7	1	13	5
Eden Foods, Aduki Beans, Dry, Organic 3 tbsp	120	0	0	0	22	5	0	7	0
Eden Foods, Baked Beans with Sorghum & Mustard, Organic 1/2 cup	150	0	0	NA	27	7	6	8	130
Eden Foods, Black Beans, Organic 1/2 cup	110	1	0	NA	18	6	NA	7	15
Eden Foods, Black Eyed Peas, Organic 1/2 cup	90	1	0	0	16	4	<1	6	25
Eden Foods, Black Soybean, Dry, Organic 3 tbsp	140	5	0.5	0	11	8	NA	13	0
Eden Foods, Black Soybeans, Organic 1/2 cup	120	6	1	0	8	7	1	11	30
Eden Foods, Black Turtle Beans, Dry, Organic 3 tbsp	110	1	0	NA	18	6	NA	7	15
Eden Foods, Brown Rice & Kidney Beans, Organic 1/2 cup	110	1	0	NA	23	3	0	3	135
Eden Foods, Brown Rice & Lentils, Organic 1/2 cup	120	1	0	NA	23	2	0	4	120
Eden Foods, Brown Rice & Mugwort Mochi, 100% Whole Grain 1 square	110	1	0	0	24	2	0	2	10
Eden Foods, Brown Rice & Pinto Beans, Organic 1/2 cup	120	1	0	NA	24	3	<1	4	140
Eden Foods, Butter Beans (Baby Lima), Organic 1/2 cup	100	1	0	0	17	4	NA	5	35
Eden Foods, Cannellini (White Kidney) Beans, Organic 1/2 cup	100	1	0	0	17	5	1	6	40
Eden Foods, Caribbean Black Beans, Organic 1/2 cup	90	0.5	0	NA	20	7	1	7	135

Food Serving size	Cal.	(g) Total Fat	(g) Sat. Fat	(mg) Chol.	(g) Carb.	(g) Fiber	(g) Sug.	(g) Prot.	(mg) Sod.
Eden Foods, Dark Red Kidney Beans, Dry, Organic									
3 tbsp	120	0	0	0	21	5	<1	8	0
Eden Foods, Garbanzo Beans (chick peas), Organic									
1/2 cup	120	1.5	0	0	19	5	NA	7	110
Eden Foods, Great Northern Beans, Organic									
1/2 cup	110	1	0	0	20	8	1	5	45
Eden Foods, Green Lentils, Dry, Organic									
3 tbsp	120	0	0	0	21	11	<1	9	0
Eden Foods, Green Split Peas, Dry, Organic									
3 tbsp	120	0	0	0	21	9	3	9	5
Eden Foods, Kidney (dark red) Beans, Organic									
1/2 cup	100	0	0	NA	18	10	<1	8	15
Eden Foods, Lentils with Onion & Bay Leaf, Organic									
1/2 cup	90	0	0	NA	13	4	0	8	210
Eden Foods, Navy Beans, Dry, Organic									
3 tbsp	120	0.5	0	0	21	9	1	8	0
Eden Foods, Navy Beans, Organic									
1/2 cup	110	0	0	0	20	7	NA	7	15
Eden Foods, Organic Shiro Miso (Aged and Fermented Rice and Soybeans)									
1 tbsp	30	0.5	0	0	6	<1	4	1	330
Eden Foods, Pinto Beans, Dry, Organic									
3 tbsp	120	0	0	0	22	5	<1	7	0
Eden Foods, Pinto Beans, Organic									
1/2 cup	100	0	0	0	18	6	0	6	110
Eden Foods, Refried Black Beans, Organic									
1/2 cup	110	1.5	0	NA	18	7	NA	6	180
Eden Foods, Refried Black Soy & Black Beans, Organic									
1/2 cup	90	3	0.5	NA	13	6	1	8	170
Eden Foods, Refried Kidney Beans, Organic									
1/2 cup	80	1	0	15	15	6	NA	7	180
Eden Foods, Refried Pinto Beans, Organic									
1/2 cup	90	1	0	NA	19	7	1	6	180
Eden Foods, Small Red Beans, Dry, Organic									
3 tbsp	120	0	0	0	22	3	<1	8	5

Food Serving size	Cal.	(g) Total Fat	(g) Sat. Fat	(mg) Chol.	(g) Carb.	(g) Fiber	(g) Sug.	(g) Prot.	(mg) Sod.
Eden Foods, Small Red Beans, Organic									
1/2 cup	100	0.5	0	0	17	5	<1	6	25
Eden Foods, Spicy Refried Black Beans, Organic									
1/2 cup	110	1.5	0	NA	18	7	NA	6	180
Frieda's, Edamame									
1/2 cup	100	3	NA	NA	10	3	2	8	10
Gopicnic Gluten Free, Ready-to-Eat Hummus + Crackers									
1 box	400	18	3	0	39	12	15	25	350
Sabra Hummus Singles, Classic Hummus									
1/4 cup	150	11	1.5	0	9	3	1	4	260
Sabra, Asian Fusion Garden Hummus									
2 tbsp	70	5	0.5	0	5	2	1	2	120
Sabra, Basil Pesto Hummus									
2 tbsp	90	7	1	0	6	2	1	2	125
Sabra, Buffalo Style Hummus									
2 tbsp	90	6	1	0	6	2	1	2	130
Sabra, Chipotle Hummus									
2 tbsp	70	6	1	0	4	1	1	2	135
Sabra, Classic Hummus									
2 tbsp	70	6	1	0	4	1	0	2	120
Sabra, Greek Olive Hummus									
2 tbsp	70	6	1	0	4	1	0	2	130
Sabra, Jalapeno Hummus									
2 tbsp	70	6	1	0	3	<1	1	1	170
Sabra, Luscious Lemon Hummus									
2 tbsp	70	6	1	0	4	1	1	2	120
Sabra, Roasted Garlic Hummus									
2 tbsp	70	6	1	0	4	1	1	2	120
Sabra, Roasted Garlic Hummus with Pretzels									
1 cup	250	22	3	0	13	3	2	6	420
Sabra, Roasted Pine Nut Hummus									
2 tbsp	80	7	1	0	4	1	0	2	125
Sabra, Roasted Red Pepper Hummus									
2 tbsp	70	6	1	0	4	1	0	2	120

Food Serving size	Cal.	(g) Total Fat	(g) Sat. Fat	(mg) Chol.	(g) Carb.	(g) Fiber	(g) Sug.	(g) Prot.	(mg) Sod.
Sabra, Roasted Red Pepper Hummus with Pretzels									
1 cup	250	22	3	0	13	3	2	6	420
Sabra, Southwest Garden Hummus									
2 tbsp	70	4.5	0.5	0	5	2	0	2	125
Sabra, Spinach and Artichoke Hummus									
2 tbsp	70	6	1	0	4	1	0	1	150
Sabra, Sun Dried Tomato Hummus									
2 tbsp	70	6	1	0	4	1	0	2	120
Sabra, Supremely Spicy Hummus									
2 tbsp	70	6	1	0	4	1	0	2	130
Sabra, Tahini Hummus									
2 tbsp	80	6	1	0	4	1	0	2	120
Sabra, Tuscan Garden Hummus									
2 tbsp	70	5	1	0	5	1	1	2	110
Simply Organic Foods, Chipotle Black Bean Dip									
1 tsp	15	0	0	0	2	1	0	1	140
Tasty Bite, Bangkok Beans									
1/2 pack	150	5	0	0	20	5	4	7	480
Tasty Bite, Bengal Lentils									
1/2 pack	160	6	0.5	0	20	7	4	7	480
Tasty Bite, Channa Masala									
1/2 pack	180	8	1	0	20	6	5	6	400
Tasty Bite, Chunky Chickpeas									
1/2 pack	210	7	0.5	0	30	10	5	9	350

Meats (Beef, Lamb, Pork)

Food Serving size	Cal.	(g) Total Fat	(g) Sat. Fat	(mg) Chol.	(g) Carb.	(g) Fiber	(g) Sug.	(g) Prot.	(mg) Sod.
Aidell's, Carmelized Onion Meatballs									
3 meatballs	130	9	2.5	55	3	0	2	10	480
Aidell's, Zesty Italian Style with Mozzarella Cheese Meatballs									
3 meatballs	140	10	3	60	2	0	<1	12	490
Amy's, Bistro Veggie Burger									
2.5 oz	110	3	0	0	15	2	1	5	330
Amy's, Sonoma Veggie Burger									
1 burger	140	5	0.5	0	18	3	2	5	450

Food Serving size	Cal.	(g) Total Fat	(g) Sat. Fat	(mg) Chol.	(g) Carb.	(g) Fiber	(g) Sug.	(g) Prot.	(mg) Sod.
Applegate Farms, Antibiotic Free Canadian Bacon 2 slices	90	4	1.5	35	1	0	1	12	500
Applegate Farms, Antibiotic Free Honey Ham 2 oz	70	1.5	0.5	30	3	0	3	10	450
Applegate Farms, Antibiotic Free Roast Beef 2 oz	80	3	1	35	0	0	0	12	320
Applegate Farms, Antibiotic Free Slow Cooked Ham 2 oz	60	1.5	0.5	35	0	0	0	11	480
Applegate Farms, Antibiotic Free Sunday Bacon 2 pan fried slices	60	5	2	10	0	0	0	4	290
Applegate Farms, Antibiotic Free Uncured Black Forest Ham 2 oz	50	1.5	0.5	35	0	0	0	10	480
Applegate Farms, Black Forest Ham 2 oz	60	2.5	1	30	0	0	0	9	320
Applegate Farms, Hand-Tied Maple Ham 2 oz	60	1.5	0.5	35	2	0	2	10	520
Applegate Farms, Organic Beef Burgers 1 cooked	195	12	5	70	0	0	0	21	85
Applegate Farms, Organic Roast Beef 2 oz	80	3	1	35	0	0	0	12	320
Applegate Farms, Organic Sunday Bacon 2 pan fried slices	60	5	2	10	0	0	0	4	290
Applegate Farms, Organic Uncured Ham 2 oz	50	1.5	0.5	35	0	0	0	10	530
Applegate Farms, Peppered Eye Round Roast Beef 2 oz	80	3	1	30	0	0	0	12	200
Applegate Farms, Roast Beef 2 oz	80	3	1	30	0	0	0	12	200
Applegate Farms, Slow Cooked Ham 2 oz	60	1.5	0.5	35	0	0	0	11	480
Applegate Farms, Uncured Cooked Capicola Ham 2 oz	60	2.5	1	30	1	0	0	9	370
Applegate Farms, Virginia-Brand Ham 2 oz	50	1.5	0.5	30	1	0	1	9	480

Food Serving size	Cal.	(g) Total Fat	(g) Sat. Fat	(mg) Chol.	(g) Carb.	(g) Fiber	(g) Sug.	(g) Prot.	(mg) Sod.
Beef, Bottom Round, Roast, Lean Only, 0" Fat, Choice, Roasted 1 roast (yield from 627g raw meat) (515g)									
	953	39	14	402	0	0	0	140	185
Beef, Bottom Sirloin, Tri-tip Roast, Lean and Fat, 0" Fat, All Grades, Cooked, Roasted 1 roast (yield from 690g raw meat) (569g)									
	1201	63	23	472	0	0	0	148	302
Beef, Bottom Sirloin, Tri-tip Roast, Lean and Fat, 0" Fat, Choice, Cooked, Roasted 1 roast (yield from 714g raw meat) (591g)									
	1306	73	27	502	0	0	0	152	296
Beef, Bottom Sirloin, Tri-tip Roast, Lean and Fat, 0" Fat, Select, Cooked, Roasted 1 roast (yield from 666g raw meat) (547g)									
	1099	53	20	443	0	0	0	145	306
Beef, Bottom Sirloin, Tri-tip Roast, Lean, 0" Fat, Choice, Cooked, Roasted 1 roast (591g)	1141	58	21	473	0	0	0	156	319
Beef, Bottom Sirloin, Tri-tip Roast, Lean, 0" Fat, Select, Cooked, Roasted 1 roast (yield from 666g raw meat) (547g)									
	979	38	14	416	0	0	0	149	317
Beef, Bottom Sirloin, Tri-tip Steak, Lean, 0" fat, All Grades, Cooked, Broiled 1 lb (453.6g)	1134	60	22	485	0	0	0	139	331
Beef, Brisket, Flat Half, Lean and Fat, 0" Fat, All Grades, Cooked, Braised 1 steak (yield from 418g raw meat) (270g)									
	575	22	9	248	0	0	0	89	146
Beef, Brisket, Flat Half, Lean and Fat, 0" Fat, Select, Cooked, Braised 1 steak (yield from 388g raw meat) (247g)									
	506	17	7	230	0	0	0	83	141
Beef, Brisket, Flat Half, Lean and Fat, 1/8" Fat, All Grades, Cooked, Braised 3 oz (85g)	246	16	6	90	0	0	0	24	41
Beef, Brisket, Whole, Lean and Fat, 1/8" Fat, All Grades, Cooked, Braised 3 oz (85g)	281	21	8	79	0	0	0	22	54
Beef, Chuck Eye Country-style Ribs, Boneless, Lean, 0" Fat, Choice, Cooked 1 piece (224g)	524	27	12	224	0	0	8	69	155
Beef, Chuck Eye Roast, Boneless, America's Beef Roast, Lean, 0" Fat, All Grades, Cooked 1 roast (609g)	1114	52	21	512	0	0	0	162	487

Food Serving size	Cal.	(g) Total Fat	(g) Sat. Fat	(mg) Chol.	(g) Carb.	(g) Fiber	(g) Sug.	(g) Prot.	(mg) Sod.
Beef, Chuck, Short Ribs, Boneless, Lean and Fat, 0" Fat, All Grades, Cooked, Braised									
1 piece (289g)	881	65	29	289	0	0	14	74	202
Beef, Composite of Retail Cuts, Lean, 0" Fat, All Grades, Cooked									
3 oz (85g)	179	8	3	73	0	0	0	25	56
Beef, Flank, Steak, Lean and Fat, 0" Fat, All Grades, Cooked, Broiled									
1 steak (yield from 475g raw meat) (383g)	735	32	13	303	0	0	0	106	214
Beef, Ground, 70% Lean Meat/30% Fat, Crumbles, Cooked, Pan-browned									
1 portion (yield from 1/2 lb raw meat) (139g)	375	25	10	122	0	0	0	36	133
Beef, Ground, 75% Lean Meat, 25% Fat, Patty, Cooked, Broiled									
1 patty (yield from 1/4 lb raw meat) (70g)	195	13	5	62	0	0	1	18	55
Beef, Ground, 75% Lean Meat, 25% Fat, Patty, Cooked, Pan-broiled									
1 patty (yield from 1/4 lb raw meat) (77g)	191	13	5	64	0	0	4	18	67
Beef, Loin, Porterhouse Steak, Lean and Fat, 0" Fat, USDA Choice, Cooked, Broiled									
1 lb (453.6g)	1284	91	34	313	0	0	0	107	295
Beef, Loin, T-bone Steak, Lean & Fat, 0" Fat, USDA Choice, Cooked, Broiled									
1 lb (453.6g)	1170	78	29	277	0	0	0	109	304
Beef, Rib Eye, Small End (Ribs 10-12), Lean and Fat, 0" Fat, All Grades, Cooked, Broiled									
1 steak (yield from 295g raw meat) (233g)	580	34	13	207	0	0	0	64	130
Beef, Rib, Large End (Ribs 6-9), Lean and Fat, 1/8" Fat, All Grades, Cooked, Broiled									
3 oz (85g)	287	23	9	68	0	0	NA	18	54
Beef, Rib, Small End (Ribs 10-12), Lean and Fat, 0" Fat, All Grades, Cooked, Broiled									
3 oz (85g)	212	13	5	76	0	0	0	23	48
Beef, Rib, Whole (Ribs 6-12), Lean and Fat, 1/8" Fat, All Grades, Cooked, Roasted									
3 oz (85g)	298	24	10	71	0	0	NA	19	54
Beef, Round, Bottom Round Roast, Lean, 1/8" Fat, Select, Cooked, Roasted									
1 lb (453.6g)	744	21	7	336	0	0	19	129	172

Food Serving size	Cal.	(g) Total Fat	(g) Sat. Fat	(mg) Chol.	(g) Carb.	(g) Fiber	(g) Sug.	(g) Prot.	(mg) Sod.
Beef, Short Loin, Porterhouse Steak, Lean and Fat, 1/8" Fat, All Grades, Cooked, Broiled									
3 oz (85g)	252	19	7	60	0	0	3	20	54
Beef, Short Loin, T-bone Steak, Lean, 0" Fat, Choice, Cooked, Broiled									
1 serving (85g)	168	8	3	71	0	0	0	22	60
Beef, Short Loin, Top Loin, Steak, Lean and Fat, 0" Fat, All Grades, Cooked, Broiled									
1 steak, excluding refuse (yield from 1 raw steak, with refuse, weighing 223 g) (155g)	299	12	5	126	0	0	0	45	91
Beef, Shoulder Pot Roast, Boneless, Lean and Fat, 0" Fat, All Grades, Cooked, Braised									
1 roast (787g)	1605	70	24	763	0	0	0	244	480
Beef, Sirloin, Tri-tip Steak, Lean and Fat, 0" Fat, All Grades, Cooked, Broiled									
1 lb (453.6g)	1202	69	26	308	0	0	NA	136	327
Beef, Tenderloin, Lean and Fat, 0" Fat, Select, Cooked, Broiled									
1 steak (yield from 136g raw meat) (108g)	221	11	4	90	0	0	0	29	63
Beef, Top Sirloin, Steak, Lean and Fat, 0" Fat, Choice, Cooked, Broiled									
1 steak (yield from 532g raw meat) (393g)	861	41	16	350	0	0	0	114	228
Beef, Variety Meats and By-products, Thymus, Cooked, Braised									
3 oz (85g)	271	21	7	250	0	0	NA	19	99
Boar's Head, All Natural Cap-Off Top Round Oven Roasted Beef									
2 oz	80	3	1	40	0	0	0	14	140
Boar's Head, All Natural Smoked Uncured Ham									
2 oz	60	1.5	0.5	35	<1	0	1	12	340
Boar's Head, All Natural Uncured Ham									
2 oz	70	1	0	35	1	0	1	12	340
Boar's Head, Diced Pancetta									
1 oz	110	9	4.5	20	1	NA	NA	4	450
Boar's Head, Pancetta									
5 oz	50	4.5	2	10	0	0	0	2	230
Boar's Head, Porketta									
2 oz	70	2	1	25	1	NA	1	11	470
Hormel Natural, Bacon									
15g	80	7	2.5	20	0	0	0	5	360

Food Serving size	Cal.	(g) Total Fat	(g) Sat. Fat	(mg) Chol.	(g) Carb.	(g) Fiber	(g) Sug.	(g) Prot.	(mg) Sod.
Jones Dairy Farms, Bacon, Old Fashioned Slab 2 oz	240	24	9	35	0	0	0	6	500
Jones Dairy Farms, Bacon, Sliced, Regular 2 slices	90	8	3	15	0	0	0	4	350
Jones Dairy Farms, Bacon, Sliced, Regular, Cherry Hardwood Smoked 1 slice	50	4	1.5	10	0	0	0	3	130
Jones Dairy Farms, Bacon, Sliced, Thick 1 slice	70	6	2.5	15	0	0	0	3	290
Jones Dairy Farms, Ham Slices 2 slices	50	1.5	0	30	1	0	0	8	500
Jones Dairy Farms, Ham Steak 3 oz	100	4	1	50	1	0	0	14	760
Jones Dairy Farms, Ham Steaks, All Natural Cherry Hardwood Smoked, Uncured 3 oz	120	4	1	50	3	0	2	18	760
Jones Dairy Farms, Ham, Dainty, Hickory Smoked, Fully Cooked 2 oz	100	4	1	50	2	0	0	15	760
Jones Dairy Farms, Ham, Half Family, Fully Cooked 2 oz	70	3	0.5	30	2	0	0	9	730
Jones Dairy Farms, Ham, Whole Family, Fully Cooked 2 oz	70	3	0.5	30	2	0	0	9	500
Jones Dairy Farms, Ham, Whole Short Shanked, Fully Cooked Hickory 3 oz	180	13	5	80	1	0	0	15	950
Jones Dairy Farms, Ham, Whole, Country Club, Fully Cooked 2 oz	70	3	0.5	30	2	0	0	9	730
Jones Dairy Farms, Ham, Whole-Old Fashioned, Hickory Smoked 3 oz	200	15	5	60	0	0	0	15	1200
Lamb, Domestic, Composite of Retail Cuts, Fat, 1/4" Fat, Choice, Cooked 3 oz (85g)	498	50	23	97	0	0	0	10	49
Lamb, Domestic, Leg, Shank Half, Lean and Fat, 1/4" Fat, Choice, Cooked, Roasted 3 oz (85g)	191	11	4	77	0	0	NA	22	55
Pork, Fresh, Composite (Leg, Loin, Shoulder and Spareribs), Lean and Fat, Cooked 3 oz (85g)	202	12	4	75	0	0	0	22	48

Food Serving size	Cal.	(g) Total Fat	(g) Sat. Fat	(mg) Chol.	(g) Carb.	(g) Fiber	(g) Sug.	(g) Prot.	(mg) Sod.
Pork, Fresh, Composite of Retail Cuts (Leg, Loin and Shoulder), Lean, Cooked									
3 oz (85g)	171	8	3	71	0	0	0	23	47
Pork, Fresh, Loin, Center Loin (Chops), Bone-in, Lean and Fat, Cooked, Broiled									
3 oz (85g)	178	9	3	71	0	0	0	22	47
Pork, Fresh, Loin, Sirloin (Roasts), Boneless, Lean and Fat, Cooked, Roasted									
3 oz (85g)	176	8	3	73	0	0	0	24	48
Pork, Fresh, Loin, Top Loin (Chops), Boneless, Lean and Fat, Cooked, Broiled									
3 oz (85g)	167	8	3	62	0	0	0	23	37
Pork, Fresh, Variety Meats and By-products, Liver, Cooked, Braised									
3 oz (85g)	140	4	1	302	3	0	NA	22	42
Thumann's, Hickory Smoked Sliced Bacon									
2 oz	80	7	3	15	0	0	0	4	280
Veal, Loin, Lean and Fat, Cooked, Roasted									
3 oz (85g)	184	10	4	88	0	0	0	21	79
Veal, Loin, Lean, Cooked, Braised									
1 chop, excluding refuse (yield from 1 raw chop, with refuse, weighing 195g) (69g)									
	156	6	2	86	0	0	0	23	58

Nuts & Seeds, Including Nut Butters

Food Serving size	Cal.	(g) Total Fat	(g) Sat. Fat	(mg) Chol.	(g) Carb.	(g) Fiber	(g) Sug.	(g) Prot.	(mg) Sod.
Acorns, Raw									
1 oz (28.35g)	110	7	1	0	12	NA	NA	2	0
Arrowhead Mills, Flax Seeds									
3 tbsp	140	9	1	0	9	7	0	6	0
Arrowhead Mills, Gluten Free Nut Butters, Cashew Butter, Creamy									
2 tbsp	160	13	2.5	NA	9	<1	2	4	0
Arrowhead Mills, Gluten Free Nut Butters, Creamy Almond Butter, Roasted									
2 tbsp	200	17	1.5	NA	6	4	2	7	0
Arrowhead Mills, Gluten Free Nut Butters, Creamy Peanut Butter									
2 tbsp	190	17	2.5	0	6	2	1	8	0
Arrowhead Mills, Gluten Free Nut Butters, Crunchy Peanut Butter									
2 tbsp	190	17	2.5	0	6	2	1	8	0
Arrowhead Mills, Gluten Free Nut Butters, Organic Peanut Butter, Creamy									
2 tbsp	190	17	2.5	0	6	2	1	8	0
Arrowhead Mills, Gluten Free Nut Butters, Organic Peanut Butter, Crunchy									
2 tbsp	190	17	2.5	0	6	2	1	8	0

Food Serving size	Cal.	(g) Total Fat	(g) Sat. Fat	(mg) Chol.	(g) Carb.	(g) Fiber	(g) Sug.	(g) Prot.	(mg) Sod.
Arrowhead Mills, Gluten Free Nut Butters, Sesame Tahini, Organic									
2 tbsp	190	18	2.5	0	3	<1	1	8	10
Arrowhead Mills, Mechanically Hulled Sesame Seeds									
1/4 cup	210	19	2.5	0	3	1	0	9	15
Arrowhead Mills, Organic Flax Seed Meal									
2 tbsp	80	4.5	0.5	0	5	4	0	3	0
Arrowhead Mills, Organic Golden Flax Seeds									
3 tbsp	160	10	1	0	10	9	0	8	10
Arrowhead Mills, Sunflower Seeds									
1/4 cup	170	15	1.5	0	6	3	1	7	0
Arrowhead Mills, Unhulled Sesame Seeds									
1/4 cup	190	17	2.5	0	8	4	0	6	0
Betty Crocker, Bhuja Fruit and Nut Mix									
25g	123	7	1	0	10	3	6	5	71
Bhuja, Fruit and Nut Mix									
.88 oz	123	7	1	0	10	3	6	5	71
Bhuja, Nut Mix									
.88 oz	156	12	2	0	5	2	2	5	165
Bhuja, Seasoned Almonds									
.88 oz	156	13	1	0	4.9	2	2	5.45	168
Bhuja, Seasoned Cashews									
.88 oz	158	13	2	0	5	1	1	4	128
Bhuja, Seasoned Peanuts									
.88 oz	155	12	2	0	4	2	1	6	132
Bob's Red Mill, Brown Flaxseeds									
2 tbsp	90	8	0.5	0	7	6	0	4	5
Bob's Red Mill, Flaxseed Meal									
2 tbsp	60	4.5	0	0	4	4	0	3	0
Bob's Red Mill, Golden Flaxseed									
2 tbsp	90	8	0.5	0	7	6	0	4	5
Bob's Red Mill, Golden Flaxseed Meal									
2 tbsp	60	4.5	0	0	4	4	0	3	0
Bob's Red Mill, Organic Brown Flaxseed Meal									
2 tbsp	60	4.5	0	0	4	4	0	3	0

Food Serving size	Cal.	(g) Total Fat	(g) Sat. Fat	(mg) Chol.	(g) Carb.	(g) Fiber	(g) Sug.	(g) Prot.	(mg) Sod.
Bob's Red Mill, Organic Brown Flaxseeds									
2 tbsp	90	8	0.5	0	7	6	0	4	5
Bob's Red Mill, Organic Golden Flaxseed Meal									
2 tbsp	60	4.5	0	0	4	4	0	3	0
Bob's Red Mill, Organic Golden Flaxseeds									
2 tbsp	90	8	0.5	0	7	6	0	4	5
Borage, Raw									
1 cup (1″ pieces) (89g)	19	1	0	0	3	NA	NA	2	71
Breadfruit Seeds, Raw									
1 oz (28.35g)	54	2	0	0	8	1.5	NA	2	7
Breadfruit, Raw									
.25 fruit, small (96g)	99	0	0	0	26	4.7	11	1	2
Broadbeans (Fava Beans), Mature Seeds, Raw									
1 tbsp (9.4g)	32	0	0	0	5	2.4	1	2	1
Broadbeans, Immature Seeds, Raw									
1 broadbean (8g)	6	0	0	0	1	0.3	NA	0	4
Chestnuts, Chinese, Raw									
1 oz (28.35g)	64	0	0	0	14	NA	NA	1	1
Chestnuts, European, Raw, Peeled									
1 oz (28.35g)	56	0	0	0	13	NA	NA	0	1
Chestnuts, European, Raw, Unpeeled									
1 oz (28.35g)	60	1	0	0	13	2.3	NA	1	1
Chestnuts, Japanese, Raw									
1 oz (28.35g)	44	0	0	0	10	NA	NA	1	4
Coconut Cream, Raw (Liquid Expressed from Grated Meat)									
1 tbsp (15g)	50	5	5	0	1	0.3	NA	1	1
Coconut Meat, Raw									
1 medium (397g)	1405	133	118	0	60	35.7	25	13	79
Earth Balance, Creamy Almond Nut Butter									
2 tbsp	170	16	1	0	6	4	2	7	110
Earth Balance, Creamy Coconut Nut Butter									
2 tbsp	190	17	5	0	7	2	2	6	95
Earth Balance, Creamy Peanut Nut Butter									
2 tbsp	190	17	3	0	7	3	2	7	110

Food Serving size	Cal.	(g) Total Fat	(g) Sat. Fat	(mg) Chol.	(g) Carb.	(g) Fiber	(g) Sug.	(g) Prot.	(mg) Sod.
Earth Balance, Crunchy Coconut Nut Butter 2 tbsp	190	17	5	0	7	2	2	6	95
Earth Balance, Crunchy Peanut Nut Butter 2 tbsp	190	17	3	0	7	3	2	7	110
Eden Foods, All Mixed Up (Nuts and Dried Fruit) 3 tbsp	160	12	2	0	7	4	2	8	70
Eden Foods, All Mixed Up Too (Nuts, Seeds and Dried Fruits) 3 tbsp	140	11	1.5	0	10	4	3	5	15
Eden Foods, Pistachios, Shelled, Dry Roasted, Organic 3 tbsp	160	12	1.5	0	7	3	1	6	60
Eden Foods, Pumpkin Seeds – Dry Roasted & Sea Salted, Organic 1/4 cup	200	16	3	0	5	5	0	10	100
Eden Foods, Spicy Pumpkin Seeds – Tamari Dry Roasted, Organic 1/4 cup	200	16	3	0	5	5	0	10	75
Eden Foods, Tamari Roasted Almonds, Organic 3 tbsp	160	11	1	0	8	4	<1	8	65
Eden Foods, Tamari Roasted Spicy Pumpkin Seeds, Organic 1/4 cup	200	16	3	0	5	5	1	10	75
Enjoy Life Foods, Beach Bash Seed & Fruit Mix 28g	130	7	1	0	13	2	9	4	45
Enjoy Life Foods, Mountain Mambo Seed & Fruit Mix 28g	140	8	1.5	0	12	2	9	5	45
Enjoy Life, Not Nuts! Seed and Fruit Mix – Mountain Mambo 28g	140	8	1.5	0	12	2	9	5	45
Frieda's, BBQ Soy Nuts 1 serving	140	7	1	NA	11	5	2	10	110
Frieda's, Honey Roasted Soy Nuts 1 serving	140	7	1	NA	11	5	3	10	110
Frieda's, Pine Nuts 1/4 cup	150	15	2	NA	4	1	NA	7	NA
Frieda's, Roasted Salted Soy Nuts 1/3 cup	140	7	1	NA	9	1	NA	11	50
Frieda's, Unsalted Soy Nuts 1/3 cup	140	7	1	NA	9	1	NA	NA	NA

Food Serving size	Cal.	(g) Total Fat	(g) Sat. Fat	(mg) Chol.	(g) Carb.	(g) Fiber	(g) Sug.	(g) Prot.	(mg) Sod.
Frieda's, Wasabi Flavored Soy Nuts 1 serving	140	7	1	NA	11	5	2	10	110
Frito-Lay, Cashews, Salted 1 package	240	20	4	0	12	2	3	6	180
Frito-Lay, Deluxe Mixed Nuts About 1/4 cup	170	16	2.5	0	6	2	1	4	115
Frito-Lay, Munchies Wasabi Almonds 1 package	260	23	2.5	0	8	5	2	9	150
Frito-Lay, Nut Harvest Natural Lightly Roasted Almonds About 2 tbsp	180	15	1.5	0	6	3	1	6	150
Frito-Lay, Nut Harvest Natural Nut & Fruit Mix About 1/4 cup	150	9	1.5	0	12	2	7	4	80
Frito-Lay, Nut Harvest Natural Sea Salted Whole Cashews About 2 tbsp	170	13	2.5	0	9	1	2	4	150
Frito-Lay, Praline Pecans 1 package	350	26	2.5	0	26	4	9	4	230
Frito-Lay, Ranch Sunflower Seeds 1 package	200	17	2	0	7	3	3	5	1400
Frito-Lay, Salted In-Shell Peanuts 1 oz	160	14	2	0	6	2	1	7	170
Frito-Lay, Sunflower Seed Kernels 1 package	380	33	4.5	0	10	4	3	12	230
Frito-Lay, Sunflower Seeds 1 oz	190	16	2	0	5	3	<1	6	90
Frito-Lay, Trail Mix Nut & Chocolate 28g	160	10	2.5	0	13	2	11	4	65
Frito-Lay, Trail Mix Nut & Fruit 1 oz	150	9	1.5	0	12	2	7	4	80
Ginkgo Nuts, Raw 1 oz (28.35g)	52	0	0	0	11	NA	NA	1	2
Hodgson Mill, Milled Flax Seed 2 tbsp	60	5	0	0	4	4	0	3	0
Hodgson Mill, Milled Flax Seed "Travel Flax" 1 packet	30	2	0	0	2	2	0	1	0

Food Serving size	Cal.	(g) Total Fat	(g) Sat. Fat	(mg) Chol.	(g) Carb.	(g) Fiber	(g) Sug.	(g) Prot.	(mg) Sod.
Hodgson Mill, Organic Golden Milled Flax Seed 2 tbsp	65	4	0	0	4	4	0	3	0
Hodgson Mill, Organic Golden Milled Flax Seed "Travel Flax" 1 packet	30	2	0	0	2	2	0	1	0
Hodgson Mill, Whole Grain Flax Seed 3 tbsp	160	11	1	0	9	9	0	6	9
I.M. Healthy, Chocolate SoyNut Butter 2 tbsp	190	14	2	0	12	3	8	6	0
I.M. Healthy, Honey Creamy SoyNut Butter 2 tbsp	190	14	2	0	10	3	4	7	100
I.M. Healthy, Original Chunky SoyNut Butter 2 tbsp	190	14	2.5	0	10	3	3	7	100
I.M. Healthy, Original Creamy SoyNut Butter 2 tbsp	190	14	2.5	0	10	3	3	7	100
I.M. Healthy, Unsweetened Creamy SoyNut Butter 2 tbsp	190	15	2	0	6	5	1	9	100
Justin's, Chocolate Almond Butter 2 tbsp	180	14	2.5	0	11	3	7	5	75
Justin's, Chocolate Hazelnut Butter 2 tbsp	180	15	3	0	12	3	7	4	65
Justin's, Chocolate Peanut Butter 2 tbsp	170	13	3	0	11	2	7	5	75
Justin's, Classic Almond Butter 2 tbsp	200	18	2	0	6	4	2	7	0
Justin's, Classic Peanut Butter 2 tbsp	200	17	3	0	7	2	1	7	0
Justin's, Honey Almond Butter 2 tbsp	190	17	1.5	0	8	3	3	6	65
Justin's, Honey Peanut Butter 2 tbsp	190	16	3	0	8	2	3	6	65
Justin's, Maple Almond Butter 2 tbsp	200	17	2	0	8	3	3	6	70
Lotus Seeds, Raw 1 oz (28.35g)	25	0	0	0	5	NA	NA	1	0

Food Serving size	Cal.	(g) Total Fat	(g) Sat. Fat	(mg) Chol.	(g) Carb.	(g) Fiber	(g) Sug.	(g) Prot.	(mg) Sod.
Macadamia Nuts, Raw									
1 oz (10-12 kernels) (28.35g)	204	21	3	0	4	2.4	1	2	1
Maple Grove Farms, No Salt Added Natural Crunchy Peanut Butter									
2 tbsp	190	15	2	NA	6	2	2	8	15
MaraNatha Nut Butters, All Natural Almond Butter – No Salt (Creamy)									
2 tbsp	190	16	1.5	0	6	4	2	7	0
MaraNatha Nut Butters, All Natural Almond Butter – No Salt (Crunchy)									
2 tbsp	190	16	1.5	0	6	4	NA	7	0
MaraNatha Nut Butters, All Natural Honey Almond Butter									
2 tbsp	180	14	1	0	9	3	5	6	70
MaraNatha Nut Butters, All Natural Raw Almond Butter									
2 tbsp	195	16	1	0	6	4	2	7	0
MaraNatha Nut Butters, Almond Butter – Hint of Sea Salt (Creamy)									
2 tbsp	180	16	1	0	6	4	2	7	60
MaraNatha Nut Butters, Almond Butter – Hint of Sea Salt (Crunchy)									
2 tbsp	180	16	1	0	6	4	2	7	60
MaraNatha Nut Butters, Natural Peanut Butter – With Hint of Sea Salt (Creamy)									
2 tbsp	190	16	2	0	7	3	1	8	80
MaraNatha Nut Butters, Natural Peanut Butter – With Hint of Sea Salt (Crunchy)									
2 tbsp	190	16	2	0	7	3	1	8	80
MaraNatha Nut Butters, No Stir Almond Butter (Creamy)									
2 tbsp	190	17	2.5	0	7	3	3	6	65
MaraNatha Nut Butters, No Stir Almond Butter (Crunchy)									
2 tbsp	190	17	2.5	0	7	3	3	6	65
MaraNatha Nut Butters, No Stir Natural Peanut Butter (Creamy)									
2 tbsp	190	16	2.5	0	8	2	3	7	70
MaraNatha Nut Butters, No Stir Natural Peanut Butter (Crunchy)									
2 tbsp	190	16	2.5	0	8	2	3	7	70
MaraNatha Nut Butters, No Stir Natural Peanut Spread, with Omega-3's and Calcium (Creamy)									
2 tbsp	180	15	3	0	7	3	3	7	65
MaraNatha Nut Butters, No Stir Organic Peanut Butter (Creamy)									
2 tbsp	190	16	2.5	0	8	2	3	7	70
MaraNatha Nut Butters, No Stir Organic Peanut Butter (Crunchy)									
2 tbsp	190	16	2.5	0	8	2	3	7	70

Food Serving size	Cal.	(g) Total Fat	(g) Sat. Fat	(mg) Chol.	(g) Carb.	(g) Fiber	(g) Sug.	(g) Prot.	(mg) Sod.
MaraNatha Nut Butters, No Stir Raw Maple Almond Butter									
2 tbsp	180	15	1.5	0	9	3	3	6	50
MaraNatha Nut Butters, Organic Almond Butter, No Salt Added (Creamy)									
2 tbsp	190	16	1.5	0	6	4	2	7	0
MaraNatha Nut Butters, Organic Almond Butter, No Salt Added (Crunchy)									
2 tbsp	190	16	1.5	0	6	4	2	7	0
MaraNatha Nut Butters, Organic Peanut Butter, No Salt Added (Creamy)									
2 tbsp	190	16	2	0	7	3	1	8	0
MaraNatha Nut Butters, Organic Peanut Butter, No Salt Added (Crunchy)									
2 tbsp	190	16	2	0	7	3	1	8	0
MaraNatha Nut Butters, Organic Peanut Butter, with Hint of Sea Salt (Creamy)									
2 tbsp	190	16	2	0	7	3	1	8	80
MaraNatha Nut Butters, Organic Peanut Butter, with Hint of Sea Salt (Crunchy)									
2 tbsp	190	16	2	0	7	3	1	8	80
MaraNatha Nut Butters, Organic Raw Almond Butter, No Salt (Creamy)									
2 tbsp	190	17	1.5	0	6	4	2	7	0
MaraNatha Nut Butters, Organic Raw Almond Butter, No Salt (Crunchy)									
2 tbsp	190	17	1.5	0	6	4	2	7	0
MaraNatha Nut Butters, Original Natural Sesame Tahini Butter, with Salt									
2 tbsp	190	17	2.5	0	7	1	0	6	75
MaraNatha Nut Butters, Roasted Natural Sesame Tahini Butter, with Salt									
2 tbsp	190	17	2.5	0	7	1	0	6	75
MaraNatha Nut Butters, Specialty Nut Butters, Dark Chocolate Almond Spread									
2 tbsp	180	14	3	0	12	2	9	4	15
MaraNatha Nut Butters, Specialty Nut Butters, Dark Chocolate Peanut Spread									
2 tbsp	180	13	2	0	12	1	8	5	30
MaraNatha Nut Butters, Specialty Nut Butters, Natural Cashew Butter (Roasted)									
2 tbsp	190	15	3	0	10	2	2	5	0
MaraNatha Nut Butters, Specialty Nut Butters, Sunflower Seed Butter									
2 tbsp	180	12	1.5	0	8	4	<1	9	65
Nuts, Cashew Nuts, Raw									
1 oz (28.35g)	157	12	2	0	9	0.9	2	5	3
Peanuts, All Types, Raw									
1 oz (28.35g)	161	14	2	0	5	2.4	1	7	5

Food Serving size	Cal.	(g) Total Fat	(g) Sat. Fat	(mg) Chol.	(g) Carb.	(g) Fiber	(g) Sug.	(g) Prot.	(mg) Sod.
Peanuts, Spanish, Raw 1 oz (28.35g)	162	14	2	0	4	2.7	NA	7	6
Peanuts, Valencia, Raw 1 oz (28.35g)	162	13	2	0	6	2.5	NA	7	0
Peanuts, Virginia, Raw 1 oz (28.35g)	160	14	2	0	5	2.4	1	7	3
Pecans 1 cup, halves (99g)	684	71	6	0	14	9.5	4	9	0
Pistachio Nuts, Raw 1 oz (49 kernels) (28.35g)	159	13	2	0	8	2.9	2	6	0
Smart Balance, Rich Roast Chunky Peanut Butter and Omega-3 from Flax Oil 2 tbsp	190	16	3	0	8	2	3	7	145
Smart Balance, Rich Roast Creamy Peanut Butter and Omega-3 from Flax Oil 2 tbsp	190	16	3	0	8	2	3	7	145
SunButter, 1.5 Ounce Cup 1 1.5 oz cup	266	21	3	0	9	5	4	9	160
SunButter, Creamy (5 lb pail) 2 tbsp	200	16	2	0	7	4	3	7	120
SunButter, Natural No-Stir (Creamy) 2 tbsp	200	16	2	0	7	4	3	7	120
SunButter, Natural Omega-3 2 tbsp	203	16	1	0	7	3	4	8	100
SunButter, On-The-Go Snack Pack, SunButter Natural, and SunButter Natural Crunch 2 tbsp	200	16	2	0	7	4	3	7	120
SunButter, Organic Unsweetened 2 tbsp	220	20	2	0	5	2	1	6	30
Walnuts, English 1 cup, ground (80g)	523	52	5	0	11	5.4	2	12	2

Poultry

Food Serving size	Cal.	(g) Total Fat	(g) Sat. Fat	(mg) Chol.	(g) Carb.	(g) Fiber	(g) Sug.	(g) Prot.	(mg) Sod.
Applegate Farms, Antibiotic Free Herb Turkey 2 oz	50	0	0	30	0	0	0	12	360
Applegate Farms, Antibiotic Free Honey & Maple Turkey Breast 2 oz	60	0.5	0	25	2	0	2	11	450

Food Serving size	Cal.	(g) Total Fat	(g) Sat. Fat	(mg) Chol.	(g) Carb.	(g) Fiber	(g) Sug.	(g) Prot.	(mg) Sod.
Applegate Farms, Antibiotic Free Roasted Chicken Breast									
2 oz	60	1.5	0.5	30	1	0	1	10	360
Applegate Farms, Antibiotic Free Roasted Turkey Breast									
2 oz	50	0	0	30	0	0	0	12	360
Applegate Farms, Antibiotic Free Smoked Turkey Breast									
2 oz	50	0	0	30	0	0	0	12	360
Applegate Farms, Antibiotic Free Turkey Bacon									
1 pan fried slice	35	1.5	0	25	0	0	0	6	200
Applegate Farms, Barbecue Chicken Breast									
2 oz	70	1	0	25	2	0	1	12	300
Applegate Farms, Chipotle Chicken									
2 oz	60	0.5	0	30	1	0	0	12	400
Applegate Farms, Gluten-Free Chicken Breast Tenders									
2 pieces	130	4.5	1	30	10	0	0	11	350
Applegate Farms, Gluten-Free Chicken Nuggets									
7 nuggets	170	9	1.5	35	11	0	0	12	350
Applegate Farms, Grilled Chicken Breast Strips									
3 oz	100	1	0	40	0	0	0	24	290
Applegate Farms, Herb Turkey Breast									
2 oz	50	0	0	30	0	0	0	12	400
Applegate Farms, Honey Maple Turkey Breast									
2 oz	50	0	0	25	3	0	2	12	450
Applegate Farms, Lemon Rosemary Turkey Breast									
2 oz	70	1.5	0	40	1	0	0	13	330
Applegate Farms, No Salt Turkey									
2 oz	60	0	0	35	0	0	0	15	30
Applegate Farms, Organic Herb Turkey Breast									
2 oz	50	0	0	25	0	0	0	10	360
Applegate Farms, Organic Roasted Chicken Breast									
2 oz	60	1.5	0.5	30	1	0	1	10	360
Applegate Farms, Organic Roasted Turkey Breast									
2 oz	50	0	0	25	0	0	0	10	360
Applegate Farms, Organic Smoked Chicken Breast									
2 oz	60	1.5	0.5	30	1	0	1	10	360

Food Serving size	Cal.	(g) Total Fat	(g) Sat. Fat	(mg) Chol.	(g) Carb.	(g) Fiber	(g) Sug.	(g) Prot.	(mg) Sod.
Applegate Farms, Organic Smoked Turkey Breast									
2 oz	50	0	0	25	0	0	0	10	360
Applegate Farms, Organic Turkey Bacon									
1 pan fried slice	35	1.5	0	25	0	0	0	6	200
Applegate Farms, Organic Turkey Burgers									
1 cooked	140	7	2	60	0	0	0	17	55
Applegate Farms, Organic Uncured Turkey Bologna									
2 oz	90	5.5	1.5	30	0	0	0	9	400
Applegate Farms, Oven Roasted Chicken Breast									
2 oz	70	1.5	0	30	1	0	1	12	310
Applegate Farms, Oven Roasted Turkey Breast									
2 oz	50	0	0	30	0	0	0	12	400
Applegate Farms, Oven Roasted Turkey Breast Layout									
2 oz	50	0	0	30	0	0	0	12	400
Applegate Farms, Peppered Turkey Breast									
2 oz	50	0	0	30	0	0	0	12	360
Applegate Farms, Smoked Chicken Breast									
2 oz	60	1.5	0	30	2	0	1	12	310
Applegate Farms, Smoked Turkey Breast									
2 oz	50	0	0	30	0	0	0	12	400
Applegate Farms, Southwestern Grilled Chicken Breast Strips									
3 oz	90	2	0	45	2	0	0	15	340
Applegate Farms, Southwestern Turkey Breast									
2 oz	50	0	0	25	1	0	0	11	420
Applegate Farms, Turkey Pastrami									
2 oz	50	0	0	30	0	0	0	12	360
Applegate Farms, Uncured Turkey Bologna									
2 oz	90	5.5	1.5	30	0	0	0	9	400
Applegate Farms, Uncured Turkey Salami									
2 oz	70	2	1	30	0	0	0	11	360
Boar's Head, All Natural Roasted Turkey Breast									
2 oz	60	1	0	30	1	0	0	13	330
Boar's Head, All Natural Roasted Turkey Breast with Lemon & Herb									
2 oz	60	1	0	30	0	0	1	12	400

Food Serving size	Cal.	(g) Total Fat	(g) Sat. Fat	(mg) Chol.	(g) Carb.	(g) Fiber	(g) Sug.	(g) Prot.	(mg) Sod.
Boar's Head, All Natural Smoked Turkey Breast									
2 oz	60	1	0	30	0	0	0	14	390
Boar's Head, All Natural Tuscan Brand Roasted Turkey Breast									
2 oz	60	1	0	30	0	0	0	15	380
Chicken, Broilers or Fryers, Breast, Meat Only, Cooked, Roasted									
1 unit (yield from 1 lb ready-to-cook chicken) (52g)	86	2	1	44	0	0	0	16	38
Chicken, Broilers or Fryers, Dark Meat, Meat Only, Cooked, Roasted									
1 unit (yield from 1 lb ready-to-cook chicken) (81g)	166	8	2	75	0	0	0	22	75
Chicken, Broilers or Fryers, Leg, Meat and Skin, Cooked, Roasted									
1 unit (yield from 1 lb ready-to-cook chicken) (69g)	160	9	3	63	0	0	0	18	60
Chicken, Broilers or Fryers, Light Meat, Meat Only, Cooked, Roasted									
1 unit (yield from 1 lb ready-to-cook chicken) (64g)	111	3	1	54	0	0	0	20	49
Chicken, Roasting, Meat Only, Cooked, Roasted									
1 unit (yield from 1 lb ready-to-cook chicken) (171g)	286	11	3	128	0	0	NA	43	128
Duck, Domesticated, Meat Only, Cooked, Roasted									
1 unit (yield from 1 lb ready-to-cook duck) (100g)	201	11	4	89	0	0	0	23	65
Ground Turkey, 93% Lean, 7% Fat, Patties, Broiled									
3 oz (85g)	176	10	3	90	0	0	0	22	77
Hormel Natural, Grilled Carved Chicken Breast									
56g	60	1.5	0.5	35	0	0	0	12	390
Hormel Natural, Oven Roasted Carved Chicken Breast									
56g	60	1.5	0.5	35	0	0	0	12	390
Ian's Natural Foods, Allergy Friendly Chicken Nuggets									
5 nuggets	200	10	1	35	13	<1	0	13	310
Ian's Natural Foods, Allergy Friendly Chicken Patties									
1 patty	210	10	0.5	40	15	<1	0	15	370
Ian's Natural Foods, Allergy Friendly Chicken Tenders									
3 oz	160	6	0.5	30	7	<1	0	20	210

Food Serving size	Cal.	(g) Total Fat	(g) Sat. Fat	(mg) Chol.	(g) Carb.	(g) Fiber	(g) Sug.	(g) Prot.	(mg) Sod.
Turkey, Young Hen, Meat Only, Cooked, Roasted 1 unit (yield from 1 lb ready-to-cook turkey) (212g)									
	371	12	4	155	0	0	NA	62	142
Turkey, Young Tom, Breast, Meat and Skin, Cooked, Roasted .5 breast, bone removed (1329g)									
	2512	98	28	997	0	0	NA	380	890

Protein Alternatives, Including Vegetable Proteins (Soy & Tofu Products)

Food Serving size	Cal.	(g) Total Fat	(g) Sat. Fat	(mg) Chol.	(g) Carb.	(g) Fiber	(g) Sug.	(g) Prot.	(mg) Sod.
Arrowhead Mills, Soybeans 1/4 cup	160	8	1	0	11	4	3	14	0
Bob's Red Mill, Organic Textured Soy Protein 1/4 cup	80	1.5	0	0	5	3	1.5	7	0
Bob's Red Mill, TVP (Textured Vegetable Protein) 1/4 cup	80	0	0	0	7	4	3	12	2
Dr. Praeger's Sensible Foods, Gluten Free California Veggie Burgers 1 burger	120	6	0.5	0	13	4	3	5	180
Earthbound Farm, Blueberry Quinoa, Protein Balance PowerMeal 1 container	360	22	3	0	34	6	7	9	520
Earthbound Farm, Tomatillo Black Bean, Protein Energy PowerMeal 1 container	350	23	3	0	31	6	4	8	550
Eden Foods, Dried Tofu 1 piece	50	2.5	0	0	0	2	0	5	0
Eden Foods, Genmai (Brown Rice) Miso, Organic 1 tbsp	25	0.5	0	0	3	2	1	2	780
Frieda's, Extra Firm Tofu 3 oz	90	5	NA	NA	1	NA	NA	10	10
Frieda's, Firm Tofu 3 oz	70	4	NA	NA	1	NA	NA	7	10
Frieda's, Meatless Taco Filling 30g	50	3	0	0	3	2	0	4	180
Frieda's, Soft Tofu 3.8 oz	45	2.5	NA	NA	1	NA	NA	5	15
Frieda's, Soyrizo Meatless Soy Chorizo 2 oz	90	4	1	0	7	2	3	6	450

Food Serving size	Cal.	(g) Total Fat	(g) Sat. Fat	(mg) Chol.	(g) Carb.	(g) Fiber	(g) Sug.	(g) Prot.	(mg) Sod.

Sausages & Luncheon Meats

Food Serving size	Cal.	Total Fat	Sat. Fat	Chol.	Carb.	Fiber	Sug.	Prot.	Sod.
Aidell's, Artichoke & Garlic Dinner Sausage									
1 link	150	11	3	75	1	<1	0	13	650
Aidell's, Awesome Apple Hot Dog									
1 link	110	7	2	50	2	<1	2	8	420
Aidell's, Cajun Style Andouille Dinner Sausage									
1 link	160	11	4	50	1	0	1	15	600
Aidell's, Cajun Style Andouille Sausage Minis									
5 links	100	6	2	45	1	1	0	11	490
Aidell's, Chicken & Apple Breakfast Sausage Links									
2 oz	110	8	2	50	2	0	1	8	410
Aidell's, Chicken & Apple Dinner Sausage									
1 link	150	10	3	85	3	<1	2	13	680
Aidell's, Chicken & Apple Sausage Minis									
5 links	110	7	2	60	2	0	2	9	500
Aidell's, Fresh Chicken & Apple Sausage									
1 link	150	10	3	85	3	<1	2	13	680
Aidell's, Fresh Italian Style Sausage									
1 link	150	10	3	85	3	<1	2	13	680
Aidell's, Fresh Roasted Garlic with Gruyere Cheese Sausage									
1 link	150	10	3	85	3	<1	2	13	680
Aidell's, Fresh Spicy Mango Jalapeno Sausage									
1 link	150	10	3	85	3	<1	2	13	680
Aidell's, Habanero & Green Chile Dinner Sausage									
1 link	160	11	3	70	2	<1	<1	12	650
Aidell's, Hawaiian Style Pineapple Sausage Minis									
5 links	120	8	2.5	50	6	<1	6	7	420
Aidell's, Italian Style Dinner Sausage with Mozzarella Cheese									
1 link	170	12	3.5	70	2	<1	<1	14	580
Aidell's, Mango Dinner Sausage									
1 link	170	12	3.5	85	4	<1	4	13	650
Aidell's, Maple and Smoked Bacon Breakfast Sausage									
2 oz	100	6	2	45	2	<1	2	10	490

Food Serving size	Cal.	(g) Total Fat	(g) Sat. Fat	(mg) Chol.	(g) Carb.	(g) Fiber	(g) Sug.	(g) Prot.	(mg) Sod.
Aidell's, Organic Cajun Style Andouille Sausage									
1 link	160	10	3	90	2	0	2	13	700
Aidell's, Organic Chicken & Apple Breakfast Links Sausage									
2 oz	120	8	2.5	50	2	<1	1	9	440
Aidell's, Organic Chicken & Apple Sausage									
1 link	150	10	3	85	3	<1	2	13	680
Aidell's, Organic Chicken and Apple Breakfast Sausage Links									
2 oz	120	8	2.5	50	2	<1	1	9	440
Aidell's, Organic Spinach & Feta Sausage									
1 link	140	9	2.5	90	2	<1	<1	13	600
Aidell's, Organic Sun-Dried Tomato Sausage									
1 link	150	9	2.5	85	3	<1	2	13	770
Aidell's, Organic Sweet Basil & Roasted Garlic Sausage									
1 link	160	11	3	65	2	<1	1	13	700
Aidell's, Pineapple & Bacon Dinner Sausage									
1 link	210	14	4	80	8	<1	8	12	630
Aidell's, Pineapple Paradise Hot Dog									
1 link	120	7	2	50	5	<1	5	9	490
Aidell's, Portobello Mushroom Dinner Sausage									
1 link	160	11	3.5	70	1	<1	1	14	610
Aidell's, Roasted Garlic & Gruyere Cheese Dinner Sausage									
1 link	190	14	5	85	2	2	<1	14	700
Aidell's, Spinach & Feta Dinner Sausage									
1 link	160	11	3	95	2	1	<1	14	600
Aidell's, Sun-Dried Tomato Dinner Sausage with Mozzarella Cheese									
1 link	170	12	3.5	70	2	<1	<1	14	670
Applegate Farms, Antibiotic Free Big Apple Hot Dog									
1 hot dog	110	9	3.5	30	1	0	0	7	360
Applegate Farms, Antibiotic Free Coppa									
1 oz	100	7	2.5	20	0	0	0	8	510
Applegate Farms, Antibiotic Free Genoa Salami									
1 oz	100	7	3	20	0	0	0	8	480
Applegate Farms, Antibiotic Free Hot Genoa Salami									
1 oz	100	7	3	20	0	0	0	8	480

Food Serving size	Cal.	(g) Total Fat	(g) Sat. Fat	(mg) Chol.	(g) Carb.	(g) Fiber	(g) Sug.	(g) Prot.	(mg) Sod.
Applegate Farms, Antibiotic Free Hot Soppressata									
1 oz	100	7	3	20	0	0	0	8	480
Applegate Farms, Antibiotic Free Pancetta									
1 oz	100	8	3	20	0	0	0	6	550
Applegate Farms, Antibiotic Free Pepperoni									
1 oz	80	7	2.5	20	1	0	1	4	260
Applegate Farms, Antibiotic Free Prosciutto									
1 oz	70	4	1.5	25	0	0	0	8	520
Applegate Farms, Antibiotic Free Soppressata									
1 oz	100	7	3	20	0	0	0	8	480
Applegate Farms, Antibiotic Free Turkey Salami									
2 oz	60	2	0.5	40	0	0	0	10	480
Applegate Farms, Antibiotic Free Uncured Turkey Bologna									
2 oz	90	5.5	1.5	30	0	0	0	9	400
Applegate Farms, Chicken & Apple Breakfast Sausage									
2 links	100	7	2	35	2	0	2	7	260
Applegate Farms, Chicken & Maple Breakfast Sausage									
2 links	100	7	2	40	1	0	1	7	270
Applegate Farms, Chicken & Sage Breakfast Sausage									
2 links	90	7	2	35	0	0	0	7	270
Applegate Farms, Classic Pork Breakfast Sausage									
2 links	130	11	4	30	0	0	0	8	300
Applegate Farms, Genoa Salami									
1 oz	100	7	3	20	0	0	0	8	480
Applegate Farms, Great Organic Beef Hot Dog									
1 hot dog	110	8	3	30	0	0	0	7	330
Applegate Farms, Great Organic Chicken Hot Dog									
1 hot dog	70	3.5	1	35	0	0	0	8	360
Applegate Farms, Great Organic Hotdog, Original Beef									
1 hot dog	90	6	2.5	25	0	0	0	6	380
Applegate Farms, Great Organic Stadium Hot Dog									
1 hot dog	110	8	3	30	0	0	0	7	330
Applegate Farms, Great Organic Turkey Hot Dog									
1 hot dog	60	3.5	1	25	1	0	0	7	370

Food Serving size	Cal.	(g) Total Fat	(g) Sat. Fat	(mg) Chol.	(g) Carb.	(g) Fiber	(g) Sug.	(g) Prot.	(mg) Sod.
Applegate Farms, Greatest Little Organic Uncured Smoky Cocktail Pork Franks									
7 links	120	9	3.5	35	1	0	1	8	390
Applegate Farms, Organic Andouille Poultry Sausage									
1 link	140	6	2	60	3	1	1	13	620
Applegate Farms, Organic Chicken & Apple Sausage									
1 link	140	7	1.5	65	6	1	3	14	500
Applegate Farms, Organic Fire Roasted Red Pepper Poultry Sausage									
1 link	120	6	1.5	65	2	1	0	14	500
Applegate Farms, Organic Genoa Salami									
1 oz	100	7	3	20	0	0	0	8	480
Applegate Farms, Organic Spinach & Feta Poultry Sausage									
1 link	120	7	2.5	60	2	0	0	13	470
Applegate Farms, Organic Sweet Italian Poultry Sausage									
1 link	130	6	2	70	2	1	0	15	500
Applegate Farms, Pepper Salami									
1 oz	100	7	1.5	20	1	0	0	8	440
Applegate Farms, Pepperoni (Sliced)									
1 oz	80	7	2.5	20	1	0	1	4	260
Applegate Farms, Pepperoni (Stick)									
1 oz	60	5	1.5	20	0	0	0	5	320
Applegate Farms, Prosciutto									
1 oz	70	4	1.5	25	0	0	0	8	520
Applegate Farms, Salametti									
1 oz	100	7	3	20	0	0	0	8	480
Applegate Farms, Savory Turkey Breakfast Sausage									
2 links	90	6	1.5	35	0	0	0	8	320
Applegate Farms, Smoked Pork Bratwurst									
1 link	170	12	4	45	2	0	1	12	660
Applegate Farms, Smoked Pork Kielbasa									
1 link	190	14	5	50	2	0	1	12	600
Applegate Farms, Soppressata									
1 oz	100	7	3	15	0	0	0	8	480
Applegate Farms, Super Natural Uncured Beef Hot Dog									
1 hot dog	70	6	2	20	0	0	0	6	330

Food Serving size	Cal.	(g) Total Fat	(g) Sat. Fat	(mg) Chol.	(g) Carb.	(g) Fiber	(g) Sug.	(g) Prot.	(mg) Sod.
Applegate Farms, Super Natural Uncured Chicken Hot Dog									
1 hot dog	60	3	1	35	0	0	0	7	370
Applegate Farms, Super Natural Uncured Turkey Hot Dog									
1 hot dog	50	3.5	1	25	0	0	0	5	260
Applegate Farms, Wheat-Free Beef Corn Dogs									
1 corn dog	180	8	2.5	30	21	1	6	7	410
Boar's Head, 1st Cut Cooked Corned Beef Brisket									
2 oz	80	4	1.5	40	0	0	0	12	460
Boar's Head, 1st Cut Pastrami Brisket									
2 oz	90	4	1.5	30	2	0	0	12	670
Boar's Head, 28% Lower Sodium Bologna									
2 oz	150	13	5	30	0	0	0	8	410
Boar's Head, All American BBQ Seasoned Roasted Chicken Breast									
2 oz	60	0.5	0	35	2	0	2	13	340
Boar's Head, Beef Bologna									
2 oz	150	13	4	35	0	0	0	7	520
Boar's Head, Beef Frankfurters (Natural Casing)									
1 frank	160	14	6	30	1	0	0	7	440
Boar's Head, Beef Frankfurters (Skinless)									
1 frank	120	11	4.5	20	0	0	0	6	350
Boar's Head, Bianco D'Oro, Italian Dry Salame									
2 oz	110	8	3.5	25	1	0	0	7	470
Boar's Head, Black Forest Brand Boneless Smoked Ham, 25% Lower Sodium									
2 oz	60	1	0	30	2	0	2	10	440
Boar's Head, Blazing Buffalo Style, Roasted Chicken Breast									
2 oz	60	1	0	35	0	0	0	13	460
Boar's Head, Bologna (Pork & Beef)									
2 oz	150	13	4.5	35	1	0	1	7	530
Boar's Head, Boneless, Shankless, Prosciutto de Parma									
2 slices	70	4	1	30	0	0	0	9	750
Boar's Head, Branded Deluxe Ham									
2 oz	60	1	0	25	2	0	2	9	590
Boar's Head, Branded Deluxe Ham, 42% Lower Sodium									
2 oz	60	1	0	25	2	0	2	10	460

Food Serving size	Cal.	(g) Total Fat	(g) Sat. Fat	(mg) Chol.	(g) Carb.	(g) Fiber	(g) Sug.	(g) Prot.	(mg) Sod.
Boar's Head, Bratwurst									
1 wurst	300	25	11	75	0	0	0	19	650
Boar's Head, Cajun Style Seasoned, Cap-Off Top Round									
2 oz	80	3	1	35	0	0	0	12	330
Boar's Head, Cajun Style Smoked, Oven Roasted Turkey Breast									
2 oz	60	0.5	0	25	1	0	0	13	650
Boar's Head, Capocollo (Hot & Sweet)									
1 oz	80	7	2.5	25	0	0	0	7	590
Boar's Head, Cap-Off Top Round Pastrami									
2 oz	70	2.5	1	30	1	0	0	13	600
Boar's Head, Cappy Brand Ham									
2 oz	60	1.5	0.5	15	3	0	2	10	590
Boar's Head, Chipotle Chicken Breast									
2 oz	60	1	0	40	1	0	0	13	420
Boar's Head, Chorizo Espanol									
1 oz	80	6	2	15	1	0	1	6	430
Boar's Head, Cooked Corned Beef Top Round, Cap-Off									
2 oz	80	2.5	1	30	0	0	0	14	490
Boar's Head, Cracked Pepper Mill, Smoked Turkey Breast									
2 oz	60	1	0	30	0	0	1	13	460
Boar's Head, Cream Havarti Cheese									
1 oz	110	10	1	35	0	NA	NA	6	210
Boar's Head, Deluxe Low Sodium Oven Roasted Beef, Cap-Off Round									
2 oz	80	2.5	1	30	<1	0	0	15	80
Boar's Head, Dry Sausage Hot									
1 oz	100	7	3	25	0	NA	NA	8	500
Boar's Head, Dry Sausage Sweet									
1 oz	100	7	3	25	0	NA	NA	8	500
Boar's Head, EverRoast, Oven Roasted Chicken Breast									
2 oz	50	0.5	0	30	1	0	1	13	440
Boar's Head, Garlic Bologna									
2 oz	150	13	4.5	35	1	0	1	7	530
Boar's Head, Genoa Salami									
2 oz	190	15	5	50	1	0	0	12	920

Food Serving size	Cal.	(g) Total Fat	(g) Sat. Fat	(mg) Chol.	(g) Carb.	(g) Fiber	(g) Sug.	(g) Prot.	(mg) Sod.
Boar's Head, Golden Catering Style, Oven Roasted Turkey Breast, 47% Lower Sodium									
2 oz	60	1	0	25	0	0	0	13	340
Boar's Head, Golden Classic, Oven Roasted Chicken Breast, 42% Lower Sodium									
2 oz	60	1	0	35	0	0	0	13	350
Boar's Head, Gourmet Pepper Brand Ham									
2 oz	60	1	0	20	2	0	1	10	500
Boar's Head, Hard Salami									
1 oz	110	9	3.5	30	1	0	0	6	490
Boar's Head, Hickory Smoked Black Forest Turkey Breast, 40% Lower Sodium									
2 oz	60	1	0	25	0	0	0	13	390
Boar's Head, Hickory Smoked Chicken Breast									
2 oz	60	1	0	35	0	0	0	13	360
Boar's Head, Honey Smoked Turkey Breast, Skinless									
2 oz	70	1	0	25	2	0	2	13	480
Boar's Head, Hot Smoked Sausage									
1 sausage	250	22	9	55	1	0	0	12	740
Boar's Head, Italian Style Seasoned Beef with Braciole Seasoning									
2 oz	70	2	1	35	0	0	0	13	370
Boar's Head, Jerk Turkey									
2 oz	60	1	0	25	0	0	0	12	370
Boar's Head, Lemon Pepper, Roasted Chicken Breast									
2 oz	60	1	0	35	1	0	0	13	360
Boar's Head, Lite Beef Frankfurters, Skinless & Natural Casing									
1 frank	90	6	2.5	25	0	0	0	7	270
Boar's Head, Lite Braunschweiger Liverwurst									
2 oz	120	8	5	50	1	0	0	9	450
Boar's Head, London Broil									
2 oz	70	3	1	25	0	0	0	12	310
Boar's Head, Londonport, Top Round Seasoned Roast Beef									
2 oz	80	2.5	1	40	2	0	2	13	350
Boar's Head, Maple Glazed Honey Coat, Cured Turkey Breast									
2 oz	70	0.5	0	30	2	0	2	14	440
Boar's Head, Maple Glazed, Honey Coat Ham									
2 oz	60	1	0	20	3	0	3	10	570

Food Serving size	Cal.	(g) Total Fat	(g) Sat. Fat	(mg) Chol.	(g) Carb.	(g) Fiber	(g) Sug.	(g) Prot.	(mg) Sod.
Boar's Head, Maple Glazed, Roasted Chicken Breast									
2 oz	70	1	0	35	2	0	2	13	310
Boar's Head, Mesquite Wood Smoked, Roasted Turkey Breast									
2 oz	60	1	0	25	0	0	0	12	440
Boar's Head, No Salt Added, Oven Roasted Turkey Breast									
2 oz	70	1	0	40	0	0	0	15	55
Boar's Head, Olive Loaf									
2 oz	130	12	4.5	20	<1	0	<1	6	630
Boar's Head, Our Premium 47% Lower Sodium, Roasted Turkey Breast, Skinless									
2 oz	60	0.5	0	20	0	0	0	12	340
Boar's Head, Ovengold, Roasted Breast of Turkey, Skinless									
2 oz	60	1	0	20	0	0	0	13	350
Boar's Head, Pastrami Seasoned, Turkey Breast									
2 oz	60	0.5	0	25	1	0	0	13	440
Boar's Head, Pesto Parmesan Ham									
2 oz	70	2.5	1	30	1	0	0	12	550
Boar's Head, Pickle & Pepper Loaf									
2 oz	150	13	7	30	2	0	1	6	500
Boar's Head, Pork & Beef Frankfurter, Natural Casing									
1 frank	150	14	5	25	0	0	0	7	460
Boar's Head, Pork & Beef Frankfurter, Skinless									
1 frank	150	14	5	25	0	0	0	7	460
Boar's Head, Prosciutto di Parma									
1 oz	60	3.5	1	25	0	0	0	8	660
Boar's Head, Rosemary & Sundried Tomato Ham									
2 oz	70	2.5	1	10	2	0	0	10	500
Boar's Head, Rotisserie Seasoned Roasted Chicken Breast									
2 oz	60	1	0	35	0	0	0	13	400
Boar's Head, Salsalito, Roasted Turkey Breast									
2 oz	60	0.5	0	25	1	0	0	13	480
Boar's Head, Sandwich Style Pepperoni									
1 oz	130	11	4.5	25	1	0	1	6	480
Boar's Head, Seasoned Filet of Roast Beef, Cap-Off Top Round									
2 oz	80	2.5	1	40	0	0	0	14	230

Food Serving size	Cal.	(g) Total Fat	(g) Sat. Fat	(mg) Chol.	(g) Carb.	(g) Fiber	(g) Sug.	(g) Prot.	(mg) Sod.
Boar's Head, Serrano Ham 1 oz	60	3	0.5	15	0	0	0	9	550
Boar's Head, Smoked Sausage, Natural Casing 1 link	310	27	11	65	2	0	0	15	920
Boar's Head, Smoked Virginia Ham 2 oz	60	1	0	25	2	0	2	9	590
Boar's Head, Sopressata Grande, Hot & Sweet 1 oz	90	7	3	20	1	0	0	7	510
Boar's Head, Strassburger Brand, Liverwurst 2 oz	170	15	6	85	1	0	1	8	470
Boar's Head, Sweet Slice, Boneless Smoked Ham 2 oz	60	2.5	1	20	1	0	0	10	520
Boar's Head, Tavern Ham 2 oz	60	1.5	0.5	30	2	0	2	10	540
Boar's Head, Virginia Brand Ham 2 oz	60	1	0	25	3	0	3	9	590
Buddig Organic, Deli Cuts, Baked Honey Ham 2 oz	60	1.5	NA	NA	1	NA	NA	10	NA
Buddig Organic, Deli Cuts, Brown Sugar Baked Ham 2 oz	80	2.5	NA	NA	0	NA	NA	15	NA
Buddig Organic, Deli Cuts, Honey Roasted Turkey 2 oz	60	1.5	NA	NA	1	NA	NA	10	NA
Buddig Organic, Deli Cuts, Oven-Roasted Turkey 2 oz	80	2.5	NA	NA	0	NA	NA	15	NA
Buddig Organic, Deli Cuts, Pastrami 2 oz	90	2.5	NA	NA	2	NA	NA	15	NA
Buddig Organic, Deli Cuts, Roast Beef 2 oz	80	2.5	NA	NA	0	NA	NA	15	NA
Buddig Organic, Deli Cuts, Rotisserie Chicken 2 oz	60	1.5	NA	NA	1	NA	NA	10	NA
Buddig Organic, Deli Cuts, Smoked Ham 2 oz	60	1.5	NA	NA	1	NA	NA	10	NA
Buddig Organic, Deli Cuts, Smoked Turkey 2 oz	60	1.5	NA	NA	1	NA	NA	10	NA

Food Serving size	Cal.	(g) Total Fat	(g) Sat. Fat	(mg) Chol.	(g) Carb.	(g) Fiber	(g) Sug.	(g) Prot.	(mg) Sod.
Buddig Organic, Fix Quix, Chicken									
1.75 oz	60	1	0.5	30	1	NA	1	11	310
Buddig Organic, Fix Quix, Smoked Ham									
2 oz	70	2.5	1	20	1	NA	1	10	460
Buddig Organic, Fix Quix, Turkey									
2 oz	70	2.5	1	20	2	NA	1	10	460
Buddig Organic, Old Wisconsin Festival Bratwurst									
1 link	280	25	9	50	3	0	0	0	820
Buddig Organic, Old Wisconsin Natural Casing Weiners									
1 link	140	12	4	30	1	0	0	6	440
Buddig Organic, Old Wisconsin Smoked Polish Sausage									
1 link	250	23	8	45	1	0	1	9	780
Buddig Organic, Old Wisconsin Smoked Sausage with Cheddar									
1 link	210	21	8	45	2	0	1	9	750
Buddig Organic, Old Wisconsin Snack Bites, Beef									
6 pieces	120	10	4	25	1	0	1	5	380
Buddig Organic, Old Wisconsin Snack Bites, Turkey									
6 pieces	80	5	1.5	25	0.5	0	0	7	300
Buddig Organic, Old Wisconsin Summer Sausage, Beef									
2 oz	200	18	7	40	0	0	0	9	710
Buddig Organic, Old Wisconsin Summer Sausage, Beef Garlic									
2 oz	200	18	7	40	0	0	0	9	710
Buddig Organic, Old Wisconsin Summer Sausage, Garlic									
2 oz	200	18	7	40	1	0	1	9	710
Buddig Organic, Old Wisconsin Summer Sausage, Original									
2 oz	220	20	9	45	1	0	0	10	680
Buddig Organic, Original Beef									
2 oz	90	5	NA	NA	1	NA	NA	10	NA
Buddig Organic, Original Brown Sugar Ham									
2 oz	90	5	NA	NA	3	NA	NA	9	NA
Buddig Organic, Original Chicken									
2 oz	90	5	NA	NA	2	NA	NA	10	NA
Buddig Organic, Original Corned Beef									
2 oz	90	5	NA	NA	2	NA	NA	10	NA

Food Serving size	Cal.	(g) Total Fat	(g) Sat. Fat	(mg) Chol.	(g) Carb.	(g) Fiber	(g) Sug.	(g) Prot.	(mg) Sod.
Buddig Organic, Original Ham 2 oz	90	5	NA	NA	2	NA	NA	10	NA
Buddig Organic, Original Honey Ham 2 oz	90	5	NA	NA	2	NA	NA	10	NA
Buddig Organic, Original Honey Roasted Turkey 2 oz	90	5	NA	NA	3	NA	NA	9	NA
Buddig Organic, Original Mesquite Turkey 2 oz	90	5	NA	NA	2	NA	NA	10	NA
Buddig Organic, Original Oven Roasted Turkey 2 oz	90	5	NA	NA	2	NA	NA	9	NA
Buddig Organic, Original Pastrami 2 oz	90	5	NA	NA	1	NA	NA	10	NA
Buddig Organic, Original Turkey 2 oz	90	5	NA	NA	2	NA	NA	10	NA
Hormel Natural, Apple Gouda Chicken Sausage 85g	170	9	3.5	60	7	0	7	14	580
Hormel Natural, Beef Sausage 56g	150	13	6	30	0	0	0	8	470
Hormel Natural, Jalapeno Cheddar Chicken Sausage 85g	160	11	4	75	1	0	0	15	680
Hormel Natural, Original Smoked Sausage 56g	160	15	5	35	0	0	0	7	540
Hormel Natural, Packaged Deli Sandwich Meats, Brown Sugar Deli Ham 56g	70	1.5	0.5	30	3	0	3	10	570
Hormel Natural, Packaged Deli Sandwich Meats, Cooked Deli Ham 56g	60	1.5	0.5	30	1	0	1	10	520
Hormel Natural, Packaged Deli Sandwich Meats, Hard Salami 28g	110	10	4	30	0	0	0	6	450
Hormel Natural, Packaged Deli Sandwich Meats, Honey Deli Ham 56g	70	1.5	0.5	30	3	0	3	10	520
Hormel Natural, Packaged Deli Sandwich Meats, Honey Deli Turkey 56g	60	1	0	25	2	0	2	11	450
Hormel Natural, Packaged Deli Sandwich Meats, Mesquite Deli Turkey 56g	60	1	0	25	1	0	1	11	450

Food Serving size	Cal.	(g) Total Fat	(g) Sat. Fat	(mg) Chol.	(g) Carb.	(g) Fiber	(g) Sug.	(g) Prot.	(mg) Sod.
Hormel Natural, Packaged Deli Sandwich Meats, Oven Roasted Deli Turkey									
56g	60	1	0	25	1	0	1	11	460
Hormel Natural, Packaged Deli Sandwich Meats, Roast Beef									
56g	60	2	1	25	0	0	0	11	520
Hormel Natural, Packaged Deli Sandwich Meats, Rotisserie Style Chicken Breast									
56g	50	1	0	35	0	0	0	11	470
Hormel Natural, Packaged Deli Sandwich Meats, Smoked Deli Ham									
56g	60	1.5	0.5	30	1	0	1	10	520
Hormel Natural, Packaged Deli Sandwich Meats, Smoked Deli Turkey									
56g	60	1	0	25	1	0	1	11	450
Hormel Natural, Spinach Asiago Chicken Sausage									
85g	140	9	3	60	1	0	1	14	570
Hormel Natural, Turkey Smoked Sausage									
56g	80	5	2	35	1	0	1	8	470
Jones Dairy Farms, All Natural Golden Brown Light Sausage & Rice Links									
3 links	130	9	3.5	35	3	0	0	10	350
Jones Dairy Farms, All Natural Golden Brown Made from Beef Sausage Links									
3 links	200	28	40	50	2	0	1	7	470
Jones Dairy Farms, All Natural Golden Brown Maple Pork Sausage Links									
3 links	240	22	8	45	0	0	1	7	420
Jones Dairy Farms, All Natural Golden Brown Maple Pork Sausage Patties									
1 patty	130	12	4.5	25	1	0	1	4	230
Jones Dairy Farms, All Natural Golden Brown Mild Pork Sausage Links									
3 links	250	24	8	45	1	0	0	7	380
Jones Dairy Farms, All Natural Golden Brown Mild Pork Sausage Patties									
1 patty	120	12	4	25	0	0	0	4	220
Jones Dairy Farms, All Natural Golden Brown Pork and Uncured Bacon Sausage Links									
3 links	230	21	8	40	1	0	0	8	480
Jones Dairy Farms, All Natural Golden Brown Spicy Pork Sausage Links									
3 links	250	24	8	45	1	0	0	7	380
Jones Dairy Farms, All Natural Golden Brown Turkey Sausage Links									
3 links	90	4.5	1.5	40	2	0	0	10	420

Food Serving size	Cal.	(g) Total Fat	(g) Sat. Fat	(mg) Chol.	(g) Carb.	(g) Fiber	(g) Sug.	(g) Prot.	(mg) Sod.
Jones Dairy Farms, All Natural Pork Sausage & Rice, Light Links									
2 links	110	80	2.5	30	3	0	0	8	440
Jones Dairy Farms, All Natural Pork Sausage, Hearty Links									
1 link	210	19	6	35	2	0	0	7	320
Jones Dairy Farms, All Natural Pork Sausage, Little Links									
3 links	260	24	8	50	0	0	0	10	460
Jones Dairy Farms, All Natural Pork Sausage, Little Links, Maple									
2 links	180	16	5	300	2	0	1	7	300
Jones Dairy Farms, All Natural Pork Sausage, Patties									
1 patty	120	11	4	30	0	0	0	6	250
Jones Dairy Farms, All Natural Pork Sausage, Roll									
2 oz	230	21	8	50	1	0	0	9	430
Jones Dairy Farms, Braunschweiger (Liverwurst), Chunk, Light									
2 oz	90	5	2	125	0	0	0	10	430
Jones Dairy Farms, Braunschweiger (Liverwurst), Chunk, Regular									
2 oz	180	16	5	110	1	0	0	8	460
Jones Dairy Farms, Braunschweiger (Liverwurst), Club, Bacon & Onion									
2 oz	160	13	5	110	2	0	0	8	560
Jones Dairy Farms, Braunschweiger (Liverwurst), Club, Light									
2 oz	90	5	2	140	1	0	0	10	500
Jones Dairy Farms, Braunschweiger (Liverwurst), Sliced, Cracker Size Slices									
2 oz	150	13	4	90	1	0	0	6	370
Jones Dairy Farms, Braunschweiger (Liverwurst), Sliced, Sandwich Size Slices									
2 oz	120	10	3.5	75	1	0	0	7	410
Jones Dairy Farms, Canadian Bacon Slices									
3 slices	60	1.5	0.5	30	1	0	0	11	460
Thumann's, "Chef's Slice" Smoked Ham – Boneless									
2 oz	60	1	0	21	0	0	0	10	510
Thumann's, All Natural Black Angus Cooked Corned Beef Round									
2 oz	70	2	1	32	0	0	0	12	450
Thumann's, All Natural Black Forest Brand Ham									
2 oz	60	1	0	21	<1	0	<1	10	400
Thumann's, All Natural Oven Roasted Gourmet Chicken Breast									
2 oz	40	0.5	0	25	0	0	0	13	350

Food Serving size	Cal.	(g) Total Fat	(g) Sat. Fat	(mg) Chol.	(g) Carb.	(g) Fiber	(g) Sug.	(g) Prot.	(mg) Sod.
Thumann's, All Natural Oven Roasted Gourmet Turkey Breast									
2 oz	40	0.5	0	25	0	0	0	13	350
Thumann's, All Natural Oven Roasted Top Round									
2 oz	70	1	0.5	25	0	0	0	15	160
Thumann's, Barbeque Style Chicken Breast									
2 oz	60	1	0	30	0	0	0	13	260
Thumann's, Beef Bologna									
2 oz	140	11	6	30	1	0	1	13	470
Thumann's, Beef Frankfurters Pushcart Style, Natural Casings									
1 frank	150	14	6	30	0	0	0	8	460
Thumann's, Beef Frankfurters, Skinless									
1 frank	130	11	5	24	0	0	0	6	440
Thumann's, Black Forest Brand Ham									
2 oz	60	1	0	21	<1	0	<1	10	510
Thumann's, Bologna, Pork and Beef									
2 oz	150	13	5	28	1	0	<1	7	470
Thumann's, Bone in Smoked Ham									
3 oz	120	5	2	45	1	0	1	11	635
Thumann's, Bratwurst, Natural Casing, Cooked and Raw									
1 link	290	25	10	65	0	0	0	19	750
Thumann's, Braunschweiger, Regular or Natural Casing									
2 oz	160	12	5	80	3	0	2	9	580
Thumann's, Brown Sugar Cured Ham									
2 oz	60	1	0	21	<1	0	<1	10	510
Thumann's, Buffalo Style, Oven Roasted Chicken Breast									
2 oz	60	1	0	30	0	0	0	13	260
Thumann's, Cajun Style Roast Beef									
2 oz	100	2.5	1.5	32	0	0	0	12	250
Thumann's, Cajun Style Turkey Breast, 99% Fat Free									
2 oz	40	0.5	0	25	0	0	0	13	350
Thumann's, Cap Corned Beef									
2 oz	150	1.5	5	30	0	0	0	14	560
Thumann's, Cap Pastrami									
2 oz	80	3	1.5	30	0	0	0	14	520

Food Serving size	Cal.	(g) Total Fat	(g) Sat. Fat	(mg) Chol.	(g) Carb.	(g) Fiber	(g) Sug.	(g) Prot.	(mg) Sod.
Thumann's, Capless Corned Beef 2 oz	150	1.5	5	30	0	0	0	14	560
Thumann's, Capless Roast Beef 2 oz	70	1.5	0.5	20	0	0	0	14	160
Thumann's, Cocktail Franks, Natural Casings 2 oz	150	14	5	30	1	0	<1	14	480
Thumann's, Cooked Salami 2 oz	110	7	2.5	30	1	0	NA	9	440
Thumann's, Corned Beef Bottom Round, Cooked 2 oz	80	3	1.5	30	0	0	0	14	520
Thumann's, Corned Beef Brisket, Cooked 2 oz	70	2	1	32	0	0	0	14	500
Thumann's, Cracked Pepper & Paprika Turkey Breast, 99% Fat Free 2 oz	40	0.5	0	25	0	0	0	13	350
Thumann's, Deluxe Cooked Ham, 98% Fat Free 2 oz	60	1	0	21	<1	0	<1	10	510
Thumann's, Deluxe Cooked Ham, Lower Sodium 2 oz	60	1	0	21	<1	0	<1	10	400
Thumann's, Deluxe Flat Smoked Ham, Tavern Ham 2 oz	60	1	0	21	0	0	<1	10	510
Thumann's, Deluxe Hot Ham 2 oz	60	1	0	21	<1	0	<1	10	510
Thumann's, Deluxe Virginia Brand Ham 2 oz	60	1	0	21	<1	0	<1	10	510
Thumann's, Filet of Turkey, Caramel Color Coated 2 oz	40	0.5	0	25	0	0	0	13	350
Thumann's, Filet of Turkey, Rotisserie Flavor 2 oz	40	0.5	0	25	0	0	0	13	350
Thumann's, First Cut Corned Beef, Cooked and Raw 2 oz	150	1.5	0.5	30	0	0	0	14	560
Thumann's, First Cut Pastrami 2 oz	70	2	1	32	0	0	0	12	520
Thumann's, Garlic Bologna 2 oz	150	13	5	28	1	0	<1	7	470

Food Serving size	Cal.	(g) Total Fat	(g) Sat. Fat	(mg) Chol.	(g) Carb.	(g) Fiber	(g) Sug.	(g) Prot.	(mg) Sod.
Thumann's, Genoa Salami, Natural Casing									
1 oz	120	10	4	45	0	0	0	6	450
Thumann's, Golden Roasted Gourmet, Turkey Breast									
2 oz	40	0.5	0	25	0	0	0	13	280
Thumann's, Hard Salami									
1 oz	110	9	4	25	1	0	1	6	490
Thumann's, Head Cheese									
2 oz	100	2	0	21	<1	0	<1	12	460
Thumann's, Hickory Smoked Turkey Breast, 99% Fat Free									
2 oz	40	0.5	0	25	0	0	0	13	350
Thumann's, Home Style Oven Roasted, Fresh Ham – Roast Pork									
2 oz	150	14	6	30	0	0	0	10	75
Thumann's, Honey & Molasses Coated, Turkey Breast									
2 oz	60	0.5	0	20	1	0	1	13	320
Thumann's, Honey Cured, Baked Ham									
2 oz	100	2	0	21	<1	0	<1	10	510
Thumann's, Hot & Sweet Italian Sausage, Natural Casing									
1 link	290	25	10	65	0	0	<1	19	750
Thumann's, Italian Style Turkey Breast, 99% Fat Free									
2 oz	40	0.5	0	25	0	0	0	13	350
Thumann's, Italian Style, Roast Beef									
2 oz	100	4	2	38	0	0	0	13	400
Thumann's, Jumbo Pork & Beef Franks, Skinless									
1 frank	300	27	10	55	1.5	0	<1	13	955
Thumann's, Kielbasa Loaf									
2 oz	150	13	5	28	<1	0	<1	9	470
Thumann's, Knockwurst, Natural Casing									
1 link	300	27	10	55	2	0	<1	13	960
Thumann's, Lemon Pepper Turkey Breast, 99% Fat Free									
2 oz	40	0.5	0	25	0	0	0	13	350
Thumann's, London Broil, Roast Beef									
2 oz	100	3	1.5	32	0	0	0	13	400
Thumann's, Lower Sodium, Bologna									
2 oz	150	13	5	28	1	0	<1	7	370

Food Serving size	Cal.	(g) Total Fat	(g) Sat. Fat	(mg) Chol.	(g) Carb.	(g) Fiber	(g) Sug.	(g) Prot.	(mg) Sod.
Thumann's, Maple Glazed, Smoked Ham									
2 oz	60	1	0	21	<1	0	1	14	510
Thumann's, Maple Glazed, Turkey Breast, 99% Fat Free									
2 oz	60	0.5	0	20	1	0	0	13	320
Thumann's, Mesquite Smoked, Turkey Breast, 99% Fat Free									
2 oz	40	0.5	0	25	0	0	0	13	350
Thumann's, Mortadella									
2 oz	170	14	5	3	<1	0	0	8	660
Thumann's, Mortadella with Pistachios									
2 oz	170	15	6	35	<1	0	0	8	610
Thumann's, Olive Loaf									
2 oz	130	12	4	18	<1	0	<1	8	580
Thumann's, Oval Minced Loaf									
2 oz	150	13	5	28	1	0	<1	7	470
Thumann's, Oven Roasted Premium Chicken Breast									
2 oz	60	1	0	30	0	0	0	13	260
Thumann's, Pastrami									
2 oz	80	3	1.5	30	0	0	0	14	520
Thumann's, Pastrami Bottom Round									
2 oz	80	3	1.5	30	0	0	0	14	520
Thumann's, Pastrami Turkey Breast, 99% Fat Free									
2 oz	40	0.5	0	25	0	0	0	13	350
Thumann's, Pepperoni Sticks									
2 oz	130	11	4	30	1	0	0	5	540
Thumann's, Petite Filet of Turkey, Smoked, Skinless									
2 oz	40	0.5	0	25	0	0	0	13	350
Thumann's, Pickle & Pimento Loaf									
2 oz	130	12	4	18	<1	0	<1	8	470
Thumann's, Pork & Beef Frankfurters, Skinless									
1 frank	115	10	4	21	0	0	<1	5	360
Thumann's, Pork and Beef Frankfurters, Natural Casings									
1 frank	240	21	8	45	2	0	0	9	720

Food Serving size	Cal.	(g) Total Fat	(g) Sat. Fat	(mg) Chol.	(g) Carb.	(g) Fiber	(g) Sug.	(g) Prot.	(mg) Sod.
Thumann's, Pork Sausage Links, Natural Casing									
3 links	270	27	9	50	4	0	0	5	600
Thumann's, Pork Shoulder Butt									
3 oz	225	18	9	45	0	0	0	21	765
Thumann's, Premium Turkey Breast, Browned in Cotton Seed Oil									
2 oz	60	2.5	1	30	0	0	0	13	400
Thumann's, Premium White Turkey Breast, Lower Sodium									
2 oz	60	0.5	0	25	0	0	0	13	280
Thumann's, Premium White Turkey Breast, Skinless									
2 oz	40	0.5	0	25	0	0	0	13	350
Thumann's, Prosciuttini Ham, Peppered Ham									
2 oz	60	1	0	21	<1	0	<1	10	510
Thumann's, Prosciutto									
1 oz	60	2.5	1	25	0	0	1	10	770
Thumann's, Ring Bologna									
2 oz	150	13	5	28	1	0	<1	7	470
Thumann's, Ring Kielbasa									
2 oz	150	13	5	28	1	0	<1	7	470
Thumann's, Ripple Roast Beef									
2 oz	80	3	1.5	30	0	0	1	14	150
Thumann's, Sandwich Style Pepperoni									
1 oz	150	14	5	55	0	0	0	5	420
Thumann's, Santa Fe Style Turkey Breast, 99% Fat Free									
2 oz	40	0.5	0	25	0	0	0	13	350
Thumann's, Smoked Liverwurst, Natural Casing									
2 oz	160	12	5	80	3	0	2	9	580
Thumann's, Sopressata, Sweet									
1 oz	90	6	2	20	1	0	<1	8	510
Thumann's, Top Round Corned Beef, Cooked									
2 oz	70	2	1	32	0	0	0	14	500
Thumann's, Top Round Roast Beef									
2 oz	80	3	1.5	30	0	0	0	14	150

Food Serving size	Cal.	(g) Total Fat	(g) Sat. Fat	(mg) Chol.	(g) Carb.	(g) Fiber	(g) Sug.	(g) Prot.	(mg) Sod.

Seafood (Fish, Shellfish, Misc. Seafood)

Food Serving size	Cal.	Total Fat	Sat. Fat	Chol.	Carb.	Fiber	Sug.	Prot.	Sod.
Bass, Fresh Water, Mixed Species, Cooked, Dry Heat 3 oz (85g)	124	4	1	74	0	0	NA	21	77
Bass, Striped, Cooked, Dry Heat 3 oz (85g)	105	3	1	88	0	0	NA	19	75
Bluefish, Cooked, Dry Heat 3 oz (85g)	135	5	1	65	0	0	NA	22	65
Burbot, Cooked, Dry Heat 3 oz (85g)	98	1	0	65	0	0	NA	21	105
Butterfish, Cooked, Dry Heat 3 oz (85g)	159	9	NA	71	0	0	NA	19	97
Carp, Cooked, Dry Heat 3 oz (85g)	138	6	1	71	0	0	NA	19	54
Catfish, Channel, Wild, Cooked, Dry Heat 3 oz (85g)	89	2	1	61	0	0	NA	16	43
Clam, Mixed Species, Cooked, Moist Heat 20 small (190g)	281	4	0	127	10	0	NA	49	213
Cod, Atlantic, Cooked, Dry Heat 3 oz (85g)	89	1	0	47	0	0	0	19	66
Cod, Pacific, Cooked, Dry Heat 3 oz (85g)	72	0	0	48	0	0	0	16	316
Crab, Alaska King, Cooked, Moist Heat 3 oz (85g)	82	1	0	45	0	0	NA	16	911
Crab, Blue, Cooked, Moist Heat 1 cup (not packed) (135g)	112	1	0	131	0	0	0	24	533
Crab, Dungeness, Cooked, Moist Heat 1 crab (127g)	140	2	0	97	1	0	NA	28	480
Crab, Queen, Cooked, Moist Heat 3 oz (85g)	98	1	0	60	0	0	NA	20	587
Crayfish, Mixed Species, Wild, Cooked, Moist Heat 3 oz (85g)	70	1	0	113	0	0	0	14	80
Cusk, Cooked, Dry Heat 3 oz (85g)	95	1	NA	45	0	0	NA	21	34

Food Serving size	Cal.	(g) Total Fat	(g) Sat. Fat	(mg) Chol.	(g) Carb.	(g) Fiber	(g) Sug.	(g) Prot.	(mg) Sod.
Cuttlefish, Mixed Species, Cooked, Moist Heat									
3 oz (85g)	134	1	0	190	1	0	NA	28	632
Dolphinfish, Cooked, Dry Heat									
3 oz (85g)	93	1	0	80	0	0	NA	20	96
Dr. Praeger's Sensible Foods, Potato Crusted Fish Fillets (Gluten Free)									
1 fillet	90	6	0.5	45	5	1	0	5	210
Dr. Praeger's Sensible Foods, Potato Crusted Fish Sticks (Gluten Free)									
3 fish sticks	120	6	1	25	7	<1	0	6	220
Dr. Praeger's Sensible Foods, Potato Crusted Fishies (Gluten Free)									
4 fishies	80	4	0.5	25	7	1	0	4	220
Drum, Fresh Water, Cooked, Dry Heat									
3 oz (85g)	130	5	1	70	0	0	NA	19	82
Eden Foods, Bonito Flakes									
2 tbsp	5	0	0	1	0	0	0	1	4
Eel, Mixed Species, Cooked, Dry Heat									
1 oz, with bone (yield after bone removed) (22g)	52	3	1	35	0	0	NA	5	14
Flatfish (Flounder and Sole Species), Cooked, Dry Heat									
3 oz (85g)	73	2	0	48	0	0	0	13	309
Grouper, Mixed Species, Cooked, Dry Heat									
3 oz (85g)	100	1	0	40	0	0	NA	21	45
Haddock, Cooked, Dry Heat									
3 oz (85g)	77	0	0	56	0	0	0	17	222
Halibut, Atlantic and Pacific, Cooked, Dry Heat									
3 oz (85g)	94	1	0	51	0	0	0	19	70
Halibut, Greenland, Cooked, Dry Heat									
3 oz (85g)	203	15	3	50	0	0	NA	16	88
Herring, Atlantic, Cooked, Dry Heat									
3 oz (85g)	173	10	2	65	0	0	0	20	98
Herring, Pacific, Cooked, Dry Heat									
3 oz (85g)	213	15	4	84	0	0	NA	18	81
Ian's Natural Foods, Allergy Friendly Fish Sticks									
6 sticks	190	5	0	35	24	<1	0	11	170

Food Serving size	Cal.	(g) Total Fat	(g) Sat. Fat	(mg) Chol.	(g) Carb.	(g) Fiber	(g) Sug.	(g) Prot.	(mg) Sod.
Lobster, Northern, Cooked, Moist Heat									
3 oz (85g)	76	1	0	124	0	0	0	16	413
Mackerel, Atlantic, Cooked, Dry Heat									
3 oz (85g)	223	15	4	64	0	0	NA	20	71
Mackerel, King, Cooked, Dry Heat									
3 oz (85g)	114	2	0	58	0	0	NA	22	173
Mackerel, Pacific and Jack, Mixed Species, Cooked, Dry Heat									
1 cubic inch, boneless (17g)	34	2	0	10	0	0	0	4	19
Mackerel, Spanish, Cooked, Dry Heat									
3 oz (85g)	134	5	2	62	0	0	NA	20	56
Milkfish, Cooked, Dry Heat									
3 oz (85g)	162	7	NA	57	0	0	NA	22	78
Monkfish, Cooked, Dry Heat									
3 oz (85g)	82	2	NA	27	0	0	NA	16	20
Mullet, Striped, Cooked, Dry Heat									
3 oz (85g)	128	4	1	54	0	0	NA	21	60
Mussel, Blue, Cooked, Moist Heat									
3 oz (85g)	146	4	1	48	6	0	NA	20	314
Oyster, Eastern, Wild, Cooked, Dry Heat									
6 medium (59g)	47	2	0	37	2	0	1	5	78
Oyster, Eastern, Wild, Cooked, Moist Heat									
6 medium (42g)	43	1	0	33	2	0	1	5	70
Oyster, Pacific, Cooked, Moist Heat									
3 oz (85g)	139	4	1	85	8	0	0	16	180
Oyster, Pacific, Raw									
3 oz (85g)	69	2	0	43	4	0	NA	8	90
Perch, Mixed Species, Cooked, Dry Heat									
3 oz (85g)	99	1	0	98	0	0	NA	21	67
Pike, Northern, Cooked, Dry Heat									
3 oz (85g)	96	1	0	43	0	0	NA	21	42
Pike, Walleye, Cooked, Dry Heat									
3 oz (85g)	101	1	0	94	0	0	NA	21	55
Pollock, Atlantic, Cooked, Dry Heat									
3 oz (85g)	100	1	0	77	0	0	NA	21	94

Food Serving size	Cal.	(g) Total Fat	(g) Sat. Fat	(mg) Chol.	(g) Carb.	(g) Fiber	(g) Sug.	(g) Prot.	(mg) Sod.
Pollock, Walleye, Cooked, Dry Heat 3 oz (85g)	94	1	0	73	0	0	0	20	88
Sablefish, Cooked, Dry Heat 3 oz (85g)	213	17	3	54	0	0	NA	15	61
Salmon, Atlantic, Wild, Cooked, Dry Heat 3 oz (85g)	155	7	1	60	0	0	NA	22	48
Salmon, Coho, Wild, Cooked, Dry Heat 3 oz (85g)	118	4	1	47	0	0	0	20	49
Salmon, Coho, Wild, Cooked, Moist Heat 3 oz (85g)	156	6	1	48	0	0	NA	23	45
Salmon, Pink, Cooked, Dry Heat .5 fillet (124g)	190	7	1	68	0	0	0	30	112
Salmon, Sockeye, Cooked, Dry Heat 3 oz (85g)	144	6	1	54	0	0	0	22	114
Sea Bass, Mixed Species, Cooked, Dry Heat 3 oz (85g)	105	2	1	45	0	0	NA	20	74
Sea Trout, Mixed Species, Cooked, Dry Heat 3 oz (85g)	113	4	1	90	0	0	NA	18	63
Shrimp, Mixed Species, Cooked, Moist Heat 4 large (22g)	26	0	0	46	0	0	0	5	208
Snapper, Mixed Species, Cooked, Dry Heat 3 oz (85g)	109	1	0	40	0	0	NA	22	48
Spiny Lobster, Mixed Species, Cooked, Moist Heat 3 oz (85g)	122	2	0	77	3	0	NA	22	193
Swordfish, Cooked, Dry Heat 3 oz (85g)	146	7	2	66	0	0	0	20	82
Thumann's, Tuna Salad 100g	270	22	3	40	4	0	2	14	480
Trout, Mixed Species, Cooked, Dry Heat 3 oz (85g)	162	7	1	63	0	0	NA	23	57
Trout, Rainbow, Wild, Cooked, Dry Heat 3 oz (85g)	128	5	1	59	0	0	NA	19	48
Tuna, Fresh, Bluefin, Cooked, Dry Heat 3 oz (85g)	156	5	1	42	0	0	NA	25	43

Food Serving size	Cal.	(g) Total Fat	(g) Sat. Fat	(mg) Chol.	(g) Carb.	(g) Fiber	(g) Sug.	(g) Prot.	(mg) Sod.
Tuna, Skipjack, Fresh, Cooked, Dry Heat									
3 oz (85g)	112	1	0	51	0	0	NA	24	40
Tuna, Yellowfin, Fresh, Cooked, Dry Heat									
3 oz (85g)	111	1	0	40	0	0	0	25	46
Whitefish, Mixed Species, Cooked, Dry Heat									
3 oz (85g)	146	6	1	65	0	0	NA	21	55
Whiting, Mixed Species, Cooked, Dry Heat									
3 oz (85g)	99	1	0	71	0	0	0	20	112
Yellowtail, Mixed Species, Cooked, Dry Heat									
3 oz (85g)	159	6	NA	60	0	0	NA	25	43

Fats & Oils

Why Eat Fats & Oils?

Fats and oils are not a food group, but they do provide essential nutrients and are gluten-free. Most of the fats you eat should be polyunsaturated (PUFA) or monounsaturated (MUFA) fats. PUFAs contain some fatty acids that are necessary for health—called "essential fatty acids." The MUFAs and PUFAs found in fish, nuts, and vegetable oils do not raise LDL ("bad") cholesterol levels in the blood. In addition to the essential fatty acids they contain, oils are the major source of vitamin E, a potent antioxidant.

Daily Goal

Six teaspoons for an adult on a 2,000 calorie diet.
One teaspoon equivalents:
   1 tbsp oil = 2.5 teaspoons
   1 tbsp mayonnaise = 2.5 teaspoons
   2 tbsp Italian dressing = 2 teaspoons
   4 large olives = ½ teaspoon
   1 oz nuts = 3 teaspoons
   2 tbsp peanut butter = 4 teaspoons

Gluten-Free Shopping Tips

- Choose fats and oils high in monounsaturated and polyunsaturated fatty acids, such as fish, nuts, seeds, and vegetable oils.
- Limit solid fats such as butter, stick margarine, shortening, and animal fats.
- Choose fats high in omega-3s, such as olive oil, soy oil, and flaxseed oil.

Gluten-Free Shopping List Essentials

Olive oil
Canola Oil
Soybean Oil
Margarine
Avocados

Approved Fats & Oils and Those to Avoid on a Gluten-Free Diet

Gluten-Free

- Butter, margarine, lard, shortening, and vegetable oil
- Salad dressing with approved ingredients
- Nuts and seeds

May Contain Gluten

- Salad dressings made with ingredients to avoid
- Suet (hard fat that occurs in loins of beef and mutton)
- Cooking spray made with ingredients to avoid
- Seasoned nuts and seeds.

Caution

While consuming some oil is needed for health, oils still contain calories. In fact, oils and solid fats both contain about 120 calories per tablespoon. Therefore, the amount of oil consumed needs to be limited to balance total calorie intake.

Food Serving size	Cal.	(g) Total Fat	(g) Sat. Fat	(mg) Chol.	(g) Carb.	(g) Fiber	(g) Sug.	(g) Prot.	(mg) Sod.
Butter / Margarine									
Earth Balance, Olive Oil Spread									
1 tbsp	80	9	2.5	0	0	NA	NA	0	75
Earth Balance, Organic Coconut Spread									
1 tbsp	100	11	5	0	0	NA	0	0	70
Earth Balance, Original Spread									
1 tbsp	100	11	3	0	0	NA	NA	0	100
Earth Balance, Shortening Baking Sticks									
1 tbsp	130	14	5	0	0	NA	NA	0	0
Earth Balance, Soy Free Spread									
1 tbsp	100	11	3	0	0	NA	NA	0	110
Earth Balance, Soy Garden Spread									
1 tbsp	100	11	3.5	0	0	NA	NA	0	120
Earth Balance, Vegan Buttery Baking Sticks									
1 tbsp	100	11	4	0	0	NA	NA	0	120
Earth Balance, Whipped Spread									
1 tbsp	80	9	2.5	0	0	NA	NA	0	100
Smart Balance, Butter & Canola and Extra Virgin Olive Oil Blend, Spreadable Butter									
1 tbsp	100	11	4	15	0	NA	NA	0	85
Smart Balance, Butter & Canola Oil Blend, Spreadable Butter									
1 tbsp	100	11	4	15	0	NA	NA	0	85
Smart Balance, Buttery Burst Spray									
5 sprays as topping	0	0	0	0	0	NA	NA	0	0
Smart Balance, Buttery Spread with Calcium									
1 tbsp	80	9	2.5	0	0	NA	NA	0	90
Smart Balance, Buttery Spread with Extra Virgin Olive Oil									
1 tbsp	60	7	2	NA	0	NA	NA	0	70
Smart Balance, Buttery Sticks with Extra Virgin Olive Oil									
1 tbsp	100	11	5	15	0	NA	NA	0	100
Smart Balance, HeartRight, Light Buttery Spread									
1 tbsp	45	5	1.5	0	0	NA	NA	0	80
Smart Balance, Light Butter & Canola Oil Blend, Spreadable Butter									
1 tbsp	50	5	2	10	0	NA	NA	0	90

Food Serving size	Cal.	(g) Total Fat	(g) Sat. Fat	(mg) Chol.	(g) Carb.	(g) Fiber	(g) Sug.	(g) Prot.	(mg) Sod.
Smart Balance, Light Buttery Spread with Extra Virgin Olive Oil									
1 tbsp	50	5	1.5	NA	0	NA	NA	0	70
Smart Balance, Light Buttery Spread with Flax Oil									
1 tbsp	50	5	1.5	0	0	NA	NA	0	90
Smart Balance, Light Original Buttery Spread									
1 tbsp	50	5	1.5	0	0	NA	0	0	85
Smart Balance, Omega-3 Buttery Spread									
1 tbsp	80	8	2.5	NA	0	NA	NA	0	85
Smart Balance, Omega-3 Buttery Sticks									
1 tbsp	100	11	5	15	0	NA	NA	0	100
Smart Balance, Omega-3 Light Buttery Spread									
1 tbsp	50	5	1.5	NA	0	NA	NA	0	80
Smart Balance, Organic Whipped Buttery Spread									
1 tbsp	80	9	2.5	0	0	NA	NA	0	100
Smart Balance, Original Buttery Spread									
1 tbsp	80	9	2.5	0	0	NA	NA	0	90
Smart Balance, Whipped Low Sodium Buttery Spread									
1 tbsp	60	7	2	0	0	NA	NA	0	30

Oils

Food Serving size	Cal.	(g) Total Fat	(g) Sat. Fat	(mg) Chol.	(g) Carb.	(g) Fiber	(g) Sug.	(g) Prot.	(mg) Sod.
Eden Foods, Hot Pepper Sesame Oil, Imported									
1 tbsp	120	14	2	0	0	0	0	0	0
Eden Foods, Olive Oil, Extra Virgin, Spanish									
1 tbsp	120	14	1.5	0	0	0	0	0	0
Eden Foods, Safflower Oil, High Oleic, Organic									
1 tbsp	120	14	1	0	0	0	0	0	0
Eden Foods, Sesame Oil, Extra Virgin, Organic									
1 tbsp	120	14	2	0	0	0	0	0	0
Eden Foods, Soybean Oil, Organic									
1 tbsp	120	14	2	0	NA	NA	NA	0	0
Eden Foods, Toasted Sesame Oil									
1 tbsp	120	14	2	0	0	0	0	0	0
Lucini, Delicate Lemon, Extra Virgin Olive Oil									
1 tbsp	120	14	2	NA	0	NA	NA	0	0

Food Serving size	Cal.	(g) Total Fat	(g) Sat. Fat	(mg) Chol.	(g) Carb.	(g) Fiber	(g) Sug.	(g) Prot.	(mg) Sod.
Lucini, Estate Select, Extra Virgin Olive Oil									
1 tbsp	120	14	2	NA	0	NA	NA	0	0
Lucini, Fiery Chili, Extra Virgin Olive Oil									
1 tbsp	120	14	2	NA	0	NA	NA	0	0
Lucini, Limited Reserve, Premium Select Extra Virgin Olive Oil, 100% Organic									
1 tbsp	120	14	2	NA	0	NA	NA	0	0
Lucini, Premium Select Extra Virgin Olive Oil									
1 tbsp	120	14	2	NA	0	NA	NA	0	0
Lucini, Premium Select, White Truffle, Extra Virgin Olive Oil									
1 tbsp	120	14	2	NA	0	NA	NA	0	0
Lucini, Robust Garlic, Extra Virgin Olive Oil									
1 tbsp	120	14	2	NA	0	NA	NA	0	0
Lucini, Tuscan Basil, Extra Virgin Olive Oil									
1 tbsp	120	14	2	NA	0	NA	NA	0	0
Mezzetta, Extra Virgin Olive Oil									
1 tbsp	120	2	0	0	0	0	0	0	0
Smart Balance, Cooking Oil									
1 tbsp	120	14	1.5	0	0	NA	NA	0	0
Smart Balance, Omega Non-Stick Cooking Spray									
1 sec spray	10	1.5	0	0	0	NA	NA	0	0
Smart Balance, Omega Plus, Light Mayonnaise Dressing									
1 tbsp	50	5	0	5	2	NA	NA	0	125

Olives

Food Serving size	Cal.	(g) Total Fat	(g) Sat. Fat	(mg) Chol.	(g) Carb.	(g) Fiber	(g) Sug.	(g) Prot.	(mg) Sod.
Mezzetta, Anchovy Stuffed Olives									
4 olives	40	4	0	0	0	NA	NA	0	240
Mezzetta, Blue Cheese Stuffed Olives									
1 olive	10	1	0	0	1	0	0	0	170
Mezzetta, Feta Cheese Stuffed Olives									
1 olive	10	1	0	0	0	0	0	0	170
Mezzetta, Garlic Stuffed Olives									
1 olive	10	1	0	0	1	0	0	0	140
Mezzetta, Habanero Jack Cheese Stuffed Olives									
1 olive	10	1	0	0	1	NA	NA	0	170

Food Serving size	Cal.	(g) Total Fat	(g) Sat. Fat	(mg) Chol.	(g) Carb.	(g) Fiber	(g) Sug.	(g) Prot.	(mg) Sod.
Mezzetta, Jalapeno Stuffed Olives									
1 olive	10	1	0	0	1	0	0	0	140
Mezzetta, Kalamata Olive Sandwich Spread									
1 tbsp	50	4	0	0	5	0	3	0	90
Mezzetta, Kalamata Olives									
4 olives	40	4	0	0	1	0	0	0	240
Mezzetta, Martini Olives									
1 olive	10	1	0	0	1	0	0	0	170
Mezzetta, Mediterranean Olive Sandwich Spread									
15g	35	4	0	0	1	0	1	0	150
Mezzetta, Pimiento Stuffed Olives									
1 olive	10	0	0	0	0	0	0	0	165
Mezzetta, Salad Olives									
10 olives	20	2.5	0.5	0	0	1	NA	0	270
Mezzetta, Smoked Gouda Stuffed Olives									
1 olive	10	1	0	0	1	NA	NA	NA	170

Salad Dressings

Food Serving size	Cal.	(g) Total Fat	(g) Sat. Fat	(mg) Chol.	(g) Carb.	(g) Fiber	(g) Sug.	(g) Prot.	(mg) Sod.
Annie's, Artichoke Parmesan Dressing									
2 tbsp	90	9	1.5	5	1	NA	NA	1	290
Annie's, Balsamic Vinaigrette									
2 tbsp	100	10	1	NA	2	NA	2	0	55
Annie's, Cowgirl Ranch Dressing									
1 tbsp	110	11	1	10	3	NA	2	1	240
Annie's, Fat Free Mango Vinaigrette									
2 tbsp	20	0	NA	NA	5	NA	5	0	5
Annie's, Fat Free Raspberry Balsamic Vinaigrette									
2 tbsp	30	0	NA	NA	7	NA	7	0	10
Annie's, Lemon & Chive Dressing									
2 tbsp	110	12	1	NA	1	NA	NA	0	170
Annie's, Lite Goddess Dressing									
2 tbsp	60	6	0.5	NA	2	NA	NA	1	240
Annie's, Lite Herb Balsamic									
2 tbsp	50	5	NA	NA	2	NA	2	0	230

Food Serving size	Cal.	(g) Total Fat	(g) Sat. Fat	(mg) Chol.	(g) Carb.	(g) Fiber	(g) Sug.	(g) Prot.	(mg) Sod.
Annie's, Lite Honey Mustard Vinaigrette									
2 tbsp	40	3	NA	NA	4	NA	NA	0	125
Annie's, Lite Poppy Seed Dressing									
2 tbsp	70	4	1	5	10	NA	9	0	210
Annie's, Lite Raspberry Vinaigrette									
2 tbsp	40	3	NA	NA	4	NA	4	0	55
Annie's, Organic Balsamic Vinaigrette									
2 tbsp	100	10	1	NA	1	NA	1	0	55
Annie's, Organic Buttermilk Dressing									
2 tbsp	70	6	1	250	1	NA	1	1	250
Annie's, Organic Caesar Dressing									
2 tbsp	110	11	1	10	3	NA	2	1	240
Annie's, Organic Cowgirl Ranch Dressing									
2 tbsp	110	11	1	10	3	NA	2	1	240
Annie's, Organic Creamy Asiago Cheese Dressing									
2 tbsp	80	8	1	5	1	NA	NA	1	320
Annie's, Organic French Dressing									
2 tbsp	110	11	1	NA	3	NA	3	0	200
Annie's, Organic Green Garlic Dressing									
2 tbsp	80	8	0.5	NA	2	NA	1	0	170
Annie's, Organic Green Goddess Dressing									
2 tbsp	110	11	1.5	5	1	NA	1	0	260
Annie's, Organic Oil & Vinegar									
2 tbsp	120	13	1	NA	1	NA	NA	0	220
Annie's, Organic Papaya Poppy Seed Dressing									
2 tbsp	90	8	1	NA	5	NA	4	0	180
Annie's, Organic Pomegranate Vinaigrette Dressing									
2 tbsp	70	7	0.5	NA	2	NA	1	0	220
Annie's, Organic Red Wine & Olive Oil Vinaigrette									
2 tbsp	130	14	2	NA	0	NA	NA	0	190
Annie's, Organic Roasted Garlic Vinaigrette									
2 tbsp	110	11	1	NA	3	NA	2	0	220
Annie's, Organic Sesame Ginger Vinaigrette									
2 tbsp	90	8	1	NA	4	NA	3	1	250

Food Serving size	Cal.	(g) Total Fat	(g) Sat. Fat	(mg) Chol.	(g) Carb.	(g) Fiber	(g) Sug.	(g) Prot.	(mg) Sod.
Annie's, Organic Thousand Island Dressing									
2 tbsp	90	8	1	NA	5	NA	5	0	360
Annie's, Roasted Red Pepper Vinaigrette									
2 tbsp	60	6	NA	NA	3	NA	2	0	240
Annie's, Tuscany Italian Dressing									
2 tbsp	100	9	0.5	NA	3	NA	2	0	250
Boar's Head, Deli Dressing									
1 tbsp	100	11	1	50	0	0	0	0	50
Earth Balance, Olive Oil Dressing									
1 tbsp	90	9	0.5	0	0	NA	NA	0	70
Earth Balance, Organic Dressing									
1 tbsp	90	9	0.5	0	0	NA	NA	0	65
Earth Balance, Original Dressing									
1 tbsp	90	9	0.5	0	0	NA	NA	0	70
Lucini, Bold Parmesan & Garlic Vinaigrette									
2 tbsp	130	13	1.5	5	2	NA	1	0	240
Lucini, Charma Vi Balsamico Artisan Vinegar									
1 tbsp	30	0	NA	NA	7	NA	7	0	3
Lucini, Cherry Balsamic & Rosemary Vinaigrette									
2 tbsp	120	12	1	NA	3	NA	3	1	105
Lucini, Dark Cherry Balsamico Artisan Vinegar									
1 tbsp	30	0	0	NA	7	NA	7	0	3
Lucini, Delicate Cucumber & Shallot Vinaigrette									
2 tbsp	120	12	1	NA	2	NA	1	0	170
Lucini, Fig & Walnut Savory Balsamic Vinaigrette									
2 tbsp	110	10	1	NA	4	NA	3	0	180
Lucini, Roasted Hazelnut & Extra Virgin Vinaigrette									
2 tbsp	120	11	1	NA	3	NA	2	1	190
Lucini, Tuscan Balsamic & Extra Virgin Vinaigrette									
2 tbsp	120	12	1.5	NA	3	NA	3	0	180
Maple Grove Farms, All Natural Dressing, Aged Parmesan Peppercorn									
2 tbsp	110	11	1	NA	3	NA	3	0	390
Maple Grove Farms, All Natural Dressing, Champagne Vinaigrette									
2 tbsp	100	11	1	NA	2	NA	1	0	130

Food Serving size	Cal.	(g) Total Fat	(g) Sat. Fat	(mg) Chol.	(g) Carb.	(g) Fiber	(g) Sug.	(g) Prot.	(mg) Sod.
Maple Grove Farms, All Natural Dressing, Citrus Vinaigrette									
2 tbsp	80	6	NA	NA	6	NA	5	0	70
Maple Grove Farms, All Natural Dressing, Creamy Balsamic									
2 tbsp	120	12	1	NA	5	NA	4	0	230
Maple Grove Farms, All Natural Dressing, Ginger Pear									
2 tbsp	40	3	NA	NA	3	NA	2	0	40
Maple Grove Farms, All Natural Dressing, Sesame Ginger									
2 tbsp	45	2	NA	NA	6	NA	5	<1	260
Maple Grove Farms, All Natural Dressing, Strawberry Balsamic									
2 tbsp	30	0	NA	NA	6	NA	6	0	160
Maple Grove Farms, Fat Free Dressing, Balsamic Vinaigrette									
2 tbsp	15	0	NA	NA	3	NA	2	0	95
Maple Grove Farms, Fat Free Dressing, Caesar									
2 tbsp	10	0	NA	NA	2	<1	<1	0	320
Maple Grove Farms, Fat Free Dressing, Cranberry Balsamic									
2 tbsp	30	0	NA	NA	7	NA	6	0	180
Maple Grove Farms, Fat Free Dressing, Greek									
2 tbsp	10	0	NA	NA	3	<1	2	0	240
Maple Grove Farms, Fat Free Dressing, Honey Dijon									
2 tbsp	35	0	NA	NA	9	<1	8	0	200
Maple Grove Farms, Fat Free Dressing, Lime Basil									
2 tbsp	25	0	NA	NA	6	NA	5	0	130
Maple Grove Farms, Fat Free Dressing, Poppyseed									
2 tbsp	35	0	NA	NA	7	NA	7	0	160
Maple Grove Farms, Fat Free Dressing, Raspberry Vinaigrette									
2 tbsp	35	0	NA	NA	7	NA	7	0	160
Maple Grove Farms, Fat Free Dressing, Vidalia Onion									
2 tbsp	20	0	NA	NA	5	NA	4	0	140
Maple Grove Farms, Fat Free Dressing, Wasabi Dijon									
2 tbsp	40	0	NA	NA	9	<1	8	0	190
Maple Grove Farms, Lite Dressing, Caesar									
2 tbsp	50	4.5	NA	NA	4	NA	3	0	260
Maple Grove Farms, Lite Dressing, Honey Mustard									
2 tbsp	70	4	NA	NA	8	NA	7	0	260

Food Serving size	Cal.	(g) Total Fat	(g) Sat. Fat	(mg) Chol.	(g) Carb.	(g) Fiber	(g) Sug.	(g) Prot.	(mg) Sod.
Maple Grove Farms, Original Dressing, Asiago and Garlic									
2 tbsp	40	3.5	NA	NA	2	NA	1	0	260
Maple Grove Farms, Original Dressing, Balsamic Vinaigrette with Maple									
2 tbsp	50	3	NA	NA	5	NA	5	0	35
Maple Grove Farms, Original Dressing, Honey Mustard									
2 tbsp	100	8	0.5	NA	8	NA	7	<1	260
Maple Grove Farms, Original Dressing, Sweet 'n Sour									
2 tbsp	90	6	NA	NA	10	NA	9	0	150
Maple Grove Farms, Sugar Free Dressing, Balsamic Vinaigrette									
2 tbsp	5	0	NA	NA	1	NA	NA	0	90
Maple Grove Farms, Sugar Free Dressing, Creamy Ranch									
2 tbsp	100	12	1	NA	<1	NA	NA	0	110
Maple Grove Farms, Sugar Free Dressing, Italian White Balsamic									
2 tbsp	100	11	1	NA	<1	NA	NA	0	70
Maple Grove Farms, Sugar Free Dressing, Raspberry Vinaigrette									
2 tbsp	5	0	NA	NA	1	NA	NA	0	160
Newman's Own, Balsamic Vinaigrette Salad Dressing									
2 tbsp	90	9	1	0	3	0	1	0	290
Newman's Own, Caesar Salad Dressing									
2 tbsp	150	16	2.5	0	1	0	1	1	420
Newman's Own, Creamy Balsamic Salad Dressing									
2 tbsp	110	10	1.5	0	6	0	5	0	200
Newman's Own, Creamy Caesar Salad Dressing									
2 tbsp	150	16	2.5	20	1	0	1	1	420
Newman's Own, Greek Vinaigrette Salad Dressing									
2 tbsp	100	10	1.5	0	2	0	1	0	270
Newman's Own, Honey French Salad Dressing									
2 tbsp	130	11	1.5	0	6	0	5	0	170
Newman's Own, Lite Balsamic Vinaigrette Salad Dressing									
2 tbsp	45	4	0.5	0	2	0	2	0	350
Newman's Own, Lite Caesar Salad Dressing									
2 tbsp	70	6	1	5	3	0	2	1	420
Newman's Own, Lite Cranberry Walnut Salad Dressing									
2 tbsp	70	4	0.5	0	8	0	7	1	230

Food Serving size	Cal.	(g) Total Fat	(g) Sat. Fat	(mg) Chol.	(g) Carb.	(g) Fiber	(g) Sug.	(g) Prot.	(mg) Sod.
Newman's Own, Lite Honey Mustard Salad Dressing									
2 tbsp	70	4	0.5	0	7	0	5	0	280
Newman's Own, Lite Italian Salad Dressing									
2 tbsp	60	6	1	0	1	0	0	0	260
Newman's Own, Lite Lime Vinaigrette Salad Dressing									
2 tbsp	60	6	1	0	4	0	4	0	320
Newman's Own, Lite Raspberry Walnut Salad Dressing									
2 tbsp	70	5	10	0	7	0	5	0	120
Newman's Own, Lite Red Wine Vinegar & Olive Oil Salad Dressing									
2 tbsp	50	4.5	0.5	0	2	0	2	0	390
Newman's Own, Lite Roasted Garlic Balsamic Salad Dressing									
2 tbsp	50	4	0.5	0	3	0	3	0	420
Newman's Own, Lite Sun Dried Tomato Italian Salad Dressing									
2 tbsp	60	4	0.5	0	5	0	3	0	380
Newman's Own, Olive Oil & Vinegar Salad Dressing									
2 tbsp	150	16	2.5	0	1	0	1	0	150
Newman's Own, Organic Lite Balsamic Salad Dressing									
2 tbsp	45	4	0.5	0	2	0	2	0	450
Newman's Own, Organic Tuscan Italian Salad Dressing									
2 tbsp	100	11	1.5	0	2	0	1	0	380
Newman's Own, Parmesan & Roasted Garlic Salad Dressing									
2 tbsp	110	11	2	0	2	0	1	1	340
Newman's Own, Poppy Seed Salad Dressing									
2 tbsp	140	13	2	0	5	0	5	0	220
Newman's Own, Ranch Salad Dressing									
2 tbsp	150	16	2.5	10	2	0	1	0	310
Newman's Own, Three Cheese Balsamic Vinaigrette Salad Dressing									
2 tbsp	110	11	1.5	0	2	0	2	0	380
San-J, Tamari Ginger Salad Dressing									
2 tbsp	25	0	0	0	5	0	4	<1	490
San-J, Tamari Peanut Salad Dressing									
2 tbsp	70	2	0	0	9	<1	7	3	230
San-J, Tamari Sesame Salad Dressing									
2 tbsp	40	2	0	0	5	0	3	2	570

Food Serving size	Cal.	(g) Total Fat	(g) Sat. Fat	(mg) Chol.	(g) Carb.	(g) Fiber	(g) Sug.	(g) Prot.	(mg) Sod.
Seeds of Change, Balsamic Vinaigrette Salad Dressing									
2 tbsp	60	4	0	0	6	0	3	0	105
Seeds of Change, French Tomato Salad Dressing									
2 tbsp	60	3	0	0	8	0	6	0	210
Seeds of Change, Greek Feta Vinaigrette Salad Dressing									
2 tbsp	60	4.5	0.5	0	5	0	2	1	270
Seeds of Change, Italian Herb Vinaigrette Salad Dressing									
2 tbsp	60	4.5	0	0	5	0	3	0	260
Seeds of Change, Roasted Red Pepper Vinaigrette Salad Dressing									
2 tbsp	50	3.5	0	0	5	0	3	0	240
Simply Organic Foods, Classic Caesar Dressing									
3/4 tsp	15	0	0	0	3	0	1	0	240
Simply Organic Foods, Garlic Vinaigrette Dressing									
3/4 tsp	10	0	0	0	2	0	1	0	230
Simply Organic Foods, Italian Dressing									
3/4 tsp	5	0	0	0	2	0	1	0	150
Simply Organic Foods, Orange Ginger Vinaigrette									
1 tsp	5	0	0	0	2	0	0	0	170
Simply Organic Foods, Pineapple Cilantro Vinaigrette									
1 tsp	10	0	0	0	2	0	0	0	150
Simply Organic Foods, Ranch Dressing									
1 tsp	10	0	0	0	1	0	1	1	140

Spreads & Dips

Food Serving size	Cal.	(g) Total Fat	(g) Sat. Fat	(mg) Chol.	(g) Carb.	(g) Fiber	(g) Sug.	(g) Prot.	(mg) Sod.
Frito-Lay, Fritos Bean Dip									
2 tbsp	35	1	0	0	5	2	0	2	190
Frito-Lay, Fritos Chili Cheese Dip									
2 tbsp	45	3	1	0	3	<1	1	1	290
Frito-Lay, Fritos Hot Bean Dip									
2 tbsp	35	1	0	0	5	2	0	2	230
Frito-Lay, Fritos Jalapeno & Cheddar Flavored Cheese Dip									
2 tbsp	50	3.5	0.5	<5mg	3	0	<1	1	320
Frito-Lay, Fritos Mild Cheddar Flavored Cheese Dip									
2 tbsp	50	3.5	0.5	<5mg	4	0	<1	1	340

Food Serving size	Cal.	(g) Total Fat	(g) Sat. Fat	(mg) Chol.	(g) Carb.	(g) Fiber	(g) Sug.	(g) Prot.	(mg) Sod.
Frito-Lay, Fritos Southwest Enchilada Black Bean Flavored Dip									
2 tbsp	30	0	0	0	5	2	<1	2	200
Frito-Lay, Lay's Dip Creations, Country Ranch Dry Dip Mix, Prepared with Sour Cream									
2 tbsp	70	6	3.5	10	2	0	0	1	160
Frito-Lay, Lay's Dip Creations, Garden Onion Dry Dip Mix, Prepared with Sour Cream									
2 tbsp	70	6	3.5	10	2	0	0	1	160
Frito-Lay, Lay's French Onion Dip									
2 tbsp	60	5	0	<5mg	2	0	0	1	230
Frito-Lay, Lay's Smooth Ranch Dip									
2 tbsp	60	5	0	<5mg	2	0	<1	1	210
Frito-Lay, Tostitos Creamy Southwestern Ranch Dip									
2 tbsp	60	5	0.5	<5mg	2	<1	<1	1	160
Frito-Lay, Tostitos Dip Creations, Freshly Made Guacamole Dry Dip Mix, Prepared									
2 tbsp	50	4	0.5	0	3	2	0	1	120
Frito-Lay, Tostitos Monterey Jack Queso Dip									
2 tbsp	40	2.5	0.5	<5mg	4	0	0	1	210
Frito-Lay, Tostitos Salsa Con Queso									
2 tbsp	40	2.5	1	<5mg	5	<1	<1	<1	280
Frito-Lay, Tostitos Smooth & Cheesy Dip									
2 tbsp	50	3.5	1	5	4	0	0	1	200
Frito-Lay, Tostitos Spicy Nacho Cheese Dip									
2 tbsp	35	3	1	<5mg	2	0	<1	0	170
Frito-Lay, Tostitos Zesty Bean & Cheese Dip									
2 tbsp	45	2	0.5	0	5	2	<1	2	230
Mezzetta, Peperoncini & Feta Sandwich Spread									
1 tbsp	35	3	1	0	2	0	1	1	180
Mezzetta, Roasted Red Bell Pepper & Chipotle Spread									
1 tbsp	45	4	0	0	1	0	1	1	180
Newman's Own, Salsa Con Queso									
2 tbsp	40	3	0.5	5	3	0	1	0	200
Simply Organic Foods, Creamy Dill Dip									
1/2 tsp	5	0	0	0	<1	0	0	0	90

Food Serving size	Cal.	(g) Total Fat	(g) Sat. Fat	(mg) Chol.	(g) Carb.	(g) Fiber	(g) Sug.	(g) Prot.	(mg) Sod.
Simply Organic Foods, Fruit Dip									
2 tsp	15	0	0	0	4	0	3	0	0
Simply Organic Foods, Guacamole Dip									
1/2 tsp	5	0	0	0	1	0	0	0	90
Simply Organic Foods, Ranch Dip									
1 tsp	10	0	0	0	1	0	1	1	140
Simply Organic Foods, Spinach Dip									
3/4 tsp	10	0	0	0	2	0	0	0	105

Snacks & Sweets

Why Eat Snacks?

Snacks are important to keep you energized throughout the day, especially when the time between meals is longer than 4 hours. This is the amount of time it takes for the food you eat to be digested, metabolized, and assimilated into your body cells where it is used for energy and other maintenance tasks. After about 4 hours, your body will start sending hunger messages and may start slowing down. So, a snack between meals can help you stay alert and not hungry. The important thing is to make nutritious gluten-free snack choices that don't contain empty calories.

Daily Goal

Plan two healthy snacks each day.
Avoid "empty calories" in added sugar and solid fats.

Shopping Tips

- Keep raw nuts and seeds handy
- Prepare cut up fruits and vegetables and store in the refrigerator
- Air-popped corn is a gluten-free whole grain snack
- Gluten-free whole grain cereal makes a great snack

Shopping List Essentials

Popcorn
Fruits
Vegetables

Approved Snacks & Sweets and Those to Avoid on a Gluten-Free Diet

Gluten-Free

- Plain popcorn
- Plain rice crackers, rice cakes, and popped corn cakes
- Baked chips

Contain Gluten

Seasoned (flavored) chips, rice cakes, and popped corn cakes made with ingredients to avoid

Caution

Avoid "empty calories" in added sugar and solid fats. "Empty calorie" foods and beverages provide calories but few or no nutrients. Solid fats can be butter or shortening used in baking or fried foods or they can be other fats added in processing that result in trans fats. Check ingredient lists for the term "partially hydrogenated fats." This term means the presence of "trans fats" even when the Nutrition Facts say "0 grams trans fat."

Food Serving size	Cal.	(g) Total Fat	(g) Sat. Fat	(mg) Chol.	(g) Carb.	(g) Fiber	(g) Sug.	(g) Prot.	(mg) Sod.

Candies (Including Brand-name Bars)

Enjoy Life Foods, Boom Choco Boom, Dark Chocolate Bar
1 bar	200	15	9	0	22	3	17	2	0

Enjoy Life Foods, Boom Choco Boom, Ricemilk Chocolate Bar
1 bar	230	17	11	0	21	1	17	1	25

Enjoy Life Foods, Boom Choco Boom, Ricemilk Crunch Bar
1 bar	220	15	10	0	22	1	16	1	30

Justin's, Dark Chocolate Peanut Butter Cup
2 cups	200	16	7	0	20	2	14	4	120

Justin's, Dark Chocolate Peanut Candy Bar
1 bar	260	14	6	0	32	2	21	5	130

Justin's, Mik Chocolate Peanut Candy Bar
1 bar	270	14	6	5	32	2	23	6	150

Justin's, Milk Chocolate Almond Candy Bar
1 bar	280	16	5	5	31	2	22	5	125

Justin's, Milk Chocolate Peanut Butter Cup
2 cups	200	14	6	0	18	2	14	4	120

Let's Do — Organic, Organic Classic Gummi Bears
1 packet	100	0	0	0	23	0	18	0	15

Let's Do — Organic, Organic Jelly Gummi Bears
1 packet	100	0	0	0	23	0	19	0	15

Let's Do — Organic, Organic Super Sour Gummi Bears
1 packet	100	0	0	0	23	0	19	0	15

Maple Grove Farms, Fancies & Leaf Tray Blend Candy
1 large or 4 small pieces	160	0	NA	NA	42	NA	37	0	0

Maple Grove Farms, Large Leaf Blend Maple Candy
1 piece	170	0	NA	NA	44	NA	39	0	0

Maple Grove Farms, Large Leaf Pure Maple Candy
1 piece	170	0	NA	NA	44	NA	42	0	0

Maple Grove Farms, Massachusetts Box Blend Candy
5 pieces	160	0	NA	NA	42	NA	37	0	0

Maple Grove Farms, New Hampshire State Box Blend Candy
5 pieces	160	0	NA	NA	42	NA	37	0	0

Food Serving size	Cal.	(g) Total Fat	(g) Sat. Fat	(mg) Chol.	(g) Carb.	(g) Fiber	(g) Sug.	(g) Prot.	(mg) Sod.
Maple Grove Farms, Pilgrims, Blend Candy									
2 pieces	220	0	NA	NA	57	NA	50	0	0
Maple Grove Farms, Pocket Pack, Fancies Blend Candy									
5 pieces	140	0	NA	NA	36	NA	32	0	0
Maple Grove Farms, Pocket Pack, Fancies Pure Candy									
5 pieces	140	0	NA	NA	36	NA	34	0	0
Maple Grove Farms, Santa Claus, Blend Candy									
1 piece	170	0	NA	NA	44	NA	39	0	0
Maple Grove Farms, Vermont State Box, Blend Candy									
5 pieces	160	0	NA	NA	42	NA	37	0	0
Maple Grove Farms, Vermont State Box, Pure Candy									
5 pieces	160	0	NA	NA	42	NA	40	0	5
Maple Grove Farms, Will Moses Art Box, Blend Candy									
5 pieces	160	0	NA	NA	42	NA	37	0	0
Maple Grove Farms, Will Moses Art Box, Pure Candy									
5 pieces	160	0	NA	NA	42	NA	40	0	5
Nestlé, Baby Ruth									
1 bar	280	14	8	0	39	1	33	4	130
Nestlé, Bit-O-Honey									
6 pieces	150	3	2	0	32	0	19	1	120
Nestlé, Butterfinger									
1 bar	270	11	6	0	43	1	28	4	135
Nestlé, Cranberry Raisinets									
1/4 cup	200	8	5	5	32	0	30	1	15
Nestlé, Dark Chocolate Raisinets									
1 bag or 1/4 cup	190	8	5	5	31	2	27	2	5
Nestlé, Goobers									
1/4 cup	210	14	5	5	22	2	18	5	15
Nestlé, Milk Chocolate Raisinets									
1 bag or 1/4 cup	190	8	5	5	32	1	28	2	15
Nestlé, Nips Butter Rum									
2 pieces	60	1.5	1.5	NA	12	NA	8	0	45
Nestlé, Nips Caramel									
2 pieces	60	1.5	1.5	NA	12	NA	8	0	45

Food Serving size	Cal.	(g) Total Fat	(g) Sat. Fat	(mg) Chol.	(g) Carb.	(g) Fiber	(g) Sug.	(g) Prot.	(mg) Sod.
Nestlé, Nips Chocolate Parfait									
2 pieces	60	2	2	NA	11	NA	8	0	35
Nestlé, Nips Coffee									
2 pieces	60	1.5	1.5	NA	NA	NA	8	0	45
Nestlé, Nips Peanut Butter Parfait									
2 pieces	60	2	2	NA	11	NA	8	0	45
Nestlé, Nips, Sugar Free Nips Caramel									
2 pieces	60	1.5	1	5	12	NA	0	0	10
Nestlé, Nips, Sugar Free Nips Coffee									
2 pieces	60	1.5	1	5	12	NA	0	0	10
Nestlé, Oh Henry!									
1 package	230	11	5	<5	33	1	24	3	100
Nestlé, Sno-Caps									
1/4 cup	180	8	5	<5	30	2	24	1	0
Nestlé, Wonka Laffy Taffy Bags									
All flavors, 4 bars	140	2	1.5	0	30	0	19	0	50
Nestlé, Wonka Laffy Taffy Rope									
All flavors, 1 rope	80	1.5	1	0	18	0	11	0	40
Nestlé, Wonka Laffy Taffy Stretchy and Tangy									
All flavors, 1 bar	150	3.5	3.5	0	29	0	19	0	20
Nestlé, Wonka Lik-M-Aid Fun Dip									
1 packet	50	0	0	0	13	0	13	0	0
Nestlé, Wonka Pixy Stix, Giant									
1 stick	100	0	0	0	26	NA	26	0	0
Nestlé, Wonka Pixy Stix, Peg Bag									
7 straws	60	0	0	0	15	0	15	0	0
Sharkies Kids, Organic Sport Chews, Berry Bites and Fruit Splash									
1 package	70	0	0	0	18	0	10	0	40
Sharkies Kids, Organic Sport Chews, Berry Surf and Tropical Wave									
1 twist	70	0	0	0	16	1	13	0	15
Sharkies Kids, Organic Sport Chews, Tropical Splash and Berry Blasters									
12 pieces	140	0	0	0	35	0	26	0	60
Sharkies, Organic Sports Chew: Citrus Squeeze, Fruit Splash, Berry Blast, Watermelon Scream									
1 package	140	0	0	0	36	1	17	0	110

Food Serving size	Cal.	(g) Total Fat	(g) Sat. Fat	(mg) Chol.	(g) Carb.	(g) Fiber	(g) Sug.	(g) Prot.	(mg) Sod.
Yamate Chocolatier, Gluten Free Dark Chocolate Bars, 70% Cacao									
40g	180	18	11	0	18	14	0	3	0
Yamate Chocolatier, Gluten Free Masterpiece Almonds and Caramel Chocolate Bar									
1.34 oz	170	13	4.5	10	14	2	1	4	10

Chips, Pretzels & Popcorn

Food Serving size	Cal.	(g) Total Fat	(g) Sat. Fat	(mg) Chol.	(g) Carb.	(g) Fiber	(g) Sug.	(g) Prot.	(mg) Sod.
Annie Chun's, Brown Sugar & Sea Salt Seaweed Snacks									
10 sheets	25	1.5	NA	NA	2	NA	NA	1	60
Annie Chun's, Cracked Pepper & Herbs Seaweed Snacks									
10 sheets	25	2	NA	NA	1	NA	NA	1	70
Annie Chun's, Sesame Seaweed Snacks									
10 sheets	30	2.5	NA	NA	1	NA	NA	1	70
Annie Chun's, Wasabi Seaweed Snacks									
10 sheets	30	2	NA	NA	1	NA	NA	1	65
Bachman Gluten-Free Puzzle Pretzels									
16 pretzels	120	3	1.5	0	22	4	0	1	250
Beanitos, Black Bean Chips									
1 oz	140	7	0.5	0	15	5	0	4	55
Beanitos, Cheddar Cheese Pinto Bean & Flax Chips									
1 oz	140	8	1	0	14	5	0	4	140
Beanitos, Chipotle BBQ Chips									
1 oz	140	7	0.5	0	15	5	<1	4	150
Beanitos, Pinto Bean & Flax Chips									
1 oz	140	8	0.5	0	15	5	0	4	55
Bhuja, Cracker Mix									
.88 oz	113	4	1	0	16	<1	<1	4	167
Bhuja, Original Mix									
.88 oz	129	6	1	0	12	2	1	5	171
Blue Diamond, Baked Nut Chips, Nacho Flavor									
14 chips	130	4	0.5	0	21	1	1	3	210
Blue Diamond, Baked Nut Chips, Sea Salt Flavor									
15 chips	130	3.5	0	0	22	1	0	3	170
Blue Diamond, Baked Nut Chips, Sour Cream & Chive Flavor									
14 chips	130	4.5	0	0	21	1	1	3	160

Food Serving size	Cal.	(g) Total Fat	(g) Sat. Fat	(mg) Chol.	(g) Carb.	(g) Fiber	(g) Sug.	(g) Prot.	(mg) Sod.
Boulder Canyon, 60% Reduced Sodium, Totally Natural Kettle Chips									
1 oz, approx 14 chips	140	7	1	0	17	2	<1	2	70
Boulder Canyon, Balsamic Vinegar & Rosemary, Kettle Chips									
1 oz, approx 14 chips	150	7	1	0	17	2	1	2	334
Boulder Canyon, Garden Select Vegetable Crisps, Red Ripe Tomato									
15 chips	120	7	1	0	16	3	2	2	165
Boulder Canyon, Hickory Barbeque, Kettle Chips									
1 oz, approx 14 chips	140	7	1	0	17	1	1	2	175
Boulder Canyon, Hummus Chips, Lightly Salted									
14 chips	140	7	0.5	0	17	1	<1	2	270
Boulder Canyon, Hummus Chips, Lightly Salted with Sesame									
14 chips	140	7	0.5	0	17	1	<1	2	270
Boulder Canyon, Jalapeno Cheddar, Kettle Chips									
1.5 oz, approx 14 chips	210	11	1	0	25	2	2	4	330
Boulder Canyon, Lightly Salted Tortilla Chips, with Hummus and Sesame Chips									
14 chips	140	7	0.5	0	17	1	<1	2	270
Boulder Canyon, Olive Oil, Totally Natural Kettle Chips									
1 oz, approx 14 chips	140	7	1	0	16	0	0	3	120
Boulder Canyon, Parmesan & Garlic, Kettle Chips									
1 oz, approx 14 chips	130	7	1	0	17	1	0	2	170
Boulder Canyon, Red Wine Vinegar, Kettle Chips									
1 oz, approx 14 chips	140	7	1	0	18	2	1	2	270
Boulder Canyon, Rice & Bean Chipotle Cheese, Artisan Snack Chips									
20 chips	120	7	1	0	17	3	1	2	185
Boulder Canyon, Rice & Bean Natural Salt, Artisan Snack Chips									
20 chips	120	7	1	0	17	3	1	2	130
Boulder Canyon, Sea Salt & Cracked Pepper, Kettle Chips									
1 oz, approx 14 chips	130	7	1	0	17	1	0	2	150
Boulder Canyon, Spinach & Artichoke, Kettle Chips									
1 oz, approx 16 chips	130	7	1	0	17	1	0	2	280
Boulder Canyon, Totally Natural Kettle Chips									
1 oz, approx 14 chips	130	7	1	0	17	1	0	2	120
Boulder Canyon, Vegetable Crisps, Hearty Cheddar									
15 chips	120	7	1	0	16	3	2	2	140

Food Serving size	Cal.	(g) Total Fat	(g) Sat. Fat	(mg) Chol.	(g) Carb.	(g) Fiber	(g) Sug.	(g) Prot.	(mg) Sod.
Boulder Canyon, Vegetable Crisps, Sour Cream & Chive									
15 chips	120	7	1	0	16	3	2	2	180
Boulder Canyon, Wavy Canyon Cut, Honey BBQ Potato Chips									
1 oz, about 14 chips	130	6	1	0	18	2	2	2	220
Boulder Canyon, Wavy Canyon Cut, Sour Cream & Chive Potato Chips									
1 oz, about 14 chips	150	8	1	0	17	2	1	2	205
Boulder Canyon, Wavy Canyon Cut, Totally Natural Potato Chips									
1 oz, about 14 chips	130	7	1	0	17	1	0	2	120
Eden Foods, Popcorn, 100% Whole Grain, Organic									
2 tbsp	80	1	0	NA	20	5	0	2	0
El's Kitchen Gluten Free, Cheddar Snack Medleys									
1 oz	150	8	1	NA	18	2	<1	2	210
El's Kitchen Gluten Free, Original Snack Medleys									
1 oz	140	8	1	NA	18	2	2	2	310
El's Kitchen Gluten Free, Sour Cream & Onion Snack Medley's									
1 oz	140	7	1	NA	18	2	<1	2	190
Ener-G, Ener-G Pretzels									
25 pretzels	140	6	1	0	21	<1	<1	<1	480
Ener-G, Sesame Pretzel Rings									
19 pretzels	150	8	3	0	19	0	0	1	390
Enjoy Life Foods, Dill & Sour Cream, Plentils Chips									
1 oz, 31 pieces	130	6	0	0	18	1	1	3	400
Enjoy Life Foods, Garlic & Parmesan, Plentils Chips									
1 oz, 31 pieces	130	6	0	0	17	1	0	3	410
Enjoy Life Foods, Light Sea Salt, Plentils Chips									
1 oz, 31 pieces	130	6	0	0	17	1	0	3	420
Enjoy Life Foods, Margherita Pizza, Plentils Chips									
1 oz, 31 pieces	130	6	0	0	17	1	0	3	370
Food Should Taste Good, Barbeque Sweet, Potato Chips									
About 14 chips	150	8	0.5	0	17	3	4	1	140
Food Should Taste Good, Blue Corn, Tortilla Chips									
About 9 chips	140	7	0.5	0	18	3	1	2	80
Food Should Taste Good, Blue Corn, Tortilla Dipping Chips									
About 14 chips	140	7	0.5	0	19	3	0	2	100

Food Serving size	Cal.	(g) Total Fat	(g) Sat. Fat	(mg) Chol.	(g) Carb.	(g) Fiber	(g) Sug.	(g) Prot.	(mg) Sod.
Food Should Taste Good, Cantina, Tortilla Chips									
About 9 chips	140	7	0.5	0	18	3	0	2	140
Food Should Taste Good, Cheddar, Tortilla Chips									
About 10 chips	140	7	1	0	17	3	1	3	135
Food Should Taste Good, Chocolate, Tortilla Chips									
About 10 chips	140	7	1	0	17	3	4	2	80
Food Should Taste Good, Hatch Chile, Tortilla Chips									
About 12 chips	140	6	0.5	0	18	3	1	2	140
Food Should Taste Good, Hemp, Tortilla Chips									
About 12 chips	140	7	0.5	0	17	3	0	3	80
Food Should Taste Good, Jalapeno & Cheddar, Tortilla Chips									
About 12 chips	140	6	1	0	16	3	1	2	190
Food Should Taste Good, Jalapeno, Tortilla Chips									
About 12 chips	140	6	0.5	0	18	3	0	2	140
Food Should Taste Good, Kettle Corn, Tortilla Chips									
About 12 chips	140	7	0.5	0	18	3	2	2	120
Food Should Taste Good, Lime, Tortilla Chips									
About 12 chips	140	6	0.5	0	19	4	0	2	95
Food Should Taste Good, Multigrain, Tortilla Chips									
About 10 chips	140	6	0.5	0	18	3	1	3	80
Food Should Taste Good, Olive, Tortilla Chips									
About 10 chips	140	6	0.5	0	18	3	0	2	140
Food Should Taste Good, Original Sweet, Potato Chips									
About 15 chips	150	8	0.5	0	17	3	3	1	140
Food Should Taste Good, Salt & Pepper, Sweet Potato Chips									
About 14 chips	150	8	0.5	0	17	3	3	1	140
Food Should Taste Good, Sweet Potato, Tortilla Chips									
About 12 chips	140	6	0.5	0	18	3	2	2	80
Food Should Taste Good, The Works!, Tortilla Chips									
About 9 chips	140	6	0.5	0	18	3	2	2	120
Food Should Taste Good, Toasted Sesame, Tortilla Chips									
About 11 chips	150	8	1	0	17	3	0	2	100
Food Should Taste Good, White Cheddar, Tortilla Chips									
About 10 chips	140	7	1	0	17	3	1	3	135

Food Serving size	Cal.	(g) Total Fat	(g) Sat. Fat	(mg) Chol.	(g) Carb.	(g) Fiber	(g) Sug.	(g) Prot.	(mg) Sod.
Food Should Taste Good, White Corn, Tortilla Dipping Chips									
About 10 chips	140	7	0.5	0	19	3	0	2	100
Frito-Lay, Baked Lay's, Southwestern Ranch Flavored, Potato Crisps									
1 oz	120	3	0.5	0	21	2	2	2	160
Frito-Lay, Baked! Cheetos Crunchy Cheese Flavored Snacks									
About 34 pieces	130	5	1	0	20	<1	<1	2	150
Frito-Lay, Baked! Cheetos Flamin' Hot, Cheese Flavored Snacks									
About 34 pieces	120	5	1	0	17	<1	<1	2	220
Frito-Lay, Baked! Doritos Nacho Cheese Flavored Tortilla Chips									
1 oz	120	3.5	0.5	0	21	2	1	2	230
Frito-Lay, Baked! Lay's Original Potato Crisps									
About 15 crisps	120	2	0	0	23	2	2	2	135
Frito-Lay, Baked! Lay's, Sour Cream & Onion Artificially Flavored Potato Crisps									
1 oz	120	3	0.5	0	21	2	3	2	210
Frito-Lay, Baked! Lay's, Southwestern Ranch Flavored Potato Crisps									
1 oz	120	3	0.5	0	21	2	2	2	160
Frito-Lay, Baked! Ruffles, Cheddar & Sour Cream Flavored Potato Crisps									
1 oz	120	3.5	0.5	0	21	2	2	2	270
Frito-Lay, Baked! Ruffles, Original Potato Crisps									
About 9 crisps	120	3	0	0	22	2	1	2	135
Frito-Lay, Baked! Tostitos Scoops! Tortilla Chips									
About 16 crisps	120	3	0.5	0	22	2	0	2	140
Frito-Lay, Baken-Ets, Hot 'N Spicy Flavored Fried Pork Cracklins									
8 pieces	80	5	2	20	<1	<1	0	7	330
Frito-Lay, Baken-Ets, Hot 'N Spicy Flavored Pork Skins									
9 pieces	80	5	2	20	0	0	0	7	470
Frito-Lay, Baken-Ets, Tangy BBQ Flavored Fried Pork Skins									
9 pieces	80	5	2.5	20	1	0	0	7	400
Frito-Lay, Baken-Ets, Traditional Fried Pork Skins									
9 pieces	80	5	2.5	20	0	0	0	7	310
Frito-Lay, Cheetos, Crunchy Cheddar Jalapeno Cheese Flavored Snacks									
About 21 pieces	170	11	2	0	15	<1	<1	2	290
Frito-Lay, Cheetos, Crunchy Cheese Flavored Snacks									
About 21 pieces	150	10	1.5	0	13	<1	1	2	250

Food Serving size	Cal.	(g) Total Fat	(g) Sat. Fat	(mg) Chol.	(g) Carb.	(g) Fiber	(g) Sug.	(g) Prot.	(mg) Sod.
Frito-Lay, Cheetos, Crunchy Flamin Hot, Cheese Flavored Snacks									
About 21 pieces	160	11	1.5	0	13	<1	0	1	250
Frito-Lay, Cheetos, Crunchy Flamin' Hot, Limon Cheese Flavored Snacks									
About 21 pieces	160	11	1.5	0	13	<1	0	1	260
Frito-Lay, Cheetos, Crunchy Salsa Con Queso, Cheese Flavored Snacks									
About 21 pieces	150	10	1.5	0	13	<1	<1	2	220
Frito-Lay, Cheetos, Fantastix!, Chili Cheese Flavored Baked Corn/ Potato Snacks									
1 package	130	5	1	0	19	1	<1	2	200
Frito-Lay, Cheetos, Fantastix!, Flamin' Hot Flavored Baked Corn/ Potato Snacks									
1 package	120	4.5	0.5	0	18	1	<1	2	200
Frito-Lay, Cheetos, Puffs, Cheese Flavored Snacks									
About 13 pieces	160	10	2	0	13	0	1	2	350
Frito-Lay, Cheetos, Puffs, Flamin' Hot Cheese Flavored Snacks									
1 oz	150	10	1.5	0	13	1	1	1	300
Frito-Lay, Cheetos, Puffs, Simply Natural, White Cheddar Cheese Flavored Snacks									
About 32 pieces	150	9	1.5	0	16	<1	1	2	290
Frito-Lay, Cheetos, Puffs, Twisted Cheese Flavored Snacks									
About 7 pieces	150	10	1.5	0	13	<1	1	2	300
Frito-Lay, Chester's, Butter Flavored Puffcorn Snacks									
1 oz	160	11	1.5	0	14	<1	0	1	300
Frito-Lay, Chester's, Cheddar Cheese Flavored Popcorn									
1 serving	150	10	1.5	0	15	3	<1	2	200
Frito-Lay, Chester's, Cheese Flavored Puffcorn Snacks									
1 oz	160	11	1.5	0	14	0	1	2	290
Frito-Lay, Chester's, Flamin' Hot Flavored Fries									
1 package	260	14	2.5	<5	30	1	1	3	490
Frito-Lay, Chester's, Flamin' Hot Flavored Puffcorn Snacks									
1 oz	150	10	1.5	0	13	1	1	2	320
Frito-Lay, Cracker Jack, Original Caramel Coated Popcorn & Peanuts									
1/2 cup	120	2	0	0	23	1	15	2	70
Frito-Lay, Doritos, Blazin' Buffalo & Ranch Flavored Tortilla Chips									
About 12 chips	140	7	1.5	0	18	1	<1	2	260

Food Serving size	Cal.	(g) Total Fat	(g) Sat. Fat	(mg) Chol.	(g) Carb.	(g) Fiber	(g) Sug.	(g) Prot.	(mg) Sod.
Frito-Lay, Doritos, Cool Ranch Flavored Tortilla Chips									
About 12 chips	150	8	1	0	18	2	<1	2	180
Frito-Lay, Doritos, Dinamita Chile Limon Flavored Rolled Tortilla Chips									
About 15 pieces	140	8	1	0	16	1	0	2	200
Frito-Lay, Doritos, Dinamita Nacho Picoso Flavored Rolled Tortilla Chips									
About 15 pieces	140	9	1.5	0	15	1	0	2	230
Frito-Lay, Doritos, Fiery Habanero Flavored Tortilla Chips									
About 11 chips	150	8	1	0	18	1	1	2	240
Frito-Lay, Doritos, Flamas Flavored Tortilla Chips									
About 11 chips	140	8	1	0	16	1	0	2	200
Frito-Lay, Doritos, Jacked Enchilada Supreme Flavored Tortilla Chips									
About 6 chips	140	7	1	0	17	1	0	2	170
Frito-Lay, Doritos, Jacked Smoky Chipotle BBQ Flavored Tortilla Chips									
About 6 chips	130	7	1	0	17	1	<1	2	160
Frito-Lay, Doritos, Reduced Fat Cool Ranch Flavored Tortilla Chips									
1 package	130	5	1	0	19	2	1	2	160
Frito-Lay, Doritos, Reduced Fat Nacho Cheese Flavored Tortilla Chips									
1 package	130	5	0.5	0	20	2	0	2	200
Frito-Lay, Doritos, Salsa Verde Flavored Tortilla Chips									
About 12 chips	140	7	1	0	19	1	1	2	210
Frito-Lay, Doritos, Spicy Nacho Flavored Tortilla Chips									
12 chips	140	7	1	0	19	1	1	2	210
Frito-Lay, Doritos, Taco Flavored Tortilla Chips									
About 10 chips	140	8	1	0	16	1	0	2	170
Frito-Lay, Doritos, Tapatio Flavored Tortilla Chips									
About 11 chips	140	8	1.5	0	16	1	0	2	170
Frito-Lay, Doritos, Toasted Corn Tortilla Chips									
About 13 chips	140	7	1	0	18	1	0	2	120
Frito-Lay, El Isleno, Plantain Chips									
1 oz	150	9	1	0	17	2	0	<1	35
Frito-Lay, Fritos Tapatio Flavored Corn Chips									
About 16 pieces	140	8	1	0	15	1	0	1	160
Frito-Lay, Fritos, Flamin' Hot Flavored Corn Chips									
1 oz	160	10	1.5	0	15	1	<1	2	160

Food Serving size	Cal.	(g) Total Fat	(g) Sat. Fat	(mg) Chol.	(g) Carb.	(g) Fiber	(g) Sug.	(g) Prot.	(mg) Sod.
Frito-Lay, Fritos, Flavor Twists, Honey BBQ Flavored Corn Chips									
1 oz	150	9	1.5	0	16	1	1	2	180
Frito-Lay, Fritos, Lightly Salted Corn Chips									
1 oz	160	10	1.5	0	16	1	0	2	80
Frito-Lay, Fritos, Original Corn Chips									
About 32 chips	160	10	1.5	0	15	1	<1	2	170
Frito-Lay, Fritos, Scoops! Corn Chips									
About 10 chips	160	10	1.5	0	16	1	0	2	110
Frito-Lay, Funyuns, Flamin' Hot Onion Flavored Rings									
About 13 pieces	130	7	1	0	17	<1	<1	2	300
Frito-Lay, Funyuns, Onion Flavored Rings									
About 13 pieces	140	7	1	0	18	<1	<1	2	240
Frito-Lay, Lay's, Cheddar & Sour Cream Flavored Potato Chips									
About 15 chips	160	10	1	0	15	1	1	2	170
Frito-Lay, Lay's, Chile Limon Potato Chips									
About 15 chips	160	10	1	0	15	1	<1	2	160
Frito-Lay, Lay's, Classic BLT Potato Chips									
About 15 chips	160	10	1.5	0	15	1	1	2	150
Frito-Lay, Lay's, Classic Potato Chips									
About 15 chips	160	10	1	0	15	1	<1	2	170
Frito-Lay, Lay's, Deli Style Original Potato Chips									
About 17 chips	160	10	1	0	15	1	<1	2	140
Frito-Lay, Lay's, Dill Pickle Flavored Potato Chips									
About 17 chips	160	10	1	0	15	1	1	2	210
Frito-Lay, Lay's, Garden Tomato & Basil Flavored Potato Chips									
About 15 chips	160	10	1	0	16	1	2	2	170
Frito-Lay, Lay's, Honey BBQ Flavored Potato Chips									
About 15 chips	160	10	1	0	16	1	2	2	105
Frito-Lay, Lay's, Honey Mustard Flavored Potato Chips									
About 15 chips	160	10	1	0	16	1	2	2	80
Frito-Lay, Lay's, Kettle Cooked, Creamy Mediterranean Herb Flavored Potato Chips									
About 16 chips	150	9	1	0	16	1	1	2	140

Food Serving size	Cal.	(g) Total Fat	(g) Sat. Fat	(mg) Chol.	(g) Carb.	(g) Fiber	(g) Sug.	(g) Prot.	(mg) Sod.
Frito-Lay, Lay's, Kettle Cooked, Crinkle Cut Spice Rubbed BBQ Flavored Potato Chips									
About 15 chips	140	8	1	0	17	1	2	2	130
Frito-Lay, Lay's, Kettle Cooked, Harvest Ranch Flavored Potato Chips									
About 18 chips	150	9	1	0	16	1	1	2	140
Frito-Lay, Lay's, Kettle Cooked, Jalapeno Flavored Potato Chips									
About 15 chips	150	9	1.5	0	16	1	1	2	130
Frito-Lay, Lay's, Kettle Cooked, Maui Onion Flavored Potato Chips									
About 18 chips	150	9	1.5	0	17	1	1	2	115
Frito-Lay, Lay's, Kettle Cooked, Original Potato Chips									
About 16 chips	160	9	1.5	0	16	1	<1	2	90
Frito-Lay, Lay's, Kettle Cooked, Reduced Fat Original Potato Chips									
About 18 chips	140	6	1	0	19	2	1	2	135
Frito-Lay, Lay's, Kettle Cooked, Sea Salt & Cracked Pepper Flavored Potato Chips									
About 18 chips	150	9	1.5	0	16	1	<1	2	110
Frito-Lay, Lay's, Kettle Cooked, Sea Salt & Vinegar Flavored Potato Chips									
About 18 chips	150	9	1.5	0	17	1	1	2	170
Frito-Lay, Lay's, Kettle Cooked, Sharp Cheddar Flavored Potato Chips									
About 18 chips	150	9	1.5	0	16	1	1	2	130
Frito-Lay, Lay's, Kettle Cooked, Spicy Cayenne & Cheese Flavored Potato Chips									
About 16 chips	150	9	1	0	16	1	1	2	140
Frito-Lay, Lay's, Light Original Potato Chips									
About 15 chips	75	0	0	0	17	1	0	2	200
Frito-Lay, Lay's, Lightly Salted Potato Chips									
About 15 chips	160	10	1	0	16	1	<1	2	85
Frito-Lay, Lay's, Limon Flavored Potato Chips									
About 15 chips	150	10	1	0	15	1	<1	2	210
Frito-Lay, Lay's, Salt & Vinegar Flavored Potato Chips									
About 17 chips	160	10	1	0	15	1	<1	2	230
Frito-Lay, Lay's, Simply Natural, Sea Salt Flavored Thick Cut Potato Chips									
About 17 chips	150	10	1	0	15	1	0	2	150
Frito-Lay, Lay's, Sour Cream & Onion Flavored Potato Chips									
About 17 chips	160	10	1	0	15	1	<1	2	160

Food Serving size	Cal.	(g) Total Fat	(g) Sat. Fat	(mg) Chol.	(g) Carb.	(g) Fiber	(g) Sug.	(g) Prot.	(mg) Sod.
Frito-Lay, Lay's, Stax, Cheddar Flavored Potato Crisps									
About 12 crisps	150	9	2.5	0	16	1	1	2	200
Frito-Lay, Lay's, Stax, Hot'n Spicy BBQ Flavored Potato Crisps									
About 12 crisps	150	9	2.5	0	16	1	2	1	190
Frito-Lay, Lay's, Stax, Mesquite Barbecue Flavored Potato Crisps									
About 12 crisps	150	9	2.5	0	16	1	1	1	180
Frito-Lay, Lay's, Stax, Original Potato Crisps									
About 12 crisps	150	9	2.5	0	16	1	1	1	140
Frito-Lay, Lay's, Stax, Pizza Flavored Potato Crisps									
About 12 crisps	150	9	2.5	0	16	1	1	1	200
Frito-Lay, Lay's, Stax, Salt & Vinegar Flavored Potato Crisps									
About 12 crisps	150	9	2.5	0	17	1	1	1	290
Frito-Lay, Lay's, Stax, Sour Cream & Onion Flavored Potato Crisps									
About 12 crisps	150	9	2.5	0	17	1	1	2	190
Frito-Lay, Lay's, Sweet Southern Heat, BBQ Flavored Potato Chips									
About 15 chips	160	10	1	0	16	1	2	2	150
Frito-Lay, Lay's, Tangy Carolina, BBQ Flavored Potato Chips									
About 15 chips	160	10	1	0	15	1	2	2	190
Frito-Lay, Lay's, Wavy Au Gratin Flavored Potato Chips									
About 13 chips	160	10	1	0	15	1	2	2	160
Frito-Lay, Lay's, Wavy Hickory BBQ Flavored Potato Chips									
About 13 chips	160	10	1	0	16	1	1	2	140
Frito-Lay, Lay's, Wavy Original Potato Chips									
About 11 chips	160	10	1	0	15	1	<1	2	140
Frito-Lay, Lay's, Wavy Ranch Flavored Potato Chips									
About 12 chips	160	10	1	0	15	1	<1	2	120
Frito-Lay, Maui Style, Regular Potato Chips									
About 14 chips	150	9	1.5	0	16	1	<1	2	140
Frito-Lay, Maui Style, Salt & Vinegar Flavored Potato Chips									
About 18 chips	150	9	1.5	0	17	1	1	2	170
Frito-Lay, Miss Vickie's, Jalapeno, Kettle Cooked Flavored Potato Chips									
About 15 chips	150	9	1.5	0	16	1	1	2	130
Frito-Lay, Miss Vickie's, Sea Salt & Cracked Pepper Flavored Potato Chips									
About 18 chips	150	9	1.5	0	16	1	<1	2	110

Food Serving size	Cal.	(g) Total Fat	(g) Sat. Fat	(mg) Chol.	(g) Carb.	(g) Fiber	(g) Sug.	(g) Prot.	(mg) Sod.
Frito-Lay, Miss Vickie's, Sea Salt & Vinegar, Kettle Cooked Flavored Potato Chips About 18 chips	150	9	1.5	0	17	1	1	2	170
Frito-Lay, Miss Vickie's, Simply Sea Salt, Kettle Cooked Potato Chips About 16 chips	160	9	1.5	0	16	1	<1	2	90
Frito-Lay, Munchos, Original Potato Crisps About 11 chips	160	10	1.5	0	16	1	0	1	230
Frito-Lay, Ruffles, Cheddar & Sour Cream Flavored Potato Chips About 11 chips	160	10	1.5	0	15	1	1	2	180
Frito-Lay, Ruffles, Light Original Potato Chips 1 oz	80	0	0	0	17	1	0	2	190
Frito-Lay, Ruffles, Loaded Bacon & Cheddar Potato Skins Flavored Potato Chips About 11 chips	160	10	1.5	0	15	1	1	2	170
Frito-Lay, Ruffles, Loaded Chili & Cheese Flavored Potato Chips About 11 chips	160	10	1	0	15	1	1	2	180
Frito-Lay, Ruffles, Original Potato Chips About 12 chips	160	10	1	0	15	1	<1	2	160
Frito-Lay, Ruffles, Queso Flavored Potato Chips About 11 chips	160	10	1	0	15	1	1	2	230
Frito-Lay, Ruffles, Queso Jalapeno Flavored Potato Chips About 11 chips	160	10	1	0	15	1	1	2	190
Frito-Lay, Ruffles, Reduced Fat Original Potato Chips About 13 chips	140	7	1	0	18	1	0	2	180
Frito-Lay, Ruffles, Simply Natural, Reduced Fat Sea Salted Potato Chips About 15 chips	140	7	0.5	0	17	1	0	2	160
Frito-Lay, Ruffles, Smokehouse Style BBQ Flavored Potato Chips About 11 chips	160	10	1	0	15	1	2	2	170
Frito-Lay, Ruffles, Sour Cream & Onion Flavored Potato Chips About 11 chips	160	10	1	0	15	1	2	2	150
Frito-Lay, Ruffles, Tapatio Limon Flavored Potato Chips About 11 chips	160	10	1.5	0	15	1	<1	2	190
Frito-Lay, Ruffles, Ultimate Kickin' Jalapeno Ranch Flavored Potato Chips About 10 chips	160	10	1.5	0	15	1	1	2	170
Frito-Lay, Ruffles, Ultimate Sweet & Smokin' BBQ Flavored Potato Chips About 10 chips	160	9	1.5	0	16	1	2	2	190

Food Serving size	Cal.	(g) Total Fat	(g) Sat. Fat	(mg) Chol.	(g) Carb.	(g) Fiber	(g) Sug.	(g) Prot.	(mg) Sod.
Frito-Lay, Ruffles, Ultimate The Original Flavored Potato Chips									
About 11 chips	160	10	1.5	0	15	1	<1	2	160
Frito-Lay, Santitas, White Corn Triangles Tortilla Chips									
9 chips	140	6	1	0	19	2	0	2	115
Frito-Lay, Santitas, Yellow Corn Rounds Tortilla Chips									
1 oz	140	6	1	0	20	1	0	2	120
Frito-Lay, Santitas, Yellow Corn Triangles Tortilla Chips									
About 9 chips	140	6	1	0	19	2	0	2	110
Frito-Lay, Tostitos, Bite Size Rounds Tortilla Chips									
About 24 chips	140	7	1	0	18	2	0	2	110
Frito-Lay, Tostitos, Crispy Rounds Tortilla Chips									
1 oz	140	7	1	0	18	2	0	2	120
Frito-Lay, Tostitos, Multigrain Scoops! Tortilla Chips									
About 12 chips	140	7	1	0	17	2	<1	2	110
Frito-Lay, Tostitos, Restaurant Style Tortilla Chips									
About 7 chips	140	7	1	0	19	1	0	2	115
Frito-Lay, Tostitos, Restaurant Style with a Hint of Lime Flavored Tortilla Chips									
About 6 chips	150	7	1	0	18	1	<1	2	125
Frito-Lay, Tostitos, Restaurant Style with a Hint of Jalapeno Flavored Tortilla Chips									
About 6 chips	140	7	1	0	17	1	0	2	130
Frito-Lay, Tostitos, Restaurant Style with a Hint of Pepper Jack Flavored Tortilla Chips									
About 6 chips	140	7	1	0	17	1	0	2	140
Frito-Lay, Tostitos, Scoops!, Tortilla Chips									
About 13 chips	140	7	1	0	19	2	0	2	120
Frito-Lay, Tostitos, Simply Natural, Blue Corn Restaurant Style Tortilla Chips									
About 6 chips	140	6	0.5	0	19	1	0	2	80
Frito-Lay, Tostitos, Simply Natural, Yellow Corn Restaurant Style Tortilla Chips									
About 6 chips	140	6	0.5	0	19	1	0	2	100
Glutino, Chocolate Covered Pretzels									
9 pretzels	160	8	5	5	19	0	8	1	200
Glutino, Gluten Free Cinnamon and Sugar Bagel Chips									
7 bagel chips	110	4.5	0	0	18	0	6	<1	120

Food Serving size	Cal.	(g) Total Fat	(g) Sat. Fat	(mg) Chol.	(g) Carb.	(g) Fiber	(g) Sug.	(g) Prot.	(mg) Sod.
Glutino, Gluten Free Original Bagel Chips									
10 bagel chips	130	4.5	0	0	21	<1	3	1	240
Glutino, Gluten Free Parmesan Garlic Bagel Chips									
About 9 bagel chips	120	4.5	0	0	20	<1	4	1	210
Glutino, Gluten Free Pretzel Sticks									
33 pretzels	140	6	2.5	0	21	0	<1	0	420
Glutino, Gluten Free Pretzel Sticks, Family Pack									
33 pretzels	140	6	2.5	0	21	0	<1	0	420
Glutino, Gluten Free Pretzel Twists									
24 pretzels	140	6	2.5	0	21	0	<1	0	420
Glutino, Gluten Free Pretzel Twists, Family Pack									
33 pretzels	140	6	2.5	0	21	0	<1	0	420
Glutino, Gluten Free Sesame Pretzel Rings									
18 pretzels	150	8	2.5	0	19	0	<1	1	390
Glutino, Snack Pack Pretzels									
24 pretzels	140	6	2.5	0	21	0	<1	0	420
Glutino, Yogurt Covered Pretzels									
9 pretzels	160	9	5	5	19	0	10	1	160
Kay's Naturals, Chili Nacho Protein Chips snack									
1.2 oz	120	2.5	1	0	15	4	1	12	240
Kay's Naturals, Cinnamon Toast Pretzel Sticks snack									
1.2 oz	120	3.5	1.5	0	15	4	3	12	160
Kay's Naturals, Crispy Parmesan Protein Chips snack									
1.2 oz	120	2.5	1	0	15	4	1	12	240
Kay's Naturals, Jalapeno Honey Mustard Pretzel Sticks snack									
1.2 oz	120	3.5	1.5	0	15	4	3	12	160
Kay's Naturals, Kruncheeze White Cheddar Cheese snacks									
1.2 oz	130	4	0.5	0	14	2	1	12	240
Kay's Naturals, Lemon Herb Protein Chips snack									
1.2 oz	120	2.5	1	0	15	4	1	12	240
Kay's Naturals, Mac & Cheese Protein Chips snack									
1.2 oz	120	2.5	1	0	15	4	1	12	240
Kay's Naturals, Original Pretzel Pretzel Sticks snack									
1.2 oz	120	3.5	1.5	0	15	4	3	12	160

Food Serving size	Cal.	(g) Total Fat	(g) Sat. Fat	(mg) Chol.	(g) Carb.	(g) Fiber	(g) Sug.	(g) Prot.	(mg) Sod.
Kay's Naturals, Protein Puffs Almond Delight snack									
1.2 oz	120	3	1	5	16	4	3	12	200
Kay's Naturals, Protein Puffs Mac & Cheese snack									
1.2 oz	120	2.5	1	0	15	4	1	12	240
Kay's Naturals, Protein Puffs Tomato Basil snack									
1.2 oz	115	2.5	1	5	17	5	3	12	268
Kay's Naturals, Protein Puffs Veggie Pizza snack									
1.2 oz	110	2.5	0.5	0	16	4	3	12	230
Kay's Naturals, Protein Snack Mix Sweet BBQ Mix snack									
1.2 oz	120	3.5	1.5	0	15	4	3	12	160
Lundberg Family Farms, Eco-Farmed Apple Cinnamon Rice Cakes									
1 cake	70	0.5	0	0	16	1	2	1	0
Lundberg Family Farms, Eco-Farmed Brown Rice, Lighty Salted Rice Cakes									
1 cake	60	0.5	0	0	14	1	0	1	35
Lundberg Family Farms, Eco-Farmed Brown Rice, Salt-Free Rice Cakes									
1 cake	60	0.5	0	0	14	1	0	1	0
Lundberg Family Farms, Eco-Farmed Buttery Caramel Rice Cakes									
1 cake	70	0.5	0	0	16	1	2	1	0
Lundberg Family Farms, Eco-Farmed Honey Nut Rice Cakes									
1 cake	80	0.5	0	0	18	1	2	2	5
Lundberg Family Farms, Eco-Farmed Sesame Tamari Rice Cakes									
1 cake	70	0.5	0	0	16	2	0	2	120
Lundberg Family Farms, Eco-Farmed Toasted Sesame Rice Cakes									
1 cake	70	0	0	0	16	1	0	2	65
Lundberg Family Farms, Fiesta Lime Rice Chips									
9 chips	140	6	0.5	0	19	1	1	2	135
Lundberg Family Farms, Honey Dijon Rice Chips									
9 chips	140	6	0.5	0	19	1	1	2	130
Lundberg Family Farms, Organic Brown Rice, Lightly Salted Rice Cakes									
1 cake	60	0.5	0	0	14	1	0	1	35
Lundberg Family Farms, Organic Brown Rice, Salt-Free Rice Cakes									
1 cake	60	0.5	0	0	14	1	0	1	0
Lundberg Family Farms, Organic Caramel Corn Rice Cakes									
1 cake	80	0.5	0	0	18	1	2	1	40

Food Serving size	Cal.	(g) Total Fat	(g) Sat. Fat	(mg) Chol.	(g) Carb.	(g) Fiber	(g) Sug.	(g) Prot.	(mg) Sod.
Lundberg Family Farms, Organic Cinnamon Toast Rice Cakes									
1 cake	80	0.5	0	0	18	1	3	1	0
Lundberg Family Farms, Organic Cracked Black Pepper Rice Chips									
9 chips	140	6	0.5	0	19	1	0	2	110
Lundberg Family Farms, Organic Koku Seaweed Rice Cakes									
1 cake	60	0.5	0	0	14	1	1	1	75
Lundberg Family Farms, Organic Mochi Sweet Rice Cakes									
1 cake	60	0.5	0	0	14	1	0	1	35
Lundberg Family Farms, Organic Popcorn Rice Cakes									
1 cake	60	0.5	0	0	14	1	0	1	35
Lundberg Family Farms, Organic Sesame Tamari Rice Cakes									
1 cake	60	1	0	0	14	1	0	1	75
Lundberg Family Farms, Organic Spicy Black Bean Rice Chips									
9 chips	140	6	0.5	0	18	1	1	2	170
Lundberg Family Farms, Organic Tamari with Seaweed Rice Cakes									
1 cake	60	0	0	0	13	1	0	1	75
Lundberg Family Farms, Organic Wild Rice Lightly Salted Rice Cakes									
1 cake	70	0	0	0	15	1	0	1	55
Lundberg Family Farms, Pico de Gallo Rice Chips									
9 chips	140	6	0.5	0	18	1	0	2	135
Lundberg Family Farms, Santa Fe Barbecue Rice Chips									
9 chips	140	6	0.5	0	19	1	1	2	120
Lundberg Family Farms, Sea Salt Rice Chips									
9 chips	140	6	0.5	0	19	1	0	2	110
Lundberg Family Farms, Sesame & Seaweed Rice Chips									
9 chips	140	6	0.5	0	19	1	1	2	140
Lundberg Family Farms, Wasabi Rice Chips									
9 chips	140	6	0.5	0	19	1	0	2	115
Mary's Gone Crackers, Chipotle Tomato Pretzel-Sticks									
15 pieces	150	5	0.5	0	21	4	0	4	160
Mary's Gone Crackers, Curry Pretzel-Sticks									
15 pieces	150	5	0.5	0	21	4	0	4	190
Mary's Gone Crackers, Sea Salt Pretzel-Sticks									
15 pieces	150	5	0.5	0	21	4	0	4	300

Food Serving size	Cal.	(g) Total Fat	(g) Sat. Fat	(mg) Chol.	(g) Carb.	(g) Fiber	(g) Sug.	(g) Prot.	(mg) Sod.
Newman's Own, 94% Fat Free Flavor Microwave Popcorn									
3.5 cup	110	1.5	0	0	20	4	0	3	250
Newman's Own, Butter Boom Flavor Microwave Popcorn									
3.5 cup	130	5	2	0	18	3	0	2	290
Newman's Own, Butter Flavor Microwave Popcorn									
3.5 cup	130	5	2	0	18	3	0	2	180
Newman's Own, Light Butter Flavor Microwave Popcorn									
3.5 cup	120	4	1.5	0	19	4	0	3	170
Newman's Own, Natural 100 Calorie Mini-Bags Microwave Popcorn									
3.5 cup	100	2.5	1	0	18	4	0	2	210
Newman's Own, Natural Flavor Microwave Popcorn									
3.5 cup	130	5	2	0	18	3	0	2	200
Newman's Own, White Kernels Microwave Popcorn									
3.5 cup	130	5	2	0	18	3	0	2	200
Pirate Brands, Pirate's Booty, Aged White Cheddar									
1 oz	130	5	1	0	19	0	0	2	140
Pirate Brands, Pirate's Booty, Barrrrrbegue									
1 oz	130	4.5	0.5	0	19	1	2	2	135
Pirate Brands, Pirate's Booty, Chocolate									
1 oz	140	8	1	0	17	1	5	1	40
Pirate Brands, Pirate's Booty, New York Pizza									
1 oz	120	5	0.5	0	18	1	1	2	120
Pirate Brands, Pirate's Booty, Sour Cream & Onion									
1 oz	130	5	1	0	18	1	1	2	140
Pirate Brands, Pirate's Booty, Veggie									
1 oz	130	5	0.5	0	17	1	1	2	90
Pirate Brands, Potato Flyers, Homestyle Barbeque									
1 oz	120	4.5	0	0	19	1	2	1	230
Pirate Brands, Potato Flyers, Original Tings Crunchy Corn Sticks									
1 oz	150	8	0.5	0	18	0	0	1	140
Pirate Brands, Potato Flyers, Sour Cream & Onion									
1 oz	120	5	0.5	0	19	1	1	1	200
Pirate Brands, Smart Puffs									
1-1/2 oz	150	8	1.5	5	18	1	2	3	290

Food Serving size	Cal.	(g) Total Fat	(g) Sat. Fat	(mg) Chol.	(g) Carb.	(g) Fiber	(g) Sug.	(g) Prot.	(mg) Sod.
Pirate Brands, The Original Potato Flyers 1 oz	120	5	0	0	18	1	0	1	240
PopChips, Barbeque 1 oz, about 20 chips	120	4	0	0	20	1	2	1	250
PopChips, Jalapeno 1 oz, about 21 chips	120	4	0	0	19	1	1	2	190
PopChips, Original 1 oz, about 23 chips	120	4	0	0	20	1	0	1	280
PopChips, Parmesan & Garlic 1 oz, about 21 chips	120	4	0	0	20	1	1	2	280
PopChips, Sea Salt & Vinegar 1 oz, about 23 chips	120	4	0	0	20	1	1	1	260
PopChips, Sour Cream & Onion 1 oz, about 22 chips	120	4	0.5	0	20	1	2	2	320
PopChips, Sweet Potato 1 oz, about 23 chips	120	4	0	0	20	<1	3	1	115
Popcorn, Indiana, Aged White Cheddar Popcorn 2.5 cups	150	9	1	5	14	2	2	3	290
Popcorn, Indiana, All Natural Bacon Ranch Popcorn 2.5 cups	150	10	1	5	13	2	0	3	270
Popcorn, Indiana, Buffalo Cheddar Kettlecorn 2.5 cups	150	11	1	0	13	2	1	2	290
Popcorn, Indiana, Chip'ins, Classic BBQ Chip'ins 1 oz, about 18 chips	130	4	0	0	21	1	1	2	220
Popcorn, Indiana, Chip'ins, Hot Buffalo Wing Chip'ins 1 oz, about 18 chips	130	4	0	0	21	1	0	2	230
Popcorn, Indiana, Chip'ins, Jalapeno Ranch Chip'ins 1 oz, about 18 chips	130	4	0	0	21	1	0	2	230
Popcorn, Indiana, Chip'ins, Sea Salt Chip'ins 1 oz, about 20 chips	120	2.5	0	0	22	1	0	2	230
Popcorn, Indiana, Chip'ins, White Cheddar Chip'ins 1 oz, about 18 chips	130	4	0	0	21	1	1	2	240
Popcorn, Indiana, Cinnamon Sugar Kettlecorn 2.5 cups	130	4.5	0	0	21	2	7	1	115

Food Serving size	Cal.	(g) Total Fat	(g) Sat. Fat	(mg) Chol.	(g) Carb.	(g) Fiber	(g) Sug.	(g) Prot.	(mg) Sod.
Popcorn, Indiana, Movie Theater Popcorn									
2 cups	160	12	2	5	13	2	0	2	170
Popcorn, Indiana, Original Kettlecorn									
2 cups	130	5	0	0	21	2	6	1	130
Popcorn, Indiana, Reserve Flavors, Wasabi Popcorn									
2.5 cups	150	9	0.5	0	15	3	0	2	260
Popcorn, Indiana, Smoked Cheddar Popcorn									
2 cups	160	12	1.5	0	12	2	1	2	260
Popcorn, Indiana, Sweet & Tangy BBQ Kettlecorn									
2.5 cups	130	4.5	0	0	21	2	7	1	160
Popcorn, Indiana, Touch of Sea Salt Popcorn									
3 cups	130	6	0	0	18	3	0	3	190
Riceworks, Gourmet Brown Rice Crisps, Parmesan & Sundried Tomatoes									
1 oz, about 10 chips	140	6	0.5	0	19	1	<1	2	200
Riceworks, Gourmet Brown Rice Crisps, Salsa Fresca									
1 oz, about 10 chips	140	6	0.5	0	19	1	<1	2	110
Riceworks, Gourmet Brown Rice Crisps, Sea Salt									
1 oz, about 10 chips	140	6	0.5	0	19	1	0	2	110
Riceworks, Gourmet Brown Rice Crisps, Sweet Chilli									
1 oz, about 10 chips	140	6	0.5	0	19	1	<1	2	170
Riceworks, Gourmet Brown Rice Crisps, Tangy BBQ									
1 oz, about 10 chips	140	6	0.5	0	19	1	1	2	120
RW Garcia, 3-Seed Blue Corn Dipping Chips									
1 oz, about 10 strips	140	8	1	0	17	2	0	2	50
RW Garcia, 3-Seed Curry & Mango Dipping Chips									
1 oz	140	7	1	0	18	2	0	2	110
RW Garcia, 3-Seed Veggie Dipping Chips (Spinach & Garlic, Red Beet & Onion, Carrot, Tomato & Sesame)									
1 oz	140	7	1	0	18	2	0	2	50
RW Garcia, 3-Seed Veggie Tortilla Dipping Chips									
1 oz, about 7 chips	140	6	1	0	19	2	1	2	50
RW Garcia, Blue, made with Organic Blue Corn Chips									
1 oz, about 15 chips	130	5	0.5	0	19	2	0	3	50
RW Garcia, Flaxseed Tortilla Chips with Soy									
1 oz, about 7 chips	140	7	1	0	14	3	1	5	50

Food Serving size	Cal.	(g) Total Fat	(g) Sat. Fat	(mg) Chol.	(g) Carb.	(g) Fiber	(g) Sug.	(g) Prot.	(mg) Sod.
RW Garcia, Flaxseed Tortilla Chips, BlueFlax Blue Corn									
1 oz, about 7 chips	140	7	1	0	17	2	0	3	50
RW Garcia, Flaxseed Tortilla Chips, Thai Sweet & Spicy									
1 oz, about 7 chips	140	7	1	0	18	2	1	2	80
RW Garcia, Gold, made with Stone Ground Corn Chips									
1 oz, about 15 chips	130	4.5	0.5	0	20	2	0	2	50
RW Garcia, Himalayan Pink Salt & Tellicherry Cracked Pepper Savory 3 Seed-Dipping Chips									
1 oz	140	7	1	0	18	2	0	2	110
RW Garcia, Red & Yellow Tortilla Chips, MixtBag, Family Value Packs									
1 oz, about 15 chips	140	6	1	0	19	2	0	2	50
RW Garcia, Spice Flaxseed Tortilla Chips with Soy									
1 oz, about 7 chips	140	7	1	0	14	3	1	5	80
RW Garcia, Yellow & Blue Corn Tortilla Chips, MixtBag, Family Value Packs									
1 oz, about 15 chips	140	6	1	0	19	2	0	2	50
Smart Balance, Light Butter Popcorn									
1 cup popped	25	4.5	1.5	0	18	4	0	3	290
Smart Balance, Light Butter Popcorn, Mini Bags									
1 cup popped	120	5	1.5	0	26	5	0	4	400
Smart Balance, Smart Movie Style, Deluxe Microwave Popcorn									
1 cup popped	35	11	4	0	16	3	0	3	420
Smart Balance, Smart 'n Healthy, Deluxe Microwave Popcorn									
1 cup popped	20	2	0.5	0	20	5	0	4	80
Snikiddy Baked Fries, Barbeque									
4.5 oz	130	4.5	0	0	21	1	2	2	190
Snikiddy Baked Fries, Bold Buffalo									
4.5 oz	130	4.5	0.5	0	20	1	2	2	180
Snikiddy Baked Fries, Cheddar Cheese									
4.5 oz	130	4.5	0.5	0	20	1	2	2	180
Snikiddy Baked Fries, Classic Ketchup									
4.5 oz	130	4.5	0	0	21	1	2	2	190
Snikiddy Baked Fries, Original Seasoning									
4.5 oz	130	4.5	0	0	20	1	1	2	190
Snikiddy Baked Fries, Sea Salt									
4.5 oz	130	4.5	0	0	21	1	2	2	210

Food Serving size	Cal.	(g) Total Fat	(g) Sat. Fat	(mg) Chol.	(g) Carb.	(g) Fiber	(g) Sug.	(g) Prot.	(mg) Sod.
Snikiddy Baked Fries, Southwest Cheddar									
4.5 oz	130	4.5	0.5	0	20	1	2	2	180
Snikiddy Cheese Puffs, Grilled Cheese									
4.0 oz	120	4.5	1	5	17	1	1	3	190
Snikiddy Cheese Puffs, Mac n' Cheese									
4.0 oz	120	4.5	1	5	17	1	1	2	190
Snikiddy Eat Your Vegetables, Italian Herb & Olive Oil									
4.5 oz	130	7	0.5	0	16	3	2	3	110
Snikiddy Eat Your Vegetables, Jalapeno Ranch									
4.5 oz	130	7	0.5	0	16	3	2	3	140
Snikiddy Eat Your Vegetables, Sea Salt									
4.5 oz	130	7	0.5	0	17	3	1	3	140
Snikiddy Eat Your Vegetables, Sour Cream & Onion									
4.5 oz	130	7	0.5	0	17	3	2	3	125
Snyder's of Hanover, Gluten-Free Mini Pretzels									
About 25 pretzels	120	2	1	0	25	1	<1	0	470
Snyder's of Hanover, Gluten-Free Pretzel Sticks									
About 30 sticks	120	1.5	0.5	0	25	<1	0	0	260
Snyder's of Hanover, MultiGrain Tortilla Chips									
About 10 chips	150	7	0.5	0	19	3	2	2	80
Wylde Pretzels									
40 pretzels	130	3	1.5	0	24	3	1	<1	230
Wylde Sesame Pretzels									
40 pretzels	130	3	1.5	0	24	2	0	<1	200

Misc. Sweets (Gums, Jellies, etc.)

Food Serving size	Cal.	(g) Total Fat	(g) Sat. Fat	(mg) Chol.	(g) Carb.	(g) Fiber	(g) Sug.	(g) Prot.	(mg) Sod.
Annie's, Organic Berry Patch Fruit Snacks									
1 pouch	70	0	NA	0	18	NA	10	0	45
Annie's, Organic Grapes Galore Fruit Snacks									
1 pouch	70	0	NA	0	18	NA	10	0	45
Annie's, Organic Orchard Apple Fruit Bites									
1 pouch	60	0	NA	0	15	1	12	0	5
Annie's, Organic Orchard Cherry Fruit Bites									
1 pouch	60	0	NA	0	15	1	12	0	5

Food Serving size	Cal.	(g) Total Fat	(g) Sat. Fat	(mg) Chol.	(g) Carb.	(g) Fiber	(g) Sug.	(g) Prot.	(mg) Sod.
Annie's, Organic Orchard Grape Fruit Bites									
1 pouch	60	0	NA	0	15	1	12	0	5
Annie's, Organic Orchard Strawberry Fruit Bites									
1 pouch	60	0	NA	0	15	1	12	0	5
Annie's, Organic Pink Lemonade Bunny Fruit Snacks									
1 pouch	70	0	NA	0	18	NA	10	0	45
Annie's, Organic Summer Strawberry Fruit Snacks									
1 pouch	70	0	NA	0	18	NA	10	0	45
Annie's, Organic Sunny Citrus Fruit Snacks									
1 pouch	70	0	NA	0	18	NA	10	0	45
Annie's, Organic Tropical Treat Bunny Fruit Snacks									
1 pouch	70	0	NA	0	18	NA	10	0	45
Betty Crocker, Gluten Free Dora the Explorer Fruit Shapes, 10 Count									
1 pouch	80	0	0	0	19	NA	12	0	30
Betty Crocker, Gluten Free Fruit Gushers Flavor Shock, 6 Count									
1 pouch	90	1	0	0	20	NA	12	0	45
Betty Crocker, Gluten Free Fruit Gushers Mood Morphers, 6 Count									
1 pouch	90	1	0	0	20	NA	12	0	45
Betty Crocker, Gluten Free Fruit Gushers Variety Pack Strawberry, Watermelon, Tropical, 6 Count									
1 pouch	90	1	0	0	20	NA	13	0	55
Betty Crocker, Gluten Free Fruit Gushers, Fruit Roll Ups & Fruit by the Foot Variety Pack, 8 Count									
1 roll	80	1	0	0	17	NA	9	0	45
Betty Crocker, Gluten Free Fruit Roll Ups Minis Strawberry Craze, 18 Count									
1 roll	40	0.5	NA	NA	9	NA	5	NA	40
Betty Crocker, Gluten Free Fruit Roll Ups Variety Pack Strawberry, Tie Dye and Wildfire, 10 Count									
1 roll	50	1	0	0	12	NA	7	0	55
Betty Crocker, Gluten Free Fruit Shapes, Comics, 10 Count									
1 pouch	80	0	0	0	21	NA	13	0	30
Betty Crocker, Gluten Free Fruit Shapes, Sunkist Mixed Fruit, 10 Count									
1 pouch	80	0	0	0	19	NA	12	0	25
Betty Crocker, Gluten Free Scooby Doo Fruit Shapes, 10 Count									
1 pouch	80	0	0	0	19	NA	12	0	30

Food Serving size	Cal.	(g) Total Fat	(g) Sat. Fat	(mg) Chol.	(g) Carb.	(g) Fiber	(g) Sug.	(g) Prot.	(mg) Sod.
Betty Crocker, Gluten Free Shark Bites Fruit Shapes, 10 Count									
1 pouch	80	0	0	0	19	NA	12	0	30
Candy Tree, Raspberry Gluten-Free Licorice Twists									
40g	143	0	0	NA	35	0	22	1	NA
Kellogg's, Disney, Fairies, Fruit Flavored Snacks									
1 pouch	70	0	0	0	17	0	11	<1	0
Kellogg's, Disney, Jake and the Never Land Pirates, Fruit Flavored Snacks									
1 pouch	70	0	0	0	17	0	11	<1	0
Kellogg's, Disney, Mickey Mouse & Friends, Fruit Flavored Snacks									
1 pouch	70	0	0	0	17	0	11	<1	0
Kellogg's, Disney, Phineas & Ferb, Fruit Flavored Snacks									
1 pouch	70	0	0	0	17	0	11	<1	0
Kellogg's, Disney, Pixar Cars, Fruit Flavored Snacks									
1 pouch	70	0	0	0	17	0	11	<1	0
Kellogg's, Disney, Pixar Finding Nemo, Fruit Flavored Snacks									
1 pouch	70	0	0	0	17	0	11	<1	0
Kellogg's, Disney, Pixar Toy Story, Fruit Flavored Snacks									
1 pouch	70	0	0	0	17	0	11	<1	0
Kellogg's, Disney, Princess, Fruit Flavored Snacks									
1 pouch	70	0	0	0	17	0	11	<1	0
Kellogg's, Fruity Snacks, Mixed Berry, Fruit Flavored Snacks									
1 pouch	70	0	0	0	17	0	11	<1	0
Kellogg's, Ice Age Continental Drift, Fruit Flavored Snacks									
(1 pouch)	70	0	0	0	17	0	11	<1	0
Kellogg's, Marvel Studios, Fruit Flavored Snacks									
1 pouch	70	0	0	0	17	0	11	<1	0
Kellogg's, Super Mario, Fruit Flavored Snacks									
1 pouch	70	0	0	0	17	0	11	<1	0
Kellogg's, The Amazing Spider-Man, Fruit Flavored Snacks									
1 pouch	70	0	0	0	17	0	11	<1	0
Maple Grove Farms, Real Mint Jelly									
1 tbsp	60	0	NA	NA	14	NA	8	0	10
Orgran, Molasses Licorice									
0.7 oz (20g)	57	1.5	0	0	14	0.5	10	0.3	6

Food Serving size	Cal.	(g) Total Fat	(g) Sat. Fat	(mg) Chol.	(g) Carb.	(g) Fiber	(g) Sug.	(g) Prot.	(mg) Sod.
Simply Fruit Roll-Up, Strawberry, 10 Count									
1 roll	50	0.5	0	0	12	1	10	0	20
Simply Fruit Roll-Up, Wildberry, 10 Count									
1 roll	50	0.5	0	0	12	1	10	0	20
Welch's, Concord Grape Jam									
1 tbsp	50	0	0	NA	13	NA	13	0	10
Welch's, Concord Grape Jelly									
1 tbsp	50	0	0	NA	13	NA	13	0	10
Welch's, Natural Grape Spread									
1 tbsp	30	0	0	NA	8	NA	8	0	15
Welch's, Natural Spreads, Concord Grape Spread									
1 tbsp	30	0	0	NA	8	NA	8	0	15
Welch's, Natural Spreads, Raspberry Spread									
1 tbsp	30	0	0	NA	8	NA	8	0	15
Welch's, Natural Spreads, Strawberry Spread									
1 tbsp	30	0	0	NA	8	NA	8	0	15
Welch's, Natural Strawberry Spread									
1 tbsp	30	0	0	NA	8	NA	8	0	15
Welch's, Reduced Sugar Concord Grape Jelly									
1 tbsp	20	0	0	NA	5	NA	5	0	15
Welch's, Reduced Sugar Strawberry Spread									
1 tbsp	20	0	0	NA	5	NA	5	0	15
Welch's, Strawberry Spread									
1 tbsp	50	0	0	NA	13	NA	13	0	10

Snack Bars

Food Serving size	Cal.	(g) Total Fat	(g) Sat. Fat	(mg) Chol.	(g) Carb.	(g) Fiber	(g) Sug.	(g) Prot.	(mg) Sod.
Betty Crocker, Nogii Super Protein Bar									
1 bar	390	14	5	0	38	3	22	30	380
Bora Bora, All Natural Bars, Exotic Coconut Almond									
1 bar	210	14	6	0	18	6	9	4	10
Bora Bora, All Natural Bars, Tropical Sesame Cranberry									
1 roll	190	11	1.5	0	20	3	11	5	10
Bora Bora, All Natural Bars, Wild Pomegranate Pecan									
1 roll	140	5	0.5	0	23	1	13	2	15

Food Serving size	Cal.	(g) Total Fat	(g) Sat. Fat	(mg) Chol.	(g) Carb.	(g) Fiber	(g) Sug.	(g) Prot.	(mg) Sod.
Bora Bora, Antioxidant Bars, Paradise Walnut Pistachio									
1 bar	180	11	1	0	21	2	13	4	50
Bora Bora, Antioxidant Bars, Tiki Blueberry Flax									
1 bar	180	10	1	0	21	4	10	5	15
Bora Bora, Energy Bars, Island Brazil Nut Almond									
1 roll	200	12	2	0	19	2	10	5	10
Bora Bora, Energy Bars, Tribal Cinnamon Oatmeal									
1 roll	160	5	1	0	27	3	13	3	25
Bora Bora, Energy Bars, Volcanic Chocolate Banana									
1 bar	190	13	5	0	20	4	12	2	40
Bora Bora, Organic Bars, Hula Cacao Hazelnut									
1 bar	200	14	4	0	19	3	11	4	80
Bora Bora, Organic Bars, Native Acai Walnut									
1 roll	160	8	1	0	24	3	16	2	10
Bora Bora, Organic Bars, Pacific Mango Macadamia									
1 roll	180	10	4.5	0	23	6	12	1	45
Bora Bora, Organic Bars, Traditional Apricot Quinoa									
1 bar	170	8	3	0	23	2	13	3	0
Bumble Bar Organic Sesame Bar, Aewsome Apricot									
1 bar	180	12	4	0	17	5	12	4	65
Bumble Bar Organic Sesame Bar, Amazing Almond									
1 bar	210	15	2	0	15	5	7	7	70
Bumble Bar Organic Sesame Bar, Amazing Almond									
1 junior bar	100	7	1	0	7	2	3	3	30
Bumble Bar Organic Sesame Bar, Chai Almond									
1 bar	200	12	1.5	0	18	4	8	7	55
Bumble Bar Organic Sesame Bar, Cherry Chocolate									
1 bar	180	12	4.5	0	19	4	14	4	75
Bumble Bar Organic Sesame Bar, Chocolate Crisp									
1 bar	190	11	2	0	21	3	10	5	60
Bumble Bar Organic Sesame Bar, Chocolate Crisp									
1 junior bar	90	5	1	0	10	1	4	2	25
Bumble Bar Organic Sesame Bar, Chunky Cherry									
1 bar	180	12	4	0	18	4	13	5	60

Food Serving size	Cal.	(g) Total Fat	(g) Sat. Fat	(mg) Chol.	(g) Carb.	(g) Fiber	(g) Sug.	(g) Prot.	(mg) Sod.
Bumble Bar Organic Sesame Bar, Classic Cashew									
1 bar	210	15	2	0	15	4	7	7	70
Bumble Bar Organic Sesame Bar, Harvest Hazelnut									
1 bar	210	15	2	0	15	5	7	7	70
Bumble Bar Organic Sesame Bar, Lushus Lemon									
1 bar	190	11	1.5	0	18	4	8	6	65
Bumble Bar Organic Sesame Bar, Mixed Nut Medley									
1 bar	210	15	2	0	15	4	7	7	70
Bumble Bar Organic Sesame Bar, Original Peanut									
1 bar	210	15	2	0	15	5	7	7	70
Bumble Bar Organic Sesame Bar, Original Peanut									
1 junior bar	100	7	1	0	7	2	3	3	30
Bumble Bar Organic Sesame Bar, Paradise Pineapple									
1 bar	190	13	4.5	0	19	4	14	5	65
Eden Foods, Agar, Agar Bars, Sea Vegetable, wild, hand harvested									
1 bar	25	0	0	0	5	5	0	0	0
Elisabeth Hasselbeck's NoGii No Gluten Bars, High Protein (20g Peanut Butter & Chocolate Bar)									
1 roll	230	8	2.5	0	20	2	10	20	230
Elisabeth Hasselbeck's NoGii No Gluten Bars, NoGii Snack Bar for Kids									
1 roll	160	5	1.5	0	21	2	10	8	200
Elisabeth Hasselbeck's NoGii No Gluten Bars, Paleo Nuts About Berries									
1 bar	180	8	1	0	24	3	17	4	0
Elisabeth Hasselbeck's NoGii No Gluten Bars, Paleo Nuts About Nuts									
1 bar	200	13	1.5	0	19	3	12	5	5
Elisabeth Hasselbeck's NoGii No Gluten Bars, Paleo Nuts About Tropical Fruit									
1 roll	190	10	2.5	0	22	3	15	4	0
Elisabeth Hasselbeck's NoGii No Gluten Bars, Protein D'lites 8g Chocolate and Caramel Bliss									
1 roll	120	4.5	2	0	12	1	7	8	105
Elisabeth Hasselbeck's NoGii No Gluten Bars, Super Protein (30g Chocolate Peanut Butter Caramel Crisp)									
1 bar	390	14	5	0	38	3	22	30	380
Ener-G, Chocolate Chip Snack Bars									
1 bar	160	3.5	1.5	0	33	1	17	<1	35

Food Serving size	Cal.	(g) Total Fat	(g) Sat. Fat	(mg) Chol.	(g) Carb.	(g) Fiber	(g) Sug.	(g) Prot.	(mg) Sod.
Gluten Free Café, Chocolate Sesame Snack Bar									
1 roll	130	8	1.5	0	14	2	7	3	40
Gluten Free Café, Cinnamon Sesame Snack Bar									
1 roll	150	11	1.5	0	9	3	5	4	50
Gluten Free Café, Lemon Sesame Snack Bar									
1 bar	130	8	1	0	12	2	6	4	45
Glutino, Gluten Free Chocolate & Banana Organic Bars									
1 bar	100	1.5	0	0	21	1	9	1	35
Glutino, Gluten Free Premium Harvest Corn Bread									
1 slice	90	2	0	0	16	<1	1	<1	200
Glutino, Gluten Free WildBerry Organic Bars									
1 roll	100	1	0	0	21	1	8	1	65
Kind Healthy Snacks, Almond & Apricot Bar									
1 bar	190	11	4.5	0	22	5	12	3	15
Kind Healthy Snacks, Almond & Coconut Bar									
1 bar	210	13	6	0	19	4	10	4	10
Kind Healthy Snacks, Almond Cashew Bar with Flax + Omega3									
1 bar	180	10	1.5	0	20	4	13	4	0
Kind Healthy Snacks, Almond Walnut Macadamia Bar + Protein									
1 bar	190	12	1.5	0	15	3	8	10	75
Kind Healthy Snacks, Almonds & Apricots in Yogurt Bar									
1 bar	220	12	6	0	26	4	17	3	15
Kind Healthy Snacks, Apple Cinnamon & Pecan Bar									
1 bar	180	10	1	0	23	2.5	13	3	25
Kind Healthy Snacks, Blueberry Pecan Bar + Fiber									
1 bar	180	10	1	0	23	5	12	3	25
Kind Healthy Snacks, Cashew & Ginger Spice Bar									
1 bar	200	14	2	0	16	5	4	6	15
Kind Healthy Snacks, Cinnamon Oat Clusters Bar with Flax Seeds									
1/3 cup	130	3.5	0	0	22	5	6	3	20
Kind Healthy Snacks, Cranberry Almond Bar + Antioxidants									
1 bar	190	13	1.5	0	20	3	12	3	20
Kind Healthy Snacks, Dark Chocolate & Cranberry Clusters Bar									
1/3 cup	130	3	0.5	0	23	3	7	3	20

Food Serving size	Cal.	(g) Total Fat	(g)* Sat. Fat	(mg) Chol.	(g) Carb.	(g) Fiber	(g) Sug.	(g) Prot.	(mg) Sod.
Kind Healthy Snacks, Dark Chocolate Cherry Cashew Bar + Antioxidants									
1 bar	180	9	2.5	0	22	3	14	4	20
Kind Healthy Snacks, Dark Chocolate Cinnamon Pecan Bar									
1 bar	200	16	3.5	0	16	7	5	5	20
Kind Healthy Snacks, Dark Chocolate Nuts & Sea Salt Bar									
1 bar	200	15	3.5	0	16	7	5	6	125
Kind Healthy Snacks, Fruit & Nut Delight Bar									
1 bar	180	11	1.5	0	20	4	11	5	15
Kind Healthy Snacks, Fruit & Nuts in Yogurt Bar									
1 bar	210	12	3.5	0	25	4	17	4	20
Kind Healthy Snacks, Macadamia & Apricot Bar									
1 bar	190	12	5	0	22	5	10	2	15
Kind Healthy Snacks, Madagascar Vanilla Almond Bar									
1 bar	210	16	2	0	14	5	4	7	15
Kind Healthy Snacks, Mango Macadamia Bar + Calcium									
1 bar	190	12	5	0	21	4	10	2	15
Kind Healthy Snacks, Maple Walnut Clusters Bar with Chia & Quinoa									
1/3 cup	130	3.5	0	0	22	3	6*	3	20
Kind Healthy Snacks, mini Almond & Apricot Bar									
1 bar	110	7	3	0	13	3	7	2	10
Kind Healthy Snacks, mini Cranberry Almond Bar + Antioxidants									
1 bar	115	8	1	0	12	2	7	2	10
Kind Healthy Snacks, mini Fruit & Nut Delight Bar									
1 bar	108	58	1	0	12	2	7	3	10
Kind Healthy Snacks, Nut Delight Bar									
1 bar	210	16	2	0	14	4	5	7	10
Kind Healthy Snacks, Oats & Honey Clusters with Toasted Coconut Bar									
1/3 cup	130	4	1.5	0	21	3	6	3	20
Kind Healthy Snacks, Peanut Butter & Strawberry Bar									
1 bar	190	11	1.5	0	18	4	10	7	30
Kind Healthy Snacks, Peanut Butter Dark Chocolate Bar + Protein									
1 bar	200	13	3.5	0	17	3	10	7	50
Kind Healthy Snacks, Peanut Butter Whole Grain Clusters Bar									
1/3 cup	130	3.5	0.5	0	20	2	5	5	80

Food Serving size	Cal.	(g) Total Fat	(g) Sat. Fat	(mg) Chol.	(g) Carb.	(g) Fiber	(g) Sug.	(g) Prot.	(mg) Sod.
Kind Healthy Snacks, Pomegranate Blueberry Pistachio Bar + Antioxidants									
1 bar	170	8	1	0	24	4	13	3	25
Kind Healthy Snacks, Sesame & Peanuts with Chocolate Bar									
1 bar	240	17	4	0	16	2	10	7	15
Kind Healthy Snacks, Vanilla Blueberry Clusters Bar with Flax Seeds									
1/3 cup	120	3	0	0	22	5	5	3	20
Kind Healthy Snacks, Walnut & Date Bar									
1 bar	170	9	1	0	22	3	16	3	10
Larabar Jocalat, Chocolate									
1 bar	200	10	2	0	27	5	21	4	0
Larabar Jocalat, Chocolate Coffee									
1 bar	190	11	2	0	24	5	19	4	0
Larabar Jocalat, Chocolate Hazelnut									
1 bar	200	10	2	0	27	5	21	4	0
Larabar Jocalat, Chocolate Mint									
1 bar	190	9	2	0	26	5	20	4	0
Larabar Uber, Apple Turnover									
1 bar	190	11	1	0	20	3	15	3	125
Larabar Uber, Bananas Foster									
1 bar	230	17	1.5	0	14	3	8	4	140
Larabar Uber, Cherry Cobbler									
1 bar	190	12	1	0	19	2	12	4	135
Larabar Uber, Roasted Nut Roll									
1 bar	220	16	2	0	14	2	7	5	140
Larabar, Apple Pie									
1 bar	190	10	1	0	24	5	18	4	5
Larabar, Banana Bread									
1 bar	230	11	1	0	30	5	20	6	0
Larabar, Blueberry Muffin									
1 bar	190	8	1.5	0	26	3	17	4	5
Larabar, Cappuccino									
1 bar	200	10	1	0	22	4	16	5	0
Larabar, Carrot Cake									
1 bar	190	8	2	0	32	4	24	3	15

Food Serving size	Cal.	(g) Total Fat	(g) Sat. Fat	(mg) Chol.	(g) Carb.	(g) Fiber	(g) Sug.	(g) Prot.	(mg) Sod.
Larabar, Cashew Cookie 1 bar	230	13	1.5	0	23	3	18	6	5
Larabar, Cherry Pie 1 bar	200	8	0.5	0	30	4	23	5	0
Larabar, Chocolate Chip Brownie 1 bar	200	9	2	0	31	4	23	4	30
Larabar, Chocolate Chip Cherry Torte 1 bar	190	12	2.5	0	28	3	22	3	40
Larabar, Chocolate Chip Cookie Dough 1 bar	210	11	3	0	28	3	16	4	55
Larabar, Chocolate Coconut Chew 1 bar	240	13	2.5	0	29	5	22	5	0
Larabar, Coconut Cream Pie 1 bar	210	10	7	0	31	5	24	3	5
Larabar, Ginger Snap 1 bar	240	13	1	0	27	5	20	5	0
Larabar, Key Lime Pie 1 bar	220	10	3.5	0	31	4	24	4	5
Larabar, Lemon Bar 1 bar	220	11	1.5	0	28	3	22	6	5
Larabar, Peanut Butter & Jelly 1 bar	210	10	1.5	0	27	4	19	6	50
Larabar, Peanut Butter Chocolate Chip 1 bar	220	11	3	0	26	3	19	6	60
Larabar, Peanut Butter Cookie 1 bar	220	12	2	0	23	4	18	7	70
Larabar, Pecan Pie 1 bar	220	13	1	0	24	4	18	3	0
Larabar, Tropical Fruit Tart 1 bar	210	11	7	0	27	4	22	3	0
Luna Protein Bar, Luna Fiber, Chocolate Raspberry 1 bar	110	3.5	0.5	0	25	7	11	2	160
Luna Protein Bar, Luna Fiber, Peanut Butter Strawberry 1 bar	120	4	0.5	0	24	7	11	2	190

Food Serving size	Cal.	(g) Total Fat	(g) Sat. Fat	(mg) Chol.	(g) Carb.	(g) Fiber	(g) Sug.	(g) Prot.	(mg) Sod.
Luna Protein Bar, Luna Fiber, Vanilla Blueberry									
1 bar	110	3	0	0	25	7	11	1	150
Luna Protein Bars, Luna Bar, Blueberry Bliss									
1 bar	180	5	2	0	27	3	13	8	115
Luna Protein Bars, Luna Bar, Caramel Nut Brownie									
1 bar	180	6	3	0	26	3	13	8	160
Luna Protein Bars, Luna Bar, Chocolate Chunk									
1 bar	180	5	1.5	0	26	3	11	9	210
Luna Protein Bars, Luna Bar, Chocolate Dipped Coconut									
1 bar	190	7	4	0	25	3	11	9	210
Luna Protein Bars, Luna Bar, Chocolate Peppermint Stick									
1 bar	180	5	2.5	0	28	4	12	8	120
Luna Protein Bars, Luna Bar, Chocolate Raspberry									
1 bar	170	5	2	0	27	5	13	8	135
Luna Protein Bars, Luna Bar, Iced Oatmeal Raisin									
1 bar	180	5	2	0	11	3	13	9	150
Luna Protein Bars, Luna Bar, LemonZest									
1 bar	180	5	2.5	0	27	3	13	9	115
Luna Protein Bars, Luna Bar, Nutz Over Chocolate									
1 bar	180	6	2.5	0	25	4	10	9	190
Luna Protein Bars, Luna Bar, Peanut Butter Cookie									
1 bar	180	6	2	0	26	3	11	9	150
Luna Protein Bars, Luna Bar, Peanut Honey Pretzel									
1 bar	190	8	2.5	0	22	3	11	9	210
Luna Protein Bars, Luna Bar, S'mores									
1 bar	180	5	2.5	0	27	3	13	9	140
Luna Protein Bars, Luna Bar, Toasted Nuts 'n Cranberry									
1 bar	170	4.5	0.5	0	26	3	11	9	180
Luna Protein Bars, Luna Bar, Vanilla Almond									
1 bar	190	6	2	0	25	3	11	10	210
Luna Protein Bars, Luna Bar, White Chocolate Macadamia									
1 bar	190	7	2.5	0	25	3	11	9	210
Luna Protein Bars, Luna Minis, LemonZest									
1 bar	80	2	1	0	11	1	6	4	50

Food Serving size	Cal.	(g) Total Fat	(g) Sat. Fat	(mg) Chol.	(g) Carb.	(g) Fiber	(g) Sug.	(g) Prot.	(mg) Sod.
Luna Protein Bars, Luna Minis, Nutz Over Chocolate									
1 bar	80	2.5	1	0	11	2	4	4	80
Luna Protein Bars, Luna Minis, S'mores									
1 bar	70	2	1	0	11	1	5	4	60
Luna Protein Bars, Luna Minis, White Chocolate Macadamia									
1 bar	80	3	1	0	10	1	5	4	85
Luna Protein Bars, Luna Protein, Chocolate									
1 bar	170	5	3.5	0	20	3	13	12	250
Luna Protein Bars, Luna Protein, Chocolate Cherry Almond									
1 bar	170	6	3	0	21	3	15	12	140
Luna Protein Bars, Luna Protein, Chocolate Peanut Butter									
1 bar	190	8	3.5	0	19	3	12	12	250
Luna Protein Bars, Luna Protein, Cookie Dough									
1 bar	170	6	3.5	0	21	3	14	12	260
Luna Protein Bars, Luna Protein, Mint Chocolate Chip									
1 bar	170	5	3.5	0	20	3	13	12	250
Mariani Premium Fruit, Cranberry HoneyBar									
1 bar	180	10	1.5	0	20	2	14	5	0
Mariani Premium Fruit, Granola HoneyBar									
1 bar	160	6	1	0	25	2	12	4	0
Mariani Premium Fruit, Sesame HoneyBar									
1 bar	200	14	2	0	16	3	9	6	0
Mariani Premium Fruit, Trail Mix HoneyBar									
1 bar	190	12	1.5	0	18	2	12	6	0
Nature Valley, Gluten Free Roasted Nut Crunch Bars, Almond Crunch									
1 bar	190	13	1.5	0	13	2	6	6	180
Nature Valley, Gluten Free Roasted Nut Crunch Bars, Peanut Crunch									
1 bar	190	13	1.5	0	13	2	6	6	180
Pamela's, Oat Blueberry Lemon Whenever Bars									
1 bar	170	7	1.5	15	26	2	10	2	120
Pamela's, Oat Chocolate Chip Coconut Whenever Bars									
1 bar	180	9	2	15	23	2	8	2	130
Pamela's, Oat Cranberry Almond Whenever Bars									
1 bar	180	9	2	15	24	2	9	2	170

Food Serving size	Cal.	(g) Total Fat	(g) Sat. Fat	(mg) Chol.	(g) Carb.	(g) Fiber	(g) Sug.	(g) Prot.	(mg) Sod.
Pamela's, Oat Raisin Walnut Spice Whenever Bars									
1 bar	190	9	1.5	15	24	2	9	2	140
Power of Fruit, Banana Berry									
1 bar	27	0.12	0	0	6.5	0.9	3.8	0.36	1.75
Power of Fruit, Cherry Berry									
1 bar	35	20	0	0	6	1	5	0.3	0.76
Power of Fruit, Orange Tango									
1 bar	33	0.9	0	0	10	1	9	0.3	2.42
Power of Fruit, Original All-Fruit									
1 bar	28	0.12	0	0	7	1	5	0.3	0.78
Power of Fruit, Tropical									
1 bar	30	0.11	0	0	7.7	0.7	6	0.31	0.66
Promax Energy Bar, Chocolate Chip Cookie Dough									
1 bar	290	7	4	0	37	1	26	20	250
Promax Energy Bar, Chocolate Coconut Crunch									
1 bar	270	12	7	0	25	2	13	18	330
Promax Energy Bar, Chocolate Fudge Lower Sugar Mini Bar									
1 bar	60	1.5	1.5	0	10	4	3	5	70
Promax Energy Bar, Chocolate Mint									
1 bar	280	6	5	10	38	2	28	20	180
Promax Energy Bar, Chocolate Peanut Crunch									
1 bar	300	8	4.5	10	37	4	22	20	160
Promax Energy Bar, Chocolate Peanut Crunch Mini Bar									
1 bar	80	2	1	5	10	1	6	5	45
Promax Energy Bar, Cookies 'n Cream									
1 bar	270	4.5	3	0	40	1	30	20	240
Promax Energy Bar, Cookies 'n Cream Promax Mini Bar									
1 bar	70	1.5	1	0	11	0	8	5	65
Promax Energy Bar, Double Fudge Brownie									
1 bar	280	7	6	10	37	2	29	20	210
Promax Energy Bar, German Chocolate Cake									
1 bar	280	6	5	10	37	2	29	20	210
Promax Energy Bar, Lemon Bar									
1 bar	280	6	3.5	5	39	4	28	20	250

Food Serving size	Cal.	(g) Total Fat	(g) Sat. Fat	(mg) Chol.	(g) Carb.	(g) Fiber	(g) Sug.	(g) Prot.	(mg) Sod.
Promax Energy Bar, Lower Sugar Chocolate Fudge									
1 bar	220	6	4.5	5	33	14	9	18	240
Promax Energy Bar, Lower Sugar Mocha Latte									
1 bar	230	6	5	10	34	11	9	18	240
Promax Energy Bar, Lower Sugar Peanut Butter Chocolate									
1 bar	220	7	4	0	32	14	9	18	250
Promax Energy Bar, Lower Sugar Peanut Butter Cookie Dough									
1 bar	240	7	4	5	34	11	9	18	360
Promax Energy Bar, Nutty Butter Crisp									
1 bar	300	8	4	0	38	2	26	20	190
Promax Energy Bar, Peanut Butter Chocolate Lower Sugar Mini Bar									
1 bar	70	2	1	0	10	4	3	5	75
Promax Energy Bar, Peanut Cherry Crunch									
1 bar	270	12	1.5	0	26	6	12	18	320
Promax Energy Bar, Rocky Road									
1 bar	300	9	7	15	37	2	28	20	150
Purefit Nutrition Bars, Almond Crunch									
1 bar	220	7	0.5	0	24	3	13	18	150
Purefit Nutrition Bars, Berry Almond Crunch									
1 bar	220	7	0.5	0	25	3	14	18	150
Purefit Nutrition Bars, Chocolate Brownie									
1 bar	210	6	1.5	0	25	4	13	18	180
Purefit Nutrition Bars, Cranola Crunch									
1 bar	220	6	1	0	26	3	10	18	180
Purefit Nutrition Bars, Peanut Butter Crunch									
1 bar	220	7	1.5	0	24	2	13	18	180
Quest Nutrition, Apple Pie									
1 bar	170	5	0	5	24	18	3	20	350
Quest Nutrition, Chocolate Brownie									
1 bar	170	6	1	5	24	19	1	20	340
Quest Nutrition, Chocolate Peanut Butter									
1 bar	160	5	1	5	25	17	1	20	270
Quest Nutrition, Cinnamon Roll									
1 bar	170	6	0	5	24	17	1	20	300

Food Serving size	Cal.	(g) Total Fat	(g) Sat. Fat	(mg) Chol.	(g) Carb.	(g) Fiber	(g) Sug.	(g) Prot.	(mg) Sod.
Quest Nutrition, Coconut Cashew									
1 bar	170	6	1.5	5	24	17	2	20	270
Quest Nutrition, Lemon Cream Pie									
1 bar	170	6	0	5	25	17	1	20	260
Quest Nutrition, Mixed Berry Bliss									
1 bar	200	8	0.5	5	22	18	2	20	340
Quest Nutrition, Peanut Butter & Jelly									
1 bar	210	10	1.5	5	21	17	2	20	340
Quest Nutrition, Peanut Butter Supreme									
1 bar	210	10	1.5	5	21	18	2	20	340
Quest Nutrition, Strawberry Cheesecake									
1 bar	160	5	0	5	25	17	2	20	105
Quest Nutrition, Vanilla Almond Crunch									
1 bar	200	9	0.5	5	22	18	1	20	360
Rise Bar, Almond Honey Protein Bar									
1 bar	280	16	1.5	0	20	4	13	20	25
Rise Bar, Apricot Goji Energy Bar									
1 bar	190	10	1.5	0	23	3	12	5	70
Rise Bar, Blueberry Coconut Energy Bar									
1 bar	190	9	5	0	27	3	16	3	70
Rise Bar, Cherry Almond Energy Bar									
1 bar	200	11	1.5	0	23	3	11	5	55
Rise Bar, Coconut Acai Energy Bar									
1 bar	210	12	4.5	0	23	4	12	4	70
Rise Bar, Crunch Cranberry Apple Breakfast Bar									
1 bar	160	7	1	0	25	3	15	3	40
Rise Bar, Crunchy Carob Chip Protein Bar									
1 bar	260	15	1	5	22	5	13	17	25
Rise Bar, Crunchy Cashew Almond Breakfast Bar									
1 bar	180	10	1	0	17	4	10	5	45
Rise Bar, Crunchy Honey Walnut Breakfast Bar									
1 bar	160	7	0	0	23	2	15	4	50
Rise Bar, Crunchy Macadamia Pineapple Breakfast Bar									
1 bar	160	10	1	0	17	2	12	2	45

Food Serving size	Cal.	(g) Total Fat	(g) Sat. Fat	(mg) Chol.	(g) Carb.	(g) Fiber	(g) Sug.	(g) Prot.	(mg) Sod.
Rise Bar, Crunchy Perfect Pumpkin Breakfast Bar									
1 bar	190	10	1	0	18	3	11	7	40
Rise Bar, Raspberry Pomegranate Energy Bar									
1 bar	200	10	5	0	26	5	14	3	90
Schar, Chocolate Hazelnut Bars									
1 bar	200	12	6	<5	21	<1	14	2	30
Soyjoy Natural Fruit & Soy Bar, Apple Walnut									
1 bar	140	6	2.5	20	16	3	10	4	50
Soyjoy Natural Fruit & Soy Bar, Banana									
1 bar	130	6	3	20	16	2	12	4	50
Soyjoy Natural Fruit & Soy Bar, Berry									
1 bar	130	4.5	2	15	17	3	12	4	50
Soyjoy Natural Fruit & Soy Bar, Blueberry									
1 bar	140	6	3	20	17	4	12	4	45
Soyjoy Natural Fruit & Soy Bar, Mango Coconut									
1 bar	140	6	3.5	20	16	3	11	4	45
Soyjoy Natural Fruit & Soy Bar, Pineapple									
1 bar	140	6	3	20	17	3	12	4	40
Soyjoy Natural Fruit & Soy Bar, Strawberry									
1 bar	130	5	2.5	20	17	3	11	4	45

Sugars, Syrups, Frostings & Toppings

Food Serving size	Cal.	(g) Total Fat	(g) Sat. Fat	(mg) Chol.	(g) Carb.	(g) Fiber	(g) Sug.	(g) Prot.	(mg) Sod.
Betty Crocker, Gluten Free Rich and Creamy Frosting Cherry									
2 tbsp	140	5	1	0	23	NA	19	0	70
Betty Crocker, Gluten Free Rich and Creamy Frosting Chocolate									
2 tbsp	130	5	1.5	0	21	<1	18	0	95
Betty Crocker, Gluten Free Rich and Creamy Frosting Coconut Pecan									
2 tbsp	140	7	3	0	19	<1	16	0	55
Betty Crocker, Gluten Free Rich and Creamy Frosting Cream Cheese									
2 tbsp	140	5	1	0	23	NA	20	0	70
Betty Crocker, Gluten Free Rich and Creamy Frosting Creamy White									
2 tbsp	140	5	1	0	23	NA	20	0	70
Betty Crocker, Gluten Free Rich and Creamy Frosting Dark Chocolate									
2 tbsp	130	5	1.5	0	20	<1	16	<1	105

Food Serving size	Cal.	(g) Total Fat	(g) Sat. Fat	(mg) Chol.	(g) Carb.	(g) Fiber	(g) Sug.	(g) Prot.	(mg) Sod.
Betty Crocker, Gluten Free Rich and Creamy Frosting Lemon									
2 tbsp	140	5	1.5	0	23	NA	19	0	70
Betty Crocker, Gluten Free Rich and Creamy Frosting Milk Chocolate									
2 tbsp	130	5	1.5	0	21	NA	17	0	95
Betty Crocker, Gluten Free Rich and Creamy Frosting Rainbow Chip									
2 tbsp	140	5	2	0	23	NA	20	0	70
Betty Crocker, Gluten Free Rich and Creamy Frosting Triple Chocolate Fudge Chip									
2 tbsp	140	5	1.5	0	22	<1	20	<1	90
Betty Crocker, Gluten Free Rich and Creamy Frosting Vanilla									
2 tbsp	140	5	1	0	23	0	19	0	70
Betty Crocker, Gluten Free Whipped Frosting Butter Cream									
2 tbsp	100	5	1.5	NA	15	NA	14	0	25
Betty Crocker, Gluten Free Whipped Frosting Chocolate									
2 tbsp	100	4.5	1.5	NA	14	<1	12	<1	60
Betty Crocker, Gluten Free Whipped Frosting Fluffy White									
2 tbsp	100	5	1.5	NA	15	NA	14	0	25
Hain Pure Foods, Organic Light Brown Sugar									
1 tsp	15	0	NA	NA	4	NA	4	0	0
Hain Pure Foods, Organic Powdered Sugar									
1/4 cup	140	0	NA	NA	37	NA	34	0	0
Hain Pure Foods, Organic Sugar									
1 tsp	10	0	NA	NA	3	NA	3	0	0
Hain Pure Foods, Turbinado Sugar									
1 tsp	15	0	NA	NA	4	NA	4	0	0
Let's Do..., Carnival Sprinkelz									
1 tsp	15	0	0	0	4	0	3	0	0
Let's Do..., Chocolatey Sprinkelz									
1 tsp	15	0	0	0	3	0	3	0	0
Let's Do..., Organic Confetti Sprinkelz									
1 tsp	25	0	0	0	7	0	6	0	0
Lundberg Family Farms, Eco-Farmed Sweet Dreams, Rice Syrup									
2 tbsp	150	0	0	0	36	0	22	0	70
Lundberg Family Farms, Organic Sweet Dreams, Rice Syrup									
2 tbsp	150	0	0	0	36	0	22	0	70

Food Serving size	Cal.	(g) Total Fat	(g) Sat. Fat	(mg) Chol.	(g) Carb.	(g) Fiber	(g) Sug.	(g) Prot.	(mg) Sod.
Maple Grove Farms, Apricot Fruit Flavored Syrup									
1/4 cup	170	0	NA	NA	42	NA	40	0	5
Maple Grove Farms, Blueberry Fruit Flavored Syrup									
1/4 cup	160	0	NA	NA	41	NA	40	0	15
Maple Grove Farms, Boysenberry Fruit Flavored Syrup									
1/4 cup	170	0	NA	NA	41	NA	41	0	5
Maple Grove Farms, Butter Flavor Sugar Free Syrup									
1/4 cup	30	0	NA	NA	11	NA	0	0	100
Maple Grove Farms, Dark Amber Pure Maple Syrup									
1/4 cup	200	0	NA	NA	53	NA	53	0	5
Maple Grove Farms, Granulated Maple Sugar									
1 tsp	15	0	NA	NA	4	NA	3	0	0
Maple Grove Farms, Honey Maple Spread									
2 tbsp	160	0	NA	NA	42	NA	37	0	60
Maple Grove Farms, Maple Flavor Sugar Free Syrup									
1/4 cup	10	0	NA	NA	3	NA	0	0	65
Maple Grove Farms, Medium Amber Pure Maple Syrup									
1/4 cup	200	0	NA	NA	53	NA	53	0	5
Maple Grove Farms, Northern Comfort Medium Amber Pure Maple Syrup									
1/4 cup	200	0	0	0	53	NA	53	0	5
Maple Grove Farms, Organic Dark Amber Maple Syrup									
1/4 cup	200	0	NA	NA	53	NA	53	0	5
Maple Grove Farms, Organic Dark Amber Syrup									
1/4 cup	200	0	NA	NA	53	NA	53	0	5
Maple Grove Farms, Red Raspberry Fruit Flavored Syrup									
1/4 cup	230	0	NA	NA	46	NA	45	0	5
Maple Grove Farms, Strawberry Fruit Flavored Syrup									
1/4 cup	170	0	NA	NA	41	NA	40	0	5
Maple Grove Farms, Tub Blended Maple Spread									
2 tbsp	170	0	NA	NA	44	NA	40	0	25
Maple Grove Farms, Vermont Maple Flavor Sugar Free Syrup									
1/4 cup	15	0	NA	NA	5	NA	0	0	110
Nestlé, Nesquik, Chocolate Syrup									
1 tbsp	50	0	0	0	13	0	12	0	30

Food Serving size	Cal.	(g) Total Fat	(g) Sat. Fat	(mg) Chol.	(g) Carb.	(g) Fiber	(g) Sug.	(g) Prot.	(mg) Sod.
Nestlé, Nesquik, Strawberry Syrup									
1 tbsp	50	0	0	0	13	0	13	0	0
Pamela's, Dark Chocolate Frosting Mix, Prepared									
1/12th of prepared frosting	160	1	0.5	0	25	0	23	2	490
Pamela's, Vanilla Frosting Mix, Prepared									
1/12th of prepared frosting	155	1	0.5	0	25	0	22	2	490
Wholesome Sweeteners, Fair Trade Certified Light Brown Sugar									
1 tsp	15	0	0	0	4	0	4	0	0
Wholesome Sweeteners, Fair Trade Certified Natural Cane Sugar									
1 tsp	15	0	0	0	4	0	4	0	0
Wholesome Sweeteners, Fair Trade Certified Organic Amber Honey									
1 tbsp	60	0	0	0	17	0	16	0	0
Wholesome Sweeteners, Fair Trade Certified Organic Blackstrap Molasses									
1 tbsp	60	0	0	0	14	0	10	0	0
Wholesome Sweeteners, Fair Trade Certified Organic Dark Brown Sugar									
1 tsp	15	0	0	0	4	0	4	0	0
Wholesome Sweeteners, Fair Trade Certified Organic Powdered Sugar									
1/4 cup	120	0	0	0	30	0	30	0	0
Wholesome Sweeteners, Fair Trade Certified Organic Raw Honey									
1 tbsp	60	0	0	0	17	0	16	0	0
Wholesome Sweeteners, Fair Trade Certified Organic Sucanat									
1 tsp	15	0	0	0	4	0	4	0	0
Wholesome Sweeteners, Fair Trade Certified Organic Sugar									
1 tsp	15	0	0	0	4	0	4	0	0
Wholesome Sweeteners, Fair Trade Certified Raw Cane Sugar									
1 tsp	15	0	0	0	4	0	4	0	0
Wholesome Sweeteners, Organic Blue Agave									
1 tbsp	60	0	0	0	16	0	16	0	0
Wholesome Sweeteners, Organic Cinnamon Flavored Blue Agave Syrup									
2 tbsp	120	0	0	0	32	0	32	0	0
Wholesome Sweeteners, Organic Coconut Palm Sugar									
1 tsp	16	0	0	0	4	0	4	NA	0
Wholesome Sweeteners, Organic Maple Flavored Blue Agave Syrup									
2 tbsp	120	0	0	0	32	0	32	0	0

Food Serving size	Cal.	(g) Total Fat	(g) Sat. Fat	(mg) Chol.	(g) Carb.	(g) Fiber	(g) Sug.	(g) Prot.	(mg) Sod.
Wholesome Sweeteners, Organic Raw Blue Agave									
1 tbsp	60	0	0	0	16	0	16	0	0
Wholesome Sweeteners, Organic Stevia									
1 packet	0	0	0	0	1	0.6	0	0	0
Wholesome Sweeteners, Organic Strawberry Flavored Blue Agave Syrup									
2 tbsp	120	0	0	0	32	0	32	0	0
Wholesome Sweeteners, Organic Turbinado Sugar									
1 tsp	15	0	0	0	4	0	4	0	0
Wholesome Sweeteners, Organic Vanilla Blue Agave									
2 tbsp	120	0	0	0	32	0	32	0	0
Wholesome Sweeteners, Zero									
6g packet	0	0	0	0	6	0	6	0	0

Beverages

Why Drink Beverages?

Beverages provide hydration and necessary nutrients. Water is the body's principal component and makes up 60% of your body weight. Every system in your body depends on water. Even mild dehydration can drain your energy and make you tired. Beverages can also provide necessary nutrients such as calcium in milk and vitamin C in orange juice.

Daily Goal

"Eight by Eight rule"—drinking eight 8-ounce glasses of fluid daily is the general rule.
Women actually need about 9 cups of total beverages daily.
Men actually need about 13 cups of total beverages daily.
Women who are expecting or breast feeding need about 10 to 13 cups of fluids daily.

Gluten-Free Shopping Tips

- Plain water is best for hydration
- Choose 100% juices rather than juice drinks
- Drink skim or fat-free milk
- Use sports drinks in moderation

Gluten-Free Shopping List Essentials

Bottled water
Milk, fat-free or skim (see *Dairy*, page 115)
Juice drinks, 100% juice (see *Fruit*, page 95)

Approved Beverages and Those to Avoid on a Gluten-Free Diet

Gluten-Free

- Tea, instant or ground coffee (regular or decaffeinated)
- Cocoa
- Soft drinks
- Most non-dairy beverages made from nut, potato, soy, and rice

May Contain Gluten

- Flavored and herbal teas
- Flavored coffees, coffee substitutes
- Hot chocolate mixes
- Cereal and malted beverages (chocolate malt and those with malt flavor)
- Non-dairy beverages (nut, potato, soy, and rice) made with barley-malt extract, barley-malt flavoring, or oats

Gluten-Free Alcoholic Beverages

- Distilled alcohol – bourbon, rum, gin, rye whiskey, scotch whiskey, vodka, and pure liquours
- Wines
- Gluten-free beers, ale, and lagers (made with rice, buckwheat, or sorghum)

Gluten-Containing Alcoholic Beverages

- Flavored alcoholic beverages (e.g., coolers, ciders, mixed drinks)
- Beer, ale, and lager (made from barley)

Caution

Drinks can be high in calories and sugars. Make sure that juice drinks don't have added sugars. A soda that only has sugar calories is an example of an "empty calories" choice. You need water for hydration, but try not to drink calories with your water.

Food Serving size	Cal.	(g) Total Fat	(g) Sat. Fat	(mg) Chol.	(g) Carb.	(g) Fiber	(g) Sug.	(g) Prot.	(mg) Sod.

Alcoholic Beverages

Bard's, American Lager Beer

12 oz	155	0	0	0	14	NA	3	0	70

Bard's, Gold Lager Beer

12 oz	155	0	0	NA	14.2	NA	3	0	70

New Planet, Gluten Free Beer, 3R Raspberry Ale

12 fl oz	160	0	0	0	17	0	0	0	0

New Planet, Gluten Free Beer, Off Grid Pale Ale

12 fl oz	170	1	0	0	17	0	0	0	0

New Planet, Gluten Free Beer, Tread Lightly Ale

12 fl oz	179	0	0	0	17	0	0	0	0

Redbridge Gluten Free Beer

12 oz	127	0	0	0	12	0	1	1	9

Woodchuck Hard Cider, 802 Dark & Dry

1 bottle, 12 oz	180	0	NA	0	16	0	16	0	15

Woodchuck Hard Cider, Amber

1 bottle, 12 oz	200	0	NA	0	21	0	21	0	15

Woodchuck Hard Cider, Crisp

1 bottle, 12 oz	120	0	0	0	10	0	9	0	5

Woodchuck Hard Cider, Fall Hard Cider

1 bottle, 12 oz	220	0	NA	0	21	0	21	0	15

Woodchuck Hard Cider, Farmhouse Select, Original '91

1 bottle, 12 oz	230	0	NA	NA	15	NA	NA	0	NA

Woodchuck Hard Cider, Granny Smith

1 bottle, 12 oz	160	0	0	0	11	0	11	0	10

Woodchuck Hard Cider, Pear

1 bottle, 12 oz	150	0	0	0	18	0	18	0	25

Woodchuck Hard Cider, Private Reserves, Belgian White (available Mar-May)

1 bottle, 12 oz	190	0	0	0	17	0	12	0	5

Woodchuck Hard Cider, Private Reserves, Ginger (available Jun-Aug)

1 bottle, 12 oz	250	0	0	0	20	0	16	0	10

Woodchuck Hard Cider, Private Reserves, Pumpkin (available Sep-Nov)

1 bottle, 12 oz	250	0	NA	NA	0	NA	NA	1	NA

Food Serving size	Cal.	(g) Total Fat	(g) Sat. Fat	(mg) Chol.	(g) Carb.	(g) Fiber	(g) Sug.	(g) Prot.	(mg) Sod.
Woodchuck Hard Cider, Raspberry									
1 bottle, 12 oz	170	0	0	0	21	0	21	0	15
Woodchuck Hard Cider, Spring Hard Cider (available Feb-Mar)									
1 bottle, 12 oz	190	0	NA	0	19	0	15	0	5
Woodchuck Hard Cider, Summer Hard Cider (available Apr-Jul)									
1 bottle, 12 oz	210	0	0	0	25	0	17	0	0
Woodchuck Hard Cider, Winter Hard Cider (available Nov-Jan)									
1 bottle, 12 oz	140	0	0	0	19	0	16	0	5

Coffees & Teas

Food Serving size	Cal.	(g) Total Fat	(g) Sat. Fat	(mg) Chol.	(g) Carb.	(g) Fiber	(g) Sug.	(g) Prot.	(mg) Sod.
AriZona Green Tea, Asia Plum Green Tea									
8 fl oz	70	0	0	0	18	0	17	0	20
AriZona Green Tea, Black Tea with Ginseng and Honey									
8 fl oz	60	0	0	0	15	0	14	0	20
AriZona Green Tea, Diet Blueberry Green Tea									
8 fl oz	5	0	0	0	2	0	0	0	20
AriZona Green Tea, Diet Decaf Green Tea									
8 fl oz	0	0	0	0	1	0	1	0	20
AriZona Green Tea, Diet Green Tea with Ginseng and Honey									
8 fl oz	0	0	0	0	1	0	1	0	20
AriZona Green Tea, Diet Lemon Tea									
8 fl oz	0	0	0	0	0	0	0	0	20
AriZona Green Tea, Diet Peach Tea									
8 fl oz	0	0	0	0	1	0	1	0	20
AriZona Green Tea, Diet Raspberry Tea									
8 fl oz	90	0	0	0	23	0	22	0	25
AriZona Green Tea, Diet White Cranapple Green Tea									
8 fl oz	5	0	0	0	2	0	0	0	20
AriZona Green Tea, Extra Sweet Green Tea									
8 fl oz	90	0	0	0	23	0	23	0	20
AriZona Green Tea, Georgia Peach Green Tea									
8 fl oz	70	0	0	0	18	0	17	0	10
AriZona Green Tea, Green Tea with Ginseng and Honey									
8 fl oz	70	0	0	0	18	0	17	0	20

Food Serving size	Cal.	(g) Total Fat	(g) Sat. Fat	(mg) Chol.	(g) Carb.	(g) Fiber	(g) Sug.	(g) Prot.	(mg) Sod.
AriZona Green Tea, Lemon Tea									
8 fl oz	90	0	0	0	25	0	24	0	20
AriZona Green Tea, Mandarin Orange Green Tea									
8 fl oz	70	0	0	0	19	0	18	0	20
AriZona Green Tea, Peach Tea									
8 fl oz	70	0	0	0	18	0	17	0	10
AriZona Green Tea, Pomegranate Green Tea									
8 fl oz	70	0	0	0	19	0	18	0	10
AriZona Green Tea, Raspberry Tea									
8 fl oz	90	0	0	0	23	0	22	0	25
AriZona Green Tea, Red Apple Green Tea									
8 fl oz	70	0	0	0	19	0	18	0	20
AriZona Green Tea, Sweet Tea									
8 fl oz	90	0	0	0	23	0	23	0	20
AriZona Herbal Tea, Rx Energy Herbal Tea									
8 fl oz	120	0	0	0	31	0	29	0	25
AriZona Herbal Tea, Rx Stress Herbal Tea									
8 fl oz	70	0	0	0	19	0	18	0	20
AriZona White Tea, Black and White Tea									
8 fl oz	50	0	0	0	14	0	14	0	10
AriZona White Tea, Blueberry White Tea									
8 fl oz	70	0	0	0	19	0	18	0	10
Bigelow Teas, Apple Cider Herb, Brewed, Prepared with Tap Water									
8 fl oz	0	0	NA	NA	0	NA	NA	0	0
Bigelow Teas, Black Tea with Pomegranate, Brewed, Prepared with Tap Water									
8 fl oz	0	0	NA	NA	0	NA	NA	0	0
Bigelow Teas, Chamomile Lemon Herb Tea, Brewed, Prepared with Tap Water									
8 fl oz	0	0	NA	NA	0	NA	NA	0	0
Bigelow Teas, Chamomile Mango Herb Tea, Brewed, Prepared with Tap Water									
8 fl oz	0	0	NA	NA	<1	NA	NA	0	0
Bigelow Teas, Chanomile Mint Herb Tea, Brewed, Prepared with Tap Water									
8 fl oz	0	0	NA	NA	0	NA	NA	0	0
Bigelow Teas, Chinese Oolong Tea, Brewed, Prepared with Tap Water									
8 fl oz	0	0	NA	NA	0	NA	NA	0	0

Food Serving size	Cal.	(g) Total Fat	(g) Sat. Fat	(mg) Chol.	(g) Carb.	(g) Fiber	(g) Sug.	(g) Prot.	(mg) Sod.
Bigelow Teas, Cinnamon Apple Herb Tea, Brewed, Prepared with Tap Water									
8 fl oz	0	0	NA	NA	0	NA	NA	0	0
Bigelow Teas, Cinnamon Stick Tea, Brewed, Prepared with Tap Water									
8 fl oz	0	0	NA	NA	<1	NA	NA	0	0
Bigelow Teas, Constant Comment Green Tea, Brewed, Prepared with Tap Water									
8 fl oz	0	0	NA	NA	0	NA	NA	0	0
Bigelow Teas, Constant Comment Tea, Brewed, Prepared with Tap Water									
8 fl oz	0	0	NA	NA	0	NA	NA	0	0
Bigelow Teas, Cozy Chamomile Herb Tea, Brewed, Prepared with Tap Water									
8 fl oz	0	0	NA	NA	0	NA	NA	0	0
Bigelow Teas, Cranberry Apple Herb Tea, Brewed, Prepared with Tap Water									
8 fl oz	0	0	NA	NA	<1	NA	NA	0	0
Bigelow Teas, Cranberry Hibiscus Herb Tea, Brewed, Prepared with Tap Water									
8 fl oz	0	0	NA	NA	0	NA	NA	0	0
Bigelow Teas, Darjeeling Tea, Brewed, Prepared with Tap Water									
8 fl oz	0	0	NA	NA	0	NA	NA	0	0
Bigelow Teas, Earl Grey Decaffeinated Tea, Brewed, Prepared with Tap Water									
8 fl oz	0	0	NA	NA	0	NA	NA	0	0
Bigelow Teas, Earl Grey Green Tea, Brewed, Prepared with Tap Water									
8 fl oz	0	0	NA	NA	0	NA	NA	0	0
Bigelow Teas, Earl Grey Tea, Brewed, Prepared with Tap Water									
8 fl oz	0	0	NA	NA	0	NA	NA	0	0
Bigelow Teas, Eggnogg'n Tea, Brewed, Prepared with Tap Water									
8 fl oz	0	0	NA	NA	0	NA	NA	0	0
Bigelow Teas, English Breakfast Tea, Brewed, Prepared with Tap Water									
8 fl oz	0	0	NA	NA	<1	NA	NA	0	0
Bigelow Teas, English Teatime Decaffeinated Tea, Brewed, Prepared with Tap Water									
8 fl oz	0	0	NA	NA	0	NA	NA	0	0
Bigelow Teas, English Teatime Tea, Brewed, Prepared with Tap Water									
8 fl oz	0	0	NA	NA	<1	NA	NA	0	0
Bigelow Teas, French Vanilla Decaffeinated Tea, Brewed, Prepared with Tap Water									
8 fl oz	0	0	NA	NA	<1	NA	NA	0	0

Food Serving size	Cal.	(g) Total Fat	(g) Sat. Fat	(mg) Chol.	(g) Carb.	(g) Fiber	(g) Sug.	(g) Prot.	(mg) Sod.
Bigelow Teas, French Vanilla Tea, Brewed, Prepared with Tap Water									
8 fl oz	0	0	NA	NA	<1	NA	NA	0	0
Bigelow Teas, Fruit & Almond Herb Tea, Brewed, Prepared with Tap Water									
8 fl oz	0	0	NA	NA	1	NA	NA	0	0
Bigelow Teas, Ginger Snappish Herb Tea, Brewed, Prepared with Tap Water									
8 fl oz	0	0	NA	NA	0	NA	NA	0	0
Bigelow Teas, Green Chai, Brewed, Prepared with Tap Water									
8 fl oz	0	0	NA	NA	0	NA	NA	0	0
Bigelow Teas, Green Tea Decaffeinated, Brewed, Prepared with Tap Water									
8 fl oz	0	0	NA	NA	0	NA	NA	0	0
Bigelow Teas, Green Tea with Lemon, Brewed, Prepared with Tap Water									
8 fl oz	0	0	NA	NA	0	NA	NA	0	0
Bigelow Teas, Green Tea with Lemon, Decaffeinated, Brewed, Prepared with Tap Water									
8 fl oz	0	0	NA	NA	0	NA	NA	0	0
Bigelow Teas, Green Tea with Mango, Brewed, Prepared with Tap Water									
8 fl oz	0	0	NA	NA	0	NA	NA	0	0
Bigelow Teas, Green Tea with Mint, Brewed, Prepared with Tap Water									
8 fl oz	0	0	NA	NA	0	NA	NA	0	0
Bigelow Teas, Green Tea with Peach, Brewed, Prepared with Tap Water									
8 fl oz	0	0	NA	NA	0	NA	NA	0	0
Bigelow Teas, Green Tea with Pomegranate Iced Tea, Brewed, Prepared with Tap Water									
8 fl oz	0	0	NA	NA	<1	NA	NA	0	0
Bigelow Teas, Green Tea with Pomegranate, Brewed, Prepared with Tap Water									
8 fl oz	0	0	NA	NA	0	NA	NA	0	0
Bigelow Teas, Green Tea with Pomegranate, Decaffeinated, Brewed, Prepared with Tap Water									
8 fl oz	0	0	NA	NA	0	NA	NA	0	0
Bigelow Teas, Green Tea with Wild Blueberry & Acai Decaffeinated, Brewed, Prepared with Tap Water									
8 fl oz	0	0	NA	NA	<1	NA	NA	0	0
Bigelow Teas, Green Tea with Wild Blueberry & Acai, Brewed, Prepared with Tap Water									
8 fl oz	0	0	NA	NA	0	NA	NA	0	0

Food Serving size	Cal.	(g) Total Fat	(g) Sat. Fat	(mg) Chol.	(g) Carb.	(g) Fiber	(g) Sug.	(g) Prot.	(mg) Sod.
Bigelow Teas, Green Tea, Brewed, Prepared with Tap Water									
8 fl oz	0	0	NA	NA	0	NA	NA	0	0
Bigelow Teas, Half Iced Tea & Half Lemonade with Pomegranate, Brewed, Prepared with Tap Water									
8 fl oz	10	0	NA	NA	3	NA	2	0	0
Bigelow Teas, Half Iced Tea & Half Lemonade, Brewed, Prepared with Tap Water									
8 fl oz	15	0	NA	NA	4	NA	3	0	0
Bigelow Teas, Herb Plus Lemon Ginger (Probiotics), Brewed, Prepared with Tap Water									
8 fl oz	0	0	NA	NA	<1	NA	NA	0	0
Bigelow Teas, I Love Lemon & C Herb Tea, Brewed, Prepared with Tap Water									
8 fl oz	0	0	NA	NA	1	NA	NA	0	0
Bigelow Teas, Jasmine Green Tea, Brewed, Prepared with Tap Water									
8 fl oz	0	0	NA	NA	0	NA	NA	0	0
Bigelow Teas, Lemon Lift Decaffeinated Tea, Brewed, Prepared with Tap Water									
8 fl oz	0	0	NA	NA	<1	NA	NA	0	0
Bigelow Teas, Lemon Lift Tea, Brewed, Prepared with Tap Water									
8 fl oz	0	0	NA	NA	<1	NA	NA	0	0
Bigelow Teas, Mint Medley Herb Tea, Brewed, Prepared with Tap Water									
8 fl oz	0	0	NA	NA	<1	NA	NA	0	0
Bigelow Teas, Orange & Spice Herb Tea, Brewed, Prepared with Tap Water									
8 fl oz	0	0	NA	NA	<1	NA	NA	0	0
Bigelow Teas, Organic Breakfast Blend Decaffeinated Tea, Brewed, Prepared with Tap Water									
8 fl oz	0	0	NA	NA	0	NA	NA	0	0
Bigelow Teas, Organic Ceylon-Fair Trade Tea, Brewed, Prepared with Tap Water									
8 fl oz	0	0	NA	NA	0	NA	NA	0	0
Bigelow Teas, Organic Chamomile Citrus Herb Tea, Brewed, Prepared with Tap Water									
8 fl oz	0	0	NA	NA	0	NA	NA	0	0
Bigelow Teas, Organic Green Decaffeinated Tea, Brewed, Prepared with Tap Water									
8 fl oz	0	0	NA	NA	0	NA	NA	0	0

Food Serving size	Cal.	(g) Total Fat	(g) Sat. Fat	(mg) Chol.	(g) Carb.	(g) Fiber	(g) Sug.	(g) Prot.	(mg) Sod.
Bigelow Teas, Organic Green Tea Pomegranate & Acai, Brewed, Prepared with Tap Water									
8 fl oz	0	0	NA	NA	0	NA	NA	0	0
Bigelow Teas, Organic Green Tea, Brewed, Prepared with Tap Water									
8 fl oz	0	0	NA	NA	0	NA	NA	0	0
Bigelow Teas, Organic Imperial Earl Grey Tea, Brewed, Prepared with Tap Water									
8 fl oz	0	0	NA	NA	0	NA	NA	0	0
Bigelow Teas, Organic Moroccan Mint Herb Tea, Brewed, Prepared with Tap Water									
8 fl oz	0	0	NA	NA	0	NA	NA	0	0
Bigelow Teas, Organic Pure Green Decaffeinated Tea, Brewed, Prepared with Tap Water									
8 fl oz	0	0	NA	NA	0	NA	NA	0	0
Bigelow Teas, Organic Pure Green Tea, Brewed, Prepared with Tap Water									
8 fl oz	0	0	NA	NA	0	NA	NA	0	0
Bigelow Teas, Organic Rooibos with Asian Pear Tea, Brewed, Prepared with Tap Water									
8 fl oz	0	0	NA	NA	0	NA	NA	0	0
Bigelow Teas, Organic White Tea with Raspberry & Chrysanthemum, Brewed, Prepared with Tap Water									
8 fl oz	0	0	NA	NA	0	NA	NA	0	0
Bigelow Teas, Peppermint Herb Tea, Brewed, Prepared with Tap Water									
8 fl oz	0	0	NA	NA	0	NA	NA	0	0
Bigelow Teas, Perfect Peach Herb Iced Tea, Brewed, Prepared with Tap Water									
8 fl oz	0	0	NA	NA	1	NA	NA	0	0
Bigelow Teas, Perfect Peach Herb Tea, Brewed, Prepared with Tap Water									
8 fl oz	0	0	NA	NA	1	NA	NA	0	0
Bigelow Teas, Plantation Mint Tea, Brewed, Prepared with Tap Water									
8 fl oz	0	0	NA	NA	0	NA	NA	0	0
Bigelow Teas, Pomegranate Pizzazz Herb Tea, Brewed, Prepared with Tap Water									
8 fl oz	0	0	NA	NA	0	NA	NA	*0	0
Bigelow Teas, Pumpkin Spice Tea, Brewed, Prepared with Tap Water									
8 fl oz	0	0	NA	NA	0	NA	NA	0	0

Food Serving size	Cal.	(g) Total Fat	(g) Sat. Fat	(mg) Chol.	(g) Carb.	(g) Fiber	(g) Sug.	(g) Prot.	(mg) Sod.
Bigelow Teas, Raspberry Royale Tea, Brewed, Prepared with Tap Water									
8 fl oz	0	0	NA	NA	<1	NA	NA	0	0
Bigelow Teas, Red Raspberry Herb Iced Tea, Brewed, Prepared with Tap Water									
8 fl oz	0	0	NA	NA	0	NA	NA	0	0
Bigelow Teas, Red Raspberry Herb Tea, Brewed, Prepared with Tap Water									
8 fl oz.	0	0	NA	NA	<1	NA	NA	0	0
Bigelow Teas, Spiced Chai Decaffeinated Tea, Brewed, Prepared with Tap Water									
8 fl oz	0	0	NA	NA	0	NA	NA	0	0
Bigelow Teas, Spiced Chai Tea, Brewed, Prepared with Tap Water									
8 fl oz	0	0	NA	NA	0	NA	NA	0	0
Bigelow Teas, Sweet Dreams Herb Tea, Brewed, Prepared with Tap Water									
8 fl oz	0	0	NA	NA	0	NA	NA	0	0
Bigelow Teas, Sweetheart Cinnamon Herb Tea, Brewed, Prepared with Tap Water									
8 fl oz	0	0	NA	NA	0	NA	NA	0	0
Bigelow Teas, Vanilla Caramel Tea, Brewed, Prepared with Tap Water									
8 fl oz	0	0	NA	NA	<1	NA	NA	0	0
Bigelow Teas, Vanilla Chai Tea, Brewed, Prepared with Tap Water									
8 fl oz	0	0	NA	NA	<1	NA	NA	0	0
Bigelow Teas, White Chocolate Obsession Tea, Brewed, Prepared with Tap Water									
8 fl oz	0	0	NA	NA	0	NA	NA	0	0
Bigelow Teas, Wild Blueberry with Acai Herb Tea, Brewed, Prepared with Tap Water									
8 fl oz	0	0	NA	NA	0	NA	NA	0	0
BiProUSA, BioZzz Alpha-lactalbumin									
1 scoop	80	0	0	0	0	0	0	18	190
BiProUSA, BiPro Whey Protein Isolate									
1 scoop	80	0	0	0	0	0	0	20	170
Bob's Red Mill, Soy Lecithin Granules									
1 tbsp	60	4	1	0	1	0	0	0	0
Bob's Red Mill, Soy Protein Powder									
1 tbsp	20	0	0	0	0	0	0	5	60

Food Serving size	Cal.	(g) Total Fat	(g) Sat. Fat	(mg) Chol.	(g) Carb.	(g) Fiber	(g) Sug.	(g) Prot.	(mg) Sod.
Coffee, Brewed from Grounds, Prepared with Tap Water									
1 fl oz (29.6g)	0	0	0	0	0	0	0	0	1
Coffee, Brewed from Grounds, Prepared with Tap Water, Decaffeinated									
1 fl oz (29.6g)	0	0	0	0	0	0	0	0	1
Coffee, Instant, Regular, Powder									
1 packet (2g)	5	0	0	0	1	0	0	0	1
Coffee, Instant, Regular, Powder, Half the Caffeine									
1 packet (2g)	7	0	0	0	1	0	0	0	1
Coffee, Instant, Regular, Prepared with Water									
1 fl oz (29.8g)	1	0	0	0	0	0	0	0	1
Eden Foods, Organic Matcha — Green Tea Powder									
1g	3	0	0	0	0	<1	0	<1	0
Hansen's Hubert's Lemonade Tea, Half & Half, Black Tea									
8 fl oz	80	0	0	NA	19	NA	18	0	0
Hansen's Hubert's Lemonade Tea, Half & Half, Green Tea									
8 fl oz	70	0	0	NA	16	NA	15	0	0
Hansen's Natural, Tea Stix, Natural Blackberry Tea									
1/2 packet (makes 8 fl oz)	5	0	NA	NA	1	NA	0	0	5
Hansen's Natural, Tea Stix, Natural Iced Tea									
1/2 packet (makes 8 fl oz)	5	0	NA	NA	1	NA	0	0	0
Honest Tea, (not too) Sweet Tea									
1 - 16.9 oz container	100	0	NA	NA	25	NA	25	0	10
Honest Tea, Assam Black Tea									
8 fl oz serving, 2 per bottle	17	0	NA	NA	5	NA	5	0	5
Honest Tea, Black Forest Berry									
8 fl oz serving, 2 per bottle	30	0	NA	NA	8	NA	8	0	5
Honest Tea, Classic Green									
8 fl oz serving, 2 per bottle	30	0	NA	NA	9	NA	9	0	5
Honest Tea, Community Green									
8 fl oz serving, 2 per bottle	17	0	NA	NA	5	NA	5	0	5
Honest Tea, Green Dragon Tea									
8 fl oz serving, 2 per bottle	30	0	NA	NA	8	NA	8	0	5
Honest Tea, Half & Half									
1 - 16.9 oz container	100	0	NA	NA	24	NA	24	0	10

Food Serving size	Cal.	(g) Total Fat	(g) Sat. Fat	(mg) Chol.	(g) Carb.	(g) Fiber	(g) Sug.	(g) Prot.	(mg) Sod.
Honest Tea, Heavenly Lemon Tulsi 8 fl oz serving, 2 per bottle	30	0	NA	NA	8	NA	8	0	5
Honest Tea, Honest Ade, Cranberry Lemonade 1 - 16.9 oz container	100	0	NA	NA	25	NA	24	0	10
Honest Tea, Honest Ade, Limeade 1 - 16.9 oz container	100	0	NA	NA	25	NA	25	0	10
Honest Tea, Honest Ade, Orange Mango 1 - 16.9 oz container	100	0	NA	NA	25	NA	25	0	10
Honest Tea, Honest Ade, Pomegranate Blue 1 - 16.9 oz container	100	0	NA	NA	25	NA	25	0	10
Honest Tea, Honest Ade, Super Fruit Punch 1 - 16.9 oz container	100	0	NA	NA	25	NA	25	0	5
Honest Tea, Honest Kids, Appley Ever After 1 - 6.75 oz pouch	40	0	NA	NA	10	NA	10	0	5
Honest Tea, Honest Kids, Berry Berry Good Lemonade 1 - 6.75 oz pouch	40	0	NA	NA	10	NA	10	0	5
Honest Tea, Honest Kids, Berry Berry Good Lemonade 8 fl oz serving	45	0	NA	NA	11	NA	11	0	5
Honest Tea, Honest Kids, Goodness Grapeness 1 - 6.75 oz pouch	40	0	NA	NA	10	NA	10	0	5
Honest Tea, Honest Kids, Just Black Tea 8 fl oz serving	0	0	NA	NA	0	NA	0	0	5
Honest Tea, Honest Kids, Just Green Tea 8 fl oz serving	0	0	NA	NA	0	NA	0	0	5
Honest Tea, Honest Kids, Super Fruit Punch 1 - 6.75 oz pouch	40	0	NA	NA	10	NA	10	0	5
Honest Tea, Honest Kids, Super Fruit Punch 8 fl oz serving	45	0	NA	NA	11	NA	11	0	5
Honest Tea, Honest Kids, Tropical Tango Punch 1 - 6.75 oz pouch	40	0	NA	NA	10	NA	10	0	5
Honest Tea, Honest Zero Classic Lemonade 8 fl oz serving, 2 per bottle	0	0	NA	NA	0	NA	0	0	5
Honest Tea, Honest Zero Passion Fruit Green Tea 1 container	0	0	NA	NA	0	NA	0	0	10

Food Serving size	Cal.	(g) Total Fat	(g) Sat. Fat	(mg) Chol.	(g) Carb.	(g) Fiber	(g) Sug.	(g) Prot.	(mg) Sod.
Honest Tea, Honey Green Tea 1 - 16.9 oz container	70	0	NA	NA	18	NA	18	0	10
Honest Tea, Jasmine Green Energy 8 fl oz serving, 2 per bottle	17	0	NA	NA	5	NA	5	0	5
Honest Tea, Just Black Tea 8 fl oz serving, 2 per bottle	0	0	NA	NA	0	NA	0	0	5
Honest Tea, Just Green Tea 8 fl oz serving, 2 per bottle	0	0	NA	NA	0	NA	0	0	5
Honest Tea, Lemon Tea 1 - 16.9 oz container	80	0	NA	NA	21	NA	20	0	5
Honest Tea, Lori's Lemon 8 fl oz serving, 2 per bottle	30	0	NA	NA	8	NA	8	0	5
Honest Tea, Mango Acai White Tea 8 fl oz serving, 2 per bottle	35	0	NA	NA	9	NA	9	0	5
Honest Tea, Moroccan Mint Tea 8 fl oz serving, 2 per bottle	17	0	NA	NA	5	NA	5	0	5
Honest Tea, Peach Oo-la-long 8 fl oz serving, 2 per bottle	30	0	NA	NA	8	NA	8	0	5
Honest Tea, Peach White Tea 1 - 16.9 oz container	80	0	NA	NA	20	NA	20	0	10
Honest Tea, Pomegranate Red Tea with Goji Berry 8 fl oz serving, 2 per bottle	35	0	NA	NA	9	NA	9	0	5
Honest Tea, Raspberry Fields 16 fl oz, 1 container	70	0	NA	NA	18	NA	0	0	10
Nestlé, Mountain Blend Instant Coffee 1 tsp	5	0	NA	NA	1	NA	0	0	5
Pacific Natural Foods, Organic Black Tea Sweetened 1 serving	60	0	0	0	15	0	15	0	NA
Pacific Natural Foods, Organic Green Iced Tea Unsweetened 1 cup	0	0	0	0	0	0	0	0	10
Pacific Natural Foods, Organic Iced Tea, Lemon 1 serving	70	0	0	0	17	0	16	0	10
Pacific Natural Foods, Organic Iced Tea, Peach 1 serving	70	0	0	0	17	0	17	0	10

Food Serving size	Cal.	(g) Total Fat	(g) Sat. Fat	(mg) Chol.	(g) Carb.	(g) Fiber	(g) Sug.	(g) Prot.	(mg) Sod.
Pacific Natural Foods, Organic Iced Tea, Raspberry 8 fl oz	70	0	0	0	18	0	17	0	10
Pacific Natural Foods, Organic Simply Coffee — Latte 8 oz	110	3	2	10	17	0	17	4	190
Pacific Natural Foods, Organic Simply Coffee — Mocha 1 cup	130	3	2	10	23	0	22	4	200
Pacific Natural Foods, Organic Simply Coffee — Vanilla Latte 8 oz	120	2	2	10	20	0	19	4	190
Pacific Natural Foods, Organic Simply Mate — Citrus Lychee Yerba Mate 8 oz	35	0	0	0	9	0	8	1	35
Pacific Natural Foods, Organic Simply Mate — Lemon Ginger Yerba Mate 1 serving	40	0	0	0	NA	NA	8	1	35
Pacific Natural Foods, Organic Simply Mate — Peach Passion Yerba Mate 1 serving	40	0	0	0	8	0	8	0	35
Pacific Natural Foods, Organic Simply Mate — Traditional Yerba Mate 1 serving	30	0	0	0	7	0	7	0	35
Pacific Natural Foods, Organic Simply Tea — Kiwi Mango Green Tea 1 serving	35	0	0	0	8	0	8	0	20
Pacific Natural Foods, Organic Simply Tea — Peach Green Tea 1 cup	35	0	0	0	8	0	8	0	20
Pacific Natural Foods, Organic Simply Tea — Tangerine Green Tea 1 serving	35	0	0	0	8	0	8	0	20
Pacific Natural Foods, Organic Simply Tea — Wild Berry Green Tea 1 serving	35	0	0	0	8	0	8	0	20
Snapple, Diet Green Tea 16 fl oz	0	0	0	NA	0	NA	NA	0	10
Snapple, Diet Half 'n Half Lemonade / Iced Tea 16 fl oz	10	0	0	NA	1	NA	NA	0	15
Snapple, Diet Lemon Tea 16 fl oz	10	0	0	NA	0	NA	NA	0	15
Snapple, Diet Peach Tea 16 fl oz	10	0	0	NA	0	NA	NA	0	15
Snapple, Diet Raspberry Tea 16 fl oz	5	0	0	NA	1	NA	NA	0	15

Food Serving size	Cal.	(g) Total Fat	(g) Sat. Fat	(mg) Chol.	(g) Carb.	(g) Fiber	(g) Sug.	(g) Prot.	(mg) Sod.
Snapple, Diet Trop-A-Rocka Tea 16 fl oz	10	0	0	NA	0	NA	NA	0	20
Snapple, Green Tea 16 fl oz	120	0	0	NA	31	NA	30	0	10
Snapple, Half 'n Half Lemonade / Iced Tea 16 fl oz	210	0	0	NA	51	NA	50	0	10
Snapple, Lemon Iced Tea 16 fl oz	160	0	0	NA	42	NA	41	0	120
Snapple, Lemon Tea 16 fl oz	150	0	0	NA	37	NA	36	0	10
Snapple, Lightly Sweetened Cherry Pomegranate Tea 16 fl oz	80	0	0	NA	19	NA	18	0	10
Snapple, Lightly Sweetened Peach Passionfruit Tea 16 fl oz	80	0	0	NA	19	NA	18	0	10
Snapple, Peach Green Tea 16 fl oz	160	0	0	NA	42	NA	41	0	120
Snapple, Peach Tea 16 fl oz	160	0	0	NA	40	NA	39	0	10
Snapple, Raspberry Tea 16 fl oz	150	0	0	NA	37	NA	36	0	10
Snapple, Refreshing Green Tea 16 fl oz	130	0	0	NA	35	NA	34	0	120
Snapple, Southern Sweet Tea 16 fl oz	170	0	0	NA	46	NA	46	0	120
Snapple, Sweet Tea 16 fl oz	190	0	0	NA	46	NA	46	0	10

Energy & Sports Drinks

Amazing Grass, Chocolate Green SuperFood 1 scoop (8g)	30	1	NA	0	4	2	0	2	8
AriZona Energy Drinks with Tea, Caution — Extreme Performance Energy Drink 8 fl oz	120	0	0	0	30	0	29	0	25
AriZona Energy Drinks with Tea, Caution — Low Carb Performance Energy Drink 8 fl oz	10	0	0	0	3	0	3	0	10

Food Serving size	Cal.	(g) Total Fat	(g) Sat. Fat	(mg) Chol.	(g) Carb.	(g) Fiber	(g) Sug.	(g) Prot.	(mg) Sod.
AriZona Energy Drinks with Tea, Diet Green Tea Energy Drink									
8 fl oz	10	0	0	0	3	0	3	0	10
AriZona Energy Drinks with Tea, Green Tea Energy Drink									
8 fl oz	100	0	0	0	16	0	25	0	10
AriZona Energy Drinks with Tea, Life Pomegranate Green Tea Energy Drink									
8 fl oz	70	0	0	0	18	0	18	0	10
Boost, Calorie Smart, Rich Chocolate									
1 bottle (237ml)	190	7	1	10	16	3	4	16	220
Boost, Calorie Smart, Very Vanilla									
1 bottle (237ml)	190	7	1	10	16	3	4	16	220
Boost, Glucose Control, Rich Chocolate									
1 bottle (8 fl oz)	190	7	1	10	16	3	4	16	180
Boost, Glucose Control, Very Vanilla									
1 bottle (8 fl oz)	190	7	1	10	16	3	4	16	180
Boost, High Protein Drink, Creamy Strawberry									
1 bottle (237ml)	240	6	1	10	33	0	18	15	200
Boost, High Protein Drink, Rich Chocolate									
1 bottle (237ml)	240	6	1	10	33	0	27	15	200
Boost, High Protein Drink, Very Vanilla									
1 bottle (237ml)	240	6	1	10	33	0	23	15	200
Boost, Original, Creamy Strawberry									
1 bottle (237ml)	240	4	1	10	41	0	23	10	150
Boost, Original, Rich Chocolate									
1 bottle (237ml)	240	4	1	10	41	0	28	10	150
Boost, Original, Very Vanilla									
1 bottle (237ml)	240	4	1	10	41	0	25	10	150
Boost Plus, Creamy Strawberry									
1 bottle (237ml)	360	14	2	10	45	3	20	14	200
Boost Plus, Rich Chocolate									
1 bottle (237ml)	360	14	2	10	45	3	24	14	200
Boost Plus, Very Vanilla									
1 bottle (237ml)	360	14	2	10	45	3	22	14	200
Ensure Clear, Blueberry Pomegranate									
8 fl oz (1 bottle)	180	0	0	5	35	0	18	9	50

Food Serving size	Cal.	(g) Total Fat	(g) Sat. Fat	(mg) Chol.	(g) Carb.	(g) Fiber	(g) Sug.	(g) Prot.	(mg) Sod.
Ensure Clear, Peach 8 fl oz (1 bottle)	180	0	0	5	35	0	18	9	50
Ensure Clinical Strength, Creamy Milk Chocolate 8 fl oz (1 bottle)	350	11	1	5	52	3	22	13	240
Ensure Clinical Strength, Homemade Vanilla 8 fl oz (1 bottle)	350	11	1	5	51	3	20	13	240
Ensure Clinical Strength, Strawberries & Cream 8 fl oz (1 bottle)	350	11	1	5	51	3	20	13	240
Ensure High Protein, Creamy Milk Chocolate 8 fl oz (1 bottle)	210	2.5	0.5	20	23	3	5	25	280
Ensure High Protein, Homemade Vanilla 8 fl oz (1 bottle)	210	2.5	0.5	20	23	3	5	25	240
Ensure Muscle Health, Banana Cream 8 fl oz (1 bottle)	250	8	1	5	32	0	23	13	240
Ensure Muscle Health, Milk Chocolate 8 fl oz (1 bottle)	250	8	1	5	32	<1	22	13	240
Ensure Muscle Health, Strawberry 8 fl oz (1 bottle)	250	8	1	5	32	0	23	13	240
Ensure Muscle Health, Vanilla 8 fl oz (1 bottle)	250	8	1	5	32	0	23	13	240
Ensure Nutrition Shake, Butter Pecan 8 fl oz (1 bottle)	250	6	1	5	40	0	23	9	200
Ensure Nutrition Shake, Coffee Latte 8 fl oz (1 bottle)	250	6	1	5	40	0	23	9	200
Ensure Nutrition Shake, Milk Chocolate 8 fl oz (1 bottle)	250	6	1	5	40	1	22	9	190
Ensure Nutrition Shake, Rich Dark Chocolate 8 fl oz (1 bottle)	250	6	1	<5	41	1	18	9	200
Ensure Nutrition Shake, Strawberry 8 fl oz (1 bottle)	250	6	1	5	40	0	23	9	200
Ensure Nutrition Shake, Vanilla 8 fl oz (1 bottle)	250	6	1	5	40	0	23	9	200
Ensure Plus, Butter Pecan 8 fl oz (1 bottle)	350	11	1	10	51	3	20	13	220

Food Serving size	Cal.	(g) Total Fat	(g) Sat. Fat	(mg) Chol.	(g) Carb.	(g) Fiber	(g) Sug.	(g) Prot.	(mg) Sod.
Ensure Plus, Dark Chocolate 8 fl oz (1 bottle)	350	11	1.5	10	49	1	18	13	230
Ensure Plus, Milk Chocolate 8 fl oz (1 bottle)	350	11	1	10	52	3	22	13	220
Ensure Plus, Strawberry 8 fl oz (1 bottle)	350	11	1	10	51	3	20	13	220
Ensure Plus, Vanilla 8 fl oz (1 bottle)	350	11	1	10	51	3	20	13	220
Hansen's PRE, Probiotics - Organic, Acai Cherry 8 fl oz	50	0	0	NA	14	2	13	NA	5
Hansen's PRE, Probiotics - Organic, Pomegranate Blueberry 8 fl oz	60	0	0	NA	14	2	11	NA	5
Hansen's PRE, Probiotics - Organic, Tropical Coconut Water 8 fl oz	40	0	0	NA	10	2	9	NA	35
Hansen's PRE, Probiotics - Zero, Cranberry Raspberry 8 fl oz	0	0	0	NA	1	2	0	NA	15
Hansen's PRE, Probiotics - Zero, Peach Mango 8 fl oz	0	0	0	NA	1	2	0	NA	15
Hansen's PRE, Probiotics - Zero, Pomegranate Blueberry 8 fl oz	0	0	0	NA	1	2	0	NA	15
Hansen's PRE, Probiotics - Zero, Pomegranate Yumberry 8 fl oz	0	0	0	NA	1	2	0	NA	15
Svelte, CalNaturale Svelte, Sustained Energy Protein Drink, Cappuccino 15.9 fl oz	260	10	1.5	0	40	8	9	16	190
Svelte, CalNaturale Svelte, Sustained Energy Protein Drink, Chocolate 15.9 fl oz	260	10	2	0	40	8	9	16	190
Svelte, CalNaturale Svelte, Sustained Energy Protein Drink, French Vanilla 15.9 fl oz	260	10	1.5	0	40	8	9	16	190
Svelte, CalNaturale Svelte, Sustained Energy Protein Drink, Spiced Chai 15.9 fl oz	260	10	1.5	0	40	8	9	16	190
Vitacoco, 100% Pure Coconut Water 8.5 fl oz	45	0	0	0	11	0	11	0	30
Vitacoco, Pure Coconut Water with Acai & Pomegranate 8.5 fl oz	60	0	0	0	16	1	15	0	45

Food Serving size	Cal.	(g) Total Fat	(g) Sat. Fat	(mg) Chol.	(g) Carb.	(g) Fiber	(g) Sug.	(g) Prot.	(mg) Sod.
Vitacoco, Pure Coconut Water with Orange									
8.5 fl oz	60	0	0	0	16	NA	16	0	30
Vitacoco, Pure Coconut Water with Peach & Mango									
8.5 fl oz	60	0	0	0	15	NA	15	0	45
Vitacoco, Pure Coconut Water with Pineapple									
8.5 fl oz	60	0	0	0	15	NA	15	0	40
Vitacoco, Pure Coconut Water with Tropical Fruit									
8.5 fl oz	55	0	0	0	13	NA	13	0	24

Flavored Drinks & Drink Mixes

Food Serving size	Cal.	Total Fat	Sat. Fat	Chol.	Carb.	Fiber	Sug.	Prot.	Sod.
AriZona Decaf Tea + 50% Juice, Apple Green Tea									
8 fl oz	80	0	0	0	20	0	19	0	20
AriZona Decaf Tea + 50% Juice, Pomegranate Green Tea									
8 fl oz	80	0	0	0	20	0	19	0	10
AriZona Decaf Tea + 50% Juice, White Grape Green Tea									
8 fl oz	80	0	0	0	21	0	19	0	10
AriZona Drink Mixes, Arnold Palmer Lite Green Tea									
8 fl oz	50	0	0	0	14	0	13	0	25
AriZona Drink Mixes, Arnold Palmer Lite Iced Tea									
8 fl oz	50	0	0	0	14	0	13	0	25
AriZona Drink Mixes, Lite Green Tea Lemonade									
8 fl oz	50	0	0	0	14	0	13	0	25
AriZona Fruit Flavored Juice Drinks, Fruit Punch									
8 fl oz	100	0	0	0	26	0	25	0	25
AriZona Fruit Flavored Juice Drinks, Grapeade									
8 fl oz	100	0	0	0	27	0	26	0	10
AriZona Fruit Flavored Juice Drinks, Kiwi Strawberry									
8 fl oz	120	0	0	0	29	0	28	0	10
AriZona Fruit Flavored Juice Drinks, Lemonade									
8 fl oz	110	0	0	0	27	0	26	0	10
Hansen's Hubert's Lemonade Tea, Half & Half, Peach									
8 fl oz	70	0	0	NA	16	NA	15	0	0
Hansen's Hubert's Lemonade Tea, Half & Half, Raspberry									
8 fl oz	45	0	0	NA	12	NA	11	0	0

Food Serving size	Cal.	(g) Total Fat	(g) Sat. Fat	(mg) Chol.	(g) Carb.	(g) Fiber	(g) Sug.	(g) Prot.	(mg) Sod.
Newman's Own, Diet Virgin Lemonade 8 fl oz	20	0	NA	NA	6	NA	4	0	5
Newman's Own, Gorilla Grape Juice Cocktail 8 fl oz	140	0	0	0	34	0	33	0	140
Newman's Own, Orange Mango Tango Juice Cocktail 8 fl oz	130	0	0	0	33	0	32	0	5
Newman's Own, Organic Lemonade 1 serving	110	0	NA	NA	27	NA	27	0	40
Newman's Own, Pink Virgin Lemonade 8 fl oz	110	0	0	0	27	0	27	0	40
Newman's Own, Pomegranate Lemonade 8 fl oz	110	0	0	NA	28	NA	26	0	15
Newman's Own, Virgin Lemon-Aided Iced Tea 8 fl oz	110	0	0	0	27	0	27	0	40
Newman's Own, Virgin Limeade 8 fl oz	140	0	0	0	34	0	34	0	35
Snapple, 100% Juiced Fruit Punch 11.5 fl oz	170	0	0	NA	42	NA	40	0	30
Snapple, 100% Juiced Grape 11.5 fl oz	170	0	0	NA	42	NA	41	0	30
Snapple, 100% Juiced Green Apple 11.5 fl oz	170	0	0	NA	41	NA	39	0	30
Snapple, Apple 16 fl oz	200	0	0	NA	48	NA	47	0	10
Snapple, Diet Cranberry Raspberry 16 fl oz	20	0	0	NA	4	NA	3	0	10
Snapple, Diet Noni Berry 16 fl oz	25	0	0	NA	3	NA	3	0	15
Snapple, Fruit Punch 16 fl oz	200	0	0	NA	48	NA	47	0	10
Snapple, Go Bananas 16 fl oz	220	0	0	NA	56	NA	55	0	15
Snapple, Grape Berry Punch 16 fl oz	210	0	0	NA	55	NA	54	0	120

Food Serving size	Cal.	(g) Total Fat	(g) Sat. Fat	(mg) Chol.	(g) Carb.	(g) Fiber	(g) Sug.	(g) Prot.	(mg) Sod.
Snapple, Grapeade 16 fl oz	190	0	0	NA	46	NA	46	0	10
Snapple, Kiwi Strawberry 16 fl oz	190	0	0	NA	46	NA	45	0	15
Snapple, Lemonade 16 fl oz	190	0	0	NA	47	NA	46	0	85
Snapple, Mango Madness 16 fl oz	190	0	0	NA	46	NA	44	0	20
Snapple, Mango Punch 16 fl oz	190	0	0	NA	49	NA	48	0	120
Snapple, Orangeade 16 fl oz	190	0	0	NA	46	NA	46	0	10
Snapple, Peach Mangosteen 16 fl oz	180	0	0	NA	41	NA	40	0	25
Snapple, Pink Lemonade 16 fl oz	210	0	0	NA	50	NA	49	0	85
Snapple, Raspberry Peach 16 fl oz	220	0	0	NA	53	NA	48	0	15
Snapple, Very Cherry Punch 16 fl oz	210	0	0	NA	55	NA	54	0	120
Snapple, Watermelon Punch 16 fl oz	190	0	0	NA	49	NA	48	0	120

Mixed Dishes

Why Eat Mixed Dishes?

Mixed dishes are a mine field for gluten-free eating. Although they are convenient and enjoyable to eat, they don't fit neatly into one food group and often contain ingredients that are not gluten-free. For example, a cheese pizza counts in several groups—the crust, which is probably made from wheat and contains gluten, is in the grains group, the tomato sauce in the vegetable group, and the cheese in the milk group. So use particular caution when choosing gluten-free frozen and shelf-stable partially-prepared foods.

Daily Goal

Compare each mixed food selection to ChooseMyPlate.

A prepared entrée should have:

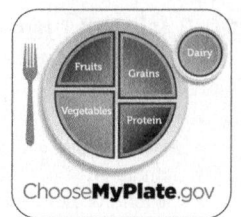

    300 to 500 calories
    10g or more protein
    30% or less fat calories (10 to 28 grams total fat)
    10% or less saturated fat (1 to 2 grams)
    480 mg or less sodium

Gluten-Free Shopping Tips

- Most prepared entrees don't include a serving of dairy. If the calcium level is below 10% of the Daily Value, plan to add milk
- Fresh fruits and vegetables are usually lacking in prepared meals—plan a side salad or vegetable
- Purchase fruit for a sweet ending to the meal
- Choose mixed dishes with sauces in separate packets so that you can decide how much to use
- Look for low-sodium soups

Gluten-Free Shopping List Essentials

Gluten-free, healthy frozen dinners and prepackaged entrees
Gluten-free low-sodium soups
Gluten-free whole grain-based entrees—brown rice, quinoa, gluten-free pasta
Vegetables
Fruits

Approved Soups and Those to Avoid on a Gluten-Free Diet

Gluten-Free

- Homemade broth
- Gluten-free bouillon cubes
- Cream soups and stocks made with approved ingredients

May Contain Gluten

- Canned soups and dried soup mixes made with ingredients to avoid
- Soup bases and bouillon cubes containing hydrolyzed wheat protein

Approved Sauces/Condiments and Those to Avoid on a Gluten-Free Diet

Gluten-Free

- Ketchup
- Plain mustard, without seasonings
- Tomato paste
- Gluten-free soy sauce and teriyaki sauce
- Gravies and sauces made with approved ingredients

May Contain Gluten

- Soy and teriyaki sauce made with wheat
- Malt vinegar
- Sauces and gravies made with wheat flour, hydrolyzed wheat protein, or other ingredients to avoid
- Worcestershire sauce made with ingredients to avoid

Approved Frozen Dinners/Meals/Pizza and Those to Avoid on a Gluten-Free Diet

Gluten-Free

Those certified gluten-free by the manufacturer

May Contain Gluten

Those not certified gluten-free by the manufacturer

Approved Meal Replacement Bars and Those to Avoid on a Gluten-Free Diet

Gluten-Free

Those certified gluten-free by the manufacturer

May Contain Gluten

Those not certified gluten-free by the manufacturer

Caution

All mixed dishes have a high probability of containing gluten. Make sure that they are certified gluten-free by the manufacturer. Additionally, some mixed foods can contain a lot of fat or sugar, which adds empty calories. Mixed dishes are also usually high in sodium. Look for those that claim "Healthy." These have limits on fat, saturated fat, and sodium, and must contain a good source of at least one positive nutrient. See the guidelines for "Healthy" on page xv.

Food Serving size	Cal.	(g) Total Fat	(g) Sat. Fat	(mg) Chol.	(g) Carb.	(g) Fiber	(g) Sug.	(g) Prot.	(mg) Sod.
Condiments									
505 Southwestern, Chipotle Honey Roasted Green Chile									
1 package	17	0	NA	NA	0	1	2	1	20
Annie's, Organic Dijon Mustard									
1 tsp	5	0	NA	NA	1	NA	NA	0	120
Annie's, Organic Honey Mustard									
1 tsp	10	0	NA	NA	2	NA	2	0	45
Annie's, Organic Horseradish Mustard									
1 tsp	5	0	0	NA	1	NA	NA	0	60
Annie's, Organic Ketchup									
1 tbsp	15	0	0	NA	5	NA	4	0	170
Annie's, Organic Yellow Mustard									
1 tsp	5	0	NA	NA	1	NA	NA	0	50
Boar's Head, Delicatessen Style Mustard									
1 tsp	0	0	0	0	0	0	0	0	40
Boar's Head, Honey Mustard									
1 tsp	10	0	0	0	2	0	1	0	25
Boar's Head, Horseradish									
1 tsp	0	0	0	0	0	0	0	0	30
Boar's Head, Pepperhouse Gourmaise									
1 tbsp	80	8	1.5	5	2	0	0	0	170
Boar's Head, Pub Style Horseradish Sauce									
1 tsp	15	1.5	0	5	1	0	1	0	15
Eden Foods, Brown Mustard, Organic Jar									
1 tsp	0	0	0	0	<1	NA	0	0	80
Eden Foods, Brown Mustard, Organic, Squeeze Bottle									
1 tsp	0	0	0	0	1	0	0	0	80
Eden Foods, Brown Rice Vinegar, Organic, Imported									
1 tbsp	2	0	NA	NA	0	NA	0	0	0
Eden Foods, Mirin (rice cooking wine)									
1 tbsp	25	0	0	0	7	0	4	0	130
Eden Foods, Red Wine Vinegar									
1 tbsp	0	0	NA	NA	0	NA	0	0	0

Food Serving size	Cal.	(g) Total Fat	(g) Sat. Fat	(mg) Chol.	(g) Carb.	(g) Fiber	(g) Sug.	(g) Prot.	(mg) Sod.
Eden Foods, Red Wine Vinegar, Raw, Unpasteurized									
1 tbsp	0	0	NA	NA	0	NA	0	0	0
Eden Foods, Shoyu Soy Sauce (Imported)									
1 tbsp	15	0	0	0	2	0	0	2	1010
Eden Foods, Shoyu Soy Sauce, Organic (Imported)									
1 tbsp	15	0	0	0	2	0	0	2	1040
Eden Foods, Tamari Soy Sauce, Brewed in U.S., Organic									
1 tbsp	15	0	0	0	2	0	0	2	860
Eden Foods, Tamari Soy Sauce, Organic (Imported)									
1 tbsp	10	0	0	0	2	0	0	2	990
Eden Foods, Tekka (Miso Condiment)									
1 tsp	5	0	0	0	<1	0	0	<1	70
Eden Foods, Ume Plum Vinegar, Raw, Unpasteurized									
1 tsp	2	0	0	0	0	NA	0	0	1050
Eden Foods, Umeboshi Paste									
1 tsp	5	0	0	0	0	0	0	0	340
Eden Foods, Yellow Mustard, Organic, Jar									
1 tsp	0	0	NA	0	0	NA	0	0	80
Eden Foods, Yellow Mustard, Organic, Squeeze Bottle									
1 tsp	0	0	0	0	0	0	0	0	80
Little Soya, Gluten Free Soy Sauce									
15ml	10	0	0	NA	2	NA	NA	<1	270
Lucini, 10-Year Gran Riserva Balsamico Vinegar									
1 tbsp	20	0	NA	NA	4	NA	4	0	0
Lucini, Estate Select Balsamic Vinegar									
1 tbsp	20	0	0	NA	4	NA	4	0	0
Lucini, Pinot Grigio Italian Wine Vinegar									
1 tbsp	0	0	0	NA	0	NA	NA	0	2
Lucini, Pinot Noir Italian Wine Vinegar									
1 tbsp	<1	0	0	NA	0	NA	NA	0	2
Lucini, Savory Fig Balsamico Artisan Vinegar									
1 tbsp	30	0	0	NA	7	NA	7	0	3
Mezzetta, Cream Style Horseradish									
1 tsp	20	2	0	1	1	0	0	0	25

Food Serving size	Cal.	(g) Total Fat	(g) Sat. Fat	(mg) Chol.	(g) Carb.	(g) Fiber	(g) Sug.	(g) Prot.	(mg) Sod.
Mezzetta, Crushed Garlic 2 tsp	20	0	0	0	4	NA	NA	NA	0
Pace, Picante Sauce, Hot 2 tbsp	10	0	NA	0	3	1	2	0	250
Pace, Picante Sauce, Medium 2 tbsp	10	0	NA	0	3	1	2	0	250
Pace, Picante Sauce, Mild 2 tbsp	10	0	NA	0	3	1	2	0	250
Premier Japan, Organic Wheat-Free Hoisin Sauce 1 tsp	15	0	0	0	3	0	2	0	160
Premier Japan, Organic Wheat-Free Teriyaki Sauce 1 tsp	15	0	0	0	3	0	2	0	250
San-J, Organic Gluten Free Tamari Travel Packs 2 packs	10	0	0	0	<1	0	0	2	940
San-J, Organic Tamari Gluten Free Reduced Sodium Soy Sauce 1 tbsp	15	0	0	0	1	0	0	2	700
San-J, Organic Tamari Gluten Free Soy Sauce 1 tbsp	10	0	0	0	<1	0	0	2	940
San-J, Tamari Gluten Free Reduced Sodium Soy Sauce (White Label) 1 tbsp	15	0	0	0	1	0	0	2	710
San-J, Tamari Gluten Free Soy Sauce (Black Label) 1 tbsp	10	0	0	0	1	0	0	2	980
Thai Kitchen, Green Curry Paste 1 tbsp	15	0	0	0	3	0	1	0	500
Thai Kitchen, Red Curry Paste 1 tbsp	15	1	0	0	3	0	1	0	390
Thai Kitchen, Roasted Red Chili Paste 1 tbsp	50	3	0	5	4	0	2	2	130
The Wizard's, Organic Wheat-Free Vegan Worcestershire 1 tsp	5	0	0	0	1	0	1	0	130
Thumann's, Creamy Horseradish Sauce 1 tsp	15	1.5	0	5	1	0	0	0	15
Thumann's, Deli Dressing 1 tsp	100	11	1	0	0	NA	NA	0	50

Food Serving size	Cal.	(g) Total Fat	(g) Sat. Fat	(mg) Chol.	(g) Carb.	(g) Fiber	(g) Sug.	(g) Prot.	(mg) Sod.
Thumann's, Dijon Wasabi 1 tsp	18	1	0	2.5	2	NA	1	0	55
Thumann's, Dill Pickles 1 tsp	3.75	0	0	0	0	0	0	0	63
Thumann's, Dusseldorf Mustard 1 tsp	3.75	0	0	0	0	0	0	0	63
Thumann's, Gourmet Onions in Sauce 1 tsp	10	0	0	0	3	0	2	0	105
Thumann's, Half Sour Pickles 1 oz	2.01	0	0	0	<1	0	1	<1	330
Thumann's, Horseradish Mustard 1 tsp	3.75	0	0	0	0	0	0	0	63
Thumann's, Real Honey Mustard 1 tsp	20	1.5	0	2	1.5	NA	1	0	28

Entrées / Meal Products

Food Serving size	Cal.	(g) Total Fat	(g) Sat. Fat	(mg) Chol.	(g) Carb.	(g) Fiber	(g) Sug.	(g) Prot.	(mg) Sod.
Against the Grain, Gourmet Three-Cheese Pizza 2 slices	410	23	7	96	34	<1	2	18	387
Amy's, Asian Noodle Stir-Fry 10 oz	300	7	1	0	50	5	16	9	630
Amy's, Baked Ziti Bowl 9.5 oz	390	12	2	0	62	6	8	9	590
Amy's, Black Bean Enchilada Whole Meal 10 oz	330	8	1	0	53	9	4	9	740
Amy's, Black Bean Tamale Verde 10.3 oz	330	10	1	0	55	12	6	7	780
Amy's, Black Bean Vegetable Enchilada 4.75 oz	160	6	0.5	0	22	4	2	5	390
Amy's, Broccoli & Cheddar Bake 9.5 oz	430	20	12	55	44	2	5	16	640
Amy's, Brown Rice & Vegetables Bowl 10 oz	260	9	1	0	36	5	7	9	550
Amy's, Brown Rice, Black-Eyed Peas & Veggies Bowl 9 oz	290	11	1.5	0	38	8	5	11	580

Food Serving size	Cal.	(g) Total Fat	(g) Sat. Fat	(mg) Chol.	(g) Carb.	(g) Fiber	(g) Sug.	(g) Prot.	(mg) Sod.
Amy's, Cheese Enchilada 4.5 oz	240	14	6	30	18	2	2	9	440
Amy's, Cheese Enchilada Whole Meal 9 oz	370	15	7	30	41	9	6	17	680
Amy's, Cheese Tamale Verde 10.3 oz	400	16	5	20	51	7	8	13	780
Amy's, Dairy Free, Rice Macaroni & Cheese 1 container	520	22	5	0	72	3	0	8	740
Amy's, Enchilada Verde Whole Meal 10 oz	400	13	6	30	54	8	5	17	780
Amy's, Garden Vegetable Lasagna 10.3 oz	290	9	4	20	41	5	7	11	720
Amy's, Gluten Free Cheddar Burrito 1 burrito	260	8	2	5	37	5	3	9	430
Amy's, Gluten Free Indian Aloo Mattar Wrap 5.5 oz	270	9	0.5	0	32	6	5	9	590
Amy's, Gluten Free Non Dairy Burrito 1 burrito	240	6	0.5	0	38	5	3	7	430
Amy's, Gluten Free Teriyaki Wrap 5.5 oz	250	6	0.5	0	38	3	7	9	540
Amy's, Gluten Free Tofu Scramble Breakfast Wrap 5.5 oz	300	13	1.5	0	35	3	4	11	460
Amy's, Gluten Free/Dairy Free Vegetable Lasagna 9 oz	300	14	3	0	39	4	7	9	680
Amy's, Indian Mattar Paneer 10 oz	370	11	4	20	54	6	8	13	780
Amy's, Indian Mattar Tofu 9.5 oz	280	8	1	0	40	5	5	12	680
Amy's, Indian Palak Paneer 10 oz	300	11	3.5	15	38	6	5	12	680
Amy's, Indian Paneer Tikka 9.5 oz	370	20	9	30	41	4	7	11	490
Amy's, Indian Vegetable Korma 9.5 oz	310	12	3.5	0	41	7	7	9	680

Food Serving size	Cal.	(g) Total Fat	(g) Sat. Fat	(mg) Chol.	(g) Carb.	(g) Fiber	(g) Sug.	(g) Prot.	(mg) Sod.
Amy's, Kids Baked Ziti Meal									
8 oz	360	12	1.5	0	57	4	15	7	460
Amy's, Kids Rice Mac n' Cheese Meal									
8 oz	390	13	7	40	58	3	11	12	510
Amy's, Light & Lean Black Bean & Cheese Enchilada									
1 enchilada	240	4.5	2	5	44	4	5	8	480
Amy's, Light & Lean Roasted Polenta									
8 oz	140	4	1.5	10	20	4	7	6	540
Amy's, Light & Lean Soft Taco Fiesta									
1 taco	220	4.5	1.5	5	40	5	6	7	560
Amy's, Light & Lean Sweet & Sour Bowl									
8 oz	250	3	0	0	46	4	10	10	610
Amy's, Light in Sodium, Black Bean Vegetable Enchilada									
4.75 oz	160	6	0.5	0	22	4	2	5	190
Amy's, Light in Sodium, Brown Rice & Vegetables Bowl									
10 oz	260	9	1	0	36	5	7	9	270
Amy's, Light in Sodium, Indian Mattar Paneer									
10 oz	370	11	4	20	54	6	8	13	390
Amy's, Light in Sodium, Mexican Casserole Bowl									
9.5 oz	370	16	5	20	48	7	4	12	390
Amy's, Light in Sodium, Shepherd's Pie									
8 oz	160	4	0	0	27	5	5	5	290
Amy's, Mexican Casserole Bowl									
9.5 oz	380	16	5	20	48	8	4	12	780
Amy's, Mexican Tamale Pie									
8 oz	150	3	0	0	27	4	2	5	590
Amy's, Mexican Tofu Scramble									
9 oz	400	18	6	15	40	6	4	20	680
Amy's, Mushroom Risotto Bowl									
269g, 1 container	240	4	8	20	35	2	2	7	590
Amy's, Rice Crust Cheese Pizza									
4 oz	320	16	4	10	34	2	5	10	590
Amy's, Rice Crust Spinach Pizza									
4.66 oz	350	19	2	0	34	4	5	8	580

Food Serving size	Cal.	(g) Total Fat	(g) Sat. Fat	(mg) Chol.	(g) Carb.	(g) Fiber	(g) Sug.	(g) Prot.	(mg) Sod.
Amy's, Rice Mac & Cheese 9 oz	400	16	10	50	47	1	6	16	640
Amy's, Roasted Vegetable Tamale 10.3 oz	280	7	0.5	0	44	10	4	9	740
Amy's, Santa Fe Enchilada Bowl 10 oz	350	11	2	5	47	9	5	16	780
Amy's, Shepherd's Pie 8 oz	160	4	0	0	27	5	5	5	590
Amy's, Single Serve, Non-Dairy Rice Crust Cheese Pizza 6 oz	460	28	3	0	46	4	7	10	680
Amy's, Single Serve, Rice Crust Margherita Pizza 6.4 oz	490	25	6	20	55	4	8	12	680
Amy's, Single Serve, Rice Crust Roasted Vegetable Pizza 6 oz	430	20	2.5	0	55	5	8	7	680
Amy's, Teriyaki Bowl 9.5 oz	290	4.5	0.5	0	52	6	15	12	780
Amy's, Thai Stir-Fry 9.5 oz	310	11	7	0	45	5	2	8	420
Amy's, Tofu Scramble 9 oz	320	19	3	0	19	4	4	22	580
Amy's, Tortilla Casserole & Black Beans Bowl 9.5 oz	390	18	6	25	41	10	6	17	780
Amy's, Vegetable Parmesan Bowl 255g, 1 container	260	13	7	30	22	6	8	15	680
Annie Chun's, Chicken & Cilantro, Mini Wontons 4 pieces	50	0.5	0	5	9	<1	1	3	160
Annie Chun's, Chicken & Garlic, Mini Wontons 4 pieces	60	0.5	0	5	9	<1	1	3	150
Annie Chun's, Kung Pao Noodle Bowl 1/2 bowl	240	5	0	0	40	1	5	7	630
Annie Chun's, Organic Chicken & Vegetable Potstickers 7 pieces	220	3.5	0.5	25	32	2	3	14	620
Annie Chun's, Organic Chow Mein, Asian Meal Starter 1/3 box	220	1.5	0	0	42	1	6	8	570

Food Serving size	Cal.	(g) Total Fat	(g) Sat. Fat	(mg) Chol.	(g) Carb.	(g) Fiber	(g) Sug.	(g) Prot.	(mg) Sod.
Annie Chun's, Organic Peanut Sesame, Asian Meal Starter									
1/3 box	250	5	0	0	41	2	5	9	360
Annie Chun's, Organic Pork & Vegetable Potstickers									
7 pieces	260	10	3	30	32	2	3	12	600
Annie Chun's, Organic Shiitake & Vegetable Potstickers									
7 pieces	240	3.5	0.5	0	44	3	4	8	640
Annie Chun's, Organic Soy Ginger, Asian Meal Starter									
1/3 box	220	1.5	0	0	41	1	5	8	600
Annie Chun's, Organic Teriyaki, Asian Meal Starter									
1/3 box	220	1.5	0	0	43	1	7	8	590
Annie Chun's, Pad Thai Noodle Bowl									
1/2 bowl	230	4.5	0	0	45	1	8	7	710
Annie Chun's, Pad Thai, Asian Meal Starter									
1/3 box	230	1	0	0	53	0	9	3	780
Annie Chun's, Peanut Sesame Noodle Bowl									
1/2 bowl	280	11	1	0	40	1	5	8	340
Annie Chun's, Pork & Ginger, Mini Wontons									
4 pieces	100	3.5	1	10	14	<1	1	4	230
Annie Chun's, Spicy Vegetable, Mini Wontons									
4 pieces	60	1	0	0	11	<1	1	2	150
Annie Chun's, Sushi Wraps, Sprouted Brown Rice									
1/2 tray	150	0.5	0	0	30	2	0	5	330
Annie Chun's, Sushi Wraps, Sticky White Rice									
1/2 tray	160	0.5	0	0	34	1	<1	4	330
Annie Chun's, Teriyaki Noodle Bowl									
1/2 bowl	200	2.5	0	0	38	1	5	6	440
Annie's, Gluten Free Deluxe Rice Pasta and Cheddar									
3.7 oz	320	4	2	10	63	2	2	8	680
Annie's, Gluten Free Rice Pasta & Cheddar									
2.5 oz	270	4	2	10	51	1	4	6	390
Annie's, Gluten-Free Microwaveable Mac & Cheese									
1 packet	240	4.5	2.5	10	43	1	4	6	540
Annie's, Gluten-Free Rice Shells with Creamy White Cheddar									
3 oz	330	4.5	2.5	10	62	2	4	7	490

Food Serving size	Cal.	(g) Total Fat	(g) Sat. Fat	(mg) Chol.	(g) Carb.	(g) Fiber	(g) Sug.	(g) Prot.	(mg) Sod.
Bold Organic, Deluxe 1/2 pizza	460	24	4.5	10	56	5	12	8	790
Bold Organic, Meat Lovers Pizza 1/2 pizza	450	24	4.5	10	54	5	11	7	790
Bold Organic, Vegan Cheese Pizza 1/2 pizza	380	18	2.5	0	54	5	11	4	580
Bold Organic, Veggie Lovers Pizza 1/2 pizza	390	18	2.5	10	55	5	12	5	580
Conte's, Cheese Ravioli 12 oz, 4 ravioli	260	9	5	100	35	2	1	9	260
Conte's, Cheese Stuffed Shells 12 oz, 2 shells	260	9	5	100	35	2	1	9	260
Conte's, Gnocchi 4 oz	250	3	0	10	53	3	1	3	920
Conte's, Gnocchi with Marinara Sauce, Microwave Meal 12 oz	390	10	2	115	81	4	13	6	760
Conte's, Margherita Pizza with Roasted Garlic and Olive Oil 1 slice	220	9	3.5	35	25	1	4	8	550
Conte's, Mushroom Florentine Pizza 1 slice	230	10	4	40	28	1	3	8	540
Conte's, Pierogies (Potato/Cheese/Onion) 4 pierogies	220	5	2	55	39	2	2	6	330
Conte's, Pierogies (Potato/Onion) 12 oz, 4 pierogies	180	1.5	0	45	39	3	1	3	110
Conte's, Spinach/Cheese Ravioli 12 oz, 4 ravioli	270	8	4.5	100	40	2	1	10	500
Eden Foods, Brown Rice & Chick Peas, Organic 1/2 cup	110	1	0	NA	23	2	0	3	135
Eden Foods, Cajun Rice & Small Red Beans, Organic 1/2 cup	110	1	0	NA	23	3	<1	3	115
Eden Foods, Caribbean Rice & Black Beans, Organic 1/2 cup	120	1	0	NA	23	4	<1	4	100
Eden Foods, Curried Rice & Lentils, Organic 1/2 cup	130	1	0	NA	21	1	<1	4	200

Food Serving size	Cal.	(g) Total Fat	(g) Sat. Fat	(mg) Chol.	(g) Carb.	(g) Fiber	(g) Sug.	(g) Prot.	(mg) Sod.
Eden Foods, Mexican Rice & Black Beans, Organic									
1/2 cup	110	1	0	NA	22	3	1	5	270
Eden Foods, Moroccan Rice & Garbanzo Beans, Organic									
1/2 cup	110	1	0	NA	22	3	<1	4	230
Eden Foods, Spanish Rice & Pinto Beans, Organic									
1/2 cup	120	1	0	NA	22	3	<1	4	260
Edward & Sons, Chreesy Mashed Potatoes, Prepared									
1/2 cup	150	0.5	0	0	18	3	1	4	190
Everybody Eats, Tomato-Mozzarella Pizza									
1/3 pizza	470	30	10	35	38	2	3	14	720
Feel Good Foods, Chicken and Vegetable Egg Rolls									
3 oz (84g)	120	3	0.5	25	14	2	1	8	350
Feel Good Foods, Chicken Dumplings (including sauce)									
4 dumplings (136g)	375	12	2	30	41	2	2	14	590
Feel Good Foods, Pork Dumplings (including sauce)									
4 dumplings (136g)	375	14	3	15	44	2	3	7	590
Feel Good Foods, Shrimp and Vegetable Egg Rolls									
3 oz (84g)	100	1.5	0	45	14	2	1	7	420
Feel Good Foods, Shrimp Dumplings (including sauce)									
4 dumplings (136g)	345	10	1.5	90	39	1	1	14	580
Feel Good Foods, Vegetable Dumplings (including sauce)									
4 dumplings (136g)	335	9	1.5	0	48	2	3	3	430
Feel Good Foods, Vegetable Egg Rolls									
3 oz (84g)	80	2	0	0	14	1	3	2	380
Garden Lites, Frozen, Low Calorie Broccoli Souffle									
7 oz container, 1 souffle	140	1.5	0	0	27	4	5	11	490
Garden Lites, Frozen, Low Calorie Butternut Squash Souffle									
7 oz container, 1 souffle	180	2	0.5	55	35	3	18	8	135
Garden Lites, Frozen, Low Calorie Carrot Raisin Souffle									
7 oz container, 1 souffle	200	0	0	0	42	5	26	9	230
Garden Lites, Frozen, Low Calorie Cauliflower Souffle									
7 oz container, 1 souffle	140	1.5	0	0	27	4	7	9	490
Garden Lites, Frozen, Low Calorie Dishes, Zucchini Marinara									
1 container	110	4	0.5	0	18	3	5	3	460

Food Serving size	Cal.	(g) Total Fat	(g) Sat. Fat	(mg) Chol.	(g) Carb.	(g) Fiber	(g) Sug.	(g) Prot.	(mg) Sod.
Garden Lites, Frozen, Low Calorie Dishes, Zucchini Portabella 1 container	110	4	0.5	0	19	4	3	3	390
Garden Lites, Frozen, Low Calorie Pizza Souffle 7 oz container, 1 souffle	200	4	1.5	5	31	3	6	12	650
Garden Lites, Frozen, Low Calorie Roasted Vegetable Souffle 7 oz container, 1 souffle	140	1.5	0	0	28	4	8	9	490
Garden Lites, Frozen, Low Calorie Southwestern Souffle 7 oz container, 1 souffle	180	2.5	0	0	30	4	4	9	650
Garden Lites, Frozen, Low Calorie Spinach Souffle 7 oz container, 1 souffle	140	1.5	0	0	26	4	6	10	490
Garden Lites, Frozen, Low Calorie Zucchini Souffle 7 oz container, 1 souffle	140	1.5	0	0	30	3	6	9	490
Gluten Free Café, Asian Noodles Entree 1 package	340	10	3	0	53	5	11	8	720
Gluten Free Café, Fettuccini Alfredo Entree 1 package	400	16	7	45	55	2	<1	4	390
Gluten Free Café, Lemon Basil Chicken Entree 1 package	340	11	5	55	42	3	1	18	720
Gluten Free Café, Pasta Primavera Entree 1 package	270	9	4.5	25	42	4	4	4	260
Glutino, Gluten Free BBQ Chicken Pizza 1 pizza	380	12	4	25	55	3	10	16	870
Glutino, Gluten Free Duo Cheese Pizza 1 pizza	310	12	5	25	37	2	4	14	700
Glutino, Gluten Free Duo Cheese Pizza, Multi Pack 1 pizza	420	12	5	25	68	2	<1	10	560
Glutino, Gluten Free Pasta Meals, Macaroni & Cheese 300g	440	15	5	25	64	3	4	14	600
Glutino, Gluten Free Pasta Meals, Penne Alfredo 1-1/4 cup	400	9	5	35	65	4	2	14	870
Glutino, Gluten Free Pepperoni Pizza 1 pizza	360	16	6	30	39	2	4	15	850
Glutino, Gluten Free Spinach & Feta Pizza 1 pizza	300	11	5	25	39	2	2	11	840

Food Serving size	Cal.	(g) Total Fat	(g) Sat. Fat	(mg) Chol.	(g) Carb.	(g) Fiber	(g) Sug.	(g) Prot.	(mg) Sod.
Gopicnic Gluten Free, Ready-to-Eat Meals, Sunbutter + Crackers									
1 box	490	26	4.5	0	63	9	28	12	260
Gopicnic Gluten Free, Ready-to-Eat Meals, Tuna + Crackers									
1 box	320	16	3	10	43	5	23	9	470
Gopicnic Gluten Free, Ready-to-Eat Meals, Turkey Pepperoni + Cheese									
1 box	290	15	6	40	29	2	15	12	890
Gopicnic Gluten Free, Ready-to-Eat Meals, Turkey Stick + Crunch									
1 box	330	12	2.5	15	44	4	27	9	400
Ian's Natural Foods, Allergy Friendly Space Nuggets									
about 5 nuggets	200	10	1	35	13	<1	0	13	310
Ian's Natural Foods, Chicken Nugget Kids Meal									
7 oz	370	17	2.5	50	38	3	10	20	580
Ian's Natural Foods, Egg & Maple Cheddar Wafflewich									
1 sandwich	350	15	4	115	46	1	5	7	580
Ian's Natural Foods, French Bread Pizza									
1 slice	180	6	0.5	0	30	3	3	2	500
Ian's Natural Foods, French Toast Sticks									
4 pieces	170	6	0	0	27	0	2	2	95
Ian's Natural Foods, Mac & No Cheese Sauce									
1 bowl	340	6	0.5	0	64	3	2	7	530
Ian's Natural Foods, Maple Sausage & Egg Wafflewich									
1 sandwich	370	18	4	120	42	1	5	9	710
Ian's Natural Foods, Pepperoni French Bread Pizza									
1 slice	180	6	0.5	0	30	3	3	2	500
Ian's Natural Foods, Popcorn Turkey Corn Dogs									
about 4 pieces	350	12	2	40	43	1	1	18	490
Joan's GF Great Bakes, Calzone									
1 calzone	480	21	10	70	51	1	8	20	280
Joan's GF Great Bakes, NY Pizza, Ready to Bake									
2 slices	450	15	6	25	60	5	5	17	860
Joan's GF Great Bakes, Sicilian Pizza									
1/2 tray	450	15	6	25	60	5	5	17	860
Lundberg Family Farms, Heat & Eat, Organic Countrywild, Brown Rice Bowl									
210g	280	3	0	0	65	6	0	6	0

Food Serving size	Cal.	(g) Total Fat	(g) Sat. Fat	(mg) Chol.	(g) Carb.	(g) Fiber	(g) Sug.	(g) Prot.	(mg) Sod.
Lundberg Family Farms, Heat & Eat, Organic Long Grain Brown Rice Bowl									
210g	290	3	0.5	0	65	6	1	6	5
Lundberg Family Farms, Heat & Eat, Organic Short Grain Brown Rice Bowl									
210g	290	2.5	0.5	0	65	5	1	5	10
Mrs. Leepers, Gluten Free Beef Stroganoff									
3/4 cup	150	2.5	1	5	30	1	2	3	830
Mrs. Leepers, Gluten Free Chicken Alfredo									
1 cup	750	3.5	2	10	27	1	2	3	590
Organic Bistro, Alaskan Salmon Cake Meal									
10 oz	370	16	2.5	55	31	8	6	22	490
Organic Bistro, Asian Style Coconut Lemongrass with Chicken Organic Bistro Bowl									
10 oz	290	6	4	30	42	7	15	18	540
Organic Bistro, Cheddar Beef Organic Bistro Bake									
8 oz	250	9	2.5	30	29	4	4	13	490
Organic Bistro, Chicken Citron Meal									
1 container	450	18	2.5	45	38	8	9	35	430
Organic Bistro, Chicken Parmesan Organic Bistro Bake									
8 oz	200	6	1	20	23	3	3	13	270
Organic Bistro, Ginger Chicken Meals									
10 oz serving	350	11	1.5	35	39	6	8	22	450
Organic Bistro, Grass-Fed Beef with Mushroom Sauce Meal									
10 oz	350	13	3.5	45	31	4	5	23	580
Organic Bistro, Savory Turkey Meals									
10.5 oz	340	11	1.5	40	35	8	5	25	480
Organic Bistro, Sesame Ginger Wild Salmon Organic Bistro Bowl									
10 oz	300	6	1	30	43	4	20	15	500
Organic Bistro, Southwest Style Grass-Fed Beef Meal									
10 oz	250	9	2	45	23	4	5	19	440
Organic Bistro, Spiced Chicken Morocco Meal									
10.75 oz	290	9	1	35	32	6	8	19	390
Organic Bistro, Thai Style Red Curry with Beef Organic Bistro Bowl									
10 oz	320	11	6	40	37	5	9	18	630

Food Serving size	Cal.	(g) Total Fat	(g) Sat. Fat	(mg) Chol.	(g) Carb.	(g) Fiber	(g) Sug.	(g) Prot.	(mg) Sod.
Organic Bistro, Thai Style Yellow Curry with Chicken Organic Bistro Bowl									
10 oz	280	7	4	30	37	4	16	17	640
Organic Bistro, Turkey Cheddar Organic Bistro Bake									
1 bake	260	9	3	30	30	3	4	14	200
Organic Bistro, Wild Alaskan Salmon Meals									
11 oz serving	380	13	2	50	49	6	11	20	240
Organic Bistro, Wild Alaskan Salmon Organic Bistro Bake									
1 bake	250	8	3	40	30	1	1	16	280
Organic Bistro, Wild Albacore Tuna Organic Bistro Bake									
1 bake	300	12	7	50	28	4	3	17	340
Organic Bistro, Wild Salmon with Pesto Meal									
10 oz	350	20	4.5	50	19	4	3	23	600
Pastariso, Gluten Free Instant Brown Rice Mac and Cheese Meal Cup									
1 container	212	4	2.5	5	38	3	6	6	670
Pastariso, Gluten Free Instant White Rice Mac and Cheese Meal Cup									
1 container	220	4	NA	5	40	<1	6	6	670
Pastariso, Gluten Free Macaroni and Yellow Cheddar Cheese (Dolphin)									
56g dry	169	1	0.5	3	32	6	2	8	152
Pastariso, Gluten Free Mini Rice Shells and Yellow Cheddar Cheese (Rhino)									
56g dry	190	2	1	10	35	3	6	8	206
Pastariso, Gluten Free Potato Macaroni and Yellow Cheese (Panda)									
56g	190	2	1	10	35	3	6	8	206
Pastariso, Gluten Free Potato Macaroni and White Cheddar Cheese (Orangutan)									
56g dry	190	2	1	10	35	3	6	8	206
Pastariso, Gluten Free Rice Macaroni Style Pasta and White Cheddar Cheese (Elephant)									
56g dry	190	2	1	10	35	3	6	8	206
Road's End Organics, Organic GF Alfredo Mac & Cheese									
1 cup prepared	330	2.5	0	0	63	5	<1	8	310
Road's End Organics, Organic GF Cheddar Penne & Cheese									
3/4 cup	330	2.5	0	0	63	5	1	8	340
Sabra, Classic Hummus with Pretzels									
1 cup	260	22	3	0	13	3	2	6	420

Food Serving size	Cal.	(g) Total Fat	(g) Sat. Fat	(mg) Chol.	(g) Carb.	(g) Fiber	(g) Sug.	(g) Prot.	(mg) Sod.
Simply Organic Foods, Fish Taco 1 tbsp	25	0	0	0	5	1	0	1	370
Tasty Bite, Jaipur Vegetables 1/2 pack	180	11	2.5	5	12	4	3	7	530
Tasty Bite, Jodhpur Lentils 1/2 pack	110	2.5	0	0	16	4	1	6	460
Tasty Bite, Kashmir Spinach 1/2 pack	90	5	1	0	7	3	1	5	510
Tasty Bite, Kerala Vegetables 1/2 pack	110	5	2	0	15	3	3	2	440
Tasty Bite, Lentil Magic 1/2 pack	240	6	0.5	0	33	9	2	12	440
Tasty Bite, Madras Lentils 1/2 pack	150	6	2.5	10	18	5	2	7	510
Tasty Bite, Mushroom Takatak 1/2 pack	120	3	0	0	17	3	5	3	420
Tasty Bite, Paneer Makhani 1/2 pack	220	17	8	35	8	1	3	10	440
Tasty Bite, Peas Paneer 1/2 pack	200	13	7	25	12	3	4	10	400
Tasty Bite, Punjab Eggplant 1/2 pack	150	9	1	0	13	4	5	3	560
Tasty Bite, Snappy Soya 1/2 pack	190	10	1	0	17	9	4	12	380
Tasty Bite, Spinach Channa 1/2 pack	130	6	0.5	0	14	6	3	6	490
Tasty Bite, Spinach Dal 1/2 pack	100	5	0.5	0	10	3	2	3	480
Tasty Bite, Tandoori Pilaf 1/2 pack	180	2.5	0	0	36	2	1	3	390
Tasty Bite, Tehari Herb Rice 1/2 pack	210	3.5	1	0	40	1	1	4	360
Tasty Bite, Tofu Corn Masala 1/2 pack	130	5	1	0	17	4	5	5	380

Food Serving size	Cal.	(g) Total Fat	(g) Sat. Fat	(mg) Chol.	(g) Carb.	(g) Fiber	(g) Sug.	(g) Prot.	(mg) Sod.
Tasty Bite, Vegetable Korma 1/2 pack	130	6	3	0	15	5	4	3	430
Tasty Bite, Zesty Lentils & Peas 1/2 pack	200	3.5	0	0	38	7	4	10	400
Thai Kitchen, Garlic & Roasted Pepper, Take Out Meal 1/2 package	240	5	0.5	0	42	2	6	6	680
Thai Kitchen, Ginger & Sweet Chili, Take Out Meal 1/2 package	250	3.5	0.5	NA	49	1	9	4	650
Thai Kitchen, Green Curry Kit 84g	210	6	5	0	35	1	4	3	310
Thai Kitchen, Original Pad Thai, Take Out Meal 4.5 oz	360	9	1	NA	80	2	20	5	720
Thai Kitchen, Pad Thai Noodle Kit 1/2 package	360	1	0	0	79.9	2	20	5	720
Thai Kitchen, Pad Thai Rice Noodle Cart 1 package	460	2	0	5	104	3	39	6	1590
Thai Kitchen, Red Curry Kit 1 cup	210	6	5	0	35	1	3	3	250
Thai Kitchen, Spicy Thai Basil Noodle Cart 1 package	430	2	0	5	97	6	25	6	1280
Thai Kitchen, Sweet Citrus Ginger Noodle Cart 1 package	440	3.5	1	5	97	6	32	6	1520
Thai Kitchen, Tangy Lemongrass Noodle Cart 1 package	450	1	0	5	105	6	31	5	1250
Thai Kitchen, Tangy Sweet & Sour, Take Out Meal 84g	260	3.5	0.5	NA	52	1	13	5	610
Thai Kitchen, Thai Basil & Chili, Take Out Meal 1/2 package	250	3	0.5	NA	50	1	10	4	730
Thai Kitchen, Thai Peanut Noodle Cart 1 package	510	9	2	5	96	6	17	10	670
Thai Kitchen, Thai Peanut Noodle Kit 1/3 package	200	4	1	0	37	1	7	5	150
Thai Kitchen, Thai Peanut, Take Out Meal 1/2 package	310	6	0.5	0	54	1	13	9	330

Food Serving size	Cal.	(g) Total Fat	(g) Sat. Fat	(mg) Chol.	(g) Carb.	(g) Fiber	(g) Sug.	(g) Prot.	(mg) Sod.
Udi's Gluten Free, Pepperoni Pizza 1/2 pizza	350	18	9	50	31	4	3	16	1010
Udi's Gluten Free, Three Cheese Pizza 1/2 pizza	320	15	7	40	32	4	3	16	880

Sauces & Gravies

Food Serving size	Cal.	(g) Total Fat	(g) Sat. Fat	(mg) Chol.	(g) Carb.	(g) Fiber	(g) Sug.	(g) Prot.	(mg) Sod.
505 Southwestern, Fajita Marinade 1 tbsp	25	0	NA	NA	6	NA	5	0	800
505 Southwestern, Green Chile Sauce 1/4 cup	25	0	NA	NA	5	0.7	2	1	40
505 Southwestern, Red Chile Sauce (Enchilada & Tamale Sauce) 1/4 cup	25	0	NA	NA	6	1	3	1	75
505 Southwestern, Roasted Green Chiles (Medium) 2 tbsp	10	0	0	0	0	0	1	1	20
Amy's, Family Marinara Pasta Sauce 1/2 cup	80	4.5	0.5	0	9	3	5	2	590
Amy's, Light in Sodium, Family Marinara Pasta Sauce .5 oz	80	4.5	0.5	0	9	2	5	2	290
Amy's, Light in Sodium, Tomato Basil Pasta Sauce 1/2 cup	90	4.5	0.5	0	11	2	6	2	290
Amy's, Tomato Basil Pasta Sauce 1/2 cup	110	6	1	0	11	3	6	2	580
Annie Chun's, Gochujang Sauce 1 tbsp	45	0.5	0	0	10	<1	5	<1	350
Annie Chun's, Korean Barbeque Sauce 1 tbsp	30	0	0	0	6	NA	6	1	380
Annie Chun's, Kung Pao Sauce 1 tbsp	30	0.5	0	0	4	0	3	1	350
Annie Chun's, Pad Thai Sauce 1 tbsp	30	0.5	0	0	7	NA	5	0	400
Annie Chun's, Shiitake Soy Ginger Sauce 1 tbsp	15	0	0	0	4	0	3	0	180
Annie Chun's, Teriyaki Sauce 1 tbsp	25	0	0	0	6	NA	5	2	300

Food Serving size	Cal.	(g) Total Fat	(g) Sat. Fat	(mg) Chol.	(g) Carb.	(g) Fiber	(g) Sug.	(g) Prot.	(mg) Sod.
Annie Chun's, Thai Peanut Sauce									
1 tbsp	60	3.5	0.5	0	5	NA	4	2	135
Annie's, Organic Annie's, Original BBQ Sauce									
2 tbsp	45	1	NA	NA	9	NA	5	0	240
Annie's, Organic Hot Chipotle BBQ Sauce									
2 tbsp	45	1	NA	NA	9	1	5	0	250
Annie's, Organic Smokey Maple BBQ Sauce									
2 tbsp	45	1	NA	NA	9	NA	5	0	240
Annie's, Organic Sweet & Spicy BBQ Sauce									
2 tbsp	40	0	NA	NA	10	1	9	0	310
Boar's Head, Brown Sugar & Spice Ham Glaze									
2 tbsp	120	0	0	0	30	0	29	0	95
Boar's Head, Savory Remoulade									
1 tbsp	90	9	1.5	5	2	0	1	0	180
Classico, Basil and Tomato Bruschetta Topping									
1 tbsp	15	1	0	0	1	0	0	0	55
Classico, Basil Pesto Sauce									
1/4 cup	240	23	4	<5	5	1	2	3	580
Classico, Creamy Alfredo Sauce									
1/4 cup	100	9	5	50	3	0	1	2	410
Classico, Extra Garlic Bruschetta Topping									
1 tbsp	15	1	0	0	1	0	0	0	55
Classico, Four Cheese Alfredo Sauce									
1/4 cup	80	6	4	40	4	0	1	2	390
Classico, Light Asiago Romano Alfredo Sauce									
1/4 cup	70	5	3	30	4	1	1	1	280
Classico, Light Creamy Alfredo Sauce									
1/4 cup	60	5	3	25	3	0	1	1	330
Classico, Mushroom Alfredo Sauce									
1/4 cup	70	5	3	35	3	2	0	2	300
Classico, Red Sauce, Cabernet Marinara with Herbs									
1/2 cup	70	1.5	0	0	11	2	6	2	330
Classico, Red Sauce, Carmelized Onion and Roasted Garlic									
1/2 cup	80	2.5	0.5	0	11	3	7	2	380

Food Serving size	Cal.	(g) Total Fat	(g) Sat. Fat	(mg) Chol.	(g) Carb.	(g) Fiber	(g) Sug.	(g) Prot.	(mg) Sod.
Classico, Red Sauce, Fire-Roasted Tomato and Garlic									
1/2 cup	60	1	0	0	10	2	5	2	380
Classico, Red Sauce, Florentino Spinach and Cheese									
1/2 cup	80	3.5	1	<5	9	3	5	2	460
Classico, Red Sauce, Four Cheese									
1/2 cup	80	3	1	<5	12	3	5	2	460
Classico, Red Sauce, Garden Vegetable									
1/2 cup	60	1.5	0	0	9	2	6	2	380
Classico, Red Sauce, Italian Sausage with Peppers and Onions									
1/2 cup	80	2.5	1	5	10	2	6	3	430
Classico, Red Sauce, Marinara with Plum Tomatoes									
1/2 cup	70	2	0	0	10	2	6	2	460
Classico, Red Sauce, Mushroom and Ripe Olives									
1/2 cup	60	1.5	0	0	10	2	6	2	360
Classico, Red Sauce, Organic Spinach and Garlic									
1/2 cup	70	1.5	0	0	11	2	7	2	330
Classico, Red Sauce, Organic Tomato, Herbs and Spices									
1/2 cup	70	1	0	0	12	2	7	2	400
Classico, Red Sauce, Portobello, Crimini & Champignon Mushroom									
1/2 cup	70	2	0	0	11	3	6	2	390
Classico, Red Sauce, Roasted Garlic									
1/2 cup	60	1.5	0	0	9	3	5	2	350
Classico, Red Sauce, Spicy Red Pepper									
1/2 cup	60	2.5	0.5	0	8	2	5	1	300
Classico, Red Sauce, Spicy Tomato and Basil									
1/2 cup	70	1.5	0	0	11	2	6	2	450
Classico, Red Sauce, Spicy Tomato and Pesto									
1/2 cup	90	5	1	0	10	3	5	2	480
Classico, Red Sauce, Sun-dried Tomato									
1/2 cup	80	4	0.5	0	9	2	5	2	420
Classico, Red Sauce, Tomato and Basil									
1/2 cup	50	1	0	0	9	1	5	2	380
Classico, Red Sauce, Traditional Sweet Basil									
1/2 cup	70	1	0	0	13	3	9	2	470

Food Serving size	Cal.	(g) Total Fat	(g) Sat. Fat	(mg) Chol.	(g) Carb.	(g) Fiber	(g) Sug.	(g) Prot.	(mg) Sod.
Classico, Red Sauce, Tuscan Olive and Garlic									
1/2 cup	70	2	0	0	10	2	6	2	410
Classico, Red Sauce, Vodka Sauce									
1/2 cup	100	5	2	10	11	3	3	3	420
Classico, Roasted Garlic Alfredo Sauce									
1/4 cup	70	6	3	30	3	1	1	1	430
Classico, Roasted Poblano Alfredo Sauce									
1/4 cup	70	7	4	35	3	0	1	1	290
Classico, Roasted Red Pepper Alfredo Sauce									
1/4 cup	60	5	3	35	3	0	1	1	310
Classico, Sun-dried Tomato Alfredo Sauce									
1/4 cup	90	7	4	35	4	0	2	2	430
Classico, Sun-dried Tomato Pesto Sauce									
1/4 cup	100	6	1.5	<5	9	2	5	2	570
Classico, Traditional Pizza Sauce									
1/4 cup	40	1	0	0	7	1	5	1	320
Eden Foods, Pizza-Pasta Sauce, Organic									
1/4 cup	35	1	0	0	4	2	2	1	150
Eden Foods, Spaghetti Sauce, No Salt Added, Organic									
1/2 cup	70	2.5	0	0	9	5	4	2	10
Eden Foods, Spaghetti Sauce, Organic									
1/2 cup	70	2.5	0	0	9	5	4	2	300
Full Flavor Foods, Gluten Free Alfredo Sauce Mix									
2 tbsp	80	5	2	20	14	0	2	10	620
Full Flavor Foods, Gluten Free Beef Gravy Mix									
1 tbsp	25	0	0	0	6	0	<1	1	275
Full Flavor Foods, Gluten Free Cheese Sauce Mix									
1-1/2 tbsp	45	2	1	6	6	0	0	1	400
Full Flavor Foods, Gluten Free Chicken Gravy Mix									
1 tbsp	25	0	0	0	6	0	<1	1	275
Full Flavor Foods, Gluten Free Pork Gravy Mix									
1 tbsp	25	0	0	0	6	0	<1	1	275
Full Flavor Foods, Gluten Free Turkey Gravy Mix									
1 tbsp	25	0	0	0	6	0	<1	1	275

Food Serving size	Cal.	(g) Total Fat	(g) Sat. Fat	(mg) Chol.	(g) Carb.	(g) Fiber	(g) Sug.	(g) Prot.	(mg) Sod.
Full Flavor Foods, Gluten Free Vegetarian Mushrooms Sauce Mix									
3 tbsp	130	8	7	0	12	0	2	1	545
Heart Smart, Traditional Italian Sauce									
1/2 cup	70	1.5	0	0	13	3	10	2	360
Lucini, Creamy Tomato Ricotta Sauce									
1/2 cup	90	5	2.4	15	7	3	4	4	330
Lucini, Pizza Sauce									
1/4 cup	50	2	0	0	7	1	4	0	280
Lucini, Robust Tomato Gorgonzola Sauce									
1/2 cup	150	10	4	20	8	3	6	7	430
Lucini, Rustic Tomato Vodka Sauce									
1/2 cup	70	2.5	1	10	10	2	2	2	230
Lucini, Savory Tomato Parmigiano Sauce									
1/2 cup	80	2.4	1.4	5	10	2	5	5	340
Lucini, Sicilian Olive & Wild Caper Tomato Sauce									
1/2 cup	50	1.5	0	0	8	2	2	1	290
Lucini, Tuscan Marinara with Roasted Garlic Sauce									
1/2 cup	60	3	0.5	0	8	2	5	2	490
Lucini, Tuscan Marinara with Roasted Garlic Sauce Pouch									
1/2 cup	60	3	0	0	7	<1	4	1	410
Mezzetta, Arrabbiata Pasta Sauce									
1/2 cup	90	5.5	9	0	5	0.9	3	0.9	490
Mezzetta, Artichoke Parmesan Marinara Pasta Sauce									
1/2 cup	100	6	1.5	5	9	2	4	3	520
Mezzetta, Creamy Vodka Style Marinara Pasta Sauce									
1/2 cup	130	7.5	4	20	8	2	5	3	700
Mezzetta, Homemade Style Marinara Pasta Sauce									
1/2 cup	90	5.5	1	0	5	1	3	1	490
Mezzetta, Pesto Sauce									
2 tbsp	150	16	2.5	5	1	1	0	2	320
Mezzetta, Porcini Mushroom Pasta Sauce									
1/2 cup	100	5	0.5	0	12	2	6	2	500
Mezzetta, Roasted Garlic Pasta Sauce									
1/2 cup	100	5	0.5	0	11	3	6	2	550

Food Serving size	Cal.	(g) Total Fat	(g) Sat. Fat	(mg) Chol.	(g) Carb.	(g) Fiber	(g) Sug.	(g) Prot.	(mg) Sod.
Mezzetta, Tomato Basil Pasta Sauce									
1/2 cup	100	5	0.5	0	11	3	6	2	550
Newman's Own, Alfredo Pasta Sauce									
1/4 cup	70	8	4.5	40	3	0	1	1	410
Newman's Own, Cabernet Marinara Pasta Sauce									
1/2 cup	70	3	0	0	10	2	9	2	590
Newman's Own, Fire Roasted Tomato & Garlic Pasta Sauce									
1/2 cup	70	3.5	0.5	0	9	2	5	2	500
Newman's Own, Five Cheese Pasta Sauce									
1/2 cup	80	3	1.5	5	10	2	9	3	610
Newman's Own, Fra Diavolo Pasta Sauce									
1/2 cup	70	3	0	0	10	2	4	0	510
Newman's Own, Garden Peppers Pasta Sauce									
1/2 cup	60	1	0	0	9	NA	5	2	440
Newman's Own, Herb & Roasted Garlic Marinade									
1 tbsp	20	1	0	0	3	0	2	0	370
Newman's Own, Italian Sausage & Peppers Pasta Sauce									
1/2 cup	90	4	1	10	11	2	9	4	630
Newman's Own, Lemon Pepper Marinade									
1 tbsp	15	0	0	0	3	0	2	0	300
Newman's Own, Marinara Pasta Sauce									
1/2 cup	70	2	0	0	12	3	8	2	460
Newman's Own, Marinara with Mushroom Pasta Sauce									
1/2 cup	70	2	0	0	12	3	11	2	520
Newman's Own, Mesquite with Lime Marinade									
1 tbsp	20	1	0	0	3	0	2	0	190
Newman's Own, Organic Marinara Pasta Sauce									
1/2 cup	70	2	0	0	12	3	8	2	550
Newman's Own, Roasted Garlic & Peppers Pasta Sauce									
1/2 cup	70	2.5	0	0	11	2	6	2	590
Newman's Own, Roasted Garlic Alfredo Pasta Sauce									
1/4 cup	90	8	4.5	40	4	0	1	1	400
Newman's Own, Sockarooni Pasta Sauce									
1/2 cup	70	2	0	0	12	3	8	2	460

Food Serving size	Cal.	(g) Total Fat	(g) Sat. Fat	(mg) Chol.	(g) Carb.	(g) Fiber	(g) Sug.	(g) Prot.	(mg) Sod.
Newman's Own, Sweet Onion & Roasted Garlic Pasta Sauce									
1/2 cup	60	1.5	0	0	12	2	10	2	530
Newman's Own, Tomato & Basil Bombolina Pasta Sauce									
1/2 cup	90	4.5	0.5	0	13	3	8	2	520
Newman's Own, Vodka Pasta Sauce									
1/2 cup	110	5	1.5	5	11	2	9	5	440
Prego, Chunky Garden Combo Italian Sauce									
1/2 cup	70	1.5	0	0	13	3	10	2	470
Prego, Chunky Garden Mushroom & Green Pepper Italian Sauce									
1/2 cup	90	3	0	0	13	3	10	2	470
Prego, Chunky Garden Mushroom Supreme with Baby Portobello Italian Sauce									
1/2 cup	90	3	0	0	13	3	10	2	460
Prego, Chunky Garden Tomato Onion & Garlic Italian Sauce									
1/2 cup	90	3	0	0	13	3	10	2	470
Prego, Fresh Mushroom Italian Sauce									
1/2 cup	70	1.5	0	0	13	3	11	2	480
Prego, Heart Smart Italian Mushroom Sauce									
1/2 cup	70	1.5	0	0	13	3	9	2	360
Prego, Heart Smart Italian Ricotta Parmesan Sauce									
1/2 cup	90	2.5	1	5	13	3	10	3	360
Prego, Heart Smart Italian Roasted Red Pepper & Garlic Sauce									
1/2 cup	70	1.5	0	0	13	3	9	2	360
Prego, Italian Sauce Flavored with Meat									
1/2 cup	80	2.5	0.5	5	13	3	10	2	480
Prego, Italian Sausage & Garlic Italian Sauce									
1/2 cup	90	3	1	5	13	3	10	3	480
Prego, Light Smart Traditional Italian Sauce									
1/2 cup	50	0	0	0	12	3	8	2	410
Prego, Marinara Italian Sauce									
1/2 cup	80	3	0.5	0	10	3	7	2	480
Prego, Pizzeria Style Pizza Sauce									
1/4 cup	40	1.5	0	0	5	1	4	1	200
Prego, Roasted Garlic & Herb Italian Sauce									
1/2 cup	90	3	0	0	13	3	9	2	460

Food Serving size	Cal.	(g) Total Fat	(g) Sat. Fat	(mg) Chol.	(g) Carb.	(g) Fiber	(g) Sug.	(g) Prot.	(mg) Sod.
Prego, Roasted Garlic Parmesan Italian Sauce									
1/2 cup	70	1	0.5	5	13	3	10	3	480
Prego, Three Cheese Italian Sauce									
1/2 cup	80	1.5	0.5	5	14	3	11	3	430
Prego, Tomato Basil Garlic Italian Sauce									
1/2 cup	80	2.5	0	0	12	3	9	2	420
Prego, Traditional Italian Sauce									
1/2 cup	70	1.5	0	0	13	3	10	2	480
Prego, Veggie Smart Pizza Sauce									
1/4 cup	45	1	0	0	8	1	6	1	220
Road's End Organics, GF Alfredo Cheese Sauce Mix									
1 tbsp	35	0.5	0	0	6	3	0	2	200
Road's End Organics, GF Cheddar Cheese Sauce Mix									
1 tbsp	30	0.5	0	0	6	2	0	2	210
Road's End Organics, Organic Golden Gravy Mix, Dry									
1 tbsp	25	0	0	0	5	0	0	<1	230
Road's End Organics, Organic Savory Herb Gravy Mix, Dry									
1 tbsp	25	0	0	0	5	0	0	<1	210
Road's End Organics, Organic Shiitake Gravy Mix, Dry									
1 tbsp	25	0	0	0	5	<1	0	<1	200
San-J, Asian BBQ Cooking Sauce									
2 tbsp	50	0	NA	NA	12	NA	10	1	420
San-J, Orange Asian Cooking Sauce									
2 tbsp	60	NA	NA	NA	14	NA	12	1	340
San-J, Sweet & Tangy Asian Cooking Sauce									
2 tbsp	50	0	NA	NA	13	NA	11	<1	320
San-J, Szechuan Asian Cooking Sauce									
1 tsp	5	0	NA	NA	<1	NA	NA	0	170
San-J, Teriyaki Asian Cooking Sauce									
1 tbsp	20	0	NA	NA	4	NA	3	<1	390
San-J, Thai Peanut Asian Cooking Sauce									
2 tbsp	80	3.5	0.5	NA	10	<1	8	3	690
Seeds of Change, Arrabiatta di Roma Pasta Sauce									
1/2 cup	80	6	0.5	0	6	2	0	1	300

Food Serving size	Cal.	(g) Total Fat	(g) Sat. Fat	(mg) Chol.	(g) Carb.	(g) Fiber	(g) Sug.	(g) Prot.	(mg) Sod.
Seeds of Change, Jalfrezi Indian Simmer Sauce									
1/3 cup	90	6	2.5	0	9	2	3	1	270
Seeds of Change, Korma Indian Simmer Sauce									
1/3 cup	140	11	7	10	9	1	4	1	290
Seeds of Change, Madras Indian Simmer Sauce									
1/3 cup	60	4	0.5	0	8	1	3	1	240
Seeds of Change, Marinara Di Venezia Pasta Sauce									
1/2 cup	60	3.5	0	0	6	2	0	1	380
Seeds of Change, Romagna Three Cheese Pasta Sauce									
1/2 cup	90	5	1.5	5	9	2	0	4	460
Seeds of Change, Tikka Masala Indian Simmer Sauce									
1/3 cup	90	7	2.5	10	8	2	2	1	280
Seeds of Change, Tomato Basil Genovese Pasta Sauce									
1/2 cup	60	3.5	0	0	9	2	0	2	350
Seeds of Change, Tuscan Tomato & Garlic Pasta Sauce									
1/2 cup	60	2.5	0	0	7	2	3	2	510
Seeds of Change, Vodka Americano Pasta Sauce									
1/2 cup	120	10	3.5	20	8	2	1	2	310
Simply Organic Foods, Alfredo Sauce									
1 tbsp	35	0	0	0	7	0	2	2	310
Simply Organic Foods, Brown Gravy Mix									
2 tsp	20	0	0	0	5	0	0	0	290
Simply Organic Foods, Enchilada Sauce									
1 tsp	15	0	0	0	3	1	0	0	340
Simply Organic Foods, Garden Vegetable Spaghetti Sauce									
1 tbsp	30	0	0	0	7	1	2	0	300
Simply Organic Foods, Hollandaise Sauce Mix									
3/4 tsp	10	0	0	10	2	0	<1	0	95
Simply Organic Foods, Italian Herb Spaghetti Sauce									
1 tbsp	30	0	0	0	7	1	1	0	310
Simply Organic Foods, Mole Sauce									
2 tsp	25	0.5	0	0	4	2	0	1	540
Simply Organic Foods, Mushroom Sauce Mix									
2 tsp	20	0	0	0	4	0	0	0	300

Food Serving size	Cal.	(g) Total Fat	(g) Sat. Fat	(mg) Chol.	(g) Carb.	(g) Fiber	(g) Sug.	(g) Prot.	(mg) Sod.
Simply Organic Foods, Roasted Garlic Spaghetti Sauce									
2 tsp	15	0	0	0	4	1	0	0	160
Simply Organic Foods, Southwest Taco									
1 tbsp	25	0.5	0	0	5	1	0	1	360
Simply Organic Foods, Tomato Basil Spaghetti Sauce									
1 tbsp	30	0	0	0	7	1	1	1	310
Simply Organic Foods, Vegetarian Brown Gravy									
2 tsp	20	0	0	0	5	0	0	0	330
Tasty Bite, Good Korma Cooking Sauce									
1/2 pack	110	8	5	0	8	1	1	2	370
Tasty Bite, Pad Thai Cooking Sauce									
1/2 pack	170	10	1	0	17	2	13	4	400
Tasty Bite, Rogan Josh Cooking Sauce									
1/2 pack	60	3.5	0	0	7	1	2	1	370
Tasty Bite, Satay Partay Cooking Sauce									
1/2 pack	150	9	2.5	0	17	2	11	3	400
Tasty Bite, Tikka Masala Cooking Sauce									
1/2 pack	90	6	2	10	9	2	5	2	420
Thai Kitchen, Green Curry 10-Minute Simmer Sauce									
1/2 cup	90	6	6	0	8	0	5	1	940
Thai Kitchen, Original Pad Thai Sauce									
2 tbsp	70	0.5	0	0	17	0	14	0	560
Thai Kitchen, Panang Curry 10-Minute Simmer Sauce									
1/2 cup	90	0	0	0	7	0	5	0	890
Thai Kitchen, Peanut Satay Sauce									
2 tbsp	80	5	0.5	NA	6	1	4	2	130
Thai Kitchen, Pineapple & Chili Sauce									
2 tbsp	25	0	0	0	7	0	6	0	160
Thai Kitchen, Premium Fish Sauce									
1 tbsp	5	0	0	NA	1	0	1	0	1190
Thai Kitchen, Red Curry 10-Minute Simmer Sauce									
1/2 cup	90	6	6	0	7	NA	5	1	900
Thai Kitchen, Spicy Thai Chili Sauce									
2 tbsp	35	0	0	0	8	0	7	0	580

Food Serving size	Cal.	(g) Total Fat	(g) Sat. Fat	(mg) Chol.	(g) Carb.	(g) Fiber	(g) Sug.	(g) Prot.	(mg) Sod.
Thai Kitchen, Spicy Thai Mango Sauce									
2 tbsp	50	0	0	0	13	0	10	0	290
Thai Kitchen, Sweet Red Chili Sauce									
1 tbsp	30	0	0	0	7	0	6	0	205
Thai Kitchen, Thai Chili & Ginger Dipping Sauce									
2 tbsp	40	0	0	0	10	0	8	0	260
Thai Kitchen, Yellow Curry Mild 10-Minute Simmer Sauce									
1 serving	90	6	5	0	8	NA	5	0	830
The Really Great Food Company, Garlic Steak Sauce									
1 tbsp	20	0	0	0	4	0	3	0	0
The Really Great Food Company, Ginger Garlic Stir Fry Sauce									
1 tbsp	15	0	0	0	4	0	3	0	0
The Really Great Food Company, Honey Barbecue Sauce									
2 tbsp	40	0	0	0	10	0	8	0	0
The Really Great Food Company, Honey Mustard Sauce									
2 tbsp	35	0	0	0	8	0	7	0	0
The Really Great Food Company, Hot Wing Sauce									
1 tbsp	15	0	0	0	3	0	2	0	0
The Really Great Food Company, Sweet and Sour Sauce									
2 tbsp	45	0	0	0	10	1	9	0	0
The Really Great Food Company, Thai Peanut Sauce (contains peanuts)									
1 tbsp	25	1	0	0	3	0	2	0	0
The Wizard's, Original Organic Hot Stuff Picante Sauce									
1 tsp	0	0	0	0	1	0	0	0	65
Thumann's, Brown Sugar & Spice Ham Glaze									
1 tsp	60	0	0	NA	15	NA	15	0	47

Soups (Including Soup-related Products)

Food Serving size	Cal.	(g) Total Fat	(g) Sat. Fat	(mg) Chol.	(g) Carb.	(g) Fiber	(g) Sug.	(g) Prot.	(mg) Sod.
Amy's, Indian Golden Lentil Soup									
1 cup	220	9	1	0	25	7	3	9	680
Amy's, Organic Black Bean Vegetable Soup									
1 cup	140	1.5	0	0	26	5	7	6	620
Amy's, Organic Chunky Tomato Bisque									
1 cup	130	3.5	2	10	21	3	14	3	680

Food Serving size	Cal.	(g) Total Fat	(g) Sat. Fat	(mg) Chol.	(g) Carb.	(g) Fiber	(g) Sug.	(g) Prot.	(mg) Sod.
Amy's, Organic Chunky Vegetable Soup									
1 cup	60	0	0	0	13	3	5	3	680
Amy's, Organic Cream of Tomato Soup									
1 cup	110	2.5	1.5	10	19	3	13	3	690
Amy's, Organic Curried Lentil Soup									
1 cup	230	8	1	0	30	11	4	9	680
Amy's, Organic Fire Roasted Southwestern Vegetable Soup									
1 cup	140	4	0.5	0	21	4	4	4	680
Amy's, Organic Hearty French Country Vegetable Soup									
1 cup	180	8	1	0	23	5	4	5	640
Amy's, Organic Hearty Rustic Italian Vegetable Soup									
1 cup	140	6	1	0	18	4	4	4	680
Amy's, Organic Hearty Spanish Rice & Red Bean Soup									
1/2 can	140	2.5	0	0	24	5	3	5	690
Amy's, Organic Lentil Soup									
1 cup	180	5	1	0	25	6	3	8	590
Amy's, Organic Lentil Vegetable Soup									
1 cup	160	4	0.5	0	24	8	5	7	680
Amy's, Organic Light in Sodium, Chunky Tomato Bisque									
1 cup	130	3.5	2	10	21	3	14	3	340
Amy's, Organic Light in Sodium, Cream of Tomato Soup									
1 cup	110	2.5	1.5	10	19	3	13	3	340
Amy's, Organic Light in Sodium, Lentil Vegetable Soup									
1 cup	160	4	0.5	0	24	8	5	7	340
Amy's, Organic Light in Sodium, Split Pea Soup									
1 cup	100	0	0	0	19	6	4	7	330
Amy's, Organic Split Pea Soup									
1 cup	100	0	0	0	19	6	4	7	670
Amy's, Organic Summer Corn & Vegetable Soup									
1 cup	150	3	2.5	15	23	2	6	4	560
Amy's, Organic Tuscan Bean & Rice Soup									
1 cup	160	4.5	0.5	0	25	5	4	5	680
Amy's, Thai Coconut Soup (Tom Kha Phak)									
1/2 can	140	10	8	0	10	2	4	4	580

Food Serving size	Cal.	(g) Total Fat	(g) Sat. Fat	(mg) Chol.	(g) Carb.	(g) Fiber	(g) Sug.	(g) Prot.	(mg) Sod.
Andean Dream, Tomato Quinoa Noodle Soup									
1 cup	130	0.5	0	0	27	2	1	3	670
Andean Dream, Vegetarian Quinoa Noodle Soup									
1 cup	100	0.5	0	0	22	1	<1	3	670
Annie Chun's, Chicken & Cilantro Wonton Soup									
1 bowl	120	2	0	20	22	3	7	2	650
Annie Chun's, Chicken & Garlic Wonton Soup									
1 bowl	140	2	0	20	22	3	4	7	630
Annie Chun's, Chinese Chicken Soup Bowl									
1 bowl	300	1.5	0	<5	61	3	3	10	710
Annie Chun's, Garlic Scallion Noodle Bowl									
1/2 bowl	310	5	0.5	0	57	2	3	8	980
Annie Chun's, Hot & Sour Soup Bowl									
1 bowl	290	1.5	0.5	0	59	2	4	11	970
Annie Chun's, Korean Kimchi Soup Bowl									
1 bowl	250	1.5	0	0	54	4	3	6	1000
Annie Chun's, Korean Sweet Chili Noodle Bowl									
1/2 bowl	320	4.5	0.5	0	60	2	7	7	830
Annie Chun's, Miso Soup Bowl									
1 bowl	240	1	0	0	50	4	3	8	990
Annie Chun's, Soy Ginger Ramen									
1 serving	230	0.5	0	0	45	1	1	12	1000
Annie Chun's, Spicy Chicken Ramen									
1 serving	230	1.5	0.5	0	45	3	1	8	980
Annie Chun's, Spicy Vegetable Wonton Soup									
1 bowl	130	1.5	0	0	25	3	5	6	990
Annie Chun's, Spring Vegetable Ramen									
1 serving	230	1	0	0	48	2	2	8	1000
Annie Chun's, Thai Tom Yum Soup Bowl									
1 bowl	310	3.5	0.5	0	60	3	7	11	990
Annie Chun's, Udon Soup Bowl									
1 bowl	240	0.5	0	0	52	4	4	7	460
Annie Chun's, Vietnamese Pho									
1 bowl	280	1	0	0	59	3	4	10	1030

Food Serving size	Cal.	(g) Total Fat	(g) Sat. Fat	(mg) Chol.	(g) Carb.	(g) Fiber	(g) Sug.	(g) Prot.	(mg) Sod.
Celifibr Gluten Free, Vegetarian Beef Boullion Soup Cubes									
3.2 serving size	5	0.1	0	0	0.8	0	0	0.2	123
Celifibr Gluten Free, Vegetarian Chicken Boullion Soup Cubes									
3.2 serving size	5	0.1	0	0	0.8	0	0	0.2	123
Eden Foods, Black Bean & Quinoa Chili									
1 cup	190	1.5	0	0	35	6	3	10	460
Edward & Sons, Garden Veggie Bouillon Cubes									
1/2 cube	20	2	1	0	0	0	0	<1	970
Edward & Sons, Low Sodium Veggie Bouillon Cubes									
1/2 cube	20	1.5	0	0	1	0	0	<1	135
Edward & Sons, Miso-Cup, Japanese Restaurant Style, Prepared									
1 cup	60	1.5	0	0	7	<1	<1	4	1170
Edward & Sons, Miso-Cup, Organic Traditional with Tofu									
1 cup	35	1	0	0	4	<1	<1	2	480
Edward & Sons, Miso-Cup, Original Golden Vegetable, Prepared									
1 cup	30	1	0	0	4	<1	3	2	740
Edward & Sons, Miso-Cup, Reduced Sodium									
1 envelope	25	1	0	0	3	<1	<1	2	270
Edward & Sons, Miso-Cup, Savory Seaweed, Prepared									
1 cup	35	1.5	0	0	3	<1	3	2	710
Edward & Sons, Not-Beef Bouillon Cubes									
1/2 cube	20	2	1	0	0	0	0	<1	930
Edward & Sons, Not-Chick'n Bouillon Cubes									
1/2 cube	20	1.5	1	0	0	0	0	<1	810
Full Flavor Foods, Gluten Free Beef Soup Stock Mix									
1 tbsp	5	0	0	0	1	0	<1	1	865
Full Flavor Foods, Gluten Free Chicken Soup Stock Mix									
1 tbsp	5	0	0	0	1	0	1	1	865
Full Flavor Foods, Gluten Free Cream Soup Mix									
3 tbsp	130	8	7	0	12	0	2	1	545
Gluten Free Café, Black Bean Soup									
1 cup	160	1.5	0	0	32	7	6	8	680
Gluten Free Café, Chicken Noodle Soup									
1 cup	90	1.5	0	5	14	2	0	4	760

Food Serving size	Cal.	(g) Total Fat	(g) Sat. Fat	(mg) Chol.	(g) Carb.	(g) Fiber	(g) Sug.	(g) Prot.	(mg) Sod.
Gluten Free Café, Cream of Mushroom Soup									
1 cup	90	6	3	20	10	2	0	2	620
Gluten Free Café, Veggie Noodle Soup									
1 cup	90	0.5	5	0	19	4	5	2	650
Kettle Cuisine, Angus Steak Chili with Beans									
1 cup	230	7	2.5	50	23	7	7	20	670
Kettle Cuisine, Aztec Chili with Ancient Grains									
1 cup	190	4	0.5	0	32	7	4	8	550
Kettle Cuisine, Beef Stew									
1 cup	200	6	2	45	19	3	4	17	740
Kettle Cuisine, Black Eyed Pea & Smoked Ham Soup									
1 cup	170	2.5	1	10	25	7	4	14	940
Kettle Cuisine, Broccoli Cheddar Soup									
1 cup	340	26	16	75	15	2	1	12	820
Kettle Cuisine, Carrot Ginger Soup									
1 cup	110	4.5	0.5	0	.18	4	7	2	320
Kettle Cuisine, Chicken Tortilla Soup									
1 cup	140	3.5	0.5	20	17	3	5	10	850
Kettle Cuisine, Chicken Vegetable Soup with Rice									
1 cup	100	2.5	1	20	12	2	2	9	630
Kettle Cuisine, Chipotle Sweet Potato Soup									
1 cup	150	7	1	0	20	3	7	2	610
Kettle Cuisine, Coconut Curry Chicken Soup									
1 cup	300	10	7	25	40	4	2	12	500
Kettle Cuisine, Loaded Potato Soup									
1 cup	280	16	10	55	22	2	2	14	650
Kettle Cuisine, Manhattan Clam Chowder									
1 cup	130	3	0	20	17	2	4	10	690
Kettle Cuisine, Roasted Vegetable Soup									
1 cup	190	11	1.5	0	22	4	3	3	750
Kettle Cuisine, Three Bean Chili									
1 cup	190	3	0.5	0	31	11	10	9	380
Kettle Cuisine, Tomato Basil Soup									
1 cup	100	4	0.5	5	14	3	7	4	860

Food Serving size	Cal.	(g) Total Fat	(g) Sat. Fat	(mg) Chol.	(g) Carb.	(g) Fiber	(g) Sug.	(g) Prot.	(mg) Sod.
Kettle Cuisine, Tomato Soup with Garden Vegetables									
1 cup	100	3.5	0.5	0	15	5	7	3	670
Kettle Cuisine, Turkey Chili with Beans									
1 cup	200	4	1	60	22	7	7	19	630
Kettle Cuisine, White Chicken Chili with Cilantro									
1 cup	310	14	5	65	24	5	3	22	710
Kettle Cuisine, Yellow Pea Soup with Roasted Red Peppers									
1 cup	240	6	0.5	0	36	15	4	11	460
Kitchen Basics, Original Beef Cooking Stock									
1 cup, 245g	20	0	0	0	1	0	0	5	430
Kitchen Basics, Original Chicken Cooking Stock									
1 cup, 245g	20	0	0	0	1	0	0	5	430
Kitchen Basics, Original Clam Cooking Stock									
1 cup, 245g	20	0	0	0	1	0	0	3	600
Kitchen Basics, Original Ham Cooking Stock									
1 cup, 245g	20	0	0	0	1	0	0	3	480
Kitchen Basics, Original Pork Cooking Stock									
1 cup, 245g	20	0	0	0	1	0	0	3	480
Kitchen Basics, Original Seafood Cooking Stock									
1 cup, 245g	10	0	0	0	0	0	1	2	480
Kitchen Basics, Original Turkey Cooking Stock									
1 cup, 245g	20	0	0	0	2	0	1	3	430
Kitchen Basics, Original Veal Cooking Stock									
1 cup, 245g	20	0	0	0	3	0	0	3	480
Kitchen Basics, Unsalted Beef Cooking Stock									
1 cup, 245g	20	0	0	0	1	0	0	5	190
Kitchen Basics, Unsalted Chicken Cooking Stock									
1 cup, 245g	20	0	0	0	1	0	0	5	150
Kitchen Basics, Unsalted Vegetable Cooking Stock									
1 cup, 245g	20	0	0	0	4	0	2	0	240
Pacific Natural Foods, All Natural Chipotle Sweet Potato Soup									
1 cup	220	4	2	15	40	3	3	4	730
Pacific Natural Foods, All Natural Rosemary Potato Chowder									
1 cup	230	8	5	30	36	2	0	1	730

Food Serving size	Cal.	(g) Total Fat	(g) Sat. Fat	(mg) Chol.	(g) Carb.	(g) Fiber	(g) Sug.	(g) Prot.	(mg) Sod.
Pacific Natural Foods, All Natural Thai Sweet Potato Soup									
1 cup	160	6	4	0	25	3	3	3	660
Pacific Natural Foods, Cashew Carrot Ginger Soup									
8 fl oz	120	5	3.5	0	19	3	8	1	650
Pacific Natural Foods, Curried Red Lentil Soup									
8 fl oz	140	5	3.5	0	20	5	8	5	720
Pacific Natural Foods, Natural Beef Broth									
8 fl oz	20	0	NA	NA	1	NA	NA	4	570
Pacific Natural Foods, Organic Beef Broth									
8 fl oz	20	1	0	5	1	0	1	2	570
Pacific Natural Foods, Organic Butternut Squash Bisque									
1 cup	110	3.5	1.5	10	18	4	5	2	510
Pacific Natural Foods, Organic Chicken and Wild Rice Soup									
1 cup	220	4	1	10	13	2	1	5	660
Pacific Natural Foods, Organic Cream of Chicken Condensed Soup									
1/2 cup	90	3.5	2	15	10	NA	NA	4	850
Pacific Natural Foods, Organic Cream of Mushroom Condensed Soup									
1/2 cup	100	2.5	1.5	10	18	1	2.9	2	740
Pacific Natural Foods, Organic Creamy Butternut Squash Soup									
8 fl oz	90	2	0	0	17	3	4	2	550
Pacific Natural Foods, Organic Creamy Tomato Soup									
8 fl oz	100	2	1.5	10	16	1	12	5	750
Pacific Natural Foods, Organic Free Range Chicken Broth									
8 fl oz	10	0	0	0	1	0	1	1	570
Pacific Natural Foods, Organic Free Range Low Sodium Chicken Broth									
8 fl oz	15	0	0	0	1	0	0	2	70
Pacific Natural Foods, Organic French Onion Soup									
8 fl oz	30	1	0.5	0	5	0	3	1	720
Pacific Natural Foods, Organic Hearty Tomato Bisque									
1 cup	150	9	5	30	17	2	10	2	750
Pacific Natural Foods, Organic Light Sodium Creamy Butternut Squash Soup									
8 fl oz	90	2	0	0	17	3	4	2	280
Pacific Natural Foods, Organic Light Sodium Creamy Tomato Soup									
8 fl oz	100	2	1.5	10	16	1	12	5	380

Food Serving size	Cal.	(g) Total Fat	(g) Sat. Fat	(mg) Chol.	(g) Carb.	(g) Fiber	(g) Sug.	(g) Prot.	(mg) Sod.
Pacific Natural Foods, Organic Light Sodium Roasted Red Pepper & Tomato Soup									
8 fl oz	110	0	1.5	10	16	1	12	5	360
Pacific Natural Foods, Organic Low Sodium Vegetable Broth									
8 fl oz	15	0	0	0	3	1	2	0	530
Pacific Natural Foods, Organic Mushroom Broth									
8 fl oz	5	0	0	0	1	0	0	0	530
Pacific Natural Foods, Organic Roasted Red Pepper & Tomato Bisque									
1 cup	110	2	1.5	10	16	1	12	5	720
Pacific Natural Foods, Organic Roasted Red Pepper & Tomato Soup									
8 fl oz	110	2	1.5	10	16	1	12	5	720
Pacific Natural Foods, Organic Savory Chicken & Wild Rice Canned Soup									
1 cup	110	4	1	10	13	2	1	5	660
Pacific Natural Foods, Organic Vegetable Broth									
8 fl oz	15	0	0	0	3	1	2	0	530
Pacific Natural Foods, Spicy Black Bean Soup									
1 cup	80	1	0	0	14	4	3	4	590
Progresso, Beef Flavored Broth									
1 cup	20	0	0	0	3	NA	1	1	850
Progresso, Gluten Free Chicken Flavored Broth									
1 cup	20	0	0	0	1	0	1	3	850
Progresso, Gluten Free Soup, High Fiber Chicken Tuscany									
1 cup	130	3	1.5	15	20	7	2	9	690
Progresso, Gluten Free Soup, Reduced Sodium Garden Vegetable									
1 cup	100	0	0	0	22	3	4	3	450
Progresso, Gluten Free Soup, Rich and Hearty Chicken Corn Chowder									
1 cup	200	9	2	15	23	2	6	7	890
Progresso, Gluten Free Soup, Rich and Hearty New England Clam Chowder									
1 cup	180	8	2	15	22	2	2	5	860
Progresso, Gluten Free Soup, Traditional, 99% Fat Free New England Clam Chowder									
1 cup	110	1.5	0	5	21	2	2	5	810
Progresso, Gluten Free Soup, Traditional, Chicken Cheese Enchilada									
1 cup	170	11	3.5	25	9	1	2	8	890

Food Serving size	Cal.	(g) Total Fat	(g) Sat. Fat	(mg) Chol.	(g) Carb.	(g) Fiber	(g) Sug.	(g) Prot.	(mg) Sod.
Progresso, Gluten Free Soup, Traditional, Manhattan Clam Chowder									
1 cup	100	2	0	5	17	2	4	3	690
Progresso, Gluten Free Soup, Traditional, New England Clam Chowder									
1 cup	180	8	2	15	20	1	2	6	890
Progresso, Gluten Free Soup, Traditional, Potato, Broccoli & Cheese Chowder									
1 cup	210	12	3.5	15	20	2	2	5	860
Progresso, Gluten Free Soup, Traditional, Southwestern-Style Chicken									
1 cup	110	2	0.5	10	18	2	2	6	690
Progresso, Gluten Free Soup, Traditional, Split Pea with Ham									
1 cup	140	1	0	5	24	4	3	9	690
Progresso, Gluten Free Soup, Vegetable Classics, 99% Fat Free Lentil									
1 cup	140	1.5	0	0	25	3	1	8	500
Progresso, Gluten Free Soup, Vegetable Classics, Creamy Mushroom									
230g	150	10	2.5	<5	11	<1	2	2	830
Progresso, Gluten Free Soup, Vegetable Classics, French Onion									
1 cup	50	1	0	0	9	1	3	2	690
Progresso, Gluten Free Soup, Vegetable Classics, Garden Vegetable									
1 cup	90	0	0	0	20	3	4	3	690
Progresso, Gluten Free Soup, Vegetable Classics, Hearty Black Bean, flavored with Bacon									
1 cup	160	1	0.5	<5mg	29	8	3	8	690
Progresso, Gluten Free Soup, Vegetable Classics, Lentil									
1 cup	160	2	0.5	0	30	5	2	9	810
Progresso, High Fiber, Chicken Tuscany Soup									
1 serving	130	3	1.5	15	20	7	2	9	690
Progresso, Reduced Sodium, Chicken Broth									
1 cup	20	0	0	0	2	NA	1	3	560
Progresso, Reduced Sodium, Garden Vegetable Soup									
1 serving	100	0	0	0	22	3	4	3	450
Progresso, Rich & Hearty, Chicken Corn Chowder Soup									
1 serving	200	9	2	15	23	2	6	7	890
Progresso, Rich & Hearty, New England Clam Chowder Soup									
1 serving	180	8	2	15	22	2	2	5	860

Food Serving size	Cal.	(g) Total Fat	(g) Sat. Fat	(mg) Chol.	(g) Carb.	(g) Fiber	(g) Sug.	(g) Prot.	(mg) Sod.
Progresso, Traditional, 99% Fat Free, New England Clam Chowder Soup									
1 serving	110	1.5	0	5	21	2	2	5	810
Progresso, Traditional, Chicken Cheese Enchilada Soup									
1 serving	170	11	3.5	25	9	1	2	8	890
Progresso, Traditional, Chicken Rice with Vegetables Soup									
1 serving	90	2	0.5	10	14	1	1	5	640
Progresso, Traditional, Manhattan Clam Chowder Soup									
1 serving	100	2	0	5	17	2	4	3	690
Progresso, Traditional, New England Clam Chowder Soup									
1 serving	180	8	2	15	20	1	2	6	890
Progresso, Traditional, Potato Broccoli & Cheese Chowder Soup									
1 serving	210	12	3.5	15	20	2	2	5	860
Progresso, Traditional, Southwestern Style Chicken Soup									
1 serving	110	2	0.5	10	18	2	2	6	690
Progresso, Vegetable Classics, Creamy Mushroom Soup									
1 serving	150	10	2.5	<5	11	<1	2	2	830
Progresso, Vegetable Classics, French Onion Soup									
1 serving	50	1	0	0	9	1	3	2	690
Progresso, Vegetable Classics, Garden Vegetable Soup									
1 serving	90	0	0	0	20	3	4	3	690
Progresso, Vegetable Classics, Hearty Black Bean Soup									
1 serving	160	1	0.5	<5	29	8	3	8	690
Progresso, Vegetable Classics, Lentil 99% Fat Free Soup									
1 serving	140	1.5	0	0	25	3	1	8	500
Progresso, Vegetable Classics, Lentil Soup									
1 serving	160	2	0.5	0	30	5	2	9	810
Savory Choice, Beef Broth Concentrate									
1 pouch	15	1	0.5	0	1	NA	NA	1	770
Savory Choice, Beef Demi Glace (Sleeved Pouch)									
2 tbsp	50	1.5	NA	5	9	0	3	1	380
Savory Choice, Chicken Broth Concentrate									
1 pouch	15	1	0.5	0	1	NA	NA	1	770
Savory Choice, Reduced Sodium, Chicken Broth Concentrate									
1 pouch	25	1	0.5	0	3	NA	NA	1	360

Food Serving size	Cal.	(g) Total Fat	(g) Sat. Fat	(mg) Chol.	(g) Carb.	(g) Fiber	(g) Sug.	(g) Prot.	(mg) Sod.
Savory Choice, Reduced Sodium, Vegetable Broth Concentrate									
1 pouch	20	0	0	0	4	NA	NA	1	360
Savory Choice, Turkey Broth Concentrate									
1 cup	15	1	0.5	0	1	NA	NA	1	770
Swanson, Beef Stock									
1 cup	30	0	0	0	3	0	3	4	500
Swanson, Chicken Broth									
1 cup	10	0.5	0	5	1	0	1	1	860
Swanson, Chicken Broth, Regular									
1 cup	10	1	0	5	1	1	1	1	860
Swanson, Chicken Stock									
1 cup	20	0	0	0	1	0	1	4	510
Swanson, Natural Goodness, Chicken Broth									
1 cup	15	0	0	0	1	0	1	2	570
Swanson, Natural Goodness, Chicken Broth									
1 cup	15	0	0	0	1	0	1	3	570
Swanson, Vegetable Broth									
1 cup	0.5	0	0	0	3	0	0	0	880
Thai Kitchen, Cocunut Ginger Soup									
7 oz	230	16	7.9	0	14.1	3	10.1	5.9	940
Thai Kitchen, Garlic & Vegetable Instant Rice Noodle Soup									
1 package	190	3	0.05	0	37	1	3	3	740
Thai Kitchen, Hot & Sour Rice Noodle Soup Bowl									
1/2 bowl	120	2.5	0	0	23	0.7	2	2	940
Thai Kitchen, Hot & Sour Soup									
7 oz	45	1	0	<5	8	1	4	1	1070
Thai Kitchen, Lemongrass & Chili, Instant Rice Noodle Soup									
1 cup	115	1.5	0.2	0	24	NA	1	2	700
Thai Kitchen, Lemongrass & Chili, Rice Noodle Soup Bowl									
1 bowl	250	4	1	0	50	1	3	4	1600
Thai Kitchen, Mushroom Rice, Noodle Soup Bowl									
1 bowl	250	3	0	0	52	1	3	5	1510
Thai Kitchen, Roasted Garlic, Rice Noodle Soup Bowl									
1 bowl	250	3	0.5	0	49	1	3	5	1170

Food Serving size	Cal.	(g) Total Fat	(g) Sat. Fat	(mg) Chol.	(g) Carb.	(g) Fiber	(g) Sug.	(g) Prot.	(mg) Sod.
Thai Kitchen, Spring Onion, Instant Rice Noodle Soup									
1.6 oz	190	3	0.5	0	37	1	3	3	730
Thai Kitchen, Spring Onion, Rice Noodle Soup Bowl									
1 bowl	250	2.5	0.5	0	50	1	3	5	1120
Thai Kitchen, Thai Ginger, Instant Rice Noodle Soup									
1 package	190	3.5	1	0	37	1	2	3	760
Thai Kitchen, Thai Ginger, Rice Noodle Soup Bowl									
1 package	170	3	1	0	33	1	1	3	950
The Really Great Food Company, Golden Pea Soup, Dry Mix									
3/4 cup	220	1	0	0	39	5	5	15	500
The Really Great Food Company, Spilt Pea Soup, Dry Mix									
3/4 cup	220	1	0	0	40	16	6	16	500
The Really Great Food Company, Sweet Corn Chowder, Dry Mix									
2/3 cup	190	1	0	0	35	5	7	13	470

Baby Foods / Formulas

Feeding Infants, Toddlers, and Children

Good nutrition is a must to support the rapid growth and development your baby will undergo in the first two years of life. Providing the right foods during this critical time will support good health and encourage enjoyment of new tastes and textures as they grow, as well as build the beginning of healthy eating habits. Use this information to help raise healthy and happy children.

Should I Start My Baby Off Gluten-Free?

Many parents worry about their babies and gluten, especially if the family has a history of celiac disease or gluten intolerance. This is a topic you should discuss with your pediatrician. There is some research that supports introducing gluten around 8 months of age and others recommend waiting until 1 to 2 years of age. The best choice for your baby is breast feeding and then introducing solid foods as recommended by your pediatrician. The guidelines and information given here are only provided as general advice. If your baby has been diagnosed with celiac disease, here are some brands that provide gluten-free products.

Baby Food Brands that provide Gluten-Free options

Beech-Nut	Ella's Kitchen	Meijer
Bright Beginnings	Gerber	Nature's Goodness
Earth's Best	Homemade Baby	O Organics (Safeway)

Baby Formula that is Gluten-Free

Bright Beginnings	Hy-Vee	Nutramigen	Similac
Earth's Best	Neocate	Pregestimil	
Enfamil	Nestle Good Start	Publix	

What Is a Healthy Diet for Your Baby, Toddler, and Child?

Here are the daily estimated calories and recommended servings of each of the major food groups for infants and children from birth to age 8. Calorie estimates are based on a moderately active child. Food portions are assumed to be nutrient-dense.

	0 to 6 months	6 months to 1 year	1 to 2 years	2 to 3 years	4 to 8 years
Calories	Variable	Variable	Variable	1,000 to 1,400	1,400 to 1,600
Milk/Dairy	18 to 45 oz (breast milk or formula)	24 to 32 oz (breast milk or formula)	24 to 32 oz (breast milk or formula) or 2 cups whole milk	2 to 2.5 cups whole milk	2.5 to 3 cups (can switch to low-fat milk)
Lean Meat/Beans	None	Begin to offer well cooked, soft, finely cut or pureed meats or cheese.	1 to 2 oz soft, finely cut meats or other protein foods	2 to 3 oz lean meat, poultry, or seafood; 1 egg; 1 tbsp peanut butter	3 to 4 oz lean meat, poultry, or seafood; 1 egg; 1 tbsp peanut butter
Fruits	None	2 to 4 oz 100% juice; begin to offer plain cooked, mashed, or strained baby food.	2 to 4 oz 100% juice or 1 cup fruit	1 cup 100% juice or 1 cup fruit	1.5 cups 100% juice or 1 cup fruit
Vegetables	None	Begin to offer plain cooked, mashed, or strained baby food.	1 cup raw or cooked	1 cup raw or cooked	1.5 cups raw or cooked
Gluten-Free Grains	None	2 to 6 tbsp iron-fortified baby cereal or other soft breads, cereals, etc.	2 oz (1 oz = 1 slice whole grain bread; ½ cup cooked cereal, rice, or pasta; 1 cup dry cereal)	3 oz (1 oz = 1 slice whole grain bread; ½ cup cooked cereal, rice, or pasta; 1 cup dry cereal)	4 to 5 oz (1 oz = 1 slice whole grain bread; ½ cup cooked cereal, rice, or pasta; 1 cup dry cereal)
Oils (g)	None	NA	NA	15 to 17 g	17 to 22 g

Adapted from 2010 US Dietary Guidelines, Appendix 7; Start Healthy Feeding Guidelines, the American Dietetic Association; and Feeding Recommendations (American Academy of Pediatrics).

Why Are Nutrition Facts for Children Different?

Because young children have unique nutritional needs for their growing bodies yet require fewer calories than the 2,000 that the regular Nutrition Facts labels are based on, the Nutrition Facts for children's foods and beverages are different. First, foods specifically for children less than 4 years do not provide % Daily Values for the macronutrients carbohydrates and fats, as well as sodium, fiber, cholesterol, saturated fat, and trans fat. Since protein is an important nutrient for growing children, a % Daily Value is provided along with % Daily Values for vitamins A and C, calcium, and iron. Unfortunately, the % Daily Values are based on a 2,000 calorie diet and are not specific to the needs of children. Also, food labels for children less than 2 years of age do not present information on calories from fat nor do they include amounts for saturated fat, polyunsaturated fat, monounsaturated fat, and cholesterol. Because fat is essential to growth, it should not be restricted during these early years. In addition, serving sizes for infant foods are based on average amounts that infants under two years usually eat.

Fruit desserts for children less than 2 years old

Nutrition Facts
Serving Size 1 jar (140g)

Amount Per Serving

Calories 110

Total Fat	0g
Trans Fat	0g
Sodium	10mg
Total Carbohydrate	27g
Dietary Fiber	4g
Sugars	0g
Protein	0g

% Daily Value

Protein 0%	•	Vitamin A 6%
Vitamin C 45%	•	Calcium 2%
Iron 2%		

Fruit desserts for children ages 2 years to 4 years

Nutrition Facts
Serving Size 1 jar (140g)

Amount Per Serving

Calories 110	Calories from Fat 0

Total Fat	0g
Saturated Fat	0g
Trans Fat	0g
Cholesterol	0mg
Sodium	10mg
Total Carbohydrate	27g
Dietary Fiber	4g
Sugars	0g
Protein	0g

% Daily Value

Protein 0%	•	Vitamin A 6%
Vitamin C 45%	•	Calcium 2%
Iron 2%		

How Do the Food Label Reference Values (Daily Values) Compare to the Nutritional Recommendations for Children (DRIs)?

Nutrient	Daily Value	2 to 3 years	4 to 8 years
Protein (grams)	50	13	19
Iron (mg)	18	7	10
Calcium (mg)	1000	700	1000
Vitamin A (IU)	5000	1000	1333
Vitamin C (mg)	60	15	25

Sources: 2010 Dietary Guidelines and IOM Dietary Reference Intakes 2006 and 2010.

Tips for Raising Healthy Children

1. **Offer a variety of healthy foods.** When children eat a variety of foods, they get the nutrients they need from every food group. They will be more likely to try new foods and to like more foods. This will make it easier to plan family meals.

2. **Start with small portions.** Offer children small, easy-to-eat amounts to make eating easy and more enjoyable. Use smaller bowls, plates, and utensils for your child to eat with. Don't insist that children finish all the food on their plate. Let your child know it is okay to only eat as much as he or she wants. We are born with an internal mechanism that signals when we are full—don't mess with it.

3. **Follow a meal and snack schedule.** Regularly scheduled meal and snack times help your child learn structure for eating. Your child is more likely to eat healthy meals and try new foods if snacks are not offered too close to mealtime.

4. **Make mealtime an enjoyable family time.** Family meals allow your child to focus on the task of eating and give you a chance to model good behaviors. You may not be able to eat together all the time, but try to plan a family meal at least once a day. It takes a little work to bring everyone together for meals, but it's worth it. Involve your child in conversation. Ask questions like:

   - What made you feel really happy today?
   - What did you have to eat at lunch today?

- What's your favorite veggie? Why?
- Tell me one thing you learned today?
- What made you laugh today?

5. **Make food fun for picky eaters.** Picky eating is temporary, so don't get discouraged. Get your child involved in planning, shopping for, and preparing the food. Let them create snacks, salads, or desserts. Be creative with the food—try fun and interesting food shapes.

6. **Set a good example.** Your child picks up all of your attitudes and behaviors—including your eating habits. Children love to copy what their parents do. They are likely to mimic your table manners, your likes and dislikes, your willingness to try new foods, and your physical activities.

Food Serving size	Cal.	(g) Total Fat	(g) Sat. Fat	(mg) Chol.	(g) Carb.	(g) Fiber	(g) Sug.	(g) Prot.	(mg) Sod.
Baby Foods / Baby Formulas									
Beech-Nut, Apple Juice 4 fl oz	60	0	NA	NA	14	0	13	0	5
Beech-Nut, Apple, Mango & Carrot 1 jar	80	0	NA	NA	20	1	14	0	10
Beech-Nut, Apple, Mango & Carrot Puree 1 pouch	70	0	0	0	18	1	12	0	10
Beech-Nut, Apple, Peach & Strawberry Puree 1 pouch	80	0	0	0	18	2	13	0	5
Beech-Nut, Apple, Sweet Potato & Pineapple Puree 1 pouch	90	0	0	0	20	1	14	0	10
Beech-Nut, Apples & Bananas 1 jar	70	0	NA	NA	17	1	13	0	5
Beech-Nut, Apples & Blueberries 1 jar	75	0	NA	NA	18	1	14	0	5
Beech-Nut, Apples & Cherries 1 jar	70	0	NA	NA	17	1	14	0	5
Beech-Nut, Apples & Chicken 1 jar	70	1	NA	NA	13	2	10	1	10
Beech-Nut, Apples, Mango & Kiwi 1 jar	100	0	NA	NA	23	2	16	0	0
Beech-Nut, Apples, Pears & Bananas 1 jar	90	0	NA	NA	21	2	17	0	5
Beech-Nut, Applesauce (Stage 1) 1 jar	45	0	NA	NA	12	1	9	0	0
Beech-Nut, Applesauce (Stage 2 1/2) 1 jar	50	0	NA	NA	12	1	8	0	0
Beech-Nut, Applesauce (Stage 2) 1 jar	70	0	NA	NA	18	1	15	0	5
Beech-Nut, Apricots with Pears & Apples (Stage 2) 1 jar	110	0	NA	NA	26	4	19	0	10
Beech-Nut, Banana Apple Yogurt 1 jar	100	1	NA	NA	22	1	13	1	15

Food Serving size	Cal.	(g) Total Fat	(g) Sat. Fat	(mg) Chol.	(g) Carb.	(g) Fiber	(g) Sug.	(g) Prot.	(mg) Sod.
Beech-Nut, Banana, Apple & Strawberry Puree									
1 pouch	90	0.5	0	0	20	2	17	0	10
Beech-Nut, Banana, Mixed Berries									
1 jar	70	0	NA	NA	18	1	13	1	5
Beech-Nut, Banana, Pear & Sweet Potato Puree									
1 pouch	80	0	NA	NA	19	1	14	0	5
Beech-Nut, Beef & Beef Broth									
1 jar	70	4	NA	NA	0	0	0	9	40
Beech-Nut, Carrots									
1 jar	30	0	NA	NA	7	2	4	0	25
Beech-Nut, Chicken & Chicken Broth									
1 jar	50	1.5	NA	NA	0	0	0	8	60
Beech-Nut, Chicken & Rice Dinner									
1 jar	45	0	NA	NA	8	1	5	2	25
Beech-Nut, Chiquita Bananas & Strawberries									
1 jar	100	0	NA	NA	23	1	19	1	0
Beech-Nut, Chiquita Bananas (Stage 1)									
1 jar	60	0	NA	NA	15	<1	11	0	0
Beech-Nut, Chiquita Bananas (Stage 2)									
1 jar	100	0	NA	NA	23	1	18	1	5
Beech-Nut, Corn & Sweet Potatoes									
1 jar	100	0	NA	NA	22	1	8	1	10
Beech-Nut, Country Garden Vegetables									
1 jar	45	0	NA	NA	10	2	2	2	10
Beech-Nut, Creamy Chicken Noodle Dinner									
1 jar	60	1.5	NA	NA	10	1	4	3	25
Beech-Nut, Green Beans									
1 jar	35	0	NA	NA	7	2	2	1	0
Beech-Nut, Ham, Pineapple & Rice									
1 jar	110	0.5	NA	NA	24	3	11	1	5
Beech-Nut, Hearty Vegetable Stew									
1 jar	90	1.5	NA	NA	17	2	3	3	20
Beech-Nut, Homestyle Apples & Bananas									
1 jar	110	0	NA	NA	27	2	18	0	5

Food Serving size	Cal.	(g) Total Fat	(g) Sat. Fat	(mg) Chol.	(g) Carb.	(g) Fiber	(g) Sug.	(g) Prot.	(mg) Sod.
Beech-Nut, Homestyle Chiquita Bananas									
1 jar	160	0	NA	NA	36	2	33	2	10
Beech-Nut, Homestyle Green Beans & Potatoes									
1 jar	70	0	NA	NA	14	4	4	3	5
Beech-Nut, Homestyle Green Beans, Corn & Rice									
1 jar	130	1	NA	NA	28	3	6	3	5
Beech-Nut, Homestyle Peaches, Apples & Bananas									
1 jar	160	0	NA	NA	38	3	31	1	10
Beech-Nut, Homestyle Pears & Blueberries									
1 jar	170	0	NA	NA	41	8	31	1	10
Beech-Nut, Homestyle Rice Cereal & Pears									
1 jar	140	0	NA	NA	32	5	19	1	5
Beech-Nut, Homestyle Squash & Zucchini									
1 jar	60	0	NA	NA	14	1	3	1	5
Beech-Nut, Homestyle Sweet Corn & Rice									
1 jar	160	2	NA	NA	33	3	10	2	10
Beech-Nut, Homestyle Sweet Potatoes									
1 jar	160	0	NA	NA	38	3	15	2	15
Beech-Nut, Homestyle Turkey Rice Dinner									
1 jar	80	1.5	NA	NA	14	1	11	3	20
Beech-Nut, Homestyle Vegetable Medley with Turkey									
1 jar	100	1.5	NA	NA	18	1	5	4	35
Beech-Nut, Homestyle Vegetables & Chicken									
1 jar	100	0.5	NA	NA	18	2	5	4	35
Beech-Nut, Macaroni & Beef with Vegetables									
1 jar	90	5	NA	NA	9	1	3	2	30
Beech-Nut, Mango									
1 jar	100	0.5	NA	NA	22	1	15	<1	0
Beech-Nut, Mixed Fruit Nibbles									
1 pouch	80	0	NA	NA	18	<1	17	0	20
Beech-Nut, Mixed Vegetables									
1 jar	45	0	NA	NA	8	2	4	1	25
Beech-Nut, Peach, Apple & Banana Puree									
1 pouch	90	0	0	0	22	2	17	0	5

Food Serving size	Cal.	(g) Total Fat	(g) Sat. Fat	(mg) Chol.	(g) Carb.	(g) Fiber	(g) Sug.	(g) Prot.	(mg) Sod.
Beech-Nut, Peaches (Stage 1)									
1 jar	45	0	NA	NA	11	1	9	0	0
Beech-Nut, Peaches (Stage 2)									
1 jar	70	0	NA	NA	18	2	14	0	0
Beech-Nut, Pear, Banana & Raspberry Puree									
1 pouch	70	0	NA	NA	16	2	12	0	5
Beech-Nut, Pear, Mango & Squash Puree									
1 pouch	70	0	0	0	17	2	11	1	5
Beech-Nut, Pears & Green Beans									
1 jar	90	0	NA	NA	21	3	14	1	5
Beech-Nut, Pears & Pineapple									
1 jar	120	0	NA	NA	29	6	22	1	10
Beech-Nut, Pears & Raspberries									
1 jar	130	0	NA	NA	30	6	23	1	10
Beech-Nut, Pears (Stage 1)									
1 jar	40	0	NA	NA	10	1	8	0	0
Beech-Nut, Pears (Stage 2 1/2)									
1 jar	90	0	NA	NA	22	3	15	0	5
Beech-Nut, Pears (Stage 2)									
1 jar	90	0	NA	NA	22	4	17	0	0
Beech-Nut, Peas & Carrots									
1 jar	60	0	NA	NA	12	4	1	3	5
Beech-Nut, Rice Cereal									
15g	50	0	NA	NA	12	NA	0	1	5
Beech-Nut, Rice Cereal & Apples with Cinnamon									
1 jar	90	0	NA	NA	23	1	12	0	5
Beech-Nut, Rice with Chiquita Bananas									
15g	60	0	NA	NA	12	0	2	1	0
Beech-Nut, Spring Water with Added Fluoride									
4 fl oz	0	0	NA	NA	0	NA	NA	0	0
Beech-Nut, Squash & Apples									
1 jar	60	0.5	NA	NA	12	1	2	2	5
Beech-Nut, Squash (Stage 1)									
1 jar	30	0	NA	NA	6	1	2	0	0

Food Serving size	Cal.	(g) Total Fat	(g) Sat. Fat	(mg) Chol.	(g) Carb.	(g) Fiber	(g) Sug.	(g) Prot.	(mg) Sod.
Beech-Nut, Squash (Stage 2) 1 jar	50	0	NA	NA	10	1	5	0	10
Beech-Nut, Strawberry Fruit Nibbles 1 pouch	80	0	NA	NA	18	0	17	0	20
Beech-Nut, Sweet Corn Casserole 1 jar	80	0	NA	NA	16	1	7	1	0
Beech-Nut, Sweet Potato & Turkey 1 jar	120	1	NA	NA	24	1	10	3	15
Beech-Nut, Sweet Potato & Zucchini 1 jar	60	0	NA	NA	13	1	9	1	0
Beech-Nut, Sweet Potatoes & Apples 1 jar	90	0	NA	NA	21	1	10	1	10
Beech-Nut, Sweet Potatoes & Chicken 1 jar	100	1	NA	NA	21	1	8	2	15
Beech-Nut, Tender Golden Sweet Potatoes (Stage 1) 1 jar	60	0	NA	NA	14	1	7	1	5
Beech-Nut, Tender Golden Sweet Potatoes (Stage 2) 1 jar	100	0	NA	NA	23	1	9	1	10
Beech-Nut, Tender Sweet Carrots (Stage 1) 1 jar	25	0	NA	NA	5	1	3	0	20
Beech-Nut, Tender Sweet Carrots (Stage 2) 1 jar	40	0	NA	NA	8	2	5	0	30
Beech-Nut, Tender Sweet Peas (Stage 1) 1 jar	40	0	NA	NA	7	2	3	2	0
Beech-Nut, Tender Sweet Peas (Stage 2) 1 jar	60	0	NA	NA	12	2	4	4	5
Beech-Nut, Tender Young Green Beans (Stage 1) 1 jar	30	0	NA	NA	6	2	2	1	0
Beech-Nut, Tender Young Green Beans (Stage 2) 1 jar	50	0	NA	NA	9	2	3	1	0
Beech-Nut, Turkey and Turkey Broth 1 jar	70	4	NA	NA	0	0	0	8	60
Beech-Nut, Turkey Rice Dinner 1 jar	100	1	NA	NA	21	1	6	2	15

Food Serving size	Cal.	(g) Total Fat	(g) Sat. Fat	(mg) Chol.	(g) Carb.	(g) Fiber	(g) Sug.	(g) Prot.	(mg) Sod.
Beech-Nut, Turkey Tetrazzini									
1 jar	110	2	NA	NA	20	1	9	4	100
Beech-Nut, Turkey Vegetable									
1 tray	130	6	NA	NA	14	NA	2	5	170
Beech-Nut, Vegetable Beef									
1 tub	120	2.5	NA	NA	18	NA	2	6	180
Beech-Nut, Vegetables & Chicken									
1 jar	50	1	NA	NA	9	1	3	2	20
Beech-Nut, White Cheddar Puffed Grain Baked Snacks									
17 pieces	30	1.5	NA	NA	5	NA	0	0	10
Beech-Nut, White Grape Juice									
4 fl oz	80	0	NA	NA	20	0	16	0	10
Bright Beginnings, Gentle, Infant Formula									
1 serving	100	5.3	NA	NA	10.8	NA	NA	2.3	NA
Bright Beginnings, Organic Formula									
1 serving	100	5.3	NA	NA	10.6	NA	NA	2.2	NA
Bright Beginnings, Premium Infant Triple Benefit Formula									
1 serving	100	5.3	NA	NA	11	NA	NA	2.1	NA
Bright Beginnings, Soy Infant Formula									
1 serving	100	5.3	NA	NA	10.6	NA	NA	2.5	NA
Bright Beginnings, Soy Pediatric Drink									
1 can (8 fl oz)	240	12	3	0	26	3	18	7	90
Ella's Kitchen, Baby Brekkie, Banana Baby Brekkie									
1 portion (3.5 oz)	130	1.5	NA	NA	25	2	12	3	0
Ella's Kitchen, Baby Brekkie, Blueberry & Pear Baby Brekkie									
1 portion (3.5 oz)	95	1	NA	NA	20	2	8	2	0
Ella's Kitchen, Baby Brekkie, Mango Baby Brekkie									
1 portion (3.5 oz)	110	2	NA	NA	20	<1	12	3	0
Ella's Kitchen, Baby Brekkie, Raisin & Prune Baby Brekkie									
1 portion (3.5 oz)	140	2	NA	NA	25	2	19	4	0
Ella's Kitchen, Ella's 1, Apples & Bananas									
1 portion (3.5 oz)	80	0	NA	NA	19	1	14	1	0
Ella's Kitchen, Ella's 1, Broccoli, Pears & Peas									
1 portion (3.5 oz)	60	0	NA	NA	14	2	7	1	20

Food Serving size	Cal.	(g) Total Fat	(g) Sat. Fat	(mg) Chol.	(g) Carb.	(g) Fiber	(g) Sug.	(g) Prot.	(mg) Sod.
Ella's Kitchen, Ella's 1, Butternut Squash, Carrots, Apples & Prunes									
1 portion (3.5 oz)	70	0	NA	NA	17	3	10	1	15
Ella's Kitchen, Ella's 1, Carrots, Apples & Parsnips									
1 portion (3.5 oz)	50	0	NA	NA	12	2	9	0	10
Ella's Kitchen, Ella's 1, Peaches & Bananas									
1 portion (3.5 oz)	60	0	NA	NA	13	1	11	1	0
Ella's Kitchen, Ella's 1, Spinach, Apples & Rutabagas									
1 portion (3.5 oz)	45	0	NA	NA	10	2	6	1	75
Ella's Kitchen, Ella's 1, Strawberries & Apples									
1 portion (3.5 oz)	50	0	NA	NA	13	1	10	0	0
Ella's Kitchen, Ella's 1, Sweet Potatoes, Pumpkin, Apples & Blueberries									
1 portion (3.5 oz)	60	0	NA	NA	14	1	8	1	5
Ella's Kitchen, First Tastes, Apples Apples Apples									
1 portion (2.5 oz)	30	0	NA	NA	8	1	7	<1	0
Ella's Kitchen, First Tastes, Bananas Bananas Bananas									
1 portion (2.5 oz)	65	0	NA	NA	16	2	14	1	0
Ella's Kitchen, First Tastes, Mangoes Mangoes Mangoes									
1 portion (2.5 oz)	40	0	NA	NA	10	2	8	<1	0
Ella's Kitchen, First Tastes, Pears Pears Pears									
1 portion (2.5 oz)	30	0	NA	NA	10	2	8	<1	0
Ella's Kitchen, Fruit + Baby Rice, Bananas, Apricots & Baby Rice									
1 portion (3.5 oz)	90	0	NA	NA	22	2	17	1	5
Ella's Kitchen, Fruit + Baby Rice, Pears, Apples & Baby Rice									
1 portion (3.5 oz)	60	0	NA	NA	12	2	10	1	0
Ella's Kitchen, Smoothie Fruits, The Green One									
1 portion (3 oz)	60	0	NA	NA	14	1	8	0	0
Ella's Kitchen, Smoothie Fruits, The Purple One									
1 portion (3 oz)	70	0	NA	NA	16	1	11	1	0
Ella's Kitchen, Smoothie Fruits, The Red One									
1 portion (3 oz)	60	0	NA	NA	13	1	11	1	0
Ella's Kitchen, Smoothie Fruits, The Yellow One									
1 portion (3 oz)	70	0	NA	NA	16	2	11	1	0
Nutramigen, with Enflora									
5 fl oz	100	5.3	NA	NA	10.3	NA	NA	2.8	NA

Restaurants & Dining

Eating Out Gluten-Free

Eating out can be a dietary danger zone, especially if you are following a gluten-free diet. But the list of restaurants and nutrition information in this book will help you plan ahead and make sensible choices. Restaurants with gluten-free menus are a good place to start, since in many cases (but not all), staff members at those restaurants receive training on how to keep food gluten-free and avoid cross contamination. Use these helpful tips to make your gluten-free dining experience a success.

DON'T START OUT HUNGRY.

This is good advice for anyone going out to eat, but it's particularly important for those on a gluten-free diet. The hungrier you are, the more likely you are to make a mistake. If you must go to a restaurant hungry, bring some gluten-free crackers to munch on while everyone else is filling up on the rolls.

SELECT THE RIGHT RESTAURANT.

The comprehensive list of restaurants in this book can assist you in choosing a restaurant that is gluten-free friendly. The restaurants included are chains that have multiple locations and have put a concerted effort into providing gluten-free menu items. For restaurants not listed, check their website or give them a phone call.

CALL AHEAD.

Don't take it for granted that each restaurant will follow all the gluten-free guidelines. Call ahead and let them know that you need a gluten-free meal and ask what the best way to handle this is when you arrive at the restaurant. There may be a specific person—manager or chef—who handles special requests.

EXPLAIN YOUR DIETARY RESTRICTIONS.

Although gluten-intolerance is not a "food allergy," this is a good term to use. Restaurants will take an allergy more seriously than if you say you are on a "special diet." The terms "celiac disease" and "gluten-free" may be unfamiliar to the server. Briefly explain that you have a serious food sensitivity and you must avoid foods containing wheat, barley, and rye in order to prevent getting sick.

Consider bringing along a gluten-free dining card to explain what you can and cannot eat. Cards are available in a wide variety of languages at *http://www.celiactravel.com/cards*. These are great when traveling in foreign countries.

CHECK THE MENU.

Look for simple dishes without coatings or sauces, or with sauces that can be left off. Don't assume that anything is gluten-free. Even if a menu item looks safe, you might not realize that the chef's secret recipe includes gluten. Egg omelets can contain pancake batter. Baked potatoes can be coated with flour to make the skins crispier. Green tea can have barley in it.

ASK QUESTIONS.

It is essential that you inquire about cooking methods, specific ingredients that are in each item, and how it is served. Here are examples of foods and the potential problems involved, along with a "Tip" for the best foods to order:

Salads and Salad Dressings – Salads may contain croutons, wheat-based Asian noodles, wontons, pasta, or taco shells. Salad dressings may contain unsafe ingredients such as wheat flour or wheat starch, hydrolyzed wheat protein, or soy sauce.

> **Tip:** Fresh salad greens and vegetables are gluten-free. Make sure they toss your salad in a clean bowl. If no safe salad dressings are available or you are unsure about the ingredients in the salad dressing, ask for oil and a lemon wedge or balsamic vinegar to be served on the side.

Marinades – Teriyaki or soy sauce (made with wheat) or beer may be used to marinade meat, fish, or poultry.

> **Tip:** Ask for a meat, fish, or poultry that has not been marinated.

Soups and Sauces – These are often made with commercial soup bases or soup cubes containing wheat flour, wheat starch, or hydrolyzed wheat protein. Roux is a combination of butter and flour which is used to thicken sauces. Soups can also contain noodles, bread, crackers, or wontons that all contain wheat. Ask if the soups are made from scratch and ask to see the recipe. If a commercially prepared product is used, ask to see the label with the ingredients listed.

> **Tip:** Choose clear broth soups with vegetables. Include sauces only if you are assured they are gluten-free.

Meat, Fish, and Poultry – Ask if these items have been dusted with flour before grilling or fying. Some hamburger patties may contain wheat flour, wheat starch, or bread crumbs. Seasonings containing wheat flour or wheat starch may be added to ground meat or sprinkled on meat, fish, or poultry. Au jus may come from a can or mix containing unsafe ingredients. Self-basting turkeys and imitation bacon bits may contain hydrolyzed wheat protein. Imitation seafood may contain wheat starch.

Tip: Order fresh cuts of meat, fish, and poultry that have not been marinated. Ask that they be grilled on a clean surface.

Fried Foods – Avoid deep-fried foods that are cooked in fryers that are used for breaded and non-breaded items.

Tip: Make sure that any gluten-free fried foods are fried in a separate fryer specified for gluten-free preparation.

Hash Brown Potatoes – Some frozen hash brown potatoes may contain wheat starch. Ask for ingredient information and whether any other ingredients have been added while cooking them— seasonings that may contain wheat flour, wheat starch, or hydrolyzed wheat protein.

Tip: Order a plain baked potato. Choose hash brown potatoes only if you are certain the potatoes have been prepared with a gluten-free recipe.

Rice Pilaf – Many restaurants use commercially packaged rice that is seasoned with unsafe ingredients—broth, soup bases, seasonings that contain wheat flour, wheat starch, or hydrolyzed wheat protein.

Tip: Ask for plain boiled rice. Choose seasoned rice dishes only if you are confident that the recipe and preparation are gluten-free.

Pasta – Ask if they provide gluten-free pasta or check to see if you can bring your own pasta. Ask that fresh water be used to avoid cross-contamination with wheat pasta.

Tip: Bring your own gluten-free pasta and make sure they boil it in fresh water. Choose a pasta entree only if you are certain that the pasta and preparation are gluten-free.

Vegetables – Avoid battered vegetables or those prepared in sauces that are usually thickened with wheat flour. Some vegetables may be sautéed or stir-fried with seasonings or soy sauce that contain wheat.

Tip: Order vegetables steamed with no seasonings or sauces. Bring your own seasonings or sprinkle with olive oil and balsamic vinegar.

CAUTION THE RESTAURANT STAFF ABOUT CROSS-CONTAMINATION.

Remind the server and the chef that your food must be prepared on a clean cooking surface with clean utensils. Many restaurant staffers will not realize the risks of cross-contamination unless they are pointed out to them. To stay safe, make sure you ask the kitchen staff for the following:

- Wash their hands and change their gloves before preparing your food
- Mix any salad in a clean bowl (many restaurants reuse bowls, and they may contain crouton fragments or unsafe salad dressings)
- Avoid using a grill surface that's shared with gluten-containing items (including hamburger buns, sauces, and breaded items)
- Use fresh water to cook gluten-free pasta or steam vegetables (some restaurants reuse pasta water for this purpose)
- Place gluten-free pizzas or rolls on a pan instead of directly on an oven surface, and cover them with foil to avoid crumbs

CONFIRM YOUR ORDER BEFORE EATING.

Ask if this is the "special meal" you ordered and confirm that all your instructions were followed.

THANK THE MANAGER, CHEF, AND FOOD SERVER.

Express your thanks for the meal if every effort was made to meet your needs. Leave a generous tip for good service and patronize this restaurant again. Tell all your gluten-free friends about your experience.

Food Serving size	Cal.	(g) Total Fat	(g) Sat. Fat	(mg) Chol.	(g) Carb.	(g) Fiber	(g) Sug.	(g) Prot.	(mg) Sod.

Applebee's
[www.applebees.com]

Appetizers

Chips & Salsa 1 serving	960	53	10	NA	107	11	NA	14	890
Potato Skins 1 serving	1340	94	46	NA	69	10	NA	58	1850
Queso Blanco Dip 1 serving	1290	77	24	NA	117	12	NA	32	2460

Desserts

Hot Fudge Sundae Shooter 1 sundae	350	18	13	NA	43	<1	NA	4	125

Salad Dressings

Champagne Vinaigrette 2 tbsp	52	5	NA	NA	NA	NA	NA	NA	NA
Creamy Bleu Cheese 1 serving	240	26	5	NA	<1	0	NA	2	260
Fat-Free Italian 2 tbsp	20	0.3	0.2	1	3.6	0.2	2.2	0.5	430
Garlic Caesar Dressing 1 serving	140	15	1	10	1	NA	1	0	120
Honey French 2 tbsp	170	14	2	0	11	0	10	0	240
Honey Mustard 1 serving	220	18	3	NA	13	<1	NA	<1	520
Mexi Ranch 1 serving	140	14	2.5	NA	2	0	NA	<1	490
Oriental Vinaigrette 1 tbsp	50	2.3	0	2.5	7.5	0	0	0	NA
Ranch 1 serving	200	21	3.5	NA	1	0	NA	<1	310

Food Serving size	Cal.	(g) Total Fat	(g) Sat. Fat	(mg) Chol.	(g) Carb.	(g) Fiber	(g) Sug.	(g) Prot.	(mg) Sod.
Red Jalapeno Caesar Dressing									
1 tbsp	61	6	1	13	1	NA	NA	0.5	78

Salads

Fiesta Chicken Chopped Salad (without dressing)									
1 salad	690	32	9	NA	65	11	NA	39	1460
Grilled Shrimp 'N Spinach Salad (without dressing)									
1 salad	630	46	7	NA	20	10	NA	45	1660
Santa Fe Chicken Salad (without dressing)									
1 salad	910	55	18	NA	52	10	NA	57	2060

Sauces

Guacamole									
1 tbsp	23	2.08	.3 oz	0	1.24	1	0.1	0.29	22
Marinara									
1/2 cup	70	5	1	0	10	NA	NA	2	470
Mayonnaise									
1 tbsp	57	4.91	0.72	4	3.51	0	0.94	0.13	105
Salsa									
1 tbsp	4	0.03	0.005	0	1	0.3	0.49	0.25	96
Sour Cream									
1 tbsp	31	3.02	1.87	6	0.61	0	0.02	0.46	8

Seafood

Blackened Tilapia (Not Including Sides)									
1 serving	410	15	4	NA	37	6	NA	34	1880
Grilled Jalapeno-Lime Shrimp (Not Including Sides)									
1 serving	300	6	1	NA	43	4	NA	22	2950

Sides

Add Grilled Shrimp									
4 large	26	0	0	46	0	0	0	5	208
Almond Rice Pilaf									
1 serving	309	13.35	5.69	23	41.42	2.3	1.7	5.98	43.95
Applesauce									
1 cup	102	0	0	0	27	2.7	23	0	5

Food Serving size	Cal.	(g) Total Fat	(g) Sat. Fat	(mg) Chol.	(g) Carb.	(g) Fiber	(g) Sug.	(g) Prot.	(mg) Sod.
Baked Potato (Loaded) 1 potato	500	35	20	NA	42	3	NA	12	500
Baked Potato (Regular) 1 potato	380	29	19	NA	28	2	NA	5	520
Celery 1 serving	18	0	0	0	3	1.8	2	1	88
Cole Slaw 1 serving	140	9	1.5	NA	15	2	NA	1	190
French Fries 1 serving	390	18	3.5	NA	53	4	NA	5	520
Fruit Side 1 serving	70	17	0	NA	17	3	NA	1	0
Garlic Mashed Potatoes (Loaded) 1 serving	430	29	12	NA	30	3	NA	13	920
Garlic Mashed Potatoes (Regular) 1 serving	330	18	3.5	NA	38	4	NA	6	900
Red Beans & Rice 1 serving	290	6	2.5	NA	48	5	NA	10	770
Seasonal Vegetables 1 serving	50	0	0	0	7	2	0	1	260

Steak Toppers

Grilled Onions 1 serving	45	2.5	0.5	NA	5	<1	NA	<1	280

Steaks

New York Strip Steak (Not Including Sides) 12 oz	480	24	10	NA	<1	0	NA	65	1120
Ribeye Steak (Not Including Sides) 12 oz	670	47	21	NA	3	0	NA	57	950

Additional Gluten-Free Menu Items
(nutritional information was not available)

Sizzling N'Awlins Skillet, Grilled Dijon Chicken & Portobello, Fiesta Lime Chicken, Bourbon Street Chicken & Shrimp, Sizzling Chicken Fundito, Tuscan Bean Soup with Chicken & Sausage, Mexi Rice,

Food Serving size	Cal.	(g) Total Fat	(g) Sat. Fat	(mg) Chol.	(g) Carb.	(g) Fiber	(g) Sug.	(g) Prot.	(mg) Sod.

Herb Potatoes, Crispy Red Potatoes, Pico de Gallo, Southern Barbecue, Bruschetta, Balsamic Glaze, Black Bean Corn Salsa, Dijon Sauce, Signature Slider Sauce, Napa Valley Red Wine Sauce, Chunky Roma Pepper Sauce, Chunky Roma Pepper Relish, Pesto Mayo, Chimichurri Sauce, Alfredo Sauce, and Honey Barbecue Sauce.

Bertucci's
[www.bertuccis.com]

Classic Entrées

Roasted Eggplant Pomodoro 1 entrée	710	50	14	NA	44	14	NA	26	1940

Desserts

Chocolate Budino 1 serving	660	50	31	NA	54	2	NA	5	0
Piccolo Chocolate Budino 1 serving	450	31	19	NA	47	5	NA	4	25

Entrées

Balsamic Chicken 1 entrée	680	44	12	NA	15	2	NA	53	790
Cod Al Forno 1 entrée	920	73	12	NA	29	3	NA	35	890
Filet Mignon with Chianti Sauce 1 entrée	980	80	30	NA	13	2	NA	48	440
Pesto Grilled Salmon 1 entrée	1030	86	17	NA	14	3	NA	49	260

Salads

Caesar Salad (serves two to four) (order without croutons) 1 serving	570	40	10	NA	33	5	NA	18	500
Farmhouse Salad (serves two to four) 1 serving	490	37	15	NA	25	7	NA	20	630
Insalata (without dressing) 1 serving	150	6	2.5	NA	21	5	NA	7	320

Food Serving size	Cal.	(g) Total Fat	(g) Sat. Fat	(mg) Chol.	(g) Carb.	(g) Fiber	(g) Sug.	(g) Prot.	(mg) Sod.
Side Caesar Salad 1 serving	260	19	4	NA	16	2	NA	7	170
Side Caesar Salad with Chicken 1 serving	280	12	5	NA	11	2	NA	31	290
Side Insalata 1 serving	80	3	1.5	NA	12	3	NA	4	180

Small Plates

Food Serving size	Cal.	(g) Total Fat	(g) Sat. Fat	(mg) Chol.	(g) Carb.	(g) Fiber	(g) Sug.	(g) Prot.	(mg) Sod.
Baked Polenta with Pomodoro (order without bread crumbs) 1 serving	550	8	3	NA	10	1	NA	6	460
Garlic and Herb Roasted Mushrooms 1 serving	290	26	5	NA	9	1	NA	5	25
Grilled Asparagus 1 serving	45	3.5	0.5	NA	2	1	NA	2	30
Roasted Green Beans 1 serving	120	10	2	NA	6	3	NA	3	15
Rosemary Roasted Red Potatoes 1 serving	220	22	4.5	NA	4	1	NA	1	10
Tuscan Roasted Vegetables 1 serving	320	27	3	0	16	6	10	6	840
Warm Assorted Olives 1 serving	330	35	7	NA	4	4	NA	0	1690

Starters

Food Serving size	Cal.	(g) Total Fat	(g) Sat. Fat	(mg) Chol.	(g) Carb.	(g) Fiber	(g) Sug.	(g) Prot.	(mg) Sod.
Eggplant Napoleone (order without crouton crumbs) 1 serving	530	38	14	NA	34	3	NA	17	780
Grilled Shrimp (order without bread crumbs) 1 serving	530	17	4	NA	14	2	NA	29	840
Sausage Soup 1 bowl	230	12	4.5	NA	20	1	NA	9	1220
Sausage Soup 1 cup	120	6	2.5	NA	10	1	NA	4	610
Vegetable Antipasto 1 serving	610	54	13	NA	21	9	NA	17	1430

Food Serving size	Cal.	(g) Total Fat	(g) Sat. Fat	(mg) Chol.	(g) Carb.	(g) Fiber	(g) Sug.	(g) Prot.	(mg) Sod.
Watermelon, Arugula and Feta Salad									
1 salad	280	24	5	NA	16	2	NA	6	380

Additional Gluten-Free Menu Items
(nutritional information was not available)

Side Caesar Salad with Shrimp

Boston Market
[www.bostonmarket.com]

Menu Item

Menu Item	Cal.	(g) Total Fat	(g) Sat. Fat	(mg) Chol.	(g) Carb.	(g) Fiber	(g) Sug.	(g) Prot.	(mg) Sod.
Cinnamon Apples 6 oz	240	3.5	0.5	0	55	4	49	0	270
Creamed Spinach 6.3 oz	280	21	12	60	11	4	2	9	530
Fresh Steamed Vegetables 4.8 oz	80	5	0	0	8	3	3	2	160
Garlic Dill New Potatoes 4.5 oz	100	2	0.5	0	20	2	1	2	80
Garlicky Lemon Spinach 6 oz	120	9	5	20	8	4	1	5	380
Green Beans 4.2 oz	90	6	2	0	9	4	2	2	200
Honey Habanero Sauce (Medium Hot) 1 oz	70	0	0	0	17	0	15	0	200
Kids Chicken 5.4 oz	310	20	6	175	1	0	1	33	670
Kids Turkey 2.5 oz	90	1.5	0.5	35	0	0	0	19	310
Loaded Mashed Potatoes 7.4 oz	310	16	9	40	31	3	3	9	840
Mashed Potatoes 7 oz	240	10	5	25	32	3	2	5	730
Poultry Gravy 1 oz	10	0	0	0	2	0	0	0	85

Food Serving size	Cal.	(g) Total Fat	(g) Sat. Fat	(mg) Chol.	(g) Carb.	(g) Fiber	(g) Sug.	(g) Prot.	(mg) Sod.
Roasted Turkey Breast - Large 7 oz	260	4.5	1.5	100	0	0	0	54	870
Roasted Turkey Breast - Regular 5 oz	180	3	1	70	0	0	0	38	620
Rotisserie Chicken - Half 12 oz	640	33	10	340	2	0	1	84	1380
Rotisserie Chicken - Quarter White 6.6 oz	320	13	4	165	1	0	1	51	710
Rotisserie Chicken - Three Piece Dark 7.3 oz	390	22	6	290	1	0	1	51	1270
Southwest Santa Fe Salad (Half Size) 9.1 oz	380	23	5	45	25	3	5	20	650
Southwest Santa Fe Salad (Whole Size) 18.3 oz	760	46	10	95	50	5	10	40	1290
Sweet Corn 4.3 oz	120	2.5	0	0	25	1	7	4	55

Bugaboo Creek Steak House
[www.bugaboocreek.com]

Bugaboo Steaks

Black Magic Steak 12 oz	827	60	22	177	0	0	0	68	228
Black Magic Steak 8 oz	551	39	14	118	0	0	0	45	152
Charlie Morgan's Ribeye 1 serving	1168	79	28	500	0	0	0	105	775
Lodge Center Cut Filet 7 oz	547	42	15	129	0	0	0	39	632
Lodge Center Cut Filet 9 oz	704	54	20	166	0	0	0	51	670
Mountain Man Strip 1 serving	890	65	24	197	0	0	0	70	730
Prime Rib (order without Au Jus sauce) 10 oz	782	63	25	188	1	0	0	50	2562

Food Serving size	Cal.	(g) Total Fat	(g) Sat. Fat	(mg) Chol.	(g) Carb.	(g) Fiber	(g) Sug.	(g) Prot.	(mg) Sod.
Prime Rib (order without Au Jus sauce)									
12 oz	938	75	30	225	1	0	0	60	3074
Prime Rib (order without Au Jus sauce)									
16 oz	1250	100	40	300	2	0	1	80	4099

Fish from the Grill

Grilled Rainbow Trout									
1 serving	322	15	3	134	0	0	0	46	106

Mountain Outfitters' Specials

Campfire Cheesesteak (order without bun or french fries)									
1 serving	663	31	10	76	64	2	1	31	2438
Moosebreath Burger (order without bun or French fries)									
1 serving	742	37	12	141	50	2	2	49	933
Roasted Half Chicken									
1 serving	518	37	10	166	4	1	2	40	704
Smoked Baby Back Ribs (order without French fries)									
1 serving	755	55	20	166	23	1	14	35	1098

Salad Dressings

Blue Cheese Dressing									
1 serving	320	34	NA	NA	2	NA	NA	2	NA
Caesar									
1 serving	560	60	NA	NA	4	NA	NA	7	NA
Lite Olive Oil Vinaigrette									
2 tbsp	60	6	0	0	3	0	2	0	240
Thousand Island									
1 serving	280	28	NA	NA	10	NA	NA	NA	NA

Sides

Baked Beans									
1 serving	212	0	0	0	47	5	26	6	652
Charlie's Smashed Potatoes									
1 serving	396	25	14	26	35	4	4	6	835

Food Serving size	Cal.	(g) Total Fat	(g) Sat. Fat	(mg) Chol.	(g) Carb.	(g) Fiber	(g) Sug.	(g) Prot.	(mg) Sod.
Fresh Steamed Vegetables									
1 serving	61	0	0	0	11	4	5	3	109
Grilled Onions									
1 serving	128	51	1	0	18	2	7	2	201
Mountain Loaded Baked Potato (real bacon only)									
1 potato	348	10	1	0	59	4	2	7	2377
Sauteed Mushrooms									
1 serving	193	10	3	0	8	2	4	4	868

The Creek's Salads

Alpine Chicken Salad									
(request no croutons on salads and to be prepared in separate bowl from other salads)									
1 salad	246	10	2	51	14	6	5	23	947
Bleu Mountain Steak Salad									
(order un-marinated steak only and without onion strings)									
1 salad	501	33	11	88	11	3	3	38	1076
Chicken Caesar Salad									
(request no croutons on salads and to be prepared in separate bowl from other salads)									
1 salad	436	22	4	102	16	8	8	44	1292
Snowbird Chicken Salad (grilled chicken only, no bacon, no croutons)									
1 salad	672	18	4	369	53	5	6	68	2724

Additional Gluten-Free Menu Items
(nutritional information was not available)

Balsamic Vinaigrette Salad Dressing, Parmesan Peppercorn Salad Dressing, Timber Creek T-Bone Steak, Mountain Man Strip, Kansas City Bone-in NY Strip Steak, Kain's Cast Iron Skillet Steak, All Moose Juices, Rocky Mountain Mudslide, Glacier Freeze Smoothies

California Pizza Kitchen
[www.cpk.com]

CPKids

CPK Salad									
1 serving	171-273	NA	0-5	NA	36	4	NA	6	1215
Fresh Fruit									
1 serving	68	NA	0	NA	16	1	NA	1	2

Food Serving size	Cal.	(g) Total Fat	(g) Sat. Fat	(mg) Chol.	(g) Carb.	(g) Fiber	(g) Sug.	(g) Prot.	(mg) Sod.
Kids Sundae 1 serving	649	NA	26	NA	58	1	NA	7	90

Desserts

Food Serving size	Cal.	(g) Total Fat	(g) Sat. Fat	(mg) Chol.	(g) Carb.	(g) Fiber	(g) Sug.	(g) Prot.	(mg) Sod.
Caramel Sundae 1 dessert	1142	NA	43	NA	91	2	NA	16	218
Hot Fudge Sundae 1 dessert	1150	NA	46	NA	80	2	NA	14	170

Salads

Food Serving size	Cal.	(g) Total Fat	(g) Sat. Fat	(mg) Chol.	(g) Carb.	(g) Fiber	(g) Sug.	(g) Prot.	(mg) Sod.
Caramelized Peach (Full) 1 salad	950	NA	18	NA	77	11	NA	20	1146
Caramelized Peach (Half) 1 salad	471	NA	9	NA	38	6	NA	10	558
CPK Cobb (Full) (with ranch dressing) 1 salad	941	NA	18	NA	22	9	NA	48	1678
CPK Cobb (Half) (with ranch dressing) 1 salad	475	NA	9	NA	12	5	NA	24	842
Field Greens (Full) 1 salad	805	NA	9	NA	56	12	NA	10	593
Field Greens (Half) 1 salad	402	NA	5	NA	28	6	NA	5	297
Moroccan Chicken (Full) 1 salad	1370	NA	12	NA	116	23	NA	43	1040
Moroccan Chicken (Half) 1 salad	685	NA	6	NA	58	11	NA	22	520
Original Chopped (Full) 1 salad	937	NA	16	NA	18	6	NA	42	1865
Original Chopped (Half) 1 salad	469	NA	8	NA	9	3	NA	21	932
Roasted Vegetable (Full) 1 salad	597	NA	6	NA	48	16	NA	11	793
Roasted Vegetable (Half) 1 salad	298	NA	3	NA	24	8	NA	5	396

Food Serving size	Cal.	(g) Total Fat	(g) Sat. Fat	(mg) Chol.	(g) Carb.	(g) Fiber	(g) Sug.	(g) Prot.	(mg) Sod.
The Original BBQ Chicken Chopped (for gluten-free, request without tortilla chips)									
1 salad	1156	NA	18	NA	98	14	NA	48	1727
Waldorf Chicken (Full) (with Dijon Balsamic Vinaigrette)									
1 salad	1293	NA	23	NA	83	13	NA	45	1945
Waldorf Chicken (Half) (with Dijon Balsamic Vinaigrette)									
1 salad	647	NA	12	NA	42	7	NA	23	972

Small Cravings & Appetizers

Food Serving size	Cal.	Total Fat	Sat. Fat	Chol.	Carb.	Fiber	Sug.	Prot.	Sod.
Asparagus & Arugula Salad									
1 salad	189	NA	2	NA	8	2	NA	4	308
The Wedge Salad									
1 salad	278	NA	6	NA	5	2	NA	6	380
White Corn Guacamole & Chips									
1 serving	363	NA	3	NA	48	7	NA	6	501

Soups

Food Serving size	Cal.	Total Fat	Sat. Fat	Chol.	Carb.	Fiber	Sug.	Prot.	Sod.
Sedona Tortilla (for gluten-free, request without tortilla chips)									
1 bowl	500	NA	20	NA	46	6	NA	7	1373
Sedona Tortilla (for gluten-free, request without tortilla chips)									
1 cup	273	NA	10	NA	27	3	NA	4	695

Specialties

Food Serving size	Cal.	Total Fat	Sat. Fat	Chol.	Carb.	Fiber	Sug.	Prot.	Sod.
Norwegian Atlantic Salmon (with vegetables)									
1 entrée	752	NA	7	NA	27	8	NA	52	1041

Carrabba's Italian Grill
[www.carrabbas.com]

Antipasto

Food Serving size	Cal.	Total Fat	Sat. Fat	Chol.	Carb.	Fiber	Sug.	Prot.	Sod.
Cozze in Bianco									
30 mussels	570	20	3	10	12	0	2	48	350
Shrimp Scampi (request no garlic toast)									
1 serving	540	0	0	0	0	0	0	0	0

Food Serving size	Cal.	(g) Total Fat	(g) Sat. Fat	(mg) Chol.	(g) Carb.	(g) Fiber	(g) Sug.	(g) Prot.	(mg) Sod.

Cucina Casuale

Mama Mandola's Sicilian Chicken Soup (request no croutons and pasta)

1 cup	161	2.2	0.6	34.1	13.7	1.3	0.9	20.6	1

Additional Gluten-Free Menu Items
(nutritional information was not available)

House Salad, Italian Salad, Caesar Salad, Insalata Carrabba Caesar, Insalata Johnny Rocco, Insalata Italian Cobb, Insalata Fiorucci, Chicken Marsala (order without grill baste), Sirloin Marsala (order without grill baste), Pork Chops Marsala (order without grill baste), The Johnny Classic (order without grill baste), Chicken Trio Combination (order without grill baste), Chicken Bryant (order without grill baste), Grilled Salmon (order without grill baste), Pollo Rosa Maria (order without baste), Grilled Chicken, Filet Florentina, John Cole, and from the Bambini Menu, Grilled Chicken Breast (order without grill baste)

Carrow's
[www.carrows.com]

Breakfast Entrées

Bacon Avocado Jack Omelette (order without toast or bread)

1 omelette	410	33	10	620	5	2	2	25	650

Breakfast Enchiladas (order without toast or bread)

1 serving	740	49	20	460	43	5	3	39	1130

Corned Beef Hash & Eggs (order without toast or bread)

1 serving	600	49	17	435	16	0	1	24	940

Denver Omelette (order without toast or bread)

1 omelette	410	29	10	630	7	1	4	29	840

Hearty Breakfast Skillet (order without toast or bread)

1 serving	970	71	26	675	42	4	4	40	1590

Joe's Special Omelette (order without toast or bread)

1 omelette	580	41	15	675	10	3	5	44	920

Migas Skillet (order without toast or bread)

1 serving	920	60	20	675	47	6	3	47	1290

Prime Ribs & Eggs (order without toast or bread)

1 serving	1000	80	30	560	1	0	1	66	730

Steak & Eggs (order without toast or bread)

1 serving	450	23	7	500	1	0	1	60	1180

Food Serving size	Cal.	(g) Total Fat	(g) Sat. Fat	(mg) Chol.	(g) Carb.	(g) Fiber	(g) Sug.	(g) Prot.	(mg) Sod.
Supreme Skillet (order without toast or bread) 1 serving	850	60	22	670	33	4	4	44	1640
Vegetable Omelette (order without toast or bread) 1 omelette	390	27	9	615	11	3	6	26	460
Vegetable Skillet (order without toast or bread) 1 serving	570	35	13	615	34	5	4	31	930

Breakfast Sides

Food Serving size	Cal.	(g) Total Fat	(g) Sat. Fat	(mg) Chol.	(g) Carb.	(g) Fiber	(g) Sug.	(g) Prot.	(mg) Sod.
Bacon Strips 4 strips	120	9	4	20	0	0	0	8	460
Country Potatoes 1 serving	250	13	6	0	27	3	1	4	300
Eggs, Whole, Cooked, Scrambled 1 tbsp	20	2	0	38	0	0	0	1	20
Fresh Seasonal Fruit 1 serving	50	0	0	0	13	1	11	1	20
Hash Browns 1 serving	340	17	3.5	0	42	4	0	4	620
Sausage Links 4 links	280	26	9	60	0	0	0	12	540
Sausage Patty 2 patties	360	32	12	80	1	0	0	16	680
Turkey Sausage Patties 2 patties	140	8	3	30	0	0	0	16	520

Desserts

Food Serving size	Cal.	(g) Total Fat	(g) Sat. Fat	(mg) Chol.	(g) Carb.	(g) Fiber	(g) Sug.	(g) Prot.	(mg) Sod.
Chocolate Ice Cream 1 scoop	150	8	5	30	16	1	15	3	35
Chocolate Ice Cream 2 scoops	300	16	10	60	32	1	30	6	70
Coffee Ice Cream 1 scoop	140	8	5	30	15	1	14	2	35
Coffee Ice Cream 2 scoops	280	16	10	60	30	1	28	4	70

Food Serving size	Cal.	(g) Total Fat	(g) Sat. Fat	(mg) Chol.	(g) Carb.	(g) Fiber	(g) Sug.	(g) Prot.	(mg) Sod.
Mini Hot Fudge Sundae 1 sundae	200	11	8	20	22	1	20	2	70
Old Fashioned Mocha Shake 1 shake	1140	50	24	140	153	18	136	16	570
Old Fashioned Strawberry Shake 1 shake	850	38	24	140	111	5	103	15	260
Old Fashioned Vanilla Shake 1 shake	700	38	24	140	73	2	68	14	230
Root Beer Float 1 float	240	8	5	30	41	0	40	2	55
Vanilla Ice Cream 1 scoop	140	8	5	30	15	1	14	2	35
Vanilla Ice Cream 2 scoops	280	16	10	60	30	1	28	4	70

Lunch / Dinner Entrées

Food	Cal.	Total Fat	Sat. Fat	Chol.	Carb.	Fiber	Sug.	Prot.	Sod.
Active & Lively Sirloin Steak Dinner (with Plain Baked Potato) (order without bread) 1 serving	310	5	2.5	85	34	6	3	32	680
Blackened Prime Rib 12 oz	1260	99	42	300	2	0	1	83	1370
Blackened Prime Rib 8 oz	860	67	29	205	2	0	1	56	1060
Charleston Chicken Salad (order without bread) 1 salad	530	32	7	120	20	7	10	40	1650
Mile High Prime Rib 16 oz	1660	131	55	395	2	0	1	111	1400
Mile High Santa Barbara Chopped Caesar Salad (order without bread) (no croutons) 1 salad	700	49	12	125	27	10	6	44	1250
Norweigan Salmon Filet (order without bread) 1 serving	320	14	2	125	1	0	0	45	450
Ribeye Steak (order without bread) 1 serving	610	33	14	165	1	0	0	72	440
Slow-Roasted BBQ Ribs (order without bread) 1 serving	1450	59	25	310	130	4	73	96	4170

Food Serving size	Cal.	(g) Total Fat	(g) Sat. Fat	(mg) Chol.	(g) Carb.	(g) Fiber	(g) Sug.	(g) Prot.	(mg) Sod.
Southwest Chicken Salad (order without bread) 1 salad	780	52	12	140	31	9	6	48	1310
T-Bone Steak (order without bread) 1 serving	620	46	18	130	0	0	0	47	470
Top Sirloin Steak (order without bread) 1 serving	290	8	3	125	7	0	0	50	1060
Traditional Prime Rib 8 oz	860	67	29	205	2	0	1	56	780

Lunch / Dinner Sides

Food Serving size	Cal.	(g) Total Fat	(g) Sat. Fat	(mg) Chol.	(g) Carb.	(g) Fiber	(g) Sug.	(g) Prot.	(mg) Sod.
Baked Potato 1 potato	110	0	0	0	26	2	1	3	0
Chicken Tortilla Soup 1 serving	220	12	5	140	20	3	4	11	730
Creamed Spinach 1/2 cup	70	2.5	1.5	0	9.1	1	4	3.1	510
Dinner Salad (no croutons) 1 salad	70	2	0	0	12	2	2	3	160
Mashed Potatoes 1 cup	714	2	1	4	155	13.2	7	22	164
Potato Cheese Soup 1 cup serving	188	7.14	4.02	20	22.3	1.7	8.41	8.98	340
Split Pea Soup 1 cup serving	165	2.93	1.4	0	26.5	5	NA	8.6	917.5

Salad Dressings

Food Serving size	Cal.	(g) Total Fat	(g) Sat. Fat	(mg) Chol.	(g) Carb.	(g) Fiber	(g) Sug.	(g) Prot.	(mg) Sod.
Honey Mustard Dressing 2 tbsp	62	3	0	0	9	0	5	0	270
Lite Italian Dressing 1 serving	70	7	1	5	1	NA	1	0	520
Ranch Dressing 1 tbsp	73	8	1	5	1	0	0	0	122
Thousand Island Dressing 1 cup	925	88	13	65	37	2	38	3	2158

Food Serving size	Cal.	(g) Total Fat	(g) Sat. Fat	(mg) Chol.	(g) Carb.	(g) Fiber	(g) Sug.	(g) Prot.	(mg) Sod.

Additional Gluten-Free Menu Items
(nutritional information was not available)

Dinner Vegetables, Broccoli Soup, and Chipotle Dressing

Chick-Fil-A
[www.chick-fil-a.com]

Beverages

Food Serving size	Cal.	Total Fat	Sat. Fat	Chol.	Carb.	Fiber	Sug.	Prot.	Sod.
100% Columbian Coffee 1 serving	5	0	0	0	0	0	0	1	10
Coca-Cola medium	170	0	0	0	47	0	47	0	15
Dasani Bottled Water 1 bottle	0	0	0	0	0	0	0	0	0
Diet Coke medium	0	0	0	0	0	0	0	0	5
Diet Lemonade medium	20	0	0	0	6	0	2	0	10
Dr Pepper medium	180	0	0	0	48	0	48	0	60
Iced Tea - Sweet medium	130	0	0	0	32	0	32	0	10
Iced Tea - Unsweet medium	0	0	0	0	0	0	0	0	10
Lemonade medium	230	0	0	0	61	0	58	0	10
Simply Orange Juice 1 serving	190	0	0	0	45	2	41	3	0

Breakfast

Food Serving size	Cal.	Total Fat	Sat. Fat	Chol.	Carb.	Fiber	Sug.	Prot.	Sod.
American cheese 1 slice	79	6.6	4.1	20	0.3	NA	0.1	4.7	313
Bacon slice .24 oz	30	2	0.5	10	NA	NA	NA	2	115

Food Serving size	Cal.	(g) Total Fat	(g) Sat. Fat	(mg) Chol.	(g) Carb.	(g) Fiber	(g) Sug.	(g) Prot.	(mg) Sod.
Egg (Jumbo) 1 egg	96	58	58	275	NA	NA	NA	8.2	NA
Hash Browns 1 order	260	17	3.5	5	25	3	0	2	380
Sausage Patty 1 patty	147	12	4	31	0	0	0	9	332

Condiments

Food Serving size	Cal.	(g) Total Fat	(g) Sat. Fat	(mg) Chol.	(g) Carb.	(g) Fiber	(g) Sug.	(g) Prot.	(mg) Sod.
Apple Jelly 1 packet	35	0	0	0	9	0	6	0	0
Grape Jelly 1 packet	35	0	0	0	9	0	6	0	0
Ketchup 1 packet	25	0	0	0	7	0	6	0	310
Mayonnaise 1 packet	90	10	1.5	10	1	0	0	0	70
Mixed Fruit Jelly 1 packet	35	0	0	0	9	0	6	0	0
Mustard 1 packet	5	0	0	0	1	0	0	0	60

Desserts

Food Serving size	Cal.	(g) Total Fat	(g) Sat. Fat	(mg) Chol.	(g) Carb.	(g) Fiber	(g) Sug.	(g) Prot.	(mg) Sod.
Icedream 1 serving	290	7	4.5	25	50	0	49	8	200

Dipping Sauces and Dressings

Food Serving size	Cal.	(g) Total Fat	(g) Sat. Fat	(mg) Chol.	(g) Carb.	(g) Fiber	(g) Sug.	(g) Prot.	(mg) Sod.
Barbecue Sauce 1 serving	45	0	0	0	11	0	9	0	180
Blue Cheese Dressing 1 serving	160	16	3	20	1	0	1	1	280
Buttermilk Ranch Dressing 1 serving	160	17	2.5	5	1	0	1	0	280
Buttermilk Ranch Sauce 1 serving	110	12	2	5	1	0	1	0	200

Food Serving size	Cal.	(g) Total Fat	(g) Sat. Fat	(mg) Chol.	(g) Carb.	(g) Fiber	(g) Sug.	(g) Prot.	(mg) Sod.
Caesar Dressing 1 serving	160	17	2.5	30	1	0	0	1	240
Chick-fil-A Buffalo Sauce 1 serving	10	0	0	0	1	0	0	0	420
Chick-fil-A Sauce 1 serving	140	13	2	10	6	0	6	0	170
Fat Free Dijon Honey Mustard Dressing 1 serving	60	0	0	0	14	1	12	0	220
Honey Mustard Sauce 1 serving	45	0	0	0	11	0	10	0	150
Honey Roasted BBQ Sauce 1 serving	60	5	1	5	2	0	2	0	70
Light Italian Dressing 1 serving	15	0.5	0	0	2	0	2	0	510
Polynesian Sauce 1 serving	110	6	1	0	14	0	5	0	210
Reduced Fat Berry Balsamic Vinaigrette Dressing 1 serving	70	2	0	0	12	0	9	0	150
Spicy Dressing 1 serving	140	14	2	5	2	0	1	0	130
Thousand Island Dressing 1 serving	150	14	2	10	5	0	4	0	230

Entrées

Chick-Fil-A Chargrilled Chicken & Fruit Salad 1 salad	230	6	3.5	60	23	5	17	22	450
Chick-Fil-A Chargrilled Chicken Filet (no bun) 1 filet	290	4	1	60	36	3	9	28	780
Chick-Fil-A Chargrilled Chicken Garden Salad 1 salad	180	6	3.5	60	11	4	6	23	450

Kid's Meals

Buddy Fruits Pure Blended Fruit to Go Applesauce 1 serving	50	0	0	0	14	1	13	0	10

Food Serving size	Cal.	(g) Total Fat	(g) Sat. Fat	(mg) Chol.	(g) Carb.	(g) Fiber	(g) Sug.	(g) Prot.	(mg) Sod.
Chick-Fil-A Grilled Nuggets									
1 serving	80	1	0	40	0	0	0	17	560

Sides

	Cal.	(g) Total Fat	(g) Sat. Fat	(mg) Chol.	(g) Carb.	(g) Fiber	(g) Sug.	(g) Prot.	(mg) Sod.
Carrot & Raisin Salad									
1 serving	260	12	2	5	40	4	31	2	160
Chick-Fil-A Waffle Potato Fries									
1 serving	390	20	3	0	48	3	0	4	150
Cole Slaw									
1 serving	360	31	5	20	19	3	16	2	280
Fruit Cup									
1 serving	70	0	0	0	17	2	14	1	0
Side Salad									
1 serving	70	4.5	3	15	5	2	2	5	110
Yogurt Parfait									
1 serving	230	3	2	10	44	0	35	6	60

Additional Gluten-Free Menu Items
(nutritional information was not available)

Tortilla Strips, Chocolate Syrup, and Blueberry Topping

Chili's
[www.chilis.com]

Beverages

	Cal.	(g) Total Fat	(g) Sat. Fat	(mg) Chol.	(g) Carb.	(g) Fiber	(g) Sug.	(g) Prot.	(mg) Sod.
Coke									
medium	170	0	0	0	47	0	47	0	15
Dasani Water									
1 bottle	0	0	0	0	0	0	0	0	0
Diet Coke									
medium	0	0	0	0	0	0	0	0	5
Dr Pepper									
medium	180	0	0	0	48	0	48	0	60
Sprite									
8 oz	100	0	0	0	26	0	26	0	45

Food Serving size	Cal.	(g) Total Fat	(g) Sat. Fat	(mg) Chol.	(g) Carb.	(g) Fiber	(g) Sug.	(g) Prot.	(mg) Sod.
Burgers									
Bacon Burger (without buns & fries) 1 burger	1570	91	28	NA	125	9	NA	61	3690
Mushroom-Swiss Burger (without buns & fries) 1 burger	1540	88	28	NA	126	10	NA	59	3710
Oldtimer Burger (without buns & fries) 1 burger	1310	65	20	NA	128	10	NA	51	3230
Chicken & Seafood									
Grilled Salmon with Garlic & Herbs 1 serving	560	25	7	NA	37	5	NA	49	1640
Monterey Chicken 1 serving	890	48	20	NA	51	8	NA	66	2920
Lighter Choices									
Classic Sirloin (without sides) 1 serving	220	9	4	NA	1	0	NA	34	810
Grilled Chicken Salad (without sides) 1 serving	430	22	6	NA	21	5	NA	38	1060
Margarita Chicken (without tortilla strips) (without sides) 1 serving	160	3	1	NA	6	1	NA	29	550
Pepper Pals									
Grilled Chicken Platter (without sides & buns) 1 serving	160	3.5	1	NA	2	0	NA	30	580
Grilled Chicken Sandwich (without sides & buns) 1 serving	230	5	0.5	NA	22	1	NA	22	440
Little Mouth Cheeseburger (without sides & buns) 1 serving	400	24	10	NA	24	1	NA	22	950
Salad Dressings									
Citrus Balsamic Vinaigrette 1 serving	250	25	4	NA	6	0	NA	0	220
Honey Lime 1 serving	200	17	3	NA	13	0	NA	0	250

Food Serving size	Cal.	(g) Total Fat	(g) Sat. Fat	(mg) Chol.	(g) Carb.	(g) Fiber	(g) Sug.	(g) Prot.	(mg) Sod.
Honey Mustard 1 serving	200	22	3	NA	1	0	NA	1	400
Low-fat Ranch 1 serving	80	5	1	NA	9	0	NA	1	360
No Fat Honey Mustard 1 serving	70	0	0	NA	11	0	NA	0	510

Salads

Food Serving size	Cal.	(g) Total Fat	(g) Sat. Fat	(mg) Chol.	(g) Carb.	(g) Fiber	(g) Sug.	(g) Prot.	(mg) Sod.
Caribbean Chicken Salad (without dressing, croutons) 1 salad	610	25	4	NA	65	6	NA	34	810
Chicken Caesar Salad (without dressing, croutons) 1 salad	680	44	9	NA	31	6	NA	42	1570
House Salad (without dressing, croutons) 1 salad	150	6	3	NA	18	3	NA	7	220

Sauces & Extras

Food Serving size	Cal.	(g) Total Fat	(g) Sat. Fat	(mg) Chol.	(g) Carb.	(g) Fiber	(g) Sug.	(g) Prot.	(mg) Sod.
Applewood Smoked Bacon 3 strips	90	7	3	NA	0	0	NA	7	370
Avocado Slices 1 serving	80	7	1	NA	4	3	NA	1	0
Guacamole 1 serving	45	4	0	NA	3	2	NA	1	140
Original BBQ Sauce 1 serving	50	0	0	NA	12	1	NA	1	500

Sides

Food Serving size	Cal.	(g) Total Fat	(g) Sat. Fat	(mg) Chol.	(g) Carb.	(g) Fiber	(g) Sug.	(g) Prot.	(mg) Sod.
Black Beans 1 serving	100	1	0	NA	18	5	NA	6	620
Cole Slaw 1 serving	240	20	4	NA	15	2	NA	1	490
Corn Kernels 1 serving	130	2	0	NA	22	6	NA	4	5
Corn on the Cob (with butter) 1 serving	200	7	1	NA	32	3	NA	5	420

Food Serving size	Cal.	(g) Total Fat	(g) Sat. Fat	(mg) Chol.	(g) Carb.	(g) Fiber	(g) Sug.	(g) Prot.	(mg) Sod.
Loaded Mashed Potatoes 1 serving	390	25	10	NA	28	3	NA	13	1160
Mandarin Oranges 1 serving	35	0	0	NA	8	0	NA	0	0
Mashed Potatoes (without gravy) 1 serving	280	15	4	NA	31	3	NA	4	1300
Rice 1 serving	190	7	2	NA	30	1	NA	3	580
Steamed Broccoli 1 serving	80	6	2	NA	6	3	NA	3	490

Slow Smoke In-House Ribs

Food Serving size	Cal.	(g) Total Fat	(g) Sat. Fat	(mg) Chol.	(g) Carb.	(g) Fiber	(g) Sug.	(g) Prot.	(mg) Sod.
Memphis Dry Rib, Original (without sides) 1/2 rack	1080	57	19	NA	82	8	NA	62	4080
Memphis Dry Rib, Original (without sides) full rack	1990	111	37	NA	137	17	NA	119	6180

Soups

Food Serving size	Cal.	(g) Total Fat	(g) Sat. Fat	(mg) Chol.	(g) Carb.	(g) Fiber	(g) Sug.	(g) Prot.	(mg) Sod.
Loaded Baked Potato 1 bowl	410	30	18	NA	22	1	NA	15	1160
Loaded Baked Potato 1 cup	210	15	9	NA	11	1	NA	8	590
Southwest Chicken & Sausage (without Tortilla Strips) 1 bowl	330	20	8	NA	25	4	NA	14	1700
Southwest Chicken & Sausage (without Tortilla Strips) 1 cup	160	10	4	NA	13	2	NA	7	850

Steaks

Food Serving size	Cal.	(g) Total Fat	(g) Sat. Fat	(mg) Chol.	(g) Carb.	(g) Fiber	(g) Sug.	(g) Prot.	(mg) Sod.
Classic Ribeye 1 serving	1270	82	33	NA	53	7	NA	86	3710
Classic Sirloin 10 oz	1050	62	22	NA	53	8	NA	74	3400
Classic Sirloin 6 oz	870	51	18	NA	53	7	NA	54	2760

Food Serving size	Cal.	(g) Total Fat	(g) Sat. Fat	(mg) Chol.	(g) Carb.	(g) Fiber	(g) Sug.	(g) Prot.	(mg) Sod.
Steak Toppers: Grilled Shrimp									
1 serving	60	3	1	NA	2	0	NA	8	340
Steak Toppers: Sauteed Mushrooms									
1 serving	70	5	3	NA	3	1	NA	3	430

Stupendously Sweet Endings

Chocolate Shake									
1 shake	690	33	21	NA	92	0	NA	8	210

Additional Gluten-Free Menu Items
(nutritional information was not available)

Mixed Cheese, Pico de Gallo, Salsa, Sauteed Mushrooms, Electric Blue Blast, IBC Root Beer, Rockin' Tropical Punch, Strawberry Lemonade, Blackberry Tea, Mango Tea, Red Wine, and White Wine.

Chipotle Mexican Grill
[www.chipotle.com]

Menu Item

Barbacoa									
4 oz	170	7	2.5	60	2	0	<1	24	510
Black Beans									
4 oz	120	1	0	0	23	11	<1	7	250
Carnitas									
4 oz	190	8	2.5	70	1	0	0	27	540
Cheese									
1 oz	100	8.5	5	30	0	0	0	8	180
Chicken									
4 oz	190	6.5	2	115	1	0	1	32	370
Chips									
4 oz	570	27	3.5	0	73	8	4	8	420
Cilantro-Lime Rice									
3 oz	130	3	0.5	0	23	0	0	2	150
Corn Salsa									
3.5 oz	80	1.5	0	0	15	3	4	3	410

Food Serving size	Cal.	(g) Total Fat	(g) Sat. Fat	(mg) Chol.	(g) Carb.	(g) Fiber	(g) Sug.	(g) Prot.	(mg) Sod.
Crispy Taco Shell 1 shell	60	2	0.5	0	9	1	<1	<1	10
Fajita Vegetables 2.5 oz	20	0.5	0	0	4	1	2	1	170
Green Tomatillo Salsa 2 fl oz	15	0	0	0	3	1	2	1	230
Guacamole 3.5 oz	150	13	2	0	8	6	1	2	190
Pinto Beans 4 oz	120	1	0	5	22	10	<1	7	330
Red Tomatillo Salsa 2 fl oz	40	1	0	0	8	4	4	2	510
Romaine Lettuce (salad) 1 serving	10	0	0	0	2	1	1	1	5
Romaine Lettuce (tacos) 1 oz	5	0	0	0	1	1	1	1	0
Soft Corn Tortilla 1 tortilla	60	0.5	0	0	13	1	0	1.5	25
Sour Cream 2 oz	120	10	7	40	2	0	2	2	30
Steak 4 oz	190	6.5	2	65	2	0	1	30	320
Tomato Salsa 3.5 oz	20	0	0	0	4	<1	3	1	470
Vinaigrette 2 fl oz	260	24.5	4	0	12	1	11	0	700

Additional Gluten-Free Menu Items
(nutritional information was not available)

Breakfast Eggs, Breakfast Relish, Breakfast Chorizo, Breakfast Potatoes, and Pozole Soup

Food Serving size	Cal.	(g) Total Fat	(g) Sat. Fat	(mg) Chol.	(g) Carb.	(g) Fiber	(g) Sug.	(g) Prot.	(mg) Sod.

Claim Jumper
[www.claimjumper.com]

Entrées

BBQ Baby Back Pork Ribs full rack	814	NA	17	148	61	3	NA	32	NA
BBQ Baby Back Pork Ribs full rack	1743	NA	39	360	111	4	NA	75	NA
Broiled Norwegian Salmon 1 entrée	543	NA	10	136	16	4	NA	42	NA
California Chicken Quesadilla 1 entrée	1141	NA	28	189	83	11	NA	61	NA
Giant Stuffed Chicken Baker (without Alfredo Sauce) 1 entrée	990	NA	18	157	118	11	NA	53	NA
Ribs & Chicken Combo 1 entrée	990	NA	18	157	118	11	NA	53	NA
Rotisserie Chicken 1 entrée	739	NA	14	452	5	1	NA	62	NA

Grilled Steaks & Lobster

Chopped Steak with Cheese 11 oz	1046	NA	33	311	13	2	NA	81	NA
Claim Jumper K-Bob (Chicken) (decline rice pilaf) 1 entrée	530	NA	2	119	45	7	NA	54	NA
Claim Jumper K-Bob (Grilled Shrimp) (decline rice pilaf) 1 entrée	654	NA	3	161	89	13	NA	34	NA
Claim Jumper K-Bob (Top Sirloin) (decline rice pilaf) 1 steak	1050	NA	15	470	90	13	NA	53	NA
Filet Mignon 7 oz	665	NA	22	491	1	0	NA	39	NA
Filet Mignon & Lobster Tail 7 oz sirloin, 8 oz tail	1083	NA	43	788	2	1	NA	67	NA
New York Strip, Blackened 1 steak	1040	NA	31	717	5	2	NA	71	NA

Food Serving size	Cal.	(g) Total Fat	(g) Sat. Fat	(mg) Chol.	(g) Carb.	(g) Fiber	(g) Sug.	(g) Prot.	(mg) Sod.
New York Strip, Broiled 1 steak	1019	NA	31	713	1	0	NA	70	NA
Porterhouse Steak 22 oz	1776	NA	56	1334	1	0	NA	102	NA
Ribeye Steak 12 oz	1131	NA	31	738	1	0	NA	91	NA
Ribeye Steak 16 oz	1475	NA	39	953	1	0	NA	121	NA
Top Sirloin 9 oz	745	NA	23	523	1	0	NA	51	NA
Top Sirloin & Lobster Tail 7 oz sirloin, 8 oz tail	1069	NA	44	773	2	1	NA	67	NA

Salads

Food Serving size	Cal.	(g) Total Fat	(g) Sat. Fat	(mg) Chol.	(g) Carb.	(g) Fiber	(g) Sug.	(g) Prot.	(mg) Sod.
BBQ Chicken Salad 1 salad	300	NA	0	56	39	6	NA	27	NA
California Citrus Chicken Salad 1 salad	865	NA	14	86	58	13	NA	39	NA

Cold Stone Creamery
[www.coldstonecreamery.com]

Fruit

Food Serving size	Cal.	(g) Total Fat	(g) Sat. Fat	(mg) Chol.	(g) Carb.	(g) Fiber	(g) Sug.	(g) Prot.	(mg) Sod.
Apple Pie Filling 3/4 oz	60	0	0	0	16	<1	14	0	25
Bananas 1/2 banana	50	0	0	0	14	2	9	<1	0
Black Cherries 3/4 oz	80	0	0	0	18	0	17	0	10
Blueberries 3/4 oz	10	0	0	0	2	<1	2	0	0
Cherry Pie Filling 3/4 oz	50	0	0	0	13	0	0	0	10
Maraschino Cherries 1 cherry	5	0	0	0	1	0	1	0	0

Food Serving size	Cal.	(g) Total Fat	(g) Sat. Fat	(mg) Chol.	(g) Carb.	(g) Fiber	(g) Sug.	(g) Prot.	(mg) Sod.
Peach Pie Filling 1 oz	60	0	0	0	16	<1	14	0	25
Pineapple Chunks 3/4 oz	15	0	0	0	4	0	4	0	0
Raspberries 3/4 oz	25	0	0	0	5	1	2	0	0
Strawberries 3/4 oz	20	0	0	0	7	<1	4	0	0

Ice Cream

Food Serving size	Cal.	(g) Total Fat	(g) Sat. Fat	(mg) Chol.	(g) Carb.	(g) Fiber	(g) Sug.	(g) Prot.	(mg) Sod.
Amaretto Ice Cream (Large) 340g	790	47	30	185	80	0	69	12	190
Amaretto Ice Cream (Medium) 227g	530	31	20	125	53	0	46	8	130
Amaretto Ice Cream (Small) 142g	330	20	12	80	33	0	29	5	80
Banana Ice Cream (Large) 340g	750	44	28	175	80	<1	68	11	170
Banana Ice Cream (Medium) 227g	500	29	18	115	53	0	46	8	115
Banana Ice Cream (Small) 142g	310	18	12	70	33	0	28	5	70
Black Cherry Ice Cream (Large) 340g	790	44	28	175	86	0	76	11	180
Black Cherry Ice Cream (Medium) 227g	530	30	19	120	58	0	51	8	120
Black Cherry Ice Cream (Small) 142g	330	19	12	75	36	0	32	5	75
Blueberry Ice Cream (Large) 340g	760	47	31	185	79	0	74	13	130
Blueberry Ice Cream (Medium) 227g	510	31	21	120	53	0	49	9	90
Blueberry Ice Cream (Small) 142g	320	20	13	75	33	0	31	5	55

Food Serving size	Cal.	(g) Total Fat	(g) Sat. Fat	(mg) Chol.	(g) Carb.	(g) Fiber	(g) Sug.	(g) Prot.	(mg) Sod.
Butter Pecan Ice Cream (Large) 340g	780	47	30	185	79	0	68	12	260
Butter Pecan Ice Cream (Medium) 227g	520	31	20	125	53	0	45	8	170
Butter Pecan Ice Cream (Small) 142g	320	19	12	75	32	0	28	5	105
Cheesecake Ice Cream (Large) 340g	760	45	30	115	86	1	76	10	210
Cheesecake Ice Cream (Medium) 227g	510	30	20	75	57	0	51	6	140
Cheesecake Ice Cream (Small) 142g	320	19	13	50	36	0	32	4	85
Cherry Vanilla Ice Cream (Large) 340g	750	45	30	115	84	1	77	9	200
Cherry Vanilla Ice Cream (Medium) 227g	500	30	20	75	56	1	51	6	135
Cherry Vanilla Ice Cream (Small) 142g	310	19	13	45	35	0	32	4	85
Chocolate Dipped Strawberry (Large) 340g	740	45	30	70	77	5	70	12	150
Chocolate Dipped Strawberry (Medium) 227g	490	30	20	45	51	3	46	8	100
Chocolate Dipped Strawberry (Small) 142g	310	19	12	30	32	2	29	5	65
Chocolate Hazelnut Ice Cream (Large) 340g	830	50	30	105	91	4	81	12	200
Chocolate Hazelnut Ice Cream (Medium) 227g	550	33	20	70	61	2	54	8	135
Chocolate Hazelnut Ice Cream (Small) 142g	340	21	12	85	38	2	34	5	38
Chocolate Ice Cream (Large) 340g	780	48	30	185	79	3	71	13	230
Chocolate Ice Cream (Medium) 227g	520	32	20	125	53	2	48	9	160

Food Serving size	Cal.	(g) Total Fat	(g) Sat. Fat	(mg) Chol.	(g) Carb.	(g) Fiber	(g) Sug.	(g) Prot.	(mg) Sod.
Chocolate Ice Cream (Small)									
142g	320	20	13	75	33	1	30	6	95
Chocolate Peanut Butter Ice Cream (Large)									
340g	990	67	31	55	86	6	74	24	480
Chocolate Peanut Butter Ice Cream (Medium)									
227g	660	45	21	35	58	4	49	16	320
Chocolate Peanut Butter Ice Cream (Small)									
142g	410	28	13	25	36	3	31	10	200
Cinnamon Ice Cream (Large)									
340g	790	47	30	185	82	2	69	35	190
Cinnamon Ice Cream (Medium)									
227g	530	32	20	125	55	1	46	8	125
Cinnamon Ice Cream (Small)									
142g	330	20	12	80	34	<1	29	5	80
Coconut Ice Cream (Large)									
340g	780	47	30	185	79	0	68	12	190
Coconut Ice Cream (Medium)									
227g	520	31	20	125	52	0	45	8	125
Coconut Ice Cream (Small)									
142g	330	20	12	75	33	0	28	5	80
Coffee Ice Cream (Large)									
340g	790	47	30	185	81	0	69	12	190
Coffee Ice Cream (Medium)									
227g	530	31	20	125	54	0	46	8	125
Coffee Ice Cream (Small)									
142g	330	20	12	80	34	0	29	5	80
Cotton Candy Ice Cream (Large)									
340g	790	47	29	185	82	0	68	12	180
Cotton Candy Ice Cream (Medium)									
227g	530	31	20	125	55	0	45	8	120
Cotton Candy Ice Cream (Small)									
142g	330	19	12	75	34	0	28	5	75
Dark Chocolate Ice Cream (Large)									
340g	800	47	30	175	77	7	68	35	230

Food Serving size	Cal.	(g) Total Fat	(g) Sat. Fat	(mg) Chol.	(g) Carb.	(g) Fiber	(g) Sug.	(g) Prot.	(mg) Sod.
Dark Chocolate Ice Cream (Medium) 227g	227	32	20	115	51	5	46	11	150
Dark Chocolate Ice Cream (Small) 142g	340	20	12	75	32	3	29	7	95
French Toast Ice Cream (Large) 340g	790	46	29	180	84	0	73	12	370
French Toast Ice Cream (Medium) 227g	530	31	19	120	56	0	49	8	250
French Toast Ice Cream (Small) 142g	330	19	12	75	35	0	30	5	150
French Vanilla Ice Cream (Large) 340g	810	46	33	240	89	0	78	12	190
French Vanilla Ice Cream (Medium) 227g	540	30	22	60	60	0	52	8	125
French Vanilla Ice Cream (Small) 142g	340	19	14	100	37	0	33	5	80
Ghirardelli Chocolate Ice Cream (Large) 340g	780	47	30	175	88	8	64	16	180
Ghirardelli Chocolate Ice Cream (Medium) 227g	520	31	20	115	59	6	43	11	125
Ghirardelli Chocolate Ice Cream (Small) 142g	330	20	12	75	37	4	27	7	75
Irish Cream Ice Cream (Large) 340g	790	47	30	190	80	0	70	12	190
Irish Cream Ice Cream (Medium) 227g	530	32	20	125	54	0	46	8	125
Irish Cream Ice Cream (Small) 142g	330	20	13	80	33	0	29	5	80
Key Lime Ice Cream (Large) 340g	820	48	31	170	94	0	87	12	120
Key Lime Ice Cream (Medium) 227g	550	32	21	115	63	0	58	8	80
Key Lime Ice Cream (Small) 142g	340	20	13	70	39	0	36	5	50

Food Serving size	Cal.	(g) Total Fat	(g) Sat. Fat	(mg) Chol.	(g) Carb.	(g) Fiber	(g) Sug.	(g) Prot.	(mg) Sod.
Macadamia Nut Ice Cream (Large) 340g	790	47	30	185	81	0	70	12	190
Macadamia Nut Ice Cream (Medium) 227g	530	31	20	125	54	0	46	8	125
Macadamia Nut Ice Cream (Small) 142g	330	20	12	80	34	0	29	5	75
Mango Ice Cream (Large) 340g	740	44	28	175	80	0	68	11	170
Mango Ice Cream (Medium) 227g	490	29	18	115	53	0	45	7	115
Mango Ice Cream (Small) 142g	310	18	12	70	33	0	28	5	70
Mint Ice Cream (Large) 340g	790	45	29	180	86	0	75	12	180
Mint Ice Cream (Medium) 227g	530	30	19	120	57	0	50	8	120
Mint Ice Cream (Small) 142g	330	19	12	75	36	0	31	5	75
Mocha Ice Cream (Large) 340g	780	47	30	180	80	3	70	14	230
Mocha Ice Cream (Medium) 227g	520	31	20	120	53	2	47	9	150
Mocha Ice Cream (Small) 142g	320	20	12	75	33	1	29	6	95
Orange Dreamsicle Ice Cream (Large) 340g	760	45	28	180	83	0	68	11	180
Orange Dreamsicle Ice Cream (Medium) 227g	510	30	19	120	55	0	45	8	120
Orange Dreamsicle Ice Cream (Small) 142g	320	19	12	75	35	0	28	5	75
Peach Ice Cream (Large) 340g	760	35	23	135	106	0	94	10	105
Peach Ice Cream (Medium) 227g	500	23	16	90	71	0	63	7	70

Food Serving size	Cal.	(g) Total Fat	(g) Sat. Fat	(mg) Chol.	(g) Carb.	(g) Fiber	(g) Sug.	(g) Prot.	(mg) Sod.
Peach Ice Cream (Small) 142g	310	15	10	55	44	0	39	4	45
Peanut Butter Ice Cream (Large) 340g	890	58	30	175	79	2	66	18	310
Peanut Butter Ice Cream (Medium) 227g	590	39	20	115	53	1	44	12	210
Peanut Butter Ice Cream (Small) 142g	370	24	13	75	33	<1	28	7	130
Pecan Praline Ice Cream (Large) 340g	800	45	28	175	88	0	73	11	220
Pecan Praline Ice Cream (Medium) 227g	530	30	19	115	58	0	49	8	150
Pecan Praline Ice Cream (Small) 142g	330	19	12	75	37	0	31	5	90
Pineapple Upside Down Cake Ice Cream (Large) 340g	740	41	26	90	90	1	76	9	350
Pineapple Upside Down Cake Ice Cream (Medium) 227g	490	27	17	60	60	1	51	6	240
Pineapple Upside Down Cake Ice Cream (Small) 142g	310	17	11	40	37	1	32	4	150
Pistachio Ice Cream (Large) 340g	780	47	30	185	80	0	70	12	200
Pistachio Ice Cream (Medium) 227g	520	31	20	125	54	0	46	8	135
Pistachio Ice Cream (Small) 142g	330	20	12	80	34	0	29	5	85
Pumpkin Ice Cream (Large) 340g	680	37	23	145	80	3	67	10	260
Pumpkin Ice Cream (Medium) 227g	460	24	15	95	53	2	45	7	170
Pumpkin Ice Cream (Small) 142g	290	15	10	60	33	1	28	4	105
Raspberry Ice Cream (Large) 340g	780	44	28	175	85	0	75	12	180

Food Serving size	Cal.	(g) Total Fat	(g) Sat. Fat	(mg) Chol.	(g) Carb.	(g) Fiber	(g) Sug.	(g) Prot.	(mg) Sod.
Raspberry Ice Cream (Medium) 227g	520	30	19	120	57	0	50	8	125
Raspberry Ice Cream (Small) 142g	330	19	12	75	36	0	31	5	75
Salted Caramel Ice Cream (Large) 340g	790	43	29	145	97	1	84	9	510
Salted Caramel Ice Cream (Medium) 227g	530	29	19	100	64	1	56	6	340
Salted Caramel Ice Cream (Small) 142g	330	18	12	60	40	35	35	4	210
Sinless Banana Ice Cream (Large) 340g	410	0.5	0.5	0	83	2	27	17	350
Sinless Banana Ice Cream (Medium) 227g	270	0	0	0	55	2	18	11	240
Sinless Banana Ice Cream (Small) 142g	170	0	0	0	35	1	11	7	150
Sinless Sans Fat Sweet Cream (Large) 340g	420	0.5	0	10	83	2	26	18	390
Sinless Sans Fat Sweet Cream (Medium) 227g	280	0	0	0	56	1	17	12	260
Sinless Sans Fat Sweet Cream (Small) 142g	170	0	0	0	35	1	11	8	160
Strawberry Cheesecake Ice Cream (Large) 340g	780	50	28	160	94	1	77	12	125
Strawberry Cheesecake Ice Cream (Medium) 227g	520	33	18	105	63	0	51	8	85
Strawberry Cheesecake Ice Cream (Small) 142g	320	21	12	65	39	0	32	5	50
Strawberry Ice Cream (Large) 340g	770	44	28	175	83	0	72	11	180
Strawberry Ice Cream (Medium) 227g	510	30	19	115	55	0	48	8	120
Strawberry Ice Cream (Small) 142g	320	18	12	75	35	0	30	5	75

Food Serving size	Cal.	(g) Total Fat	(g) Sat. Fat	(mg) Chol.	(g) Carb.	(g) Fiber	(g) Sug.	(g) Prot.	(mg) Sod.
Sweet Cream Ice Cream (Large) 340g	790	48	30	190	80	0	70	12	190
Sweet Cream Ice Cream (Medium) 227g	530	32	20	125	53	0	46	8	125
Sweet Cream Ice Cream (Small) 142g	330	20	13	80	33	0	29	5	80
Vanilla Bean Ice Cream (Large) 340g	790	46	29	180	77	0	67	12	180
Vanilla Bean Ice Cream (Medium) 227g	530	31	19	120	52	0	45	8	120
Vanilla Bean Ice Cream (Small) 142g	330	19	12	75	32	0	28	5	75
White Chocolate Ice Cream (Large) 340g	780	47	29	185	79	0	68	12	180
White Chocolate Ice Cream (Medium) 227g	520	31	20	125	53	0	45	8	125
White Chocolate Ice Cream (Small) 142g	320	19	12	75	33	0	28	5	75

Mix-Ins

Food Serving size	Cal.	(g) Total Fat	(g) Sat. Fat	(mg) Chol.	(g) Carb.	(g) Fiber	(g) Sug.	(g) Prot.	(mg) Sod.
Almond Joy Candy 1 piece	170	9	6	0	21	2	16	1	50
Butterfinger Candy Bar 1/2 bar	140	6	3	0	22	<1	15	2	65
Chocolate Chips 1 oz	130	7	4.5	0	16	1	14	1	0
Chocolate Shavings .5 oz	90	5	3	0	9	2	8	<1	0
Chocolate Sprinkles 1 oz	25	0	0	0	6	0	6	0	0
Coconut .5 oz	80	5	4.5	0	7	<1	6	0	40
Gumballs 1 oz	90	0	0	0	23	<1	24	0	0

Food Serving size	Cal.	(g) Total Fat	(g) Sat. Fat	(mg) Chol.	(g) Carb.	(g) Fiber	(g) Sug.	(g) Prot.	(mg) Sod.
Gummi Bears 1 oz	120	0	0	0	30	0	13	0	15
Heath Toffee Bar 1 bar	110	7	3.5	5	12	0	12	<1	75
M&M's Candy 1 oz	170	7	4.5	<5	25	<1	22	2	20
Marshmallows 1 oz	160	6	1.5	10	25	1	16	2	100
Peanut Butter 3/4 oz	150	13	2.5	0	5	1	2	6	125
Peanut M&M's 1 oz	150	8	3.5	<5	18	<1	14	3	30
Rainbow Sprinkles 1 oz	25	0	0	0	6	0	6	0	0
Reese's Peanut Butter Cup 1 piece	190	11	4	0	19	1	17	4	110
Reese's Pieces Candy 1 oz	180	9	6	0	21	1	19	4	70
Snickers Candy 1/2 bar	170	9	3	<5	21	<1	17	3	95
White Chocolate Chips 1 oz	160	9	8	<5	18	0	18	2	45
York Peppermint Patties 2 pieces	120	2	1.5	0	24	<1	18	<1	10

Nuts

Food Serving size	Cal.	(g) Total Fat	(g) Sat. Fat	(mg) Chol.	(g) Carb.	(g) Fiber	(g) Sug.	(g) Prot.	(mg) Sod.
Cashews 1 oz	170	14	2.5	0	9	1	2	5	90
Macadamia Nuts 1 oz	180	19	3	0	3	2	<1	2	65
Peanuts 1 oz	210	18	3	0	5	3	0	10	110
Pecan Pralines 1 oz	210	21	1.5	0	5	2	1	2	230

Food Serving size	Cal.	(g) Total Fat	(g) Sat. Fat	(mg) Chol.	(g) Carb.	(g) Fiber	(g) Sug.	(g) Prot.	(mg) Sod.
Pecans 1 oz	140	15	1.5	0	3	2	<1	2	80
Pistachios 1 oz	200	16	2	0	10	4	<1	7	0
Sliced Almonds 1 oz	210	20	2	0	6	4	0	7	0
Walnuts 1 oz	130	13	1	0	3	1	0	3	0

Sorbet and Yogurt

Food Serving size	Cal.	(g) Total Fat	(g) Sat. Fat	(mg) Chol.	(g) Carb.	(g) Fiber	(g) Sug.	(g) Prot.	(mg) Sod.
Chocolate Yogurt large	420	1	0	0	95	3	73	12	360
Chocolate Yogurt medium	280	0.5	0	0	64	2	49	8	240
Chocolate Yogurt small	180	0	0	0	40	1	31	5	150
Country Time Lemonade Sorbet large	570	0	0	0	142	0	142	0	55
Country Time Lemonade Sorbet medium	380	0	0	0	95	0	95	0	35
Country Time Lemonade Sorbet small	240	0	0	0	59	0	59	0	25
Lemon Sorbet large	370	0	0	0	96	<1	81	0	35
Lemon Sorbet medium	250	0	0	0	64	0	54	0	25
Lemon Sorbet small	150	0	0	0	40	0	34	0	15
Mojito Sorbet large	470	4.5	2.5	0	110	1	107	0	10
Mojito Sorbet medium	310	3	1.5	0	74	0	71	0	5
Mojito Sorbet small	190	2	1	0	46	0	44	0	0

Food Serving size	Cal.	(g) Total Fat	(g) Sat. Fat	(mg) Chol.	(g) Carb.	(g) Fiber	(g) Sug.	(g) Prot.	(mg) Sod.
Pineapple Sorbet large	340	0	0	0	88	1	87	0	10
Pineapple Sorbet medium	230	0	0	0	59	1	58	0	5
Pineapple Sorbet small	140	0	0	0	37	0	36	0	0
Raspberry Sorbet large	390	0	0	0	101	<1	87	0	40
Raspberry Sorbet medium	260	0	0	0	67	0	58	0	30
Raspberry Sorbet small	160	0	0	0	42	0	36	0	15
Raspberry Yogurt large	440	0	0	0	101	1	76	10	360
Raspberry Yogurt medium	290	0	0	0	67	0	51	7	240
Raspberry Yogurt small	180	0	0	0	42	0	32	4	150
Strawberry Mango Banana Sorbet large	520	0.5	0	0	131	1	125	0	35
Strawberry Mango Banana Sorbet medium	350	0	0	0	87	1	83	0	25
Strawberry Mango Banana Sorbet small	220	0	0	0	55	0	52	0	15
Vanilla Yogurt large	420	0	0	0	95	0	74	11	360
Vanilla Yogurt medium	280	0	0	0	63	0	49	7	240
Vanilla Yogurt small	170	0	0	0	40	0	31	5	150
Watermelon Sorbet large	380	0	0	90	99	<1	84	0	40
Watermelon Sorbet medium	260	0	0	0	66	0	56	0	25

Food Serving size	Cal.	(g) Total Fat	(g) Sat. Fat	(mg) Chol.	(g) Carb.	(g) Fiber	(g) Sug.	(g) Prot.	(mg) Sod.
Watermelon Sorbet small	160	0	0	0	41	0	35	0	15

Toppings

Butterscotch Fat Free 1 oz	80	0	0	0	19	0	15	<1	85
Caramel 1 oz	90	1	0.5	<5	21	0	13	<1	50
Caramel Fat Free 1 oz	80	0	0	0	19	0	14	<1	85
Cinnamon 1/8 tsp	0	0	0	0	0	0	0	0	0
Fudge 1 oz	90	2	2	0	18	0	16	1	80
Fudge Fat Free 1 oz	80	0	0	0	20	0	16	<1	15
Honey 1 oz	90	0	0	0	25	0	25	0	0
Marshmallow Crème 1 oz	100	0	0	0	24	0	20	0	20
Redi Whip Original 1 dollop	45	2.5	1	0	5	0	2	<1	15

Additional Gluten-Free Menu Items
(nutritional information was not available)

Lemon Ice Smoothie, Mango Smoothie, Orange Juice Smoothie, and Lifestyle Smoothie Mix

Dairy Queen
[www.dairyqueen.com]

Blizzard Treats

Banana Split Blizzard large	780	23	15	75	129	2	107	18	320
Banana Split Blizzard medium	570	17	11	55	93	1	77	13	230

Food Serving size	Cal.	(g) Total Fat	(g) Sat. Fat	(mg) Chol.	(g) Carb.	(g) Fiber	(g) Sug.	(g) Prot.	(mg) Sod.
Banana Split Blizzard mini	290	8	5	25	49	1	41	6	115
Banana Split Blizzard small	440	14	9	45	71	1	58	11	190
Butterfinger Blizzard large	990	35	21	70	151	0	114	21	460
Butterfinger Blizzard medium	740	26	16	55	114	0	86	16	350
Butterfinger Blizzard mini	340	12	7	30	52	0	41	8	160
Butterfinger Blizzard small	470	16	10	40	71	0	56	11	220
Hawaiian Blizzard large	820	29	22	65	125	4	103	17	330
Hawaiian Blizzard medium	600	21	15	50	92	3	75	13	240
Hawaiian Blizzard mini	300	10	7	30	45	1	37	7	125
Hawaiian Blizzard small	440	15	10	40	67	1	55	10	180
Heath Blizzard large	1260	57	36	90	173	2	153	21	680
Heath Blizzard medium	920	41	26	65	126	1	111	16	490
Heath Blizzard mini	360	14	9	30	51	0	43	8	180
Heath Blizzard small	600	26	16	50	83	1	73	11	310
M&M Chocolate Candy Blizzard large	1140	41	25	85	176	2	152	22	380
M&M Chocolate Candy Blizzard medium	840	30	19	65	127	2	110	25	270
M&M Chocolate Candy Blizzard mini	370	13	8	30	57	1	48	8	135

Food Serving size	Cal.	(g) Total Fat	(g) Sat. Fat	(mg) Chol.	(g) Carb.	(g) Fiber	(g) Sug.	(g) Prot.	(mg) Sod.
M&M Chocolate Candy Blizzard small	660	23	14	55	101	1	87	13	230
Reese's Peanut Butter Cup Blizzard large	1040	44	23	80	141	3	120	26	560
Reese's Peanut Butter Cup Blizzard medium	740	31	16	60	101	2	86	18	400
Reese's Peanut Butter Cup Blizzard mini	360	14	8	30	50	1	43	9	180
Reese's Peanut Butter Cup Blizzard small	530	21	11	45	74	1	62	13	270

Dilly Bars

Food Serving size	Cal.	Total Fat	Sat. Fat	Chol.	Carb.	Fiber	Sug.	Prot.	Sod.
Butterscotch Dilly Bar 1 bar	210	11	9	15	24	0	20	3	105
Cherry Dilly Bar 1 bar	210	12	8	15	24	0	20	3	80
Chocolate Dilly Bar 1 bar	240	15	9	15	24	1	20	4	70
Chocolate Mint Dilly Bar 1 bar	240	15	9	15	24	1	20	4	70
Heath Dilly Bar 1 bar	220	13	10	15	25	0	22	3	95
No Sugar Added Dilly Bar 1 bar	190	13	10	15	24	5	5	3	60

Drinks

Food Serving size	Cal.	Total Fat	Sat. Fat	Chol.	Carb.	Fiber	Sug.	Prot.	Sod.
Arctic Rush Slush (all flavors) large	350	0	0	0	70	0	70	0	0
Arctic Rush Slush (all flavors) medium	260	0	0	0	53	0	53	0	0
Arctic Rush Slush (all flavors) small	210	0	0	0	41	0	41	0	0

Food Serving size	Cal.	(g) Total Fat	(g) Sat. Fat	(mg) Chol.	(g) Carb.	(g) Fiber	(g) Sug.	(g) Prot.	(mg) Sod.
Food									
French Fries (request that they be fried separately) kids'	190	8	1	0	27	2	0	2	400
French Fries (request that they be fried separately) large	500	21	3.5	0	70	5	0	6	1040
French Fries (request that they be fried separately) regular	310	13	2	0	43	3	0	4	640
Grilled Chicken Patty (without bun) 1 patty	360	15	2.5	50	32	1	5	25	1040
Hamburger Patty (without bun) 1 patty	163	14	7	50	34	1	9	17	680
Hot Dog Frank (without bun) 1 frank	290	17	7	35	22	1	4	11	900

Fountain Sodas

Food Serving size	Cal.	(g) Total Fat	(g) Sat. Fat	(mg) Chol.	(g) Carb.	(g) Fiber	(g) Sug.	(g) Prot.	(mg) Sod.
Barq's large	350	0	0	0	96	0	96	0	80
Barq's medium	230	0	0	0	63	0	63	0	50
Barq's small	180	0	0	0	48	0	48	0	40
Bottled Water 1 bottle	0	0	0	0	0	0	0	0	15
Coca-Cola large	330	0	0	0	85	0	85	0	20
Coca-Cola medium	220	0	0	0	56	0	56	0	15
Coca-Cola small	160	0	0	0	43	0	43	0	10
Coffee 12 oz	0	0	0	0	0	0	0	0	5
Diet Coca-Cola large	0	0	0	0	0	0	0	0	15

Food Serving size	Cal.	(g) Total Fat	(g) Sat. Fat	(mg) Chol.	(g) Carb.	(g) Fiber	(g) Sug.	(g) Prot.	(mg) Sod.
Diet Coca-Cola medium	0	0	0	0	0	0	0	0	10
Diet Coca-Cola small	0	0	0	0	0	0	0	0	10
Diet Pepsi large	0	0	0	0	0	0	0	0	30
Diet Pepsi medium	0	0	0	0	0	0	0	0	50
Diet Pepsi small	0	0	0	0	0	0	0	0	40
Dr Pepper large	320	0	0	0	86	0	86	0	115
Dr Pepper medium	210	0	0	0	57	0	57	0	75
Dr Pepper small	160	0	0	0	43	0	43	0	55
Milk, 2% 8 oz	110	4.5	3	15	11	0	11	7	105
Mountain Dew large	360	0	0	0	98	0	98	0	150
Mountain Dew medium	240	0	0	0	64	0	64	0	100
Mountain Dew small	190	0	0	0	51	0	51	0	80
Mug large	320	0	0	0	94	0	94	0	135
Mug medium	210	0	0	0	62	0	62	0	85
Mug small	160	0	0	0	47	0	47	0	65
Pepsi large	320	0	0	0	87	0	87	0	80
Pepsi medium	210	0	0	0	57	0	57	0	50

Food Serving size	Cal.	(g) Total Fat	(g) Sat. Fat	(mg) Chol.	(g) Carb.	(g) Fiber	(g) Sug.	(g) Prot.	(mg) Sod.
Pepsi small	160	0	0	0	44	0	44	0	40
Sierra Mist large	330	0	0	0	87	0	87	0	85
Sierra Mist medium	220	0	0	0	57	0	57	0	55
Sierra Mist small	170	0	0	0	43	0	43	0	45
Sprite large	310	0	0	0	84	0	84	0	75
Sprite medium	200	0	0	0	55	0	55	0	50
Sprite small	150	0	0	0	42	0	42	0	40

MooLatte Frozen Blended Coffee

Food Serving size	Cal.	(g) Total Fat	(g) Sat. Fat	(mg) Chol.	(g) Carb.	(g) Fiber	(g) Sug.	(g) Prot.	(mg) Sod.
Caramel MooLatté large	690	23	18	55	107	0	77	13	330
Caramel MooLatté medium	650	20	15	45	103	0	81	10	250
Caramel MooLatté small	520	16	13	35	82	0	64	8	190
French Vanilla MooLatté large	780	22	16	50	129	0	108	12	240
French Vanilla MooLatté medium	630	19	14	40	101	0	84	10	190
French Vanilla MooLatté small	500	15	12	30	80	0	67	8	150
Mocha MooLatté large	820	31	18	50	121	0	105	13	310
Mocha MooLatté medium	660	25	16	40	96	0	83	11	250
Mocha MooLatté small	500	19	13	30	74	0	65	8	170

Food Serving size	Cal.	(g) Total Fat	(g) Sat. Fat	(mg) Chol.	(g) Carb.	(g) Fiber	(g) Sug.	(g) Prot.	(mg) Sod.
Novelties									
DQ Fudge Bar 1 bar	50	0	0	0	13	6	4	4	70
DQ Vanilla Orange Bar 1 bar	60	0	0	0	18	6	4	2	40
Shakes									
Caramel large	960	29	21	80	155	0	109	21	470
Caramel medium	740	24	17	65	117	0	84	16	350
Caramel small	560	20	15	50	83	0	63	13	250
Chocolate large	900	31	19	70	148	2	128	20	380
Chocolate medium	700	25	16	55	112	1	97	16	290
Chocolate small	540	20	14	45	81	1	69	12	220
Hot Fudge large	970	36	29	75	141	1	112	22	450
Hot Fudge medium	750	29	23	55	108	1	86	17	330
Hot Fudge small	560	22	17	45	79	1	64	13	240
Strawberry large	770	26	19	70	114	1	96	20	330
Strawberry medium	610	22	16	55	90	0	76	15	260
Strawberry small	490	18	14	45	70	0	59	12	200

Food Serving size	Cal.	(g) Total Fat	(g) Sat. Fat	(mg) Chol.	(g) Carb.	(g) Fiber	(g) Sug.	(g) Prot.	(mg) Sod.
Sundaes									
Caramel large	610	16	11	55	103	0	72	12	290
Caramel medium	430	11	7	35	74	0	51	9	210
Caramel small	300	8	5	25	50	0	35	6	140
Chocolate large	570	17	10	45	98	1	84	12	240
Chocolate medium	400	12	7	30	70	1	60	8	170
Chocolate small	280	8	4.5	25	48	1	41	6	115
Hot Fudge large	610	21	16	50	94	1	74	13	280
Hot Fudge medium	440	15	11	35	67	1	52	9	200
Hot Fudge small	300	10	8	25	46	0	36	6	135
Marshmallow large	580	14	9	45	103	0	85	20	220
Marshmallow medium	410	10	6	30	74	0	61	8	150
Marshmallow small	290	7	4.5	25	50	0	42	6	105
Strawberry large	480	14	9	45	76	0	63	12	200
Strawberry medium	350	10	6	30	56	0	47	8	140
Strawberry small	260	7	4.5	25	44	0	36	6	105

Food Serving size	Cal.	(g) Total Fat	(g) Sat. Fat	(mg) Chol.	(g) Carb.	(g) Fiber	(g) Sug.	(g) Prot.	(mg) Sod.

Treats

| **Vanilla and Chocolate Soft Serve** | | | | | | | | | |
| 1/2 cup | 140 | 4.5 | 3 | 15 | 22 | NA | 19 | 3 | 70 |

Denny's
[www.dennys.com]

Beverages

Apple Juice									
1 cup	117	0.3	0	0	29	0.2	27	0.1	7
Coke									
12 fl oz	140	0	0	0	39	0	39	0	45
Coke, Diet									
12 fl oz	4	0	0	0	0.5	0	NA	0.4	14
Hot Chocolate									
1 serving	100	2	2	0	28	1	24	0	219
Lemonade									
36g	66	0	0	0	17	0	16	0	1
Orange Juice									
1 cup (249g)	110	0	0	0	25	0	NA	2	2
Raspberry Tea, sweetened									
12 oz serving	70	0	0	0	18	0	18	0	45
Root Beer									
12 oz	152	0	0	0	39.2	NA	39.2	0	48
Ruby Red Grapefruit drink									
1 cup	120	0	0	0	30	NA	30	0	65

Condiments

Ketchup									
1 tbsp	15	0	0	0	3.8	0	3.4	0.3	167
Mustard, Yellow, prepared									
1 tsp	3	0.2	0	0	0.3	0.2	0	0.2	57
Pickle Slices									
2 slices	5	0	0	0	0	0	NA	0	0

Food Serving size	Cal.	(g) Total Fat	(g) Sat. Fat	(mg) Chol.	(g) Carb.	(g) Fiber	(g) Sug.	(g) Prot.	(mg) Sod.
Dressings									
Bleu Cheese 1 oz	110	11	3	20	1	0	1	1	220
Caesar 1 oz	100	10	0	5	0	0	0	1	300
Coleslaw 5 oz	260	22	4	35	15	3	12	2	520
French 1 oz	74	5	0	7	8	0	4	0	248
Honey Mustard 1 oz	160	15	0	10	5	0	4	0	140
Italian, Fat Free 1 oz	9	0	0	0	3	0	2	0	367
Low Fat Balsamic Vinaigrette 1 oz	35	1	0	0	7	0	7	0	140
Mayonnaise 1 serving	90	10	1.5	5	NA	NA	NA	NA	70
Fruits									
Strawberries cup of halves	49	0.46	0.023	0	11.67	3	7.08	1.02	2
Ice Cream									
Banana Split 15 oz	810	31	19	100	125	5	95	12	190
Chocolate 1 serving	271-309	14-17	NA	50-68	33-35	0	27	6	77-97
Mint Chocolate Chip 1/2 cup	160	8	6	25	19	0	14	2	75
Pecans, Glazed 1.25 oz	200	15	1	0	18	0	13	1	135
Strawberry 1 serving	271-309	14-17	NA	50-68	33-35	0	27	6	77-97

Food Serving size	Cal.	(g) Total Fat	(g) Sat. Fat	(mg) Chol.	(g) Carb.	(g) Fiber	(g) Sug.	(g) Prot.	(mg) Sod.
Vanilla 1 serving	271-309	14-17	NA	50-68	33-35	0	27	6	77-97
Whipped Topping 2 tbsp	25	1.5	1.5	0	2	NA	2	0	0

Margarine

Food Serving size	Cal.	(g) Total Fat	(g) Sat. Fat	(mg) Chol.	(g) Carb.	(g) Fiber	(g) Sug.	(g) Prot.	(mg) Sod.
Liquid 1 tbsp	102	11.45	1.874	0	0	0	0	0.27	111
Whipped Butter-Margarine Blend 1 tbsp	101	11	4	12	0	0	NA	0	4

Meats / Seafood

Food Serving size	Cal.	(g) Total Fat	(g) Sat. Fat	(mg) Chol.	(g) Carb.	(g) Fiber	(g) Sug.	(g) Prot.	(mg) Sod.
Bacon Strips 2 strips	70	5	2	15	1	0	0	5	230
Bacon, Turkey 2 strips	90	5	3	42	1	0	0	10	360
Chicken Sausage Patty 1 patty	110	9	3	45	0	0	1	7	260
Ham (Sliced) 1 slice	120	5	4	45	8	0	6	14	710
Prime Rib 1 serving	585	38	12.5	535	15	3	8	33	1460

Menu Item

Food Serving size	Cal.	(g) Total Fat	(g) Sat. Fat	(mg) Chol.	(g) Carb.	(g) Fiber	(g) Sug.	(g) Prot.	(mg) Sod.
American/Swiss (slice) 1 slice	106	7.8	5	26	1.5	NA	0.4	7.5	54
Applesauce 1 cup	1	0	0	0	27.5	2.9	24.6	0.4	5
Avocado 1 med	276	27.6	NA	NA	1.4	4.3	NA	1.4	NA
Black Beans 1 cup	227	1	0	0	41	15	NA	15	2
Butter, Salted 1 tbsp	102	12	7	31	0	0	0	0	101

Food Serving size	Cal.	(g) Total Fat	(g) Sat. Fat	(mg) Chol.	(g) Carb.	(g) Fiber	(g) Sug.	(g) Prot.	(mg) Sod.
Cheddar, Shredded 1 cup	455	37.45	23.834	119	1.45	0	0.59	28.14	702
Cheese Blend, Shredded 2 tbsp	14	1	NA	NA	0	NA	NA	1	NA
Cherry Topping 2 oz	57	0	0	0	14	0	12	0	12
Coffee, Decaffeinated 1 fl oz	0	0	0	0	0	0	0	0	4
Coffee, Regular 1 cup	0	0	0	0	0	0	0	0	0
Cream Cheese 1 tbsp	35	3.5	2.2	11	0.3	NA	0	0.8	30
Egg Whites (2 Whites) 4 oz	50	0	0	0	1	0	0	11	180
Pepper Jack Cheese 1 slice	80	6	4	20	0	0	0	4	140
Tortilla Chips 1 oz	138	6.6	0.8	0	18.6	1.5	0.3	2.2	119
Whole Egg Liquid 1 tbsp	8.3	0	0	0	0	0	0	1.7	25

Potatoes

Food Serving size	Cal.	(g) Total Fat	(g) Sat. Fat	(mg) Chol.	(g) Carb.	(g) Fiber	(g) Sug.	(g) Prot.	(mg) Sod.
French Fries, Salted 5 oz	430	23	5	0	50	5	0	5	95
Hash Browns 1 serving	210	12	3	0	26	2	1	2	650
Mashed Potatoes 4 oz	100	3	2	5	55	1	1	2	350
Red Skinned 4 oz	210	7	2	0	27	3	0	4	630

Sauces

Food Serving size	Cal.	(g) Total Fat	(g) Sat. Fat	(mg) Chol.	(g) Carb.	(g) Fiber	(g) Sug.	(g) Prot.	(mg) Sod.
A-1 Steak Sauce 1 tbsp	15	0	0	0	3	0	2	0	280

Food Serving size	Cal.	(g) Total Fat	(g) Sat. Fat	(mg) Chol.	(g) Carb.	(g) Fiber	(g) Sug.	(g) Prot.	(mg) Sod.
Cocktail Sauce 30g	30	0	0	0	7	0	2	0	230
Lemon Butter Sauce 2 tbsp	25	2	1.5	5	2	NA	NA	0	100
Peanut Butter Sauce 1 oz	96	8	0	0	4	0	0	4	0
Sausage Links (Breakfast) 4 links	370	34	13	70	4	3	0	9	660
Tartar Sauce 1 tbsp	74	7.39	1.109	4	2.12	0	0.56	0.15	98

Sugar Substitutes

Food Serving size	Cal.	Total Fat	Sat. Fat	Chol.	Carb.	Fiber	Sug.	Prot.	Sod.
Equal 1 packet	0	0	NA	NA	<1	NA	NA	0	0
Splenda 1 packet	0	0	0	0	<1	0	<1	0	0
Sweet & Low 1 packet	0	0	0	NA	<1	NA	<1	0	0

Syrups

Food Serving size	Cal.	Total Fat	Sat. Fat	Chol.	Carb.	Fiber	Sug.	Prot.	Sod.
Chocolate Syrup 2 tbsp	109	0.4	0.2	0	25.4	1	19.4	0.8	28
Maple Sauce (Diet) 1 serving	30	0	NA	NA	12	0.8	NA	0	115
Pancake Syrup 1/4 cup	210	0	NA	NA	52	NA	32	0	120
Peach Syrup 1 serving	120.6	1.2	0.6	2.5	28.3	1.8	26.9	1.1	7.9

Vegetables

Food Serving size	Cal.	Total Fat	Sat. Fat	Chol.	Carb.	Fiber	Sug.	Prot.	Sod.
Broccoli 3 oz	25	0	0	0	4	2	1	2	20
Corn 4 oz	120	0	0	0	21	3	4	3	45

Food Serving size	Cal.	(g) Total Fat	(g) Sat. Fat	(mg) Chol.	(g) Carb.	(g) Fiber	(g) Sug.	(g) Prot.	(mg) Sod.
Green Beans 4 oz	25-45	0-1	0	0	4-7	4.1	2	2	331
Spinach, Boiled, Drained with salt 1 cup	41	0	0	0	7	4.3	1	5	126

Vinegar

Food Serving size	Cal.	(g) Total Fat	(g) Sat. Fat	(mg) Chol.	(g) Carb.	(g) Fiber	(g) Sug.	(g) Prot.	(mg) Sod.
Red Wine Vinegar 1 cup (239g)	45	0	0	NA	1	0	0	0	19
White, Distilled 1 tbsp	0	0	0	0	0	0	0	0	0

Additional Gluten-Free Menu Items
(nutritional information was not available)

Beef Patty, Grilled Chicken Breast, Smoked Pulled Chicken, Shaved Ham, Shaved Turkey, Grilled Tilapia, Chipotle Sauce, Hickory Spread, Marinara Sauce, Pepper Jack Cheese Sauce, Salsa, Steak Sauce, Sausage Crumbles, Pineapple Syrup, Cherry Limeade Syrup, Coconut Syrup, Lime Syrup, Orange Banana Syrup, Wine, Fajita Blend Vegetables, Cappuccino Fl., Cereal, Grits, Oatmeal, Chocolate & White Chocolate Chips, Nut Topping, Chorizo, Coffee Creamer, and Low Fat Chocolate Milk

Don Pablo's
[www.DonPablos.com]

Beverages

Food Serving size	Cal.	(g) Total Fat	(g) Sat. Fat	(mg) Chol.	(g) Carb.	(g) Fiber	(g) Sug.	(g) Prot.	(mg) Sod.
Coffee 8 oz	0	0	0	NA	0	0	NA	0	0
Coke Classic 16 fl oz	150	0	0	0	40	0	40	0	10
Diet Coke 16 fl oz	0	0	0	0	0	0	0	0	20
Hi-C small	170	0	0	0	46	0	46	0	15
Iced Tea, Unsweetened medium	5	0	0	0	1	0	0	0	15
Milk 1 cup	146	7.93	4.55	24	11.03	0	12.83	7.86	98

Food Serving size	Cal.	(g) Total Fat	(g) Sat. Fat	(mg) Chol.	(g) Carb.	(g) Fiber	(g) Sug.	(g) Prot.	(mg) Sod.
Sprite 16 fl oz	150	0	0	0	39	0	39	0	40

Classic Fajitas

Grilled Shrimp Fajitas 1 serving	423	38	6	7	22	4	13	4	1209
Mesquite-Grilled Steak Fajitas 1 serving	681	36	11	128	36	3	14	59	1244
Pecos Valley Veggie Fajitas 1 serving	334	20	3	0	39	8	20	7	315
Portabella Mushroom Fajitas (request no chipotle butter on portabella) 1 serving	562	46	8	0	39	9	18	10	545
Shrimp & Steak Fajitas 1 serving	552	37	9	67	29	4	13	32	1226

Create Your Own Combos

Beef Enchiladas 1 enchilada	260	16	6	63	8	2	2	21	703
Cheese Enchiladas 1 enchilada	201	14	8	38	9	1	1	10	593
Chicken Enchiladas 1 enchilada	231	15	8	42	11	1	2	13	560
Crispy Beef Tacos 1 taco	260	13	6	51	16	3	2	18	406
Crispy Chicken Tacos 1 taco	211	10	4	32	16	2	2	15	583
Mama's Skinny Enchiladas 1 enchilada	155	7	3	25	10	1	3	12	570

Dips

Prairie Fire Bean Dip 1 bowl	717	43	16	54	53	13	4	31	1496
Prairie Fire Bean Dip 1 cup	359	21	8	27	27	7	2	16	748

Food Serving size	Cal.	(g) Total Fat	(g) Sat. Fat	(mg) Chol.	(g) Carb.	(g) Fiber	(g) Sug.	(g) Prot.	(mg) Sod.
Queso Blanco Dip 1 cup	540	44	28	130	7	1	5	30	2337
Queso Blanco Dip (Bowl) (Regular) 2 fl oz	1080	88	55	259	14	2	10	59	4673
Queso Dip 1 bowl	746	50	31	151	29	2	22	44	4916
Queso Dip 1 cup	373	25	16	76	15	1	11	22	2458
Table Salsa (Regular) 2 fl oz	15	0	0	0	3	1	2	0	361

Don's Combos

Food Serving size	Cal.	(g) Total Fat	(g) Sat. Fat	(mg) Chol.	(g) Carb.	(g) Fiber	(g) Sug.	(g) Prot.	(mg) Sod.
Cinco Combo (served with Mexican rice and GF side) 1 serving	1222	69	33	225	71	8	10	80	3300
Mexicano (served with Mexican rice and GF side) 1 serving	736	45	20	153	59	6	6	53	1728
Tejas (served with Mexican rice and GF side) 1 serving	707	43	21	130	39	5	6	42	1797

Fresh Salads

Food Serving size	Cal.	(g) Total Fat	(g) Sat. Fat	(mg) Chol.	(g) Carb.	(g) Fiber	(g) Sug.	(g) Prot.	(mg) Sod.
Red River Salad 1 serving	479	21	3	55	51	8	22	25	1842
Sizzling Fajita Salad (Chicken) 1 serving	841	45	15	87	81	14	18	36	1268
Sizzling Fajita Salad (Shrimp) 1 serving	766	50	16	57	63	14	10	24	1230
Sizzling Fajita Salad (Steak) 1 serving	895	49	19	118	69	14	11	52	1248
Taco Salad (Beef) 1 serving	1380	73	32	191	102	18	16	79	2593
Taco Salad (Chicken) 1 serving	1235	63	27	133	103	16	16	68	3126
Taco Salad (Mesquite Grilled Chicken) 1 serving	1169	49	23	184	104	15	20	77	2497

Food Serving size	Cal.	(g) Total Fat	(g) Sat. Fat	(mg) Chol.	(g) Carb.	(g) Fiber	(g) Sug.	(g) Prot.	(mg) Sod.
Taco Salad (Mesquite Grilled Steak)									
1 serving	1236	57	28	163	104	15	13	76	2457
Tortilla Salad									
1 serving	482	16	6	14	69	6	6	16	470

Gluten-Free Sauces

A-1 Steak Sauce									
1 tbsp	15	0	0	0	3	0	2	0	280
Heinz Ketchup									
2 fl oz	66	0	0	0	17	0	16	1	759
Regular Salsa									
2 fl oz	15	0	0	0	3	1	2	0	361
Sour Cream Topping									
#30 scoop	82	8	5	17	2	0	0	1	20

Gluten-Free Sides

Charra Beans									
4 fl oz	192	3	1	0	31	8	2	10	599
Chile Mashed Potatoes									
#8 scoop	182	12	4	10	16	2	2	4	604
Mexican Rice									
3 oz wt	119	2	0	1	23	1	1	2	21
Prairie Fire Beans									
4 fl oz	232	4	1	0	40	8	9	11	1138
Refritos									
5 oz wt	214	7	2	7	27	7	1	11	614
Seasoned Vegetables									
6 oz wt	110	5	1	0	16	4	5	3	83

Kids' Menu

Cheese Enchiladas									
1 serving	381	30	15	66	9	1	4	18	1066
Crispy Beef Tacos									
1 taco	260	13	6	51	16	3	2	18	406

Food Serving size	Cal.	(g) Total Fat	(g) Sat. Fat	(mg) Chol.	(g) Carb.	(g) Fiber	(g) Sug.	(g) Prot.	(mg) Sod.
Crispy Chicken Tacos									
1 taco	211	10	4	32	16	2	2	15	583
Steak Fajitas (request corn tortillas instead of flour)									
1 serving	536	34	16	108	22	2	9	38	861

Tastes of Mexico

Food Serving size	Cal.	(g) Total Fat	(g) Sat. Fat	(mg) Chol.	(g) Carb.	(g) Fiber	(g) Sug.	(g) Prot.	(mg) Sod.
Big Tex Ribeye (served with two GF sides)									
1 serving	1045	87	33	232	2	0	1	60	1958
Cadillac Enchiladas - Chicken (served with two GF sides)									
1 serving	944	47	25	157	80	3	35	49	2576
Cadillac Enchiladas - Steak (served with two GF sides)									
1 serving	1014	0	30	199	65	3	26	69	2550
Carnitas (served with two GF sides)									
1 serving	789	31	11	105	82	11	8	49	2330
Grilled Shrimp (served with two GF sides)									
1 serving	263	28	4	13	4	1	1	2	2010
Grilled Tilapia (served with two GF sides)									
1 serving	256	10	5	95	8	1	2	35	1389

Additional Gluten-Free Menu Items
(nutritional information was not available)

Ranchero Gluten-Free Sauce, Santa Fe Red Chile Gluten-Free Sauce, Sour Cream Sauce, Cholula, and the following beverages: SqueezaRita, PabloRita, LotsaRita, PrimaRita, Red Wine, White Wine, Red Sangria, and White Sangria

Dunkin' Donuts
[www.dunkindonuts.com]

Coffee

Food Serving size	Cal.	(g) Total Fat	(g) Sat. Fat	(mg) Chol.	(g) Carb.	(g) Fiber	(g) Sug.	(g) Prot.	(mg) Sod.
Blueberry Coffee (Small)									
10 fl oz	15	0	0	0	2	0	0	0	5
Caramel Coffee (Small)									
10 fl oz	10	0	0	0	5	0	0	0	5
Caramel Mocha Coffee (Large)									
20 fl oz	230	0	0	0	53	1	48	3	40

Food Serving size	Cal.	(g) Total Fat	(g) Sat. Fat	(mg) Chol.	(g) Carb.	(g) Fiber	(g) Sug.	(g) Prot.	(mg) Sod.
Caramel Mocha Coffee (Medium) 14 fl oz	170	0	0	0	39	1	36	2	30
Caramel Mocha Coffee (Small) 10 fl oz	110	0	0	0	26	1	24	2	20
Caramel Mocha Coffee (X-Large) 24 fl oz	280	0	0	5	66	2	60	4	50
Caramel Mocha Coffee with Cream (Medium) 14 fl oz	260	9	6	30	41	1	36	3	50
Caramel Mocha Iced Coffee (Large) 32 fl oz	230	0	0	0	54	1	48	4	45
Caramel Mocha Iced Coffee (Medium) 24 fl oz	180	0	0	0	41	1	36	3	35
Caramel Mocha Iced Coffee (Small) 16 fl oz	120	0	0	0	27	1	24	2	25
Caramel Mocha Iced Coffee with Cream (Large) 32 fl oz	350	12	7	40	56	1	48	5	70
Caramel Mocha Iced Coffee with Cream (Medium) 24 fl oz	260	9	6	30	42	1	36	4	50
Caramel Mocha Iced Coffee with Cream (Small) 16 fl oz	180	6	3.5	20	28	1	24	3	35
Carmel Mocha Coffee with Cream (Large) 20 fl oz	340	12	7	40	55	1	48	5	65
Carmel Mocha Coffee with Cream (Small) 10 fl oz	170	6	3.5	20	27	1	24	2	30
Carmel Mocha Coffee with Cream (X Large) 24 fl oz	430	15	9	55	68	2	60	6	80
Cinnamon Coffee (Small) 10 fl oz	15	0	0	0	2	0	0	0	5
Coconut Coffee (Small) 10 fl oz	10	0	0	0	1	0	0	0	5
Coffee (Extra Large) 24 fl oz	15	0	0	0	2	0	0	1	15
Coffee (Large) 20 fl oz	10	0	0	0	2	0	0	1	15

Food Serving size	Cal.	(g) Total Fat	(g) Sat. Fat	(mg) Chol.	(g) Carb.	(g) Fiber	(g) Sug.	(g) Prot.	(mg) Sod.
Coffee (Medium) 14 fl oz	10	0	0	0	1	0	0 .	1	10
Coffee (Small) 10 fl oz	5	0	0	0	1	0	0	0	5
Coffee with Cream (Small) 10 fl oz	60	6	4	20	2	0	0	1	20
Coffee with Cream and Sugar (Small) 10 fl oz	120	6	4	20	19	0	17	1	20
Coffee with Milk (Small) 10 fl oz	25	1	1	5	2	0	1	1	20
Coffee with Milk and Sugar (Small) 10 fl oz	80	1	1	5	20	0	19	1	20
Coffee with Skim Milk (Small) 10 fl oz	15	0	0	0	3	0	2	2	25
Coffee with Skim Milk and Splenda (Large) 20 fl oz	45	0	0	0	8	0	3	3	45
Coffee with Skim Milk and Splenda (Medium) 14 fl oz	30	0	0	0	6	0	2	2	35
Coffee with Skim Milk and Splenda (Small) 10 fl oz	25	0	0	0	5	0	2	2	25
Coffee with Skim Milk and Sugar (Small) 10 fl oz	70	0	0	0	20	0	19	2	25
Coffee with Splenda (Large) 20 fl oz	25	0	0	0	5	0	0	1	15
Coffee with Splenda (Medium) 14 fl oz	15	0	0	0	3	0	0	1	10
Coffee with Splenda (Small) 10 fl oz	15	0	0	0	3	0	0	0	5
Coffee with Sugar (Small) 10 fl oz	60	0	0	0	18	0	17	0	5
French Vanilla Coffee (Small) 10 fl oz	10	0	0	0	1	0	0	0	5
Hazelnut Coffee (Large) 20 fl oz	25	0	0	0	2	0	0	1	15

Food Serving size	Cal.	(g) Total Fat	(g) Sat. Fat	(mg) Chol.	(g) Carb.	(g) Fiber	(g) Sug.	(g) Prot.	(mg) Sod.
Hazelnut Coffee (Medium) 14 fl oz	15	0	0	0	1	0	0	1	10
Hazelnut Coffee (Small) 10 fl oz	10	0	0	0	1	0	0	0	5
Hazelnut Coffee (X Large) 24 fl oz	30	0	0	0	2	0	0	1	15
Iced Coffee (Large) 32 fl oz	20	0	0	0	3	0	0	1	15
Iced Coffee (Medium) 24 fl oz	15	0	0	0	2	0	0	1	10
Iced Coffee (Small) 16 fl oz	10	0	0	0	2	0	0	1	5
Iced Coffee with Cream (Small) 16 fl oz	70	6	4	20	3	0	0	1	20
Iced Coffee with Cream and Sugar (Small) 16 fl oz	120	6	4	20	20	0	17	1	20
Iced Coffee with Milk (Small) 16 fl oz	30	1	1	5	3	0	1	2	20
Iced Coffee with Milk and Sugar (Small) 16 fl oz	90	1	1	5	21	0	19	2	20
Iced Coffee with Skim Milk (Small) 16 fl oz	20	0	0	0	3	0	2	2	25
Iced Coffee with Skim Milk and Splenda (Large) 32 fl oz	60	0	0	0	10	0	3	3	45
Iced Coffee with Skim Milk and Splenda (Medium) 24 fl oz	40	0	0	0	8	0	2	3	35
Iced Coffee with Skim Milk and Splenda (Small) 16 fl oz	30	0	0	0	5	0	2	2	25
Iced Coffee with Skim Milk and Sugar (Small) 16 fl oz	80	0	0	0	21	0	19	2	25
Iced Coffee with Sugar (Small) 16 fl oz	70	0	0	0	19	0	17	1	5
Iced Dunkin' Dark Roast Coffee with Cream and Sugar (Large) 32 fl oz	250	12	7	40	40	0	35	3	40

Food Serving size	Cal.	(g) Total Fat	(g) Sat. Fat	(mg) Chol.	(g) Carb.	(g) Fiber	(g) Sug.	(g) Prot.	(mg) Sod.
Iced Dunkin' Dark Roast Coffee with Cream and Sugar (Medium)									
24 fl oz	190	9	5	30	30	0	26	2	30
Iced Dunkin' Dark Roast Coffee with Cream and Sugar (Small)									
16 fl oz	130	6	3.5	20	20	0	17	1	20
Iced Dunkin' Dark Roast Coffee with Skim Milk and Splenda (Large)									
32 fl oz	60	0	0	0	10	0	3	3	50
Iced Dunkin' Dark Roast Coffee with Skim Milk and Splenda (Medium)									
24 fl oz	40	0	0	0	8	0	2	3	35
Iced Dunkin' Dark Roast Coffee with Skim Milk and Splenda (Small)									
16 fl oz	30	0	0	0	5	0	1	2	25
Mocha Coffee (Extra Large)									
24 fl oz	280	1	0.5	0	65	3	57	3	50
Mocha Coffee (Large)									
20 fl oz	230	1	0	0	52	2	46	3	40
Mocha Coffee (Medium)									
14 fl oz	170	0.5	0	0	39	2	34	2	30
Mocha Coffee (Small)									
10 fl oz	110	0	0	0	26	1	23	1	20
Mocha Swirl Coffee with Cream (Extra Large)									
24 fl oz	430	16	10	50	68	3	57	5	75
Mocha Swirl Coffee with Cream (Large)									
20 fl oz	340	12	8	40	54	2	46	4	60
Mocha Swirl Coffee with Cream (Medium)									
14 fl oz	260	9	6	30	41	2	34	3	45
Mocha Swirl Coffee with Cream (Small)									
10 fl oz	170	6	4	20	27	1	23	2	30
Mocha Swirl Iced Coffee with Cream (Large)									
20 fl oz	340	12	8	40	54	2	46	4	60
Mocha Swirl Iced Coffee with Cream (Medium)									
14 fl oz	260	9	6	30	41	2	34	3	45
Mocha Swirl Iced Coffee with Cream (Small)									
10 fl oz	170	6	4	20	27	1	23	2	30

Food Serving size	Cal.	(g) Total Fat	(g) Sat. Fat	(mg) Chol.	(g) Carb.	(g) Fiber	(g) Sug.	(g) Prot.	(mg) Sod.
Raspberry Coffee (Small) 10 fl oz	15	0	0	0	2	0	0	0	5
Toasted Almond Coffee (Small) 10 fl oz	10	0	0	0	1	0	0	0	5

Coolatta

Food Serving size	Cal.	(g) Total Fat	(g) Sat. Fat	(mg) Chol.	(g) Carb.	(g) Fiber	(g) Sug.	(g) Prot.	(mg) Sod.
Orange Coolata (Large) 32 fl oz	420	0	0	0	108	0	103	2	30
Orange Coolata (Medium) 24 fl oz	310	0	0	0	81	0	77	2	20
Orange Coolata (Small) 16 fl oz	210	0	0	0	54	0	51	1	15
Strawberry Fruit Coolata (Large) 32 fl oz	470	0	0	0	115	0	114	0	70
Strawberry Fruit Coolata (Medium) 24 fl oz	350	0	0	0	86	0	85	0	55
Strawberry Fruit Coolata (Small) 16 fl oz	230	0	0	0	57	0	57	0	35
Vanilla Bean Coolata (Large) 32 fl oz	850	12	7	45	184	0	174	6	300
Vanilla Bean Coolata (Medium) 24 fl oz	630	9	5	30	138	0	130	4	220
Vanilla Bean Coolata (Small) 16 fl oz	420	6	3.5	20	92	0	87	3	150

Menu Item

Food Serving size	Cal.	(g) Total Fat	(g) Sat. Fat	(mg) Chol.	(g) Carb.	(g) Fiber	(g) Sug.	(g) Prot.	(mg) Sod.
Hash Browns 9 pieces	200	11	1.5	0	22	3	0	2	730

Other Hot Beverages

Food Serving size	Cal.	(g) Total Fat	(g) Sat. Fat	(mg) Chol.	(g) Carb.	(g) Fiber	(g) Sug.	(g) Prot.	(mg) Sod.
Caramel Hot Chocolate (Extra Large) 24 fl oz	560	18	16	0	99	4	74	5	670
Caramel Hot Chocolate (Large) 20 fl oz	460	15	14	0	82	3	62	4	560

Food Serving size	Cal.	(g) Total Fat	(g) Sat. Fat	(mg) Chol.	(g) Carb.	(g) Fiber	(g) Sug.	(g) Prot.	(mg) Sod.
Caramel Hot Chocolate (Medium) 14 fl oz	330	11	10	0	59	2	44	3	400
Caramel Hot Chocolate (Small) 10 fl oz	230	7	7	0	40	2	30	2	270
Coconut Hot Chocolate (Large) 20 fl oz	460	15	14	0	81	3	62	4	560
Coconut Hot Chocolate (Medium) 14 fl oz	330	11	10	0	58	2	44	3	400
Coconut Hot Chocolate (Small) 10 fl oz	220	7	7	0	39	2	30	2	270
Coconut Hot Chocolate (XLarge) 24 fl oz	550	18	16	0	97	4	74	5	670
Dunkaccino (Small) 10 fl oz	240	11	9	10	35	1	26	2	220
Hot Chocolate (Large) 20 fl oz	450	15	14	0	81	3	62	4	560
Hot Chocolate (Medium) 14 fl oz	320	11	10	0	58	2	44	3	400
Hot Chocolate (Small) 10 fl oz	220	7	7	0	39	2	30	2	270
Hot Chocolate (X Large) 24 fl oz	490	16	15	0	88	3	67	5	610
Mint Hot Chocolate (Large) 20 fl oz	420	13	12	0	72	3	54	3	530
Mint Hot Chocolate (Medium) 14 fl oz	310	10	9	0	52	2	39	2	390
Mint Hot Chocolate (Small) 10 fl oz	220	7	6	0	36	1	27	1	270
Mint Hot Chocolate (X Large) 24 fl oz	520	16	15	0	87	3	65	3	650
Turbo Hot Chocolate (Large) 20 fl oz	450	15	14	0	81	3	62	4	560

Food Serving size	Cal.	(g) Total Fat	(g) Sat. Fat	(mg) Chol.	(g) Carb.	(g) Fiber	(g) Sug.	(g) Prot.	(mg) Sod.
Turbo Hot Chocolate (Medium) 14 fl oz	320	11	10	0	58	2	44	3	400
Turbo Hot Chocolate (Small) 10 fl oz	220	7	7	0	39	2	30	2	270
Vanilla Chai 14 fl oz	330	8	8	10	53	1	45	11	180

Specialty Coffee

Food Serving size	Cal.	(g) Total Fat	(g) Sat. Fat	(mg) Chol.	(g) Carb.	(g) Fiber	(g) Sug.	(g) Prot.	(mg) Sod.
Cappuccino (Small) 10 fl oz	80	4	2.5	15	7	0	7	4	70
Cappuccino with Sugar (Small) 10 fl oz	140	4	2.5	15	24	0	24	4	70
Caramel Mocha Latte with Milk (Large) 20 fl oz	450	12	8	55	70	1	67	14	230
Caramel Mocha Latte with Milk (Medium) 16 fl oz	330	9	6	40	52	1	50	11	170
Caramel Mocha Latte with Milk (Small) 10 fl oz	220	6	4	25	35	1	33	7	115
Caramel Mocha Latte with Skim Milk (Large) 20 fl oz	350	1	0.5	10	70	1	68	15	200
Caramel Mocha Latte with Skim Milk (Medium) 16 fl oz	260	0.5	0	5	53	1	51	11	150
Caramel Mocha Latte with Skim Milk (Small) 10 fl oz	170	0	0	5	35	1	34	7	100
Caramel Swirl Latte (Small) 10 fl oz	220	6	3.5	25	35	0	34	8	150
Espresso 1.75 fl oz	5	0	0	0	1	0	1	0	5
Espresso with Sugar 1.75 fl oz	30	0	0	0	7	0	7	0	5
Iced Caramel Mocha Latte with Milk (Large) 32 fl oz	450	12	8	55	70	1	67	14	240
Iced Caramel Mocha Latte with Milk (Medium) 24 fl oz	330	9	6	40	52	1	50	11	180

Food Serving size	Cal.	(g) Total Fat	(g) Sat. Fat	(mg) Chol.	(g) Carb.	(g) Fiber	(g) Sug.	(g) Prot.	(mg) Sod.
Iced Caramel Mocha Latte with Milk (Small) 16 fl oz	220	6	4	25	35	1	33	7	120
Iced Caramel Mocha Latte with Skim Milk (Large) 32 fl oz	350	1	0.5	10	70	1	68	15	210
Iced Caramel Mocha Latte with Skim Milk (Medium) 24 fl oz	260	0.5	0	5	53	1	51	11	150
Iced Caramel Mocha Latte with Skim Milk (Small) 16 fl oz	170	0	0	5	35	1	34	7	105
Iced Latte Lite (Large) 32 fl oz	160	0	0	5	25	0	20	14	220
Iced Latte Lite (Medium) 24 fl oz	120	0	0	5	19	0	15	10	170
Iced Latte Lite (Small) 16 fl oz	80	0	0	0	13	0	10	7	110
Iced Latte with Skim Milk (Small) 16 fl oz	70	0	0	0	11	0	10	7	110
Iced Latte with Skim Milk and Sugar (Small) 16 fl oz	130	0	0	0	28	0	27	7	110
Iced Latte with Sugar (Small) 16 fl oz	170	6	3.5	25	27	0	27	6	100
Iced Mocha Swirl Latte (Small) 16 fl oz	220	6	4	25	35	1	32	7	115
Iced Mocha Swirl Latte with Skim Milk (Small) 16 fl oz	180	0	0	0	36	1	32	8	125
Latte (Small) 10 fl oz	120	6	3.5	25	10	0	10	6	105
Latte Lite (Large) 20 fl oz	160	0	0	5	25	0	20	14	220
Latte Lite (Medium) 16 fl oz	120	0	0	5	19	0	15	10	170
Latte Lite (Small) 10 fl oz	80	0	0	0	13	0	10	7	110
Latte with Sugar (Small) 10 fl oz	170	6	3.5	25	27	0	27	6	100

Food Serving size	Cal.	(g) Total Fat	(g) Sat. Fat	(mg) Chol.	(g) Carb.	(g) Fiber	(g) Sug.	(g) Prot.	(mg) Sod.
Mocha Swirl Latte (Small) 10 fl oz	220	6	4	25	35	1	32	7	115
Turbo Shot (Extra Large) 4 fl oz	10	0	0	0	2	0	2	0	15
Turbo Shot (Large) 3.5 fl oz	10	0	0	0	2	0	2	0	15
Turbo Shot (Medium) 2.5 fl oz	5	0	0	0	1	0	1	0	10
Turbo Shot (Small) 1.75 fl oz	5	0	0	0	1	0	1	0	5

Tea

Food Serving size	Cal.	(g) Total Fat	(g) Sat. Fat	(mg) Chol.	(g) Carb.	(g) Fiber	(g) Sug.	(g) Prot.	(mg) Sod.
Decaffeinated Tea 10 fl oz	0	0	0	0	0	0	0	0	5
Decaffeinated Tea with Milk 10 fl oz	20	1	0.5	5	1	0	1	1	20
Decaffeinated Tea with Milk and Sugar 10 fl oz	80	1	0.5	5	19	0	19	1	20
Decaffeinated Tea with Skim Milk 10 fl oz	10	0	0	0	2	0	2	1	20
Decaffeinated Tea with Skim Milk and Sugar 10 fl oz	70	0	0	0	19	0	19	1	20
Decaffeinated Tea with Sugar 10 fl oz	60	0	0	0	17	0	17	0	5
Earl Grey Tea 10 fl oz	0	0	0	0	0	0	0	0	5
Earl Grey Tea with Milk 10 fl oz	20	1	0.5	5	1	0	1	1	20
Earl Grey Tea with Milk and Sugar 10 fl oz	80	1	0.5	5	19	0	19	1	20
Earl Grey Tea with Skim Milk 10 fl oz	10	0	0	0	2	0	2	1	20
Earl Grey Tea with Skim Milk and Sugar 10 fl oz	70	0	0	0	19	0	19	1	20

Food Serving size	Cal.	(g) Total Fat	(g) Sat. Fat	(mg) Chol.	(g) Carb.	(g) Fiber	(g) Sug.	(g) Prot.	(mg) Sod.
Earl Grey Tea with Sugar 10 fl oz	60	0	0	0	17	0	17	0	5
English Breakfast Tea 10 fl oz	0	0	0	0	0	0	0	0	5
English Breakfast Tea with Milk 10 fl oz	20	1	0.5	5	1	0	1	1	20
English Breakfast Tea with Milk and Sugar 10 fl oz	80	1	0.5	5	19	0	19	1	20
English Breakfast Tea with Skim Milk 10 fl oz	10	0	0	0	2	0	2	1	20
English Breakfast Tea with Skim Milk and Sugar 10 fl oz	70	0	0	0	19	0	19	1	20
English Breakfast Tea with Sugar 10 fl oz	60	0	0	0	17	0	17	0	5
Freshly Brewed Sweetened Iced Tea 16 fl oz	80	0	0	0	20	0	19	0	0
Freshly Brewed Tea with Milk 10 fl oz	20	1	0.5	5	1	0	1	1	20
Freshly Brewed Tea with Milk and Sugar 10 fl oz	80	1	0.5	5	19	0	19	1	20
Freshly Brewed Tea with Skim Milk 10 fl oz	10	0	0	0	2	0	2	1	20
Freshly Brewed Tea with Skim Milk and Sugar 10 fl oz	70	0	0	0	19	0	19	1	20
Freshly Brewed Tea with Sugar 10 fl oz	60	0	0	0	17	0	17	0	5
Freshly Brewed Unsweetened Iced Tea 16 fl oz	5	0	0	0	1	0	0	0	0
Freshly Brewed Unsweetened Iced Tea (Large) 32 fl oz	10	0	0	0	2	0	0	0	5
Freshly Brewed Unsweetened Iced Tea (Medium) 24 fl oz	5	0	0	0	2	0	0	0	0
Freshly Brewed Unsweetened Tea 10 fl oz	0	0	0	0	0	0	0	0	5

Food Serving size	Cal.	(g) Total Fat	(g) Sat. Fat	(mg) Chol.	(g) Carb.	(g) Fiber	(g) Sug.	(g) Prot.	(mg) Sod.
Green Tea 10 fl oz	0	0	0	0	0	0	0	0	5
Green Tea with Milk 10 fl oz	20	1	0.5	5	1	0	1	1	20
Green Tea with Milk and Sugar 10 fl oz	80	1	0.5	5	19	0	19	1	20
Green Tea with Skim Milk 10 fl oz	10	0	0	0	2	0	2	1	20
Green Tea with Skim Milk and Sugar 10 fl oz	70	0	0	0	19	0	19	1	20
Green Tea with Sugar 10 fl oz	60	0	0	0	17	0	17	0	5
Peach Flavored Iced Tea 16 fl oz	15	0	0	0	2	0	0	0	0
Peach Flavored Sweetened Iced Tea 16 fl oz	90	0	0	0	21	0	19	0	0
Raspberry Flavored Iced Tea 16 fl oz	15	0	0	0	2	0	0	0	0
Raspberry Flavored Sweetened Iced Tea 16 fl oz	90	0	0	0	21	0	19	0	0
Sweet Tea 16 fl oz	120	0	0	0	29	0	28	0	0

First Watch

[www.firstwatch.com]

Fresh Spring Mix Salads

Cobb (order without ciabatta toast) 1 serving	584	44	14	276	16	9	1	35	966
Fruity Chicken (order without ciabatta toast) 1 serving	753	36	6	115	74	10	35	40	334
No. 5 Asian (order without wontons, Sesame Asian dressing and ciabatta toast) 1 serving	363	14	1	54	33	6	5	22	1263

Food Serving size	Cal.	(g) Total Fat	(g) Sat. Fat	(mg) Chol.	(g) Carb.	(g) Fiber	(g) Sug.	(g) Prot.	(mg) Sod.
Pecan Dijon (order without Honey Dijon dressing and ciabatta toast)									
1 serving	673	54	10	98	18	12	1	43	411
Santa Fe (order without croutons, Santa Fe dressing and ciabatta toast)									
1 serving	393	23	5	83	16	9	1	33	437
The Poacher (order without ciabatta toast or balsamic vinaigrette)									
1 serving	690	50	12	275	27	7	7	32	2230

Fresh Start Eggs-clusives

Food Serving size	Cal.	(g) Total Fat	(g) Sat. Fat	(mg) Chol.	(g) Carb.	(g) Fiber	(g) Sug.	(g) Prot.	(mg) Sod.
Breakfast Scramble (order without multigrain toast and Hollandaise sauce)									
1 serving	620	36	13	730	34	8	5	41	880
Burrito Vera Cruz (order without wheat tortilla and Vera Cruz sauce)									
1 serving	819	53	25	735	51	4	1	39	1135
Caps Etc. (order without English muffin)									
1 serving	804	82	53	220	14	5	5	17	1857
Casa Frittata (order without English muffin)									
1 serving	670	53	20	740	6	1	1	39	970
Chickichanga (order without flour tortilla and Vera Cruz sauce)									
1 serving	1047	74	34	601	45	6	2	53	1311
Eggs Benedict (Florentine) (order without English muffin and Hollandaise sauce)									
1 serving	626	43	16	468	41	7	1	21	540
Eggs Benedict (Ham and Tomatoes) (order without English muffin and Hollandaise sauce)									
1 serving	591	33	15	514	34	3	2	38	1922
Eggs Benedict (Smoked Turkey and Avocado) (order without English muffin and Hollandaise sauce)									
1 serving	691	43	16	502	40	7	2	38	1175
Turkey Chive Crepegg (order without Crepe, English muffin and Hollandaise sauce)									
1 serving	410	26	12	305	17	2	4	28	1150

Fresh Starts

Food Serving size	Cal.	(g) Total Fat	(g) Sat. Fat	(mg) Chol.	(g) Carb.	(g) Fiber	(g) Sug.	(g) Prot.	(mg) Sod.
The Traditional Breakfast (order without English muffin)									
1 serving	242	21	5	393	0	0	0	13	193

Kid's Menu

Food Serving size	Cal.	(g) Total Fat	(g) Sat. Fat	(mg) Chol.	(g) Carb.	(g) Fiber	(g) Sug.	(g) Prot.	(mg) Sod.
Bacon and Egg (order without sourdough toast)									
1 serving	138	12	3	224	0	0	0	7	110

Food Serving size	Cal.	(g) Total Fat	(g) Sat. Fat	(mg) Chol.	(g) Carb.	(g) Fiber	(g) Sug.	(g) Prot.	(mg) Sod.
Grilled Cheese (order without sourdough bread)									
1 serving	418	25	13	61	28	1	3	18	724
Hamwich (order without sourdough bread)									
1 serving	342	15	7	60	28	1	3	23	1341
Turkeywich (order without sourdough bread)									
1 serving	313	12	6	53	30	2	5	22	1164

Menu Item

Acapulco Express (order without English muffin)									
1 serving	782	66	20	747	16	1	1	36	675
Bacado (order without English muffin)									
1 serving	855	75	32	744	11	0	0	40	856
C'est La Vie (order without English muffin)									
1 serving	490	36	14	700	9	2	4	32	730
Greek Fetish (order without English muffin)									
1 serving	447	37	18	701	6	0	0	24	675
Killer Cajun (order without English muffin)									
1 serving	767	63	24	760	7	0	0	43	839
Swisshroom Omelet (order without English muffin)									
1 serving	630	46	20	755	6	1	4	47	680
The Forager (order without English muffin)									
1 serving	560	43	16	675	7	1	3	38	760
The Works (order without English muffin)									
1 serving	832	69	35	807	8	0	0	42	636
Veg's Out (order without English muffin)									
1 serving	577	51	26	720	7	1	5	30	524
Via Veneto (order without English muffin)									
1 serving	610	45	15	745	7	2	3	45	1110

Sandwiches

Al B. Gore (order without multigrain bread)									
1 serving	796	49	11	88	36	3	1	49	833
Baja Turkey Burger (order without bun or bread)									
1 serving	690	41	15	160	34	3	7	46	930

Food Serving size	Cal.	(g) Total Fat	(g) Sat. Fat	(mg) Chol.	(g) Carb.	(g) Fiber	(g) Sug.	(g) Prot.	(mg) Sod.
Beefeater (order without parmesan-crusted sourdough bread)									
1 serving	1049	51	31	216	71	4	3	71	1728
BLTE (order without multigrain bread)									
1 serving	793	57	19	192	34	3	2	35	887
Chicken Palermo (order without ciabatta toast)									
1 serving	720	28	9	105	64	3	5	56	2200
Chicken Salad Melt (order without multigrain bread)									
1 serving	829	55	15	147	38	4	4	46	712
Grilled Turkey (order without sourdough bread and Ranch dressing)									
1 serving	1025	56	26	151	77	4	6	53	2637
Monterey Club (order without multigrain bread)									
1 serving	738	60	20	142	42	9	6	52	2113
Not Guilty Your Honor (order without wheat tortilla)									
1 serving	433	17	5	25	54	5	2	17	1108
Pesto Roast Beef (order without bread)									
1 serving	790	43	19	115	52	4	9	49	2140
Reuben (order without rye bread)									
1 serving	945	64	28	1216	42	6	10	46	2242
Veggie Grill Sandwich (order without bread)									
1 serving	550	26	11	45	60	9	22	23	620

Sides

Food Serving size	Cal.	(g) Total Fat	(g) Sat. Fat	(mg) Chol.	(g) Carb.	(g) Fiber	(g) Sug.	(g) Prot.	(mg) Sod.
Bacon Strip									
2 strips	73	6	2	11	0	0	0	4	202
First Watch Fresh, Seasoned Potatoes									
1 serving	130	4	2	0	21	3	1	2	234
Fruit Bowl									
1 serving	206	2	0	0	51	6	41	3	10
Ham Slice									
2 slices	73	6	2	11	0	0	0	4	202
Sausage Link									
2 links	73	6	2	11	0	0	0	4	202
Turkey Sausage Link									
4 links	280	22	7	120	0	0	0	20	860

Food Serving size	Cal.	(g) Total Fat	(g) Sat. Fat	(mg) Chol.	(g) Carb.	(g) Fiber	(g) Sug.	(g) Prot.	(mg) Sod.

Skillet Hashes

Farmhouse Chicken (order without English muffin) 1 serving	790	45	17	435	43	6	9	51	2110
Market Hash (order without English muffin) 1 serving	610	38	14	355	44	7	9	31	1570
Parma Hash (order without English muffin) 1 serving	690	46	15	395	39	5	8	38	1720

The Healthier Side

Energy Bowl (order without granola) 1 serving	640	23	6	10	95	8	45	17	350
Healthy Turkey (order without English muffin) 1 serving	206	11	5	63	9	1	5	37	1367
Lean Machine (order without English muffin) 1 serving	400	25	6	90	8	1	7	35	440
Power Wrap (order without sun-dried tomato-basil tortilla) 1 serving	478	11	4	62	45	3	8	46	936
Siesta Key Cocktail (order without English muffin and granola) 1 serving	312	11	3	3	47	3	21	9	76
Tri-Athlete Omelet (order without English muffin) 1 serving	109	0	0	0	6	1	1	20	375

Additional Gluten-Free Menu Items
(nutritional information was not available)

Sunrise Select Premium Blend Coffee, Herbal Teas, Low-Fat Milk, Orange Juice, Grapefruit Juice, Cranberry Juice, V8 Vegetable Cocktail, Apple Juice, Fresh-Brewed Iced Tea, San Pellegrino Sparkling Water, and Pure Maple Syrup

Hardee's
[www.hardees.com]

Menu Item

Buttermilk Ranch Dipping Sauce 34g	140	14	2	15	3	0	2	0	300

Food Serving size	Cal.	(g) Total Fat	(g) Sat. Fat	(mg) Chol.	(g) Carb.	(g) Fiber	(g) Sug.	(g) Prot.	(mg) Sod.
Chocolate Hand-Scooped Ice Cream Shake 1 serving	705	33	23	100	86	0	68	14	260
Cole Slaw (small) 1 serving	170	10	2	10	20	2	16	1	140
Creamy Buffalo Dipping Sauce 1 serving	120	13	2	NA	3	1	NA	1	330
Fat Free Italian Salad Dressing 1 packet	25	0	0	0	7	0	5	0	360
Gluten-Sensitive 1/3 lb. Low Carb Thickburger 1 serving	420	32	12	115	5	2	3	30	1010
Gluten-Sensitive Low Carb Breakfast Bowl 1 serving	620	50	21	325	6	2	2	36	1380
Grits 142g	110	5	1	0	16	1	0	2	490
Honey Mustard Dipping Sauce 34g	180	18	3	10	6	0	5	0	190
Horseradish Packet 1 packet	25	2	NA	5	1	NA	1	NA	35
Ketchup 1 packet	10	NA	NA	NA	2	NA	2	NA	105
Mayonnaise 1 packet	90	9	1.5	5	1	NA	NA	NA	70
Natural Cut French Fries (Kids) 1 serving	200	9	2	0	28	2	0	2	450
Natural Cut French Fries (Large) 1 serving	470	21	4	5	65	5	0	5	1640
Natural Cut French Fries (Medium) 1 serving	430	19	4	5	60	4	0	5	960
Natural Cut French Fries (Small) 1 serving	320	14	3	0	45	3	0	4	710
Side Salad (no dressing) 1 serving	120	7	5	20	7	2	4	7	160
Strawberry Hand-Scooped Ice Cream Shake 1 serving	705	33	23	100	86	0	68	14	260

Food Serving size	Cal.	(g) Total Fat	(g) Sat. Fat	(mg) Chol.	(g) Carb.	(g) Fiber	(g) Sug.	(g) Prot.	(mg) Sod.
Sweet Baby Ray's BBQ Dipping Sauce									
34g	60	0	0	0	17	0	15	0	270
Texas Pete Hot Sauce									
1 tsp	0	0	0	0	1	0	0	0	160
Vanilla Hand-Scooped Ice Cream Shake									
1 serving	705	33	23	100	86	0	68	14	260

Additional Gluten-Free Menu Items
(nutritional information was not available)

Salsa Packet, Buttermilk Ranch Salad Dressing

Jamba Juice
[www.jambajuice.com]

3G Charger Boost

3G Charger Boost - Per serving									
1 boost	5	0	NA	NA	2	2	NA	NA	NA

Acai Super-Antioxidant

Acai Super-Antioxidant - Original									
24 oz	380	6	2	5	98	5	66	5	55
Acai Super-Antioxidant - Power									
30 oz	520	7	2	5	108	6	94	6	95
Acai Super-Antioxidant - Sixteen									
16 oz	260	4	1	5	54	3	46	3	45

Aloha Pineapple

Aloha Pineapple - Original									
24 oz	410	1.5	0.5	5	97	4	91	6	55
Aloha Pineapple - Power									
30 oz	550	2	1	5	130	5	123	7	70
Aloha Pineapple - Sixteen									
16 oz	290	1	0	5	67	3	63	5	50

Food Serving size	Cal.	(g) Total Fat	(g) Sat. Fat	(mg) Chol.	(g) Carb.	(g) Fiber	(g) Sug.	(g) Prot.	(mg) Sod.
Apple 'n Greens									
Apple 'n Greens - Original 16 oz	330	1.5	0	0	74	9	59	8	190
Apple 'n Greens - Power 30 oz	440	2	0	0	98	13	77	10	220
Apple 'n Greens - Sixteen 24 oz	220	1	0	0	50	6	40	5	115
Banana Berry									
Banana Berry - Original 24 oz	400	1.5	0.5	5	94	4	82	4	90
Banana Berry - Power 30 oz	560	2	0.5	5	131	5	115	6	160
Banana Berry - Sixteen 16 oz	270	1	0	0	64	3	57	3	60
Berry Fulfilling									
Berry Fulfilling - Original 24 oz	230	1	0	5	49	5	39	7	190
Berry Fulfilling - Power 30 oz	310	1	0	5	69	7	54	9	220
Berry Fulfilling - Sixteen 16 oz	140	0.5	0	5	2	2	24	6	150
Berry UpBEET									
Berry UpBeet - Original 24 oz	340	1.5	0	0	74	13	56	5	230
Berry UpBeet - Power 30 oz	430	2	0	0	93	17	70	6	280
Berry UpBeet - Sixteen 16 oz	230	1	0	0	50	8	38	3	140
Caribbean Passion									
Caribbean Passion - Original 24 oz	360	1.5	0.5	5	82	3	73	3	50

Food Serving size	Cal.	(g) Total Fat	(g) Sat. Fat	(mg) Chol.	(g) Carb.	(g) Fiber	(g) Sug.	(g) Prot.	(mg) Sod.
Caribbean Passion - Power 30 oz	490	2	1	5	112	5	101	4	70
Caribbean Passion - Sixteen 16 oz	250	1	0	5	57	2	51	2	35

Carrot Juice

Food Serving size	Cal.	(g) Total Fat	(g) Sat. Fat	(mg) Chol.	(g) Carb.	(g) Fiber	(g) Sug.	(g) Prot.	(mg) Sod.
Carrot Juice - Sixteen 16 oz	130	0.5	0	0	30	0	26	4	230
Carrot Juice - Twelve 12 oz	100	0.5	0	0	22	0	20	3	170

Chocolate Moo'd

Food Serving size	Cal.	(g) Total Fat	(g) Sat. Fat	(mg) Chol.	(g) Carb.	(g) Fiber	(g) Sug.	(g) Prot.	(mg) Sod.
Chocolate Moo'd - Original 24 oz	570	5	2.5	15	116	3	103	15	380
Chocolate Moo'd - Sixteen 16 oz	430	4	2	15	86	2	77	11	270

Classic Hot Chocolate

Food Serving size	Cal.	(g) Total Fat	(g) Sat. Fat	(mg) Chol.	(g) Carb.	(g) Fiber	(g) Sug.	(g) Prot.	(mg) Sod.
Classic Hot Chocolate - Sixteen with 2% Milk 16 oz	340	8	5	20	56	5	48	17	230
Classic Hot Chocolate - Twelve with 2% Milk 12 oz	240	6	4	15	39	3	33	13	170

Coffee Craze

Food Serving size	Cal.	(g) Total Fat	(g) Sat. Fat	(mg) Chol.	(g) Carb.	(g) Fiber	(g) Sug.	(g) Prot.	(mg) Sod.
Coffee Craze - Original 24 oz	470	0	0	5	100	1	86	13	320
Coffee Craze - Sixteen 16 oz	310	0	0	5	65	0	57	8	210

Five Fruit Frenzy

Food Serving size	Cal.	(g) Total Fat	(g) Sat. Fat	(mg) Chol.	(g) Carb.	(g) Fiber	(g) Sug.	(g) Prot.	(mg) Sod.
Five Fruit Frenzy - Original 24 oz	340	1	0	0	82	6	63	2	30
Five Fruit Frenzy - Power 30 oz	430	1.5	0	0	105	8	80	3	40

Food Serving size	Cal.	(g) Total Fat	(g) Sat. Fat	(mg) Chol.	(g) Carb.	(g) Fiber	(g) Sug.	(g) Prot.	(mg) Sod.
Five Fruit Frenzy - Sixteen 16 oz	240	0.5	0	0	58	4	44	2	25

Flax & Fiber Boost

Flax & Fiber Boost - Per serving 1 boost	30	1.5	NA	0	7	7	NA	1	NA

Mango Mantra

Mango Mantra - Original 24 oz	250	0.5	0	5	56	4	51	8	170
Mango Mantra - Power 30 oz	350	1	0	5	79	6	71	10	200
Mango Mantra - Sixteen 16 oz	160	0	0	5	33	2	30	7	170

Mango-go-go

Mango-go-go - Original 24 oz	400	1.5	0.5	5	94	3	85	3	45
Mango-go-go - Power 30 oz	550	2.5	1	5	129	4	117	4	65
Mango-go-go - Sixteen 16 oz	280	1	0	5	65	2	59	2	35

Matcha Energy Shot-Orange Juice

Matcha Energy Shot-Orange Juice - Double Shot 2 shots	60	0	0	0	13	1	13	2	0
Matcha Energy Shot-Orange Juice - Single Shot 1 shot	60	0	0	0	13	0	13	1	0

Matcha Energy Shot-Soymilk

Matcha Energy Shot-Soymilk - Double Shot 2 shots	70	0	0	0	15	1	13	3	40
Matcha Energy Shot-Soymilk - Single Shot 1 shot	70	0	0	0	15	1	13	3	40

Food Serving size	Cal.	(g) Total Fat	(g) Sat. Fat	(mg) Chol.	(g) Carb.	(g) Fiber	(g) Sug.	(g) Prot.	(mg) Sod.
Matcha Green Tea Blast									
Matcha Green Tea Blast - Original 24 oz	420	0	0	0	91	2	82	10	210
Matcha Green Tea Blast - Sixteen 16 oz	290	0	0	0	63	1	57	7	150
Mega Mango									
Mega Mango - Original 24 oz	340	0.5	0	0	85	5	78	4	10
Mega Mango - Power 30 oz	420	0.5	0	0	105	7	95	5	10
Mega Mango - Sixteen 16 oz	230	0	0	0	58	3	53	2	10
Mocha Mojo									
Mocha Mojo - Original 24 oz	510	1.5	1	5	107	1	92	13	330
Mocha Mojo - Sixteen 16 oz	350	1.5	1	5	73	1	63	9	220
Orange Carrot Karma									
Orange Carrot Karma - Original 24 oz	270	1	0	0	66	4	57	4	120
Orange Carrot Karma - Power 30 oz	360	1.5	0	0	90	6	77	5	150
Orange Carrot Karma - Sixteen 16 oz	180	0.5	0	0	43	3	38	3	90
Orange Dream Machine									
Orange Dream Machine - Original 24 oz	470	1.5	1	10	103	1	97	10	200
Orange Dream Machine - Sixteen 16 oz	350	1	1	5	76	0	71	8	150

Food Serving size	Cal.	(g) Total Fat	(g) Sat. Fat	(mg) Chol.	(g) Carb.	(g) Fiber	(g) Sug.	(g) Prot.	(mg) Sod.
Orange Juice									
Orange Juice - Sixteen 16 oz	220	1	0	0	52	1	42	3	0
Orange Juice - Twelve 12 oz	170	0.5	0	0	39	1	31	3	0
Orange-A-Peel									
Orange-A-Peel - Original 24 oz	370	0	0	0	85	3	76	7	125
Orange-A-Peel - Power 30 oz	500	1.5	0	5	115	5	104	10	200
Orange-A-Peel - Sixteen 16 oz	250	0	0	0	58	2	52	5	85
Organic House Blend									
Organic House Blend - Sixteen 16 oz	5	0	0	0	0	0	0	1	10
Organic House Blend - Twelve 12 oz	5	0	0	0	0	0	0	0	5
Organic House Blend Decaf									
Organic House Blend Decaf - Sixteen 16 oz	0	0	0	0	0	0	0	0	10
Organic House Blend Decaf - Twelve 12 oz	0	0	0	0	0	0	0	0	5
Original Spiced Chai									
Original Spiced Chai - Sixteen with 2% Milk 16 oz	240	5	3	15	38	0	35	11	210
Original Spiced Chai - Twelve with 2% Milk 12 oz	160	3	2	10	25	0	23	8	140
Peach Perfection									
Peach Perfection - Original 30 oz	300	0.5	0	0	75	5	59	2	30

Food Serving size	Cal.	(g) Total Fat	(g) Sat. Fat	(mg) Chol.	(g) Carb.	(g) Fiber	(g) Sug.	(g) Prot.	(mg) Sod.
Peach Perfection - Power 24 oz	400	0.5	0	0	99	7	80	3	35
Peach Perfection - Sixteen 16 oz	210	0	0	0	53	4	42	1	20

Peach Pleasure

Peach Pleasure - Original 24 oz	370	1.5	1	5	88	4	73	3	50
Peach Pleasure - Power 30 oz	490	2	1	5	114	5	96	4	65
Peach Pleasure - Sixteen 16 oz	260	1	0.5	5	61	3	51	2	35

Peanut Butter Moo'd

Peanut Butter Moo'd - Original 24 oz	770	20	4.5	10	126	5	109	20	490
Peanut Butter Moo'd - Sixteen 16 oz	480	10	2.5	5	83	3	72	13	300

Pomegranate Paradise

Pomegranate Paradise - Original 24 oz	340	0.5	0	0	85	5	74	2	35
Pomegranate Paradise - Power 30 oz	430	1	0	0	109	7	95	3	45
Pomegranate Paradise - Sixteen 16 oz	240	0.5	0	0	60	4	53	1	25

Pomegranate Pick-Me-Up

Pomegranate Pick-Me-Up - Original 24 oz	370	2	0.5	5	88	4	75	3	50
Pomegranate Pick-Me-Up - Power 30 oz	510	2.5	1	5	120	5	105	3	70
Pomegranate Pick-Me-Up - Sixteen 16 oz	260	1	0	5	61	3	53	2	35

Food Serving size	Cal.	(g) Total Fat	(g) Sat. Fat	(mg) Chol.	(g) Carb.	(g) Fiber	(g) Sug.	(g) Prot.	(mg) Sod.
Protein Berry Workout									
Protein Berry Workout - Original 24 oz	380	0.5	0	5	74	5	62	20	200
Protein Berry Workout - Power 30 oz	500	1	0.5	5	102	7	85	22	230
Protein Berry Workout - Sixteen 16 oz	290	0	0	5	54	3	45	17	160
Pumpkin Smash									
Pumpkin Smash - Original 24 oz	550	0.5	0	5	118	2	107	14	460
Pumpkin Smash - Sixteen 16 oz	390	0	0	5	83	1	75	10	320
Razzmatazz									
Razzmatazz - Original 24 oz	390	1.5	1	5	91	4	74	3	55
Razzmatazz - Power 30 oz	520	2.5	1	5	121	5	100	4	75
Razzmatazz - Sixteen 16 oz	270	1	0.5	5	63	3	51	2	40
Soy Protein Boost									
Soy Protein Boost - Per serving 1 boost	30	NA	NA	NA	NA	NA	NA	8	NA
Strawberries Wild									
Strawberries Wild - Original 24 oz	370	0	0	5	87	3	77	5	140
Strawberries Wild - Power 30 oz	510	0.5	0	5	118	5	104	7	210
Strawberries Wild - Sixteen 16 oz	250	0	0	0	60	2	52	3	95

Food Serving size	Cal.	(g) Total Fat	(g) Sat. Fat	(mg) Chol.	(g) Carb.	(g) Fiber	(g) Sug.	(g) Prot.	(mg) Sod.
Strawberry Lemonade									
Strawberry Lemonade - Original 24 oz	300	1	0	0	73	2	63	2	140
Strawberry Lemonade - Power 30 oz	420	1.5	1	5	101	4	88	3	190
Strawberry Lemonade - Sixteen 16 oz	230	0.5	0	0	55	3	47	1	105
Strawberry Nirvana									
Strawberry Nirvana - Original 24 oz	230	0.5	0	5	51	4	44	7	180
Strawberry Nirvana - Power 30 oz	310	0.5	0	5	69	7	59	9	220
Strawberry Nirvana - Sixteen 16 oz	150	0	0	5	32	2	27	6	150
Strawberry Surf Rider									
Strawberry Surf Rider - Original 24 oz	430	1.5	0.5	5	103	4	93	3	10
Strawberry Surf Rider - Power 30 oz	580	2	1	5	140	5	126	4	15
Strawberry Surf Rider - Sixteen 16 oz	300	1	0	5	72	2	64	2	5
Strawberry Whirl									
Strawberry Whirl - Original 24 oz	300	0.5	0	0	75	6	64	2	25
Strawberry Whirl - Power 30 oz	380	1	0	0	95	8	80	230	30
Strawberry Whirl - Sixteen 16 oz	220	0	0	0	54	4	46	1	20
The Coldbuster									
The Coldbuster - Original 24 oz	350	1.5	1	5	82	3	75	5	25

Food Serving size	Cal.	(g) Total Fat	(g) Sat. Fat	(mg) Chol.	(g) Carb.	(g) Fiber	(g) Sug.	(g) Prot.	(mg) Sod.
The Coldbuster - Power 30 oz	500	2	1	5	116	5	107	7	40
The Coldbuster - Sixteen 16 oz	250	1	0.5	5	59	2	55	4	15

Watermelon Splash

Watermelon Splash - Original 24 oz	290	0	0	0	70	3	62	2	135
Watermelon Splash - Power 30 oz	430	0	0	0	106	4	94	2	160
Watermelon Splash - Sixteen 16 oz	210	0	0	0	51	2	45	1	95

Weight Burner Boost

New! Weight Burner Boost - Sixteen 16 oz	30	3	0	0	0	0	0	0	0

Whey Protein Boost

Whey Protein Boost - Per serving 1 boost	50	0.5	NA	20	1	NA	NA	10	25

Jason's Deli ▬▬▬
[www.jasonsdeli.com]

Entrée Salads

"Lighter" Chicken Club Salad (no dressing) 1 salad	320	21	8	70	10	4	3	25	740
"Lighter" Nutty Mixed Up Salad (no dressing) 1 salad	240	6	3	45	30	3	19	17	430
"Lighter" The Big Chef Salad (no dressing) 1 salad	340	22	9	180	7	1	3	30	1100
Chicken Club Salad (no dressing) 1 salad	610	40	16	140	18	7	5	48	1370
Nutty Mixed Up Salad (no dressing) 1 salad	440	13	6	90	50	6	29	34	900

Food Serving size	Cal.	(g) Total Fat	(g) Sat. Fat	(mg) Chol.	(g) Carb.	(g) Fiber	(g) Sug.	(g) Prot.	(mg) Sod.
The Big Chef Salad (no dressing) 1 salad	500	30	13	325	13	2	5	50	1660

Gluten Free Dressing Choices

Food Serving size	Cal.	Total Fat	Sat. Fat	Chol.	Carb.	Fiber	Sug.	Prot.	Sod.
Balsamic Vinaigrette 4 tbsp	120	12	2	0	4	0	4	0	360
Blue Cheese Dressing 4 tbsp	280	28	6	20	4	0	2	2	660
Country French Dressing 4 tbsp	140	9	1	0	14	0	12	0	500
Creamy Caesar Dressing 4 tbsp	140	12	4	10	2	0	2	6	500
Extra Virgin Olive Oil 4 tbsp	480	56	8	0	0	0	0	0	0
Family Recipe Ranch 4 tbsp	253	27	3	20	3	0	0	1	493
Italian Dressing 4 tbsp	240	26	4	0	2	0	0	2	360
Low Fat Honey Mustard Dressing 4 tbsp	160	10	1	0	14	0	12	2	340
Low Fat Ranch Dressing 4 tbsp	140	14	2	10	4	0	2	2	260
Organic Balsamic Vinegar 4 tbsp	60	0	0	0	12	0	12	0	0
Thousand Island Dressing 4 tbsp	260	24	4	20	8	0	8	0	160

Potatoes

Food Serving size	Cal.	Total Fat	Sat. Fat	Chol.	Carb.	Fiber	Sug.	Prot.	Sod.
"Lighter" Pollo Mexicano Potato 1 potato	940	29	13	75	139	12	12	33	1000
"Lighter" Texas Style Spud - Beef (Limited Availablity) 1 potato	1300	69	24	135	128	9	12	36	780
"Plain" Jane Potato 1 potato	2320	150	61	190	192	13	19	56	1750

Food Serving size	Cal.	(g) Total Fat	(g) Sat. Fat	(mg) Chol.	(g) Carb.	(g) Fiber	(g) Sug.	(g) Prot.	(mg) Sod.
"Lighter Plain" Jane Potato									
1 potato	1130	55	23	85	135	9	12	29	690
Pollo Mexicano Potato									
1 potato	1520	58	25	150	196	16	18	59	1650
Texas Style Spud – Beef (Limited Availability)									
1 potato	1810	84	29	235	193	13	18	58	1010

Sides

American Potato Salad									
1 serving	350	25	4	90	28	3	3	5	500
Fresh Fruit Cup (no dip)									
1 serving	90	0	0	0	23	3	18	1	0
Fresh Made Guacamole									
1 serving	170	15	2	0	11	7	2	2	250
Fresh Made Salsa									
1 serving	27	0	0	0	6	2	3	1	296
Organic Blue Corn Tortilla Chips									
1 serving	220	11	1	0	27	3	0	3	90
Roasted Red Pepper Hummus									
1 serving	252	12	0	0	30	8	4	8	716
Steamed Veggies									
1 serving	60	0	0	0	11	4	5	3	55

Soups

Fire Roasted Tortilla Soup									
1 bowl	320	16	2	20	35	5	6	9	1300
Fire Roasted Tortilla Soup									
1 cup	160	8	1	10	18	3	3	5	680
Organic Vegetarian Vegetable Soup									
1 bowl	150	6	0	0	20	4	4	4	950
Organic Vegetarian Vegetable Soup									
1 cup	90	4	0	0	13	2	2	2	570
Red Beans and Rice with Sausage (Limited Availability)									
1 bowl	275	6	2	20	56	23	3	19	1405

Food Serving size	Cal.	(g) Total Fat	(g) Sat. Fat	(mg) Chol.	(g) Carb.	(g) Fiber	(g) Sug.	(g) Prot.	(mg) Sod.
Red Beans and Rice with Sausage (Limited Availability)									
1 cup	122	3	1	8	25	10	1	8	582
Vegetarian Tomato Basil									
1 bowl	320	25	13	65	22	4	12	3	1120
Vegetarian Tomato Basil									
1 cup	170	13	7	35	12	2	6	2	600

LongHorn Steakhouse
[www.longhornsteakhouse.com]

Burgers / Sandwiches

Bacon Cheeseburger (order without bun)									
1 burger	880	55	25	NA	47	NA	NA	51	1120
Cheeseburger (order without bun)									
1 burger	840	51	24.5	NA	44	NA	NA	49	890
Shaved Prime Rib Sandwich (order without bun or horseradish sauce)									
1 sandwich	910	50	21	NA	46	NA	NA	68	1620

Chicken

Sierra Chicken									
1 serving	410	12	3	NA	2	NA	NA	72	1240

Dressings

Balsamic Vinaigrette									
1 serving	190	20	3	NA	2	NA	NA	0	340
Bleu Cheese									
1 serving	160	15	4	NA	3	NA	NA	3	490
Caesar Dressing									
1 serving	230	24	3.5	NA	1	NA	NA	0	580
Chipotle Ranch Dressing									
1 serving	200	20	3	NA	5	NA	NA	0	320
Fat-free Ranch Dressing									
1 serving	45	0	0	NA	11	NA	NA	0	560
Honey Mustard Dressing									
1 serving	240	23	3.5	NA	7	NA	NA	0	240

Food Serving size	Cal.	(g) Total Fat	(g) Sat. Fat	(mg) Chol.	(g) Carb.	(g) Fiber	(g) Sug.	(g) Prot.	(mg) Sod.
Oil and Vinegar 1 serving	180	21	3	NA	0	NA	NA	0	0
Ranch Dressing 1 serving	200	20	3.5	NA	3	NA	NA	1	340
Thousand Island Dressing 1 serving	190	17	2.5	NA	5	NA	NA	0	400

Flavorful under 500

Food Serving size	Cal.	(g) Total Fat	(g) Sat. Fat	(mg) Chol.	(g) Carb.	(g) Fiber	(g) Sug.	(g) Prot.	(mg) Sod.
Flo's Filet (order without salmon marinade and rice) 7 oz	370	17	7	NA	10	NA	NA	44	580
Grilled Fresh Rainbow Trout 1 serving	280	15	3	NA	NA	NA	NA	NA	460
LongHorn Salmon (order without salmon marinade and rice) 7 oz	350	14	3	NA	12	NA	NA	44	560
Renegade Top Sirloin 6 oz	380	23	6	NA	0	NA	NA	43	520
Renegade Top Sirloin 8 oz	470	26	7	NA	0	NA	NA	57	680
Sierra Chicken (lighter portion) 1 serving	270	7	1.5	NA	13	NA	NA	39	1050

Kids' Meals

Food Serving size	Cal.	(g) Total Fat	(g) Sat. Fat	(mg) Chol.	(g) Carb.	(g) Fiber	(g) Sug.	(g) Prot.	(mg) Sod.
Kid's Cheeseburger (order without bun) 1 serving	510	29	13	NA	31	NA	NA	31	860
Kid's Grilled Chicken 1 serving	140	2	0	NA	0	NA	NA	30	150
Kid's Grilled Chicken Salad (order without croutons) 1 serving	270	9	3	NA	5	NA	NA	41	190
Kid's Hot Dog (order without bun) 1 serving	310	19	8	NA	23	NA	NA	11	750
Kid's Sirloin Steak 1 serving	210	9	3	NA	0	NA	NA	32	240

Food Serving size	Cal.	(g) Total Fat	(g) Sat. Fat	(mg) Chol.	(g) Carb.	(g) Fiber	(g) Sug.	(g) Prot.	(mg) Sod.
Legendary Steaks									
Bacon Wrapped Filet 9 oz	620	41	12	NA	0	NA	NA	64	880
Chop Steak (order without red wine sauce, or crisp onion straws) 1 serving	660	45	15	NA	17	NA	NA	47	1100
Fire-Grilled Bone-In Sirloin 1 steak	470	32	10	NA	1	NA	NA	45	920
Fire-Grilled T-Bone 1 steak	830	57	22	NA	1	NA	NA	78	1710
Flat Iron Steak 1 steak	440	29	10	NA	0	NA	NA	46	310
Flat Iron Steak 1 steak	620	41	15	NA	8	NA	NA	55	980
Flo's Filet 7 oz	430	30	9	NA	1	NA	NA	40	380
Flo's Filet 9 oz	520	34	11	NA	2	NA	NA	51	470
LongHorn Porterhouse Steak 1 steak	1100	79	28	NA	1	NA	NA	96	1970
New York Strip Steak 11 oz	790	60	22	NA	2	NA	NA	60	530
New York Strip Steak 14 oz	950	72	26	NA	2	NA	NA	75	650
Outlaw Ribeye Steak 18 oz	1070	79	33	NA	0	NA	NA	90	1640
Prime Rib (order without Classic Au Jus) 16 oz	980	61	28	NA	0	NA	NA	106	1300
Prime Rib (order without Classic Au Jus) 12 oz	740	46	21	NA	0	NA	NA	80	1160
Renegade Top Sirloin 12 oz	640	33	9	NA	0	NA	NA	85	990
Renegade Top Sirloin 8 oz	470	26	7	NA	0	NA	NA	59	680

Food Serving size	Cal.	(g) Total Fat	(g) Sat. Fat	(mg) Chol.	(g) Carb.	(g) Fiber	(g) Sug.	(g) Prot.	(mg) Sod.
Renegade Top Sirloin 6 oz	380	23	6	NA	0	NA	NA	43	520
Ribeye Steak 12 oz	910	68	25	NA	0	NA	NA	72	1260

Ribs, Chops, Etc.

Food Serving size	Cal.	(g) Total Fat	(g) Sat. Fat	(mg) Chol.	(g) Carb.	(g) Fiber	(g) Sug.	(g) Prot.	(mg) Sod.
Babyback Ribs (order without BBQ sauce) 1/2 rack	550	37	13	NA	2	NA	NA	51	570
Babyback Ribs (order without BBQ sauce) full rack	1090	74	25	NA	4	NA	NA	102	1140
Cowboy Pork Chops 1 serving	400	14	5	NA	1	NA	NA	67	1600

Salads

Food Serving size	Cal.	(g) Total Fat	(g) Sat. Fat	(mg) Chol.	(g) Carb.	(g) Fiber	(g) Sug.	(g) Prot.	(mg) Sod.
7-Pepper Sirloin Salad (Dinner) (request no croutons on salad, and that it is tossed in a separate mixing bowl from other salads) 1 salad	670	36	12	NA	32	NA	NA	54	1500
7-Pepper Sirloin Salad (Lunch) (request no croutons on salad, and that it is tossed in a separate mixing bowl from other salads) 1 salad	520	25	10	NA	26	NA	NA	46	1380
Caesar Side Salad (request no croutons on salad, and request that it is tossed in a separate mixing bowl from other salads) 1 salad	350	27	6	NA	18	NA	NA	7	550
Chicken Caesar Salad (request no croutons on salad, and request that it is tossed in a separate mixing bowl from other salads) 1 salad	720	47	10	NA	27	NA	NA	46	1190
Grilled Salmon Salad (Dinner) (order without Salmon Marinade and croutons, and ask that the salad be tossed in a separate mixing bowl from other salads) 1 salad	560	27	9	NA	29	NA	NA	50	690
Grilled Salmon Salad (Lunch) (order without Salmon Marinade and croutons, and ask that the salad be tossed in a separate mixing bowl from other salads) 1 salad	490	24	9	NA	28	NA	NA	40	600

Food Serving size	Cal.	(g) Total Fat	(g) Sat. Fat	(mg) Chol.	(g) Carb.	(g) Fiber	(g) Sug.	(g) Prot.	(mg) Sod.
Mixed Green Side Salad (request no croutons on salad, and request that it be tossed in a separate mixing bowl from other salads) 1 salad	110	4.5	2	NA	12	NA	NA	4	200

Seafood

Food Serving size	Cal.	Total Fat	Sat. Fat	Chol.	Carb.	Fiber	Sug.	Prot.	Sod.
Flo's Filet & LongHorn Salmon (order without salmon marinade and rice) 1 serving	740	43	11	NA	3	NA	NA	86	800
Flo's Filet and Lobster Tail (where available)(order without rice) 1 serving	500	30	8	NA	0	NA	NA	57	1000
Grilled Fresh Rainbow Trout (order without rice) 1 serving	310	13	3	NA	9	NA	NA	39	600
LongHorn Salmon (order without salmon marinade and rice) 1 serving	290	13	2.5	NA	3	NA	NA	40	300
Redrock Grilled Shrimp (order without rice) 1 serving	90	1	0	NA	2	NA	NA	18	1120

Side Items

Food Serving size	Cal.	Total Fat	Sat. Fat	Chol.	Carb.	Fiber	Sug.	Prot.	Sod.
Baked Potato 1 potato	145	0	0	0	34	2.3	3	3	376
Fresh Green Beans 1 serving	35	0	0	NA	6	NA	NA	2	230
Fresh Seasonal Vegetables 1 serving	90	4	1	NA	9	NA	NA	3	350
Fresh Steamed Asparagus 1 serving	80	4.5	1	NA	5	NA	NA	4	55
Grilled Onions 1 serving	90	4	0.5	NA	11	NA	NA	1	750
Mashed Potatoes 1 serving	340	22	12	NA	31	NA	NA	4	690
Sauteed Mushrooms 1 serving	90	5	1	NA	5	NA	NA	4	530
Sliced Tomatoes 1 slice	5	0.1	NA	NA	1.1	0.3	NA	0.2	2
Sweet Potato with Cinn-Sugar & Butter 1 potato	370	12	7	NA	58	NA	NA	7	95

Food Serving size	Cal.	(g) Total Fat	(g) Sat. Fat	(mg) Chol.	(g) Carb.	(g) Fiber	(g) Sug.	(g) Prot.	(mg) Sod.

Additional Gluten-Free Menu Items
(nutritional information was not available)

House Salad Dressing, Hot Fudge Sundae

Montana Mike's
[www.stockadecompanies.com/OurRestaurants/MMHome]

Appetizer

Potato Boat 1 serving	918	56	24	119	65	7	3	40	1824

Beverages

Cherry Pepsi 16.8 fl oz	231	0	0	0	61	0	61	0	53
Cherry Pepsi 9.6 fl oz	132	0	0	0	35	0	35	0	30
Diet Dr Pepper 16.8 fl oz	0	0	0	0	0	0	0	0	74
Diet Dr Pepper 9.6 fl oz	0	0	0	0	0	0	0	0	42
Diet Pepsi 16.8 fl oz	0	0	0	0	0	0	0	0	63
Diet Pepsi 9.6 fl oz	0	0	0	0	0	0	0	0	36
Dr Pepper 16.8 fl oz	231	0	0	0	57	0	57	0	74
Dr Pepper 9.6 fl oz	132	0	0	0	32	0	32	0	42
Mountain Dew 16.8 fl oz	231	0	0	0	65	0	65	0	105
Mountain Dew 9.6 fl oz	132	0	0	0	37	0	37	0	60
Pepsi 16.8 fl oz	210	0	0	0	57	0	57	0	53

Food Serving size	Cal.	(g) Total Fat	(g) Sat. Fat	(mg) Chol.	(g) Carb.	(g) Fiber	(g) Sug.	(g) Prot.	(mg) Sod.
Pepsi 9.6 fl oz	120	0	0	0	32	0	32	0	30
Sierra Mist 16.8 fl oz	210	0	0	0	55	0	55	0	53
Sierra Mist 9.6 fl oz	120	0	0	0	31	0	31	0	30
Tropicana Fruit Punch 16.8 fl oz	252	0	0	0	67	0	63	0	105
Tropicana Fruit Punch 9.6 fl oz	144	0	0	0	38	0	36	0	60

Condiments

Food Serving size	Cal.	(g) Total Fat	(g) Sat. Fat	(mg) Chol.	(g) Carb.	(g) Fiber	(g) Sug.	(g) Prot.	(mg) Sod.
A-1 Steak Sauce 2 tbsp	30	0	0	0	6	0	4	0	560
Hickory Sauce 3 fl oz	120	0	0	0	28	0	25	1	615
Honey Mustard 3 fl oz	373	24	3	19	36	1	31	2	964
Horseradish Sauce 2 fl oz	240	24	6	36	3	0	2	2	355
Ketchup 2 tbsp	37	0	0	0	9	0	8	0	293
Mayonnaise 1 tbsp	100	11	2	10	0	0	0	0	100
Montana Mike's Steak Sauce 2 tbsp	50	0	0	0	12	0	8	0	340
Mustard 1 tbsp	10	1	0	0	1	1	0	1	165
Peppercorn Sauce 2 fl oz	30	1	0	3	5	0	1	1	317
Ranch Dressing, for Dipping 2 fl oz	215	23	3	22	2	0	1	1	373
Tartar Sauce 2 fl oz	303	32	4	29	3	0	2	0	335

Food Serving size	Cal.	(g) Total Fat	(g) Sat. Fat	(mg) Chol.	(g) Carb.	(g) Fiber	(g) Sug.	(g) Prot.	(mg) Sod.
Entrées									
Baby Back Ribs, Dinner 1 serving	1814	131	50	448	52	0	45	91	5667
Baby Back Ribs, Lunch 1 serving	927	65	25	224	31	0	27	46	2936
Beef Tips 1 serving	420	20	7	150	13	2	3	48	874
Beef Tips with White Rice 1 serving	630	23	8	150	54	2	3	52	1705
Buffalo Sirloin 1 serving	394	14	4	117	0	0	0	67	487
Center Cut Sirloin Steak 12 oz	732	47	18	135	0	0	0	69	641
Center Cut Sirloin Steak 9 oz	551	35	13	101	0	0	0	52	570
Chicken and Ribs 1 serving	1196	79	28	324	33	0	27	81	4273
Chopped Sirloin Steak 1 serving	661	36	15	135	6	0	0	70	932
Cracked Peppercorn Sirloin 12 oz	656	36	15	135	5	2	0	70	535
Cracked Peppercorn Sirloin 9 oz	499	27	11	101	5	2	0	53	490
Filet Mignon 12 oz	979	75	29	228	0	0	0	69	765
Filet Mignon 8 oz	666	51	20	155	0	0	0	47	673
Fire Grilled Chicken Breast 1 serving	358	17	4	133	3	0	0	47	1781
Fried Catfish Strips 1 serving	777	23	4	150	84	7	0	53	4954
Fried Catfish Strips, Lunch 1 serving	389	11	2	75	42	4	0	27	2477

Food Serving size	Cal.	(g) Total Fat	(g) Sat. Fat	(mg) Chol.	(g) Carb.	(g) Fiber	(g) Sug.	(g) Prot.	(mg) Sod.
Grilled Shrimp 1 serving	303	15	3	302	2	0	0	40	451
K-Bobs 1 serving	515	27	11	101	9	2	5	53	411
KC or NY Strip Steak 14 oz	994	72	27	227	0	0	0	81	688
Mike's Big Montana Steak 22 oz	1342	87	32	248	0	0	0	127	1070
Mile High Ribeye Steak 16 oz	816	47	15	260	0	0	0	88	715
Mountain Momma Ribeye Steak 12 oz	612	35	12	195	0	0	0	66	604
Mountain Topped Chicken 1 serving	869	55	17	206	27	1	21	65	3414
Mountain Topped Chopped Sirloin 1 serving	1052	68	23	297	25	1	21	87	2084
Pork Chops, Bone In, Dinner 1 serving	659	33	12	263	2	1	0	89	2116
Pork Chops, Bone In, Lunch 1 serving	330	16	6	132	1	0	0	45	1058
Pork Chops, Dinner 1 serving	624	31	11	247	3	1	0	84	2741
Pork Chops, Lunch 1 serving	418	21	8	165	2	1	0	56	1836
Porterhouse Pork Chop 1 serving	611	39	14	195	5	1	3	60	2006
Porterhouse Steak 20 oz	1631	132	50	385	0	0	0	102	1016
Porterhouse Steak 24 oz	1957	159	60	462	0	0	0	122	1111
Ranchers T-Bone Steak 16 oz	1188	91	34	281	0	0	0	86	655
Shrimp Tejas 1 serving	717	54	21	287	9	3	2	50	1291

Food Serving size	Cal.	(g) Total Fat	(g) Sat. Fat	(mg) Chol.	(g) Carb.	(g) Fiber	(g) Sug.	(g) Prot.	(mg) Sod.
Shrimp Tejas with Garlic Butter									
1 serving	1118	97	31	287	11	3	2	50	1702
St. Louis Ribs, Dinner									
1 serving	1964	145	55	476	52	0	45	106	5707
St. Louis Ribs, Lunch									
1 serving	1002	73	27	238	31	0	27	53	2956
Steak and Catfish									
1 serving	938	47	15	176	42	4	0	78	2965
Steak and Chicken									
1 serving	819	49	16	201	2	0	0	87	1825
Steak and Grilled Shrimp									
1 serving	676	40	14	252	1	0	0	72	711
Steak and Ribs									
1 serving	1477	101	38	325	31	0	27	97	3424
The 44 Sirloin									
1 serving	2716	177	65	495	0	0	0	253	2174
Trout									
1 serving	392	23	7	140	1	0	0	44	396

Salad Dressings

Food Serving size	Cal.	(g) Total Fat	(g) Sat. Fat	(mg) Chol.	(g) Carb.	(g) Fiber	(g) Sug.	(g) Prot.	(mg) Sod.
Blue Cheese Dressing									
2 fl oz	258	27	6	37	2	0	2	3	339
Caesar Dressing									
2 fl oz	280	30	5	30	4	0	4	4	840
Chipotle Ranch Dressing									
2 fl oz	209	21	3	21	3	0	2	1	387
Golden Italian Dressing									
2 fl oz	280	28	4	0	4	0	4	0	580
Honey Mustard Dressing									
2 fl oz	248	16	2	13	24	1	21	2	643
Ranch Dressing									
2 fl oz	215	23	3	22	2	0	1	1	373
Ranch Dressing, Fat Free									
2 fl oz	60	0	0	0	16	2	10	0	620

Food Serving size	Cal.	(g) Total Fat	(g) Sat. Fat	(mg) Chol.	(g) Carb.	(g) Fiber	(g) Sug.	(g) Prot.	(mg) Sod.
Thousand Island Dressing 2 fl oz	221	20	3	18	9	0	9	0	443

Salads

Food Serving size	Cal.	Total Fat	Sat. Fat	Chol.	Carb.	Fiber	Sug.	Prot.	Sod.
Buffalo Chicken Salad 1 salad	604	40	10	49	43	9	16	19	595
Buffalo Chicken Salad with Grilled Chicken Breast 1 salad	820	48	12	149	45	9	16	54	1878
Caesar Salad 1 salad	352	33	6	33	12	2	5	8	945
Chicken Caesar Salad 1 salad	784	58	11	153	23	5	9	49	2808
Chicken Tostada Salad 1 salad	537	23	7	130	33	5	6	49	1819
Dinner Salad 1 salad	255	14	5	30	19	4	6	13	505
Garden Salad 1 salad	63	2	0	0	9	2	3	2	71
Garden Salad with Cheese and Bacon 1 salad	188	12	5	30	9	2	3	10	433
Grilled Chicken Breast Salad 1 salad	472	22	7	130	21	4	6	48	1788
Grilled Shrimp Salad 1 salad	357	16	6	181	20	4	6	33	702
Grilled Steak Salad 1 salad	570	32	13	97	19	4	6	47	595
Half Buffalo Chicken Salad 1 salad	302	20	5	24	22	4	8	9	297
Half Buffalo Chicken Salad with Grilled Chicken Breast 1 salad	411	24	6	74	23	4	8	27	939
Half Chicken Tostada Salad 1 salad	271	12	4	65	17	2	3	25	910
Half Dinner Salad 1 salad	130	7	3	15	10	2	3	6	253

Food Serving size	Cal.	(g) Total Fat	(g) Sat. Fat	(mg) Chol.	(g) Carb.	(g) Fiber	(g) Sug.	(g) Prot.	(mg) Sod.
Half Grilled Chicken Breast Salad									
1 salad	238	11	4	65	11	2	3	24	895
Half Grilled Steak Salad									
1 salad	340	19	8	60	10	2	3	29	313
Spinach and Shrimp Salad									
1 salad	292	17	3	337	8	3	3	27	302
Spinach and Shrimp Salad with Hot Bacon Dressing									
1 salad	592	45	7	337	18	3	13	27	902

Side Items

Food Serving size	Cal.	(g) Total Fat	(g) Sat. Fat	(mg) Chol.	(g) Carb.	(g) Fiber	(g) Sug.	(g) Prot.	(mg) Sod.
Authentic Mashed Potatoes									
1 serving	388	17	4	0	50	4	3	12	1069
Baked Potato									
1 serving	367	0	0	0	81	9	4	10	30
Baked Potato with Butter									
1 serving	527	18	4	0	81	9	4	10	198
Baked Potato with Butter and Sour Cream									
1 serving	575	22	7	16	83	9	6	12	234
Baked Potato with Sour Cream									
1 serving	415	4	3	16	83	9	6	12	66
Baked Sweet Potato									
1 serving	366	1	0	0	82	13	33	8	146
Cottage Cheese Salad									
1 serving	87	3	2	20	5	1	3	10	304
Green Beans									
1 serving	220	14	6	20	12	5	2	9	1263
Saucy Cinnamon Apples									
1 serving	99	5	1	0	14	1	12	0	156
Sauteed Sliced Mushrooms									
1 serving	114	7	1	0	7	2	4	5	2438
Steamed Veggies									
1 serving	202	18	4	0	7	3	3	3	465
Veggie K-Bobs									
1 serving	268	15	3	0	32	1	26	1	565

Food Serving size	Cal.	(g) Total Fat	(g) Sat. Fat	(mg) Chol.	(g) Carb.	(g) Fiber	(g) Sug.	(g) Prot.	(mg) Sod.
Soups									
Broccoli and Cheese Soup 1 bowl	213	14	6	21	9	2	3	9	882
Broccoli and Cheese Soup 1 cup	121	8	3	11	5	1	2	5	518
Chicken Tortilla Soup 1 bowl	204	10	4	34	14	1	2	14	1590
Chicken Tortilla Soup 1 cup	113	5	2	19	8	1	1	8	943

Noodles & Company
[www.noodles.com]

American

Food Serving size	Cal.	(g) Total Fat	(g) Sat. Fat	(mg) Chol.	(g) Carb.	(g) Fiber	(g) Sug.	(g) Prot.	(mg) Sod.
Buttered Noodles (regular) 1 serving	930	39	22	215	114	6	3	32	970
Buttered Noodles (small) 1 serving	460	19	11	105	57	3	2	16	530
Caesar Salad (regular) 1 salad	370	28	7	30	19	2	<1	11	940
Caesar Salad (small) 1 salad	200	15	4	15	10	1	0	6	530
Spaghetti with Marinara (regular) 1 serving	660	16	4.5	15	105	6	16	23	1040
Spaghetti with Marinara (small) 1 serving	340	9	3	10	53	3	8	13	570

Asian

Food Serving size	Cal.	(g) Total Fat	(g) Sat. Fat	(mg) Chol.	(g) Carb.	(g) Fiber	(g) Sug.	(g) Prot.	(mg) Sod.
Chinese Chop Salad (regular) 1 salad	370	200	1.5	0	39	6	20	5	880
Chinese Chop Salad (small) 1 salad	190	11	1	0	19	3	10	2	440

Food Serving size	Cal.	(g) Total Fat	(g) Sat. Fat	(mg) Chol.	(g) Carb.	(g) Fiber	(g) Sug.	(g) Prot.	(mg) Sod.
Pad Thai (regular) 1 serving	830	18	3	135	151	5	32	15	2050
Pad Thai (small) 1 serving	410	9	1.5	70	76	2	16	7	1030

Extras

Cucumber Tomato Salad 1 salad	110	0	0	0	24	2	18	1	920
Tossed Green Salad (with fat-free Asian dressing) 1 salad	45	0	0	0	11	1	9	0	420

Mediterranean

Pasta Fresca (regular) 1 serving	780	25	7	15	114	6	11	26	1030
Pasta Fresca (small) 1 serving	410	13	4.5	10	58	3	6	14	610
Penne Rosa (regular) 1 serving	790	310	19	95	97	6	13	24	950
Penne Rosa (small) 1 serving	410	18	10	50	49	3	7	13	530
Pesto Cavatappi (regular) 1 serving	800	31	13	60	102	6	10	27	890
Pesto Cavatappi (small) 1 serving	460	22	11	50	52	3	6	15	550
The Med Salad (regular) 1 salad	320	13	3	15	44	4	7	9	1000
The Med Salad (small) 1 salad	160	60	1.5	5	22	2	3	4	500
Whole Grain Tuscan Linguine (regular) 1 serving	680	32	13	55	77	13	9	22	1220
Whole Grain Tuscan Linguine (small) 1 serving	400	32	13	55	77	13	9	22	1220

Food Serving size	Cal.	(g) Total Fat	(g) Sat. Fat	(mg) Chol.	(g) Carb.	(g) Fiber	(g) Sug.	(g) Prot.	(mg) Sod.

Old Spaghetti Factory
[www.osf.com]

Beverages

Coffee 1 fl oz	0	0	0	0	0	0	0	0	1
Iced Tea (unsweetened) 12 oz	0	0	0	0	0	0	0	0	5
Italian Cream Soda 213g	140	3.5	2	10	25	0	24	1	50
Milk 1 serving	100	2.5	1.5	10	12	0	11	8	125
Tea 1 fl oz	0	0	0	0	0	0	0	0	1

Desserts

Spumoni 85g	180	9	6	40	21	0	17	3	90
Vanilla Ice Cream 85g	170	9	6	35	21	0	14	3	80

Entrée

Baked Chicken (dinner only; request gluten-free pasta) 469g	960	60	20	215	65	3	4	42	2500

House Salads

House Salad (with Balsamic Vinaigrette dressing and no croutons) 113g	190	18	1.5	0	7	1	3	1	150
House Salad (with Creamy Pesto dressing and no croutons) 128g	210	21	3	10	5	1	3	2	220

Just for Kids

Just for Kids, Kid's Clam Sauce 227g	420	16	9	70	63	1	0	8	440
Just for Kids, Kid's Marinara 227g	300	3	0	0	63	3	4	5	380

Food Serving size	Cal.	(g) Total Fat	(g) Sat. Fat	(mg) Chol.	(g) Carb.	(g) Fiber	(g) Sug.	(g) Prot.	(mg) Sod.
Just for Kids, Kid's Meat Sauce									
227g	340	6	1.5	15	63	3	3	10	530
Just for Kids, Kid's Mizithra Cheese & Browned Butter									
206g	610	35	22	105	59	1	1	15	1100
Just for Kids, Kid's Sauteed Mushroom Sauce									
284g	370	10	1	0	65	3	5	6	450
Just for Kids, Macaroni & Cheese Style Sauce									
227g	380	10	5	25	63	1	3	9	480

Pasta Classics

Food Serving size	Cal.	(g) Total Fat	(g) Sat. Fat	(mg) Chol.	(g) Carb.	(g) Fiber	(g) Sug.	(g) Prot.	(mg) Sod.
Alfredo Sauce (request gluten-free pasta)									
407g	1030	61	37	185	108	3	0	14	550
Clam Sauce (request gluten-free pasta)									
425g	800	31	18	145	115	3	1	16	870
Marinara Sauce (request gluten-free pasta)									
425g	540	5	0	0	115	5	8	9	770
Mizithra Cheese & Browned Butter Sauce (request gluten-free pasta)									
383g	1170	70	43	210	106	2	2	29	2200
Rich Meat Sauce (request gluten-free pasta)									
425g	630	11	3	35	115	5	6	19	1050
Sauteed Mushroom Sauce (request gluten-free pasta)									
510g	650	16	1	0	118	5	9	11	860

Side Orders

Food Serving size	Cal.	(g) Total Fat	(g) Sat. Fat	(mg) Chol.	(g) Carb.	(g) Fiber	(g) Sug.	(g) Prot.	(mg) Sod.
All Natural Chicken Breast									
191g	310	18	3	85	5	0	0	32	300
Marinated, diced all natural chicken									
85g	140	9	1	35	1	0	0	13	690
Sicilian Style Italian Sausage									
128g	340	27	11	70	3	2	1	15	790

Additional Gluten-Free Menu Items
(nutritional information was not available)

Soft Drinks

Food Serving size	Cal.	(g) Total Fat	(g) Sat. Fat	(mg) Chol.	(g) Carb.	(g) Fiber	(g) Sug.	(g) Prot.	(mg) Sod.

Olive Garden
[www.olivegarden.com]

Appetizers

Dipping Sauce (Marinara)									
1 serving	35	1.5	0	NA	4	1	NA	0	200

Entrées

Herb-Grilled Salmon									
1 entrée	510	26	6	NA	5	4	NA	64	760
Mixed Grill – All Chicken with Broccoli									
1 entrée	640	19	4	NA	27	7	NA	89	1260
Mixed Grill with Broccoli									
1 entrée	750	23	6	NA	24	4	NA	112	1760
Steak Toscano with Grilled Vegetables									
1 entrée	500	21	5	NA	41	0	NA	37	1030

Kids' Menu

Add Grilled Chicken									
1 serving	110	2	0	NA	0	0	NA	24	410
Add Italian Sausage									
1 serving	240	20	7	NA	1	0	NA	12	570
Add Shrimp									
1 serving	30	0	0	NA	0	0	NA	7	340
Child Sundae									
1 serving	190	8	6	NA	26	0	NA	4	50
Kids' Grilled Chicken with Penne Marinara									
1 serving	390	6	1	NA	59	4	NA	27	1040
Kids' Pasta (request gluten-free pasta)									
1 serving	250	4	0.5	NA	49	4	NA	4	750
Parmesan-Butter Sauce									
1 serving	120	10	6	NA	3	0	NA	5	260

Food Serving size	Cal.	(g) Total Fat	(g) Sat. Fat	(mg) Chol.	(g) Carb.	(g) Fiber	(g) Sug.	(g) Prot.	(mg) Sod.
Pasta									
Add Chicken 1 serving	100	2	0.5	NA	0	0	NA	20	390
Add Shrimp 1 serving	80	3.5	0	NA	1	0	NA	6	460
Penne Rigate Pomodoro (Dinner) 1 serving	490	8	1	NA	97	8	NA	9	1510
Penne Rigate Pomodoro (Lunch) 1 serving	370	6	1	NA	73	6	NA	6	1130
Penne Rigate with Marinara (Dinner) 1 serving	520	10	1.5	NA	98	9	NA	9	1570
Penne Rigate with Marinara (Lunch) 1 serving	370	7	1	NA	72	6	NA	6	1080
Salads									
Caesar Salad (no croutons) 1 salad	560	54	12	NA	10	4	NA	0	820
Garden Salad (no croutons) 1 salad	220	18	3	NA	12	4	NA	3	1360

On the Border Mexican Grill & Cantina
[www.ontheborder.com]

Appetizers

Food Serving size	Cal.	(g) Total Fat	(g) Sat. Fat	(mg) Chol.	(g) Carb.	(g) Fiber	(g) Sug.	(g) Prot.	(mg) Sod.
Chile Con Queso 1 bowl	430	31	19	NA	15	1	NA	21	2090
Chile Con Queso 1 cup	270	19	12	NA	9	1	NA	13	1310
Guacamole (without Chips) 1 serving	260	23	5	NA	16	13	NA	6	480
Guacamole Live! (without Chips) 1 serving	570	50	10	NA	34	31	NA	11	2330

Food Serving size	Cal.	(g) Total Fat	(g) Sat. Fat	(mg) Chol.	(g) Carb.	(g) Fiber	(g) Sug.	(g) Prot.	(mg) Sod.
Beverages									
Coke 12 oz	136	0	0	0	35	0	33	0	15
Diet Coke 16 fl oz	0	0	0	0	0	0	0	0	20
Dr Pepper small	160	0	0	0	43	0	43	0	40

Fajita Grill
(all listed without condiments, onions or flour tortillas) Sauces: Chile Con Queso, Red Chile-Tomatillo Salsa

Food Serving size	Cal.	(g) Total Fat	(g) Sat. Fat	(mg) Chol.	(g) Carb.	(g) Fiber	(g) Sug.	(g) Prot.	(mg) Sod.
Grilled Vegetable Fajitas with Portabello Mushrooms (not classic veggies) 1 serving	230	15	1	NA	25	4	NA	4	620
Mesquite-Grilled Chicken Fajitas 1 serving	300	16	1	NA	4	0	NA	34	730
Mesquite-Grilled Steak Fajitas 1 serving	390	28	10	NA	1	0	NA	32	830
Pork Carnita Fajitas 1 serving	920	83	16	NA	3	3	NA	43	1520

Fresh Grill

Food Serving size	Cal.	(g) Total Fat	(g) Sat. Fat	(mg) Chol.	(g) Carb.	(g) Fiber	(g) Sug.	(g) Prot.	(mg) Sod.
Chicken Salsa Fresca 1 serving	520	9	3	NA	60	12	NA	50	2410
Jalapeno BBQ Salmon 1 serving	590	21	6	NA	45	24	NA	54	1220
Queso Chicken 1 serving	1030	41	14	NA	110	8	NA	57	2300
Tomatillo Chicken 1 serving	850	24	6	NA	109	7	NA	50	1850

Kids' Menu

Food Serving size	Cal.	(g) Total Fat	(g) Sat. Fat	(mg) Chol.	(g) Carb.	(g) Fiber	(g) Sug.	(g) Prot.	(mg) Sod.
Kids Chocolate Sundae 1 serving	370	18	13	NA	51	1	NA	4	95
Kids Grilled Chicken Entrée (without sides) 1 serving	90	1	0	NA	2	0	NA	17	360

Food Serving size	Cal.	(g) Total Fat	(g) Sat. Fat	(mg) Chol.	(g) Carb.	(g) Fiber	(g) Sug.	(g) Prot.	(mg) Sod.
Kids House Salad (without dressing and sides)									
1 serving	10	0	0	NA	2	1	NA	1	5
Kids Mixed Vegetables (without sides)									
1 serving	180	14	3	NA	12	3	NA	2	10
Kids Strawberry Sundae									
1 serving	330	17	13	NA	41	1	NA	3	55

Salad Dressings

Chipotle Honey Mustard Dressing									
1 serving	320	31	5	NA	12	0	NA	0	390
Fat Free Mango Citrus Vinaigrette Dressing									
1 serving	80	0	0	NA	20	0	NA	0	135
Ranch Dressing									
1 serving	230	24	4	NA	2	0	NA	1	460
Smoked Jalapeno Vinaigrette Dressing									
1 serving	250	24	4	NA	8	0	NA	0	800

Salads

House Salad (no dressing or tortilla strips)									
1 salad	200	12	4	NA	20	5	NA	6	270
Sizzling Fajita Salad (Chicken) (no dressing, tortilla strips, sour cream or onions)									
1 salad	710	47	22	NA	23	8	NA	52	1770
Sizzling Fajita Salad (Steak) (no dressing, tortilla strips, sour cream or onions)									
1 salad	780	57	29	NA	21	8	NA	50	1850

Sauce

Chile Con Queso									
1 serving	80	6	4	NA	3	0	NA	4	390

Sides/Extras

Black Beans									
1 serving	180	3	1	NA	29	10	NA	12	830
Cilantro Lime Rice									
1 serving	390	3	0	NA	83	1	NA	8	330

Food Serving size	Cal.	(g) Total Fat	(g) Sat. Fat	(mg) Chol.	(g) Carb.	(g) Fiber	(g) Sug.	(g) Prot.	(mg) Sod.
Guacamole 1 serving	50	5	1	NA	3	3	NA	1	90
Mexican Rice 1 serving	280	5	1	NA	55	1	NA	5	630
Pico de Gallo 1 serving	10	1	0	NA	1	0	NA	0	55
Refried Beans (without Blue Corn Chip) 1 serving	220	9	4	NA	25	6	NA	10	660
Sour Cream 1 serving	60	5	3	NA	2	0	NA	1	50

Tacos

Food Serving size	Cal.	(g) Total Fat	(g) Sat. Fat	(mg) Chol.	(g) Carb.	(g) Fiber	(g) Sug.	(g) Prot.	(mg) Sod.
Achiote Chicken (without sides) 1 serving	650	12	2	NA	98	6	NA	37	1690
Street-Style (Mini) (Chicken) (without sides) 1 serving	890	40	13	NA	88	8	NA	47	1990
Street-Style (Mini) (Steak) (without sides) 1 serving	980	51	21	NA	85	8	NA	48	1530

Additional Gluten-Free Menu Items
(nutritional information was not available)

Dip Trio Appetizer, Fajita Chicken Fundido (without Flour Tortilla & Rajas Mix), Grilled Mahi Mahi, Black Bean & Corn Salsa, Cilantro Lime Rice, Corn Tortilla, House (Baja) Vegetables, Mixed Cheese, Jalapeno BBQ Sauce, Ranchero Sauce, Salsa, Borderita Grande, Grande Herradura Margarita, House Margarita, Iced Tea, Mojito, Perfect Patron Beverage, Red Wine, White Wine, Sangria, Sangria Swirl Margarita, Shaken Margarita, Skinny Margarita (Fresh Lime), Skinny Margarita (Sprite), Skinny Margarita (Strawberry Lemonade)

Outback Steakhouse
[www.outback.com]

Add Ons

Food Serving size	Cal.	(g) Total Fat	(g) Sat. Fat	(mg) Chol.	(g) Carb.	(g) Fiber	(g) Sug.	(g) Prot.	(mg) Sod.
Grilled Scallops 1 serving	210	10	5	60	8	1	NA	23	2062
Grilled Shrimp 1 serving	246	16	3	9	17	2	NA	9	736

Food Serving size	Cal.	(g) Total Fat	(g) Sat. Fat	(mg) Chol.	(g) Carb.	(g) Fiber	(g) Sug.	(g) Prot.	(mg) Sod.
Lobster Tail 1 serving	324	24	14	223	2	1	NA	22	483

After Dinner Drinks

DiSaronno Amaretto 1 serving	80	0	0	NA	12	NA	NA	0	0
Grand Marnier Straight Up 1 serving	80	0	0	NA	0	NA	NA	0	0
Kahlua 1 serving	90	0	0	NA	15	NA	NA	0	0

Aussie-tizers to Share

Grilled Shrimp on the Barbie 1 serving	147	8	2	4	12	2	NA	8	433
Seared Ahi Tuna 1 serving	181	12	2	17	12	1	NA	8	1282

Burgers & Sandwiches

Aged Cheddar Bacon Burger 1 burger	1042	75	32	207	36	2	NA	57	1652
Grilled Chicken & Swiss Sandwich 1 sandwich	709	39	13	160	41	2	NA	50	1352
The Bloomin' Burger (avoid bloomin' onion petals) 1 burger	1027	71	31	187	50	4	NA	47	1766
The Outbacker Burger 1 burger	686	40	19	141	39	3	NA	41	1001

Freshly Made Sides

Dressed Baked Potato 1 potato	230	1	0	0	49	7	NA	6	668
Fresh Seasoned Mixed Veggies (request vegetables without seasoning) 1 serving	96	3	2	0	11	6	NA	3	153
Fresh Steamed Broccoli (request vegetables without seasoning) 1 serving	109	8	4	0	9	4	NA	3	211

Food Serving size	Cal.	(g) Total Fat	(g) Sat. Fat	(mg) Chol.	(g) Carb.	(g) Fiber	(g) Sug.	(g) Prot.	(mg) Sod.
Fresh Steamed Green Beans (request vegetables without seasoning)									
1 serving	55	3	1	0	6	5	NA	2	193
Garlic Mashed Potatoes									
1 serving	305	17	7	9	32	6	NA	7	1142
Grilled Asparagus									
1 serving	52	4	1	0	3	2	NA	2	226
Sweet Potato									
1 potato	318	5	1	0	63	9	NA	5	172

Irresistible Desserts

Food Serving size	Cal.	(g) Total Fat	(g) Sat. Fat	(mg) Chol.	(g) Carb.	(g) Fiber	(g) Sug.	(g) Prot.	(mg) Sod.
Chocolate Thunder From Down Under (dessert as served serves 4)									
1 serving	389	26	13	91	33	2	NA	5	140
Sydney's Sinful Sundae (dessert as served serves 2)									
1 serving	479	31	20	76	46	2	NA	5	136

Joey Menu (Just for Kids under 10)

(Aussie fries are not gluten-free. Order with vegetables without seasoning or substitute with baked potato)
(Avoid bread. Order sandwiches without the bun. Bacon, mayonnaise, ketchup, cheeses, BBQ sauce, pickles, and honey mustard are all gluten-free.)

Food Serving size	Cal.	(g) Total Fat	(g) Sat. Fat	(mg) Chol.	(g) Carb.	(g) Fiber	(g) Sug.	(g) Prot.	(mg) Sod.
Boomerang Cheese Burger									
1 serving	526	27	12	73	41	0	NA	29	787
Grilled Chicken on the Barbie									
1 serving	147	2	0	79	0	0	NA	32	340
Joey Sirloin									
1 serving	188	6	3	82	0	0	NA	32	159
Junior Ribs									
1 serving	364	26	10	89	2	0	NA	34	249
Spotted Dog Sundae (avoid Oreo cookie crumbles)									
1 serving	157	8	4	30	19	0	NA	3	81

Outback Favorites

Food Serving size	Cal.	(g) Total Fat	(g) Sat. Fat	(mg) Chol.	(g) Carb.	(g) Fiber	(g) Sug.	(g) Prot.	(mg) Sod.
Alice Springs Chicken									
1 serving	784	49	16	209	13	1	NA	76	1724
Baby Back Ribs									
1/2 order	670	43	17	149	19	0	NA	56	846

Food Serving size	Cal.	(g) Total Fat	(g) Sat. Fat	(mg) Chol.	(g) Carb.	(g) Fiber	(g) Sug.	(g) Prot.	(mg) Sod.
Baby Back Ribs full order	1156	77	30	268	23	0	NA	101	1179
Grilled Chicken on the Barbie 1 serving	305	3	0	142	10	0	NA	57	893
New Zealand Rack of Lamb 1 serving	606	39	22	162	2	0	NA	59	1055
Sweet Glazed Pork Tenderloin 1 serving	303	9	3	102	14	0	NA	42	788
Wood-Fire Grilled Pork Chop 1 serving	381	12	4	143	17	0	NA	48	1655

Perfect Combinations

Food Serving size	Cal.	(g) Total Fat	(g) Sat. Fat	(mg) Chol.	(g) Carb.	(g) Fiber	(g) Sug.	(g) Prot.	(mg) Sod.
Filet & Grilled Shrimp on the Barbie 1 serving	563	38	11	82	17	2	NA	38	1158
Filet (6 oz) & Lobster Tail (4 oz) (order with vegetables without seasoning or substitute with baked potato) 1 serving	632	43	24	329	3	1	NA	58	989
Ribs & Chicken on the Barbie (order with vegetables without seasoning or substitute with baked potato) 1 serving	554	28	10	169	13	0	NA	66	877
Sirloin (12 oz) & Grilled Shrimp on the Barbie (order with vegetables without seasoning or substitute with baked potato) 1 serving	755	42	13	178	17	2	NA	83	1188
Sirloin (6 oz) & Grilled Shrimp on the Barbie (order with vegetables without seasoning or substitute with baked potato) 1 serving	500	29	8	93	17	2	NA	46	962
Sirloin (9 oz) & Grilled Shrimp on the Barbie (order with vegetables without seasoning or substitute with baked potato) 1 serving	627	35	10	136	17	2	NA	65	1075

Salads

Food Serving size	Cal.	(g) Total Fat	(g) Sat. Fat	(mg) Chol.	(g) Carb.	(g) Fiber	(g) Sug.	(g) Prot.	(mg) Sod.
Aussie Chicken Cobb Salad 1 salad	543	29	13	125	19	3	NA	50	899
California Chicken Salad 1 salad	690	39	9	101	52	7	NA	45	1472

Food Serving size	Cal.	(g) Total Fat	(g) Sat. Fat	(mg) Chol.	(g) Carb.	(g) Fiber	(g) Sug.	(g) Prot.	(mg) Sod.
Chicken Caesar Salad 1 salad	725	42	10	215	21	6	NA	71	1537
Filet Wedge Salad 1 salad	736	59	18	108	16	2	NA	36	1400
Shrimp Caesar Salad 1 salad	571	41	11	73	34	7	NA	26	1411

Signature Side Salads

(All salad dressings are gluten-free except the mustard vinaigrette and blue cheese dressing. Be sure to request no croutons and request that salad be mixed in a separate bowl from other salads.)

Food Serving size	Cal.	(g) Total Fat	(g) Sat. Fat	(mg) Chol.	(g) Carb.	(g) Fiber	(g) Sug.	(g) Prot.	(mg) Sod.
Blue Cheese Pecan Chopped Salad (avoid Aussie Crunch) 1 salad	561	44	12	18	28	3	NA	10	1313
Caesar Salad (to have gluten-free, avoid croutons) 1 salad	342	29	8	56	14	4	NA	11	699
Classic Blue Cheese Wedge Salad (avoid blue cheese dressing) 1 salad	419	37	10	34	16	2	NA	8	978
House Salad (to have gluten-free, avoid croutons) 1 salad	171	10	5	11	15	3	NA	6	234

Signature Steaks

Food Serving size	Cal.	(g) Total Fat	(g) Sat. Fat	(mg) Chol.	(g) Carb.	(g) Fiber	(g) Sug.	(g) Prot.	(mg) Sod.
Outback Special Steak 12 oz	508	25	10	169	0	0	NA	73	452
Outback Special Steak 9 oz	381	19	7	127	0	0	NA	55	339
Outback Special Steak 6 oz	254	13	5	85	0	0	NA	37	226
Porterhouse Steak 20 oz	1009	71	31	325	4	0	NA	88	574
Prime Rib 16 oz	690	32	13	268	3	1	NA	91	2908
Prime Rib 12 oz	519	24	10	201	3	1	NA	68	2416
Prime Rib 8 oz	349	16	6	134	2	1	NA	45	1923

Food Serving size	Cal.	(g) Total Fat	(g) Sat. Fat	(mg) Chol.	(g) Carb.	(g) Fiber	(g) Sug.	(g) Prot.	(mg) Sod.
Ribeye Steak 14 oz	762	49	21	178	0	0	NA	81	567
Ribeye Steak 10 oz	544	35	15	127	0	0	NA	58	405
Victoria's Filet Steak 8 oz	301	12	5	106	0	0	NA	50	283
Victoria's Filet Steak 6 oz	218	9	4	77	0	0	NA	36	206

Straight From the Sea

Food Serving size	Cal.	Total Fat	Sat. Fat	Chol.	Carb.	Fiber	Sug.	Prot.	Sod.
Hearts of Gold Mahi (Avoid rice garnish and Lemon Pepper Butter Sauce. Order with vegetables without seasoning or substitute with baked potato) 1 serving	616	31	18	120	32	4	NA	52	1447
Lobster Tails (4 oz) (Order with vegetables without seasoning or substitute with baked potato) 1 serving	448	27	15	389	2	1	NA	44	792
Norwegian Salmon 1 serving	387	25	4	63	2	1	NA	38	295
Wood-Fire Grilled Ahi Tuna 1 serving	529	18	4	91	49	6	NA	45	3513

Additional Gluten-Free Menu Items
(nutritional information was not available)

Outback Specialty Cocktails, including Top Shelf Patron Margarita, Naturally Skinny Margarita, Rita Trio, Sauza Gold Coast Rita, New South Wales Sangria, Captain's Mai Tai, The Wallaby Darned, Sydney's Cosmo Martini.

P. F. Chang's
[www.pfchangs.com]

Dessert

Food Serving size	Cal.	Total Fat	Sat. Fat	Chol.	Carb.	Fiber	Sug.	Prot.	Sod.
Flourless Chocolate Dome 1 serving	540	36	23	NA	69	4	NA	8	260
Triple Chocolate Mousse Mini 1 serving	300	22	13	NA	25	1	NA	3	50

Food Serving size	Cal.	(g) Total Fat	(g) Sat. Fat	(mg) Chol.	(g) Carb.	(g) Fiber	(g) Sug.	(g) Prot.	(mg) Sod.
Entrées									
Beef à la Sichuan 1 serving	680	32	7	NA	54	4	NA	47	2380
Beef with Broccoli 1 serving	670	35	8	NA	33	4	NA	56	3260
Caramel Mango Chicken 1 serving	680	24	4	NA	62	4	NA	56	1920
Chang's Spicy Chicken 1 serving	830	35	6	NA	74	0	NA	59	1380
Dali Chicken 1 serving	630	25	4	NA	47	8	NA	52	1200
Ginger Chicken with Broccoli 1 serving	470	11	2	NA	38	8	NA	59	2330
Mongolian Beef 1 serving	720	39	9	NA	31	1	NA	61	2700
Moo Goo Gai Pan 1 serving	310	9	1.5	NA	18	3	NA	39	2380
Norwegian Salmon Steamed with Ginger 1 serving	830	60	9	NA	16	5	NA	58	810
Pepper Steak 1 serving	670	37	9	NA	26	3	NA	57	3000
Philip's Better Lemon Chicken 1 serving	900	35	6	NA	91	4	NA	60	260
Shrimp with Lobster Sauce 1 serving	330	16	35	NA	17	2	NA	28	2690
Kid's Menu									
Baby Budda's Feast Steamed 1 serving	60	0	0	NA	12	5	NA	4	50
Kid's Chicken Fried Rice 1 serving	580	10	2	NA	99	2	NA	26	1120

Food Serving size	Cal.	(g) Total Fat	(g) Sat. Fat	(mg) Chol.	(g) Carb.	(g) Fiber	(g) Sug.	(g) Prot.	(mg) Sod.
Noodles									
Singapore Street Noodles									
1 serving	710	13	2	NA	105	8	NA	21	1720
Rice									
Crab Fried Rice									
1 serving	1190	44	20	NA	159	6	NA	63	2340
P. F. Chang's Fried Rice (Beef)									
1 serving	1220	26	5	NA	204	6	NA	51	2380
P. F. Chang's Fried Rice (Chicken)									
1 serving	1210	22	4	NA	206	7	NA	54	2240
P. F. Chang's Fried Rice (Pork)									
1 serving	1260	29	6	NA	208	6	NA	49	2330
P. F. Chang's Fried Rice (Shrimp)									
1 serving	1120	18	3	NA	205	6	NA	41	2350
P. F. Chang's Fried Rice Combo									
1 serving	1360	33	7	NA	209	6	NA	62	2580
Sides									
Asian Tomato-Cucumber Salad (large)									
1 serving	120	3	0	NA	18	6	NA	4	340
Asian Tomato-Cucumber Salad (small)									
1 serving	60	15	0	NA	9	3	NA	2	170
Garlic Snap Peas (large)									
1 serving	200	8	1	NA	24	7	NA	7	270
Garlic Snap Peas (small)									
1 serving	100	4	0.5	NA	12	3	NA	3	135
Lemon Scented Brussels Sprouts (large)									
1 serving	420	30	16	NA	33	14	NA	12	990
Lemon Scented Brussels Sprouts (small)									
1 serving	230	17	8	NA	17	7	NA	6	950
Spinach Stir-Fried with Garlic (large)									
1 serving	160	9	15	NA	15	9	NA	12	790

Food Serving size	Cal.	(g) Total Fat	(g) Sat. Fat	(mg) Chol.	(g) Carb.	(g) Fiber	(g) Sug.	(g) Prot.	(mg) Sod.
Spinach Stir-Fried with Garlic (small) 1 serving	110	8	1	NA	8	4	NA	6	400

Soup

Egg Drop Soup (bowl) 1 bowl	290	12	2.5	NA	39	0	NA	6	2880
Egg Drop Soup (cup) 1 cup	60	2.5	0	NA	8	0	NA	1	590

Starters

Chang's Chicken Lettuce Wraps 1 serving	540	26	6	NA	43	9	NA	35	2690
Vietnamese Crab Salad 1 salad	500	10	2	NA	81	7	NA	42	2050

Vegetarian

Buddha's Feats 1 serving	140	3	0	NA	22	8	NA	8	80

Pei Wei Asian Diner
[www.peiwei.com]

Menu Item

Gluten Free Asian Chopped Chicken Salad 1 salad	230	12	1	5	12	2	7	21	800
Gluten Free Edamame 1 serving	160	7	1.5	0	9	9	0	15	490
Gluten Free Pei Wei Spicy Chicken 1 serving	530	22	3.5	35	56	5	42	27	1400
Gluten Free Pei Wei Spicy Chicken Salad 1 salad	580	27	4	30	61	5	45	22	1570
Gluten Free Pei Wei Spicy Shrimp 1 serving	400	16	2.5	25	51	4	42	10	840

Food Serving size	Cal.	(g) Total Fat	(g) Sat. Fat	(mg) Chol.	(g) Carb.	(g) Fiber	(g) Sug.	(g) Prot.	(mg) Sod.
Gluten Free Pei Wei Spicy Shrimp Salad									
1 salad	510	26	3.5	20	61	4	45	9	1120
Gluten Free Sweet & Sour Chicken									
1 serving	380	12	2	35	43	4	28	26	1150
Gluten Free Sweet & Sour Shrimp									
1 serving	240	7	1	20	39	4	28	8	590
Gluten Free Vietnamese Rolls									
1 serving	160	6	0.5	0	18	1	5	9	430

Red Lobster
[www.redlobster.com]

Desserts

Food Serving size	Cal.	Total Fat	Sat. Fat	Chol.	Carb.	Fiber	Sug.	Prot.	Sod.
New York Style Cheesecake with Strawberries									
1 slice	520	36	21	NA	39	NA	NA	NA	270
Surf's Up Sundae									
1 sundae	170	9	6	NA	20	NA	NA	2	45

Dinner Entrées

Food Serving size	Cal.	Total Fat	Sat. Fat	Chol.	Carb.	Fiber	Sug.	Prot.	Sod.
Garlic Shrimp Scampi									
1 serving	180	11	2	NA	0	NA	NA	NA	1440
Shrimp Lover's Scampi									
1 serving	130	8	1.5	NA	0	NA	NA	NA	990
Snow Crab Legs									
1/2 lb	90	1	0	NA	0	NA	NA	NA	790
Steam Snow Crab Legs									
1 serving	90	1	0	NA	0	NA	NA	NA	790

Kids' Menu

Food Serving size	Cal.	Total Fat	Sat. Fat	Chol.	Carb.	Fiber	Sug.	Prot.	Sod.
Grilled Chicken									
1 serving	150	4.5	1	NA	0	NA	NA	NA	550

Lunch Entrées

Food Serving size	Cal.	Total Fat	Sat. Fat	Chol.	Carb.	Fiber	Sug.	Prot.	Sod.
Create Your Own Lunch – Garlic Shrimp Scampi									
1 serving	180	11	2	NA	0	NA	NA	NA	1440

Food Serving size	Cal.	(g) Total Fat	(g) Sat. Fat	(mg) Chol.	(g) Carb.	(g) Fiber	(g) Sug.	(g) Prot.	(mg) Sod.
Farm-Raised Catfish – Blackened 1 serving	190	9	1.5	NA	0	NA	NA	NA	150
Garlic Shrimp Scampi 1 serving	130	8	1.5	NA	0	NA	NA	NA	990

Regional Appetizers

Buffalo Chicken Wings 1 serving	680	39	9	NA	0	NA	NA	NA	1750

Regional Dinners

North Pacific King Crab Legs 1 serving	390	3.5	1	NA	2	NA	NA	NA	3520
Snow or King Crab Legs (with roasted corn and potatoes) 1 serving	180	2	0	NA	0	NA	NA	NA	1580

Regional Kids' Menu

Snow Crab Legs 1 serving	90	1	0	NA	0	NA	NA	NA	790

Regional Lunch Entrées

Walleye – Blackened 1 serving	150	3.5	0.5	NA	5	NA	NA	NA	200

Seaside Starters

Chilled Jumbo Shrimp Cocktail 1 serving	120	0.5	0	NA	9	NA	NA	NA	580
Shrimp Nachos 1 serving	1090	64	19	NA	94	NA	NA	NA	1680

Today's Fresh Fish

Live Maine Lobster (Steamed) 1 1/4 pound	230	1.5	0	NA	0	NA	NA	NA	840

Food Serving size	Cal.	(g) Total Fat	(g) Sat. Fat	(mg) Chol.	(g) Carb.	(g) Fiber	(g) Sug.	(g) Prot.	(mg) Sod.

Red Mango

(www.redmangousa.com]

Frozen Yogurt

Amaretto Nonfat Frozen Yogurt

1/2 cup (93g)	110	0	0	0	24	0	24	2	95

Apricot Nonfat Frozen Yogurt

1/2 cup (93g)	100	0	0	0	24	0	24	2	95

Banana Nonfat Frozen Yogurt

1/2 cup (93g)	100	0	0	0	23	0	23	2	95

Black Cherry Nonfat Frozen Yogurt

1/2 cup (93g)	80	0	0	0	18	0	18	2	105

Black Currant Nonfat Frozen Yogurt

1/2 cup (93g)	100	0	0	0	24	0	24	2	95

Blackberry Nonfat Frozen Yogurt

1/2 cup (93g)	100	0	0	0	24	0	24	2	90

Blueberry Nonfat Frozen Yogurt

1/2 cup (93g)	100	0	0	0	23	0	23	2	90

Caribbean Coconut Nonfat Frozen Yogurt

1/2 cup (93g)	100	0	0	0	24	0	24	2	90

Chai Nonfat Frozen Yogurt

1/2 cup (93g)	90	0	0	0	21	0	21	2	95

Cinnamon Nonfat Frozen Yogurt

1/2 cup (93g)	100	0	0	0	22	0	22	2	95

Cocoa Nonfat Frozen Yogurt

1/2 cup (93g)	100	0	0	0	23	0	22	2	95

Dark Chocolate Frozen Yogurt

1/2 cup (93g)	100	0.5	0	0	24	<1	23	2	110

Dulce de Leche Frozen Yogurt

1/2 cup (93g)	80	0	0	0	18	0	18	2	110

Espresso Nonfat Frozen Yogurt

1/2 cup (93g)	100	0	0	0	23	0	22	2	95

Ginger Nonfat Frozen Yogurt

1/2 cup (93g)	90	0	0	0	21	0	21	2	95

Food Serving size	Cal.	(g) Total Fat	(g) Sat. Fat	(mg) Chol.	(g) Carb.	(g) Fiber	(g) Sug.	(g) Prot.	(mg) Sod.
Golden Peach Nonfat Frozen Yogurt									
1/2 cup (93g)	100	0	0	0	24	0	23	2	90
Green Tea (Sencha) Nonfat Frozen Yogurt									
1/2 cup (93g)	80	0	0	0	18	0	18	2	105
Hazelnut Nonfat Frozen Yogurt									
1/2 cup (93g)	100	0	0	0	23	0	23	2	95
Irish Cream Nonfat Frozen Yogurt									
1/2 cup (93g)	100	0	0	0	24	0	16	2	95
Key Lime Pie Nonfat Frozen Yogurt									
1/2 cup (93g)	80	0	0	0	18	0	18	2	105
Lemon Spritzer Nonfat Frozen Yogurt									
1/2 cup (93g)	80	0	0	0	18	0	18	2	105
Madagascar Vanilla Nonfat Frozen Yogurt									
1/2 cup (93g)	80	0	0	0	18	0	18	2	105
Mandarin Orange Nonfat Frozen Yogurt									
1/2 cup (93g)	100	0	0	0	23	0	23	2	95
Mojito Nonfat Frozen Yogurt									
1/2 cup (93g)	100	0	0	0	23	0	23	2	95
Original Nonfat Frozen Yogurt									
1/2 cup (93g)	80	0	0	0	19	0	19	2	110
Peppermint Dark Chocolate Frozen Yogurt									
1/2 cup (93g)	100	0.5	0	0	24	<1	23	2	110
Peppermint Nonfat Frozen Yogurt									
1/2 cup (93g)	100	0	0	0	23	0	22	2	95
Pineapple Nonfat Frozen Yogurt									
1/2 cup (93g)	80	0	0	0	18	0	18	2	105
Pomegranate by POM Wonderful Frozen Yogurt									
1/2 cup (93g)	90	0	0	0	21	0	20	2	100
Pumpkin Spice Nonfat Frozen Yogurt (seasonal)									
1/2 cup (93g)	80	0	0	0	18	0	18	2	105
Raspberry Cheesecake Nonfat Frozen Yogurt									
1/2 cup (93g)	80	0	0	0	19	0	19	2	110
Raspberry Nonfat Frozen Yogurt									
1/2 cup (93g)	100	0	0	0	24	0	24	2	90

Food Serving size	Cal.	(g) Total Fat	(g) Sat. Fat	(mg) Chol.	(g) Carb.	(g) Fiber	(g) Sug.	(g) Prot.	(mg) Sod.
Sonoma Strawberry Nonfat Frozen Yogurt									
1/2 cup (93g)	100	0	0	0	24	0	23	3	95
Summer Melon Nonfat Frozen Yogurt									
1/2 cup (93g)	80	0	0	0	19	0	18	2	105
Tangomonium Nonfat Frozen Yogurt									
1/2 cup (93g)	80	0	0	0	18	0	18	2	105
White Peach Nonfat Frozen Yogurt									
1/2 cup (93g)	100	0	0	0	23	0	23	2	90
Wild Raspberry Nonfat Frozen Yogurt									
1/2 cup (93g)	100	0	0	0	24	0	24	2	90
Winter Caramel Nonfat Frozen Yogurt									
1/2 cup (93g)	100	0	0	0	24	0	24	2	90

Hot Chocolate Chiller

Food Serving size	Cal.	(g) Total Fat	(g) Sat. Fat	(mg) Chol.	(g) Carb.	(g) Fiber	(g) Sug.	(g) Prot.	(mg) Sod.
Dark Chocolate (Large)									
20 oz	410	2.5	1.5	<5	97	4	89	9	420
Dark Chocolate (Regular)									
16 oz	260	1.5	1	<5	60	3	55	6	260
Dark Chocolate + Banana (Large)									
20 oz	420	1.5	0.5	<5	99	4	87	7	340
Dark Chocolate + Banana (Regular)									
16 oz	270	1	0	<5	64	3	55	5	220
Dark Chocolate + Peppermint (Large)									
20 oz	430	2.5	1.5	<5	100	5	92	9	430
Dark Chocolate + Peppermint (Regular)									
16 oz	260	1.5	1	<5	62	3	57	6	260
Dark Chocolate + Strawberries (Large)									
20 oz	370	1.5	0.5	<5	86	4	80	7	340
Dark Chocolate + Strawberries (Regular)									
16 oz	230	1	0	<5	55	2	51	4	220
Dark Chocolate + Strawberries + Banana (Large)									
20 oz	420	2	0.5	<5	99	5	88	8	340
Dark Chocolate + Strawberries + Banana (Regular)									
16 oz	270	1	0	<5	64	3	56	5	220

Food Serving size	Cal.	(g) Total Fat	(g) Sat. Fat	(mg) Chol.	(g) Carb.	(g) Fiber	(g) Sug.	(g) Prot.	(mg) Sod.
Parfaits									
Key Lime Pie Frozen Yogurt Parfait (Regular)									
16 oz	310	5	0	0	63	5	42	6	180
Mixed Berry Frozen Yogurt Parfait (Regular)									
16 oz	280	4.5	0	0	57	5	38	6	150
Tropical Frozen Yogurt Parfait (Regular)									
16 oz	320	4.5	0	0	67	5	47	6	150
Smoothies									
4 Berry Blend Smoothie (Large)									
20 oz	280	1	0	<5	65	6	58	6	260
4 Berry Blend Smoothie (Regular)									
16 oz	200	0.5	0	<5	46	4	41	4	190
Acai Berry Smoothie (Large)									
20 oz	420	2.5	0.5	<5	95	2	92	5	230
Acai Berry Smoothie (Regular)									
16 oz	280	2	0	0	63	1	62	3	160
Antioxidants Smoothie (Large)									
20 oz	420	1	0	<5	98	<1	92	5	270
Antioxidants Smoothie (Regular)									
16 oz	290	0.5	0	<5	67	0	63	3	190
Berry Banana Smoothie (Large)									
20 oz	300	0.5	0	<5	69	3	61	6	260
Berry Banana Smoothie (Regular)									
16 oz	210	0.5	0	<5	49	2	43	4	190
Healthy Bones Smoothie (Large)									
20 oz	300	0	0	<5	70	3	64	5	260
Healthy Bones Smoothie (Regular)									
16 oz	210	0	0	<5	49	2	45	4	190
Mandarin Mango Smoothie (Large)									
20 oz	330	0.5	0	<5	78	3	72	6	270
Mandarin Mango Smoothie (Regular)									
16 oz	230	0	0	<5	55	2	51	4	190

Food Serving size	Cal.	(g) Total Fat	(g) Sat. Fat	(mg) Chol.	(g) Carb.	(g) Fiber	(g) Sug.	(g) Prot.	(mg) Sod.
Pomegranate by POM Wonderful Smoothie (Large)									
20 oz	380	0	0	<5	91	<1	83	5	270
Pomegranate by POM Wonderful Smoothie (Regular)									
16 oz	260	0	0	<5	62	0	57	3	190
Protein Power Smoothie (Large)									
20 oz	530	8	1	<5	95	8	65	21	360
Protein Power Smoothie (Regular)									
16 oz	380	5	0.5	<5	67	5	47	18	280
Revitalizing Energy Smoothie (Large)									
20 oz	290	0.5	0	<5	68	4	62	6	260
Revitalizing Energy Smoothie (Regular)									
16 oz	210	0.5	0	<5	48	3	44	4	190
Strawberry Banana Smoothie (Large)									
20 oz	300	0.5	0	<5	69	4	61	6	260
Strawberry Banana Smoothie (Regular)									
16 oz	210	0.5	0	<5	49	3	43	4	190
Tropical Mango Smoothie (Large)									
20 oz	330	0.5	0	<5	76	3	71	5	260
Tropical Mango Smoothie (Regular)									
16 oz	220	0	0	<5	53	2	49	4	190
Tropical Pineapple Smoothie (Large)									
20 oz	340	0.5	0	0	81	4	71	6	260
Tropical Pineapple Smoothie (Regular)									
16 oz	240	0	0	0	57	2	50	4	190

Red Robin
[www.redrobin.com]

Appetizers

Garden Fresh Hummus Plate (minus garlic bread)									
1 appetizer	444	29	NA	NA	38	12	5	14	1605

Available Sides (Adults & Kids)

Celery sticks									
1 serving	14	0	NA	NA	3	1	1	1	70

Food Serving size	Cal.	(g) Total Fat	(g) Sat. Fat	(mg) Chol.	(g) Carb.	(g) Fiber	(g) Sug.	(g) Prot.	(mg) Sod.
Freckled Fruit Salad 1 serving	97	0	NA	NA	28	3	24	1	2
Guacamole 1 serving	74	7	NA	NA	5	3	1	1	197
House Salad (no croutons) 1 serving	85	5	NA	NA	6	2	3	5	113
Mandarin oranges 1 serving	43	0	NA	NA	11	1	9	1	6
Salsa 1 serving	30	0	NA	NA	6	2	3	1	700
Steamed veggies 1 serving	32	0	NA	NA	6	3	0	3	31
Sweet Potatoes 1 serving	569	29	NA	NA	70	9	24	6	846

Chicken Burgers & Other Favorites

Bruschetta Chicken Sandwich (no ciabatta bun, no tomato-bruschetta salsa) 1 sandwich	347	21	NA	NA	2	0	0	35	710
California Chicken Sandwich (no sesame bun) 1 sandwich	491	33	NA	NA	5	1	2	40	1245
Grilled Turkey Burger (no chipotle mayo, no whole grain bun) 1 burger	262	19	NA	NA	3	0	2	20	349
Simply Grilled Chicken Sandwich (no sesame bun) 1 sandwich	159	3	NA	NA	4	0	2	29	513

Entrée

Ensenada Chicken Platter 2pcs (no tortilla strips, no ancho marinade, no baja ranch dressing) 1 platter	341	7	NA	NA	7	1	3	60	911

Fire-Grilled Burgers*

(No bun. Substitute a lettuce wedge instead or lettuce wrap your burger) *Refer to sides for available side options

Guacamole Bacon Burger (No bun. Substitute a lettuce wedge instead or lettuce wrap your burger) 1 burger	573	43	NA	NA	7	1	3	38	489
Keep It Simple Burger 1 burger	319	20	NA	NA	4	0	2	29	511

Food Serving size	Cal.	(g) Total Fat	(g) Sat. Fat	(mg) Chol.	(g) Carb.	(g) Fiber	(g) Sug.	(g) Prot.	(mg) Sod.
Red's Tavern Double									
(No bun. Substitute a lettuce wedge instead or lettuce wrap your burger) *Refer to sides for available side options									
1 burger	449	34	NA	NA	3	0	1	32	826
Royal Red Robin Burger (No bun. Substitute a lettuce wedge instead or lettuce wrap your burger)									
1 burger	942	80	NA	NA	5	0	1	51	1618
RR Bacon Cheeseburger (No bun. Substitute a lettuce wedge instead or lettuce wrap your burger)									
1 burger	749	62	NA	NA	3	0	2	41	1272
RR Gourmet Cheeseburger (No bun. Substitute a lettuce wedge instead or lettuce wrap your burger)									
1 burger	563	41	NA	NA	13	0	9	35	1246

Kid's Menu

(No bun. Substitute a lettuce wedge instead or lettuce wrap your burger)

Food Serving size	Cal.	Total Fat	Sat. Fat	Chol.	Carb.	Fiber	Sug.	Prot.	Sod.
Chick-on-a-Stick (no teriyaki sauce or ranch dressing)									
1 stick	141	3	NA	NA	0	0	0	29	250
Rad Burger (Beef Patty)									
1 burger	136	9	NA	NA	0	0	0	13	121
Rad Burger (Turkey Patty)									
1 patty	253	19	NA	NA	1	0	0	20	345

Salad Dressings

Food Serving size	Cal.	Total Fat	Sat. Fat	Chol.	Carb.	Fiber	Sug.	Prot.	Sod.
Balsamic Vinaigrette									
84g	180	15	NA	NA	9	0	NA	0	NA
Bleu Cheese Dressing									
2 oz	320	36	NA	0	0	0	0	2	520
Creamy Caesar Dressing									
84g	438	44	NA	NA	3	0	NA	3	NA
Honey Mustard Poppyseed Dressing									
89g	390	36	NA	NA	21	0	NA	0	NA

Salads

(Acceptable dressings for gluten-free diets are Balsamic Vinaigrette, Bleu Cheese, Creamy Caesar and Honey Mustard Poppyseed. Please verify with the manager since dressing may vary from restaurant location and geographic area.)

Food Serving size	Cal.	Total Fat	Sat. Fat	Chol.	Carb.	Fiber	Sug.	Prot.	Sod.
Avo-Cobb-O (no bleu cheese crumbles or garlic bread)									
1 salad	448	22	NA	NA	17	9	7	43	777

Food Serving size	Cal.	(g) Total Fat	(g) Sat. Fat	(mg) Chol.	(g) Carb.	(g) Fiber	(g) Sug.	(g) Prot.	(mg) Sod.
Crispy Chicken Tender Salad									
(no fried chicken tenders. Use grilled chicken as a substitute. No garlic bread)									
1 salad	846	58	NA	NA	33	5	25	49	1351
House Salad (no croutons)									
1 salad	115	6	NA	NA	10	2	3	6	195
Side Caesar Salad (no croutons or garlic bread)									
1 salad	196	17	NA	NA	6	2	1	4	299
Simply Grilled Chicken Salad (no croutons or garlic bread)									
1 salad	311	12	NA	NA	12	6	7	40	478

Romano's Macaroni Grill ▬▬▬▬

[www.macaronigrill.com]

Classics

Carmela's Chicken (with gluten-free penne)									
1 serving	460	16	6	NA	56	4	NA	22	770
Fettucine Alfredo (with gluten-free penne)									
1 serving	1180	73	41	NA	91	6	NA	46	2000
Pasta Milano (with gluten-free penne)									
1 serving	1010	42	15	NA	111	7	NA	47	1660
Penne Rustica (with gluten-free penne)									
1 serving	1160	49	18	NA	110	7	NA	72	2490
Shrimp Portofino (with gluten-free penne, without breadcrumbs)									
1 serving	900	60	24	NA	57	6	NA	36	760

Combinations

Caesar Salad (without croutons)									
1 salad	420	39	8	NA	11	4	NA	7	740
Capellini Pomodoro (with gluten-free penne)									
1 serving	340	11	1	NA	55	6	NA	7	760
Carmela's Chicken (with gluten-free penne)									
1 serving	460	15	6	NA	56	4	NA	22	770
Fresh Greens Salad (without croutons)									
1 salad	110	8	1	NA	9	1	NA	2	120

Food Serving size	Cal.	(g) Total Fat	(g) Sat. Fat	(mg) Chol.	(g) Carb.	(g) Fiber	(g) Sug.	(g) Prot.	(mg) Sod.
Lentil Soup 1 serving	440	12	4	NA	28	11	NA	15	790
Pomodorina Soup (without crostini) 1 serving	190	12	3	NA	16	4	NA	4	820

Create Your Own Pasta

Food Serving size	Cal.	(g) Total Fat	(g) Sat. Fat	(mg) Chol.	(g) Carb.	(g) Fiber	(g) Sug.	(g) Prot.	(mg) Sod.
Alfredo Sauce 1 serving	880	79	41	NA	14	0	NA	34	1550
Arrabbiata Sauce 1 serving	230	11	1.5	NA	21	4	NA	5	820
Artichokes 1 serving	15	0	0	NA	4	2	NA	1	15
Asparagus 1 serving	5	0	0	NA	1	1	NA	1	0
Broccolini 1 serving	10	0	0	NA	2	0	NA	1	10
Cannellini Beans 1 serving	15	0	0	NA	3	1	NA	1	55
Carmelized Onions 1 serving	25	1.5	0.5	NA	2	0	NA	0	115
Fresh Spinach 1 serving	5	0	0	NA	1	1	NA	1	20
Garlic Cream Sauce 1 serving	270	20	12	NA	14	2	NA	8	930
Garlic Olive Oil 1 serving	510	54	8	NA	5	0	NA	1	260
Gluten-Free Penne 1 serving	400	2	0	NA	91	2	NA	6	350
Italian Sausage 1 serving	430	39	10	NA	2	1	NA	17	740
Pancetta 1 serving	400	37	12	NA	2	1	NA	14	1530
Pomodoro Sauce 1 serving	190	10	1	NA	15	4	NA	4	860

Food Serving size	Cal.	(g) Total Fat	(g) Sat. Fat	(mg) Chol.	(g) Carb.	(g) Fiber	(g) Sug.	(g) Prot.	(mg) Sod.
Roasted Chicken 1 serving	290	16	1.5	NA	3	0	NA	31	560
Roasted Garlic 1 serving	40	0.5	0	NA	8	0	NA	1	35
Roasted Mushrooms 1 serving	25	2	0	NA	1	0	NA	1	40
Roasted Peppers 1 serving	5	0	0	NA	2	0	NA	0	65
Roasted Tomatoes 1 serving	15	1	0	NA	1	0	NA	0	80
Shrimp 1 serving	180	15	1	NA	0	0	NA	13	360
Snap Peas 1 serving	10	0	0	NA	2	1	NA	1	0
Sun-Dried Tomatoes 1 serving	20	2	0	NA	1	0	NA	0	10

Dolce

Food Serving size	Cal.	(g) Total Fat	(g) Sat. Fat	(mg) Chol.	(g) Carb.	(g) Fiber	(g) Sug.	(g) Prot.	(mg) Sod.
Gelato: Dark Chocolate (without biscotti) 1 serving	260	12	8	NA	36	3	NA	2	40
Gelato: Double Vanilla (without biscotti) 1 serving	290	12	9	NA	40	0	NA	6	40
Sorbet: White Peach 1 serving	160	0	0	NA	39	0	NA	0	0

Fresh Pasta

Food Serving size	Cal.	(g) Total Fat	(g) Sat. Fat	(mg) Chol.	(g) Carb.	(g) Fiber	(g) Sug.	(g) Prot.	(mg) Sod.
Carbonara (with gluten-free penne) 1 serving	1260	68	29	NA	101	4	NA	62	3640
Pasta di Mare (with gluten-free penne) 1 serving	1310	57	16	NA	118	7	NA	11	1900

Kids' Menu

Food Serving size	Cal.	(g) Total Fat	(g) Sat. Fat	(mg) Chol.	(g) Carb.	(g) Fiber	(g) Sug.	(g) Prot.	(mg) Sod.
Fettuccine Alfredo (with gluten-free penne) 1 serving	550	32	17	NA	45	3	NA	24	1030

Food Serving size	Cal.	(g) Total Fat	(g) Sat. Fat	(mg) Chol.	(g) Carb.	(g) Fiber	(g) Sug.	(g) Prot.	(mg) Sod.
Grilled Chicken & Broccolini (with gluten-free penne)									
1 serving	350	6	1	NA	43	5	NA	30	840
Mac & Cheese (with gluten-free penne)									
1 serving	630	29	16	NA	66	4	NA	27	1540
Broccolini									
1 serving	10	0	0	NA	2	0	NA	1	10
Spaghetti & Pomodoro Sauce (with gluten-free penne)									
1 serving	310	9	1.5	NA	46	5	NA	8	670

Pantry

Food Serving size	Cal.	(g) Total Fat	(g) Sat. Fat	(mg) Chol.	(g) Carb.	(g) Fiber	(g) Sug.	(g) Prot.	(mg) Sod.
Bibb & Blue (without crispy onion)									
1 serving	680	56	14	NA	23	4	NA	22	2020
Caesar Salad (without croutons & breadstick)									
1 salad	420	39	8	NA	11	4	NA	7	740
Caprese Salad									
1 salad	480	40	15	NA	10	2	NA	17	740
Fresh Greens Salad (without croutons)									
1 salad	110	8	1	NA	9	1	NA	2	120
Market Chop (without breadstick)									
1 salad	480	37	10	NA	11	4	NA	26	1200
Warm Spinach & Shrimp Salad									
1 salad	440	26.5	5	NA	18	6	NA	34	1600

Principale

Food Serving size	Cal.	(g) Total Fat	(g) Sat. Fat	(mg) Chol.	(g) Carb.	(g) Fiber	(g) Sug.	(g) Prot.	(mg) Sod.
Chicken Under a Brick (without potatoes)									
1 serving	1440	115	23	NA	24	3	NA	76	3640
Grilled Chicken Spiedini (without vegetables)									
1 serving	410	11	2	NA	38	10	NA	39	990
Grilled King Salmon (without orzo)									
1 serving	1110	68	25	NA	71	4	NA	54	1220
Grilled Shrimp Spiedini (without vegetables)									
1 serving	380	9	1.5	NA	41	9	NA	31	1830
Pan-Roasted Pork Chop (without risotto)									
1 serving	1370	91	39	NA	58	7	NA	76	1900

Food Serving size	Cal.	(g) Total Fat	(g) Sat. Fat	(mg) Chol.	(g) Carb.	(g) Fiber	(g) Sug.	(g) Prot.	(mg) Sod.
Pollo Caprese (with gluten-free penne) 1 serving	560	22	7	NA	31	5	NA	60	1530

Salad Dressings

Balsamic Vinaigrette 2 tbsp	100	9	1.5	NA	4	0	4	0	340
Caesar Dressing 2 tbsp	160	17	2.5	30	1	0	0	1	240
Mediterranean Vinaigrette Dressing 2 tbsp	90	9	1	0	2	1	2	0	350
Parmesan Peppercorn Ranch Dressing 2 oz	321	30	5	19	4	0	2	2	586

Sides

Bibb & Blue (without crispy onions) 1 serving	680	56	14	NA	23	4	NA	22	2020
Caesar Salad (without croutons) 1 serving	160	13	3	NA	8	2	NA	3	330
Fresh Greens Salad (without croutons) 1 serving	110	8	1	NA	9	1	NA	2	120
Grilled Asparagus 1 serving	30	1	NA	NA	4	2	NA	2	590
Spinach Garlic 1 serving	35	1	0	0	5	3	1	3	105

Soups

Lentil Soup 1 serving	440	12	4	NA	28	11	NA	15	790
Pomodorina Soup (without crostini) 1 serving	190	12	3	NA	16	4	NA	4	820

Tapas & Antipasto

Baked Prosciutto & Mozzarella (without bread) 1 serving	800	46	21	NA	53	3	NA	42	1990

Food Serving size	Cal.	(g) Total Fat	(g) Sat. Fat	(mg) Chol.	(g) Carb.	(g) Fiber	(g) Sug.	(g) Prot.	(mg) Sod.
Mediterranean Olives (without bread)									
1 serving	150	16	3	NA	4	3	NA	1	910

Additional Gluten-Free Menu Items
(nutritional information was not available)

Crisp Salad (without croutons)

Rubio's Fresh Mexican Grill ▬▬▬▬
[www.rubios.com]

Chips & Tortilla

Chips (Large)									
	570	29	2.5	0	74	9	0	7	650
Chips (Regular)									
	260	13	1	0	33	4	0	3	290

Dressings, Salsas & Sauces

Chipotle Ranch Dressing									
1 oz	110	11	2	5	1	0	1	0	180
Light Balsamic Vinaigrette Dressing									
1 oz	45	3	1	0	4	0	4	0	190

Menu Item

Balsamic & Roasted Veggie Salad (with dressing)									
14.4 oz	310	11	3.5	40	29	7	14	20	950
Blackened Ono Taco									
1 taco	149	10	1.5	20	26	4	1	12	360
Chipotle Orange Shrimp Salad									
332g	380	21	3.5	110	33	5	12	16	1120
Chipotle Ranch Salad									
(with dressing) (Choose blackened or grilled salmon or mahi machi or grilled steak, or request without chicken)									
1 salad	450	31	6	50	22	8	8	20	1220
Chopped Salad									
(with dressing) (Substitute grilled chicken with chile-lime salmon, grilled ono)									
1 salad	460	24	6	70	36	10	10	28	1250

Food Serving size	Cal.	(g) Total Fat	(g) Sat. Fat	(mg) Chol.	(g) Carb.	(g) Fiber	(g) Sug.	(g) Prot.	(mg) Sod.
Classic Grilled Steak Taco 1 taco	143	8	3	30	22	4	2	12	340
Grilled Chile-Lime Wild Salmon Taco 1 taco	149	9	1.5	25	25	4	2	13	190
Grilled Gourmet Taco (with Garlic Herb Shrimp) 1 taco	163	19	7	80	23	4	2	19	570
Grilled Gourmet Taco (with Steak) 1 taco	163	19	7	55	24	3	2	19	610
Grilled Grande Bowl (with dressing) 1 salad	630	27	8	80	62	10	9	34	1490
Grilled Ono Taco 1 taco	149	8	1.5	20	26	4	2	13	240
Rubio's Street Tacos (Carnitas) 1 taco	67	4	1	20	8	2	1	7	160
Rubio's Street Tacos (Steak) 1 taco	70	4	1	20	9	2	1	8	190
Salsa Verde Pan-Seared Shrimp Taco (Request the taco on a corn tortilla.) 1 taco	141	13	3.5	60	22	4	1	12	310
Side Salad 1 salad	145	3	1	0	12	2	7	3	380

Others

Black Beans (Large)	280	1	0	0	50	7	7	17	950
Black Beans (Regular)	100	1	0	0	17	2	2	6	340
Pinto Beans (Large) 343g	300	3	NA	0	65	24	1	5	940
Pinto Beans (Regular) 116g	110	2	0.5	0	22	8	0	2	340

Additional Gluten-Free Menu Items
(nutritional information was not available)

Wild Planet Tuna Salad, Creamy Chipotle Sauce, Creamy Wasabi Sauce, Fire-Roasted Corn Sauce, Habanero Citrus Salsa, Mild Salsa, Picante Salsa, Roasted Chipotle Salsa, Salsa Fresca, Salsa Verde,

Food Serving size	Cal.	(g) Total Fat	(g) Sat. Fat	(mg) Chol.	(g) Carb.	(g) Fiber	(g) Sug.	(g) Prot.	(mg) Sod.

Sesame Soy Sauce, Tomatillo Salsa, White Sauce, Corn Tortilla, Applesauce, Bacon, Carnitas, Cheese, Chicken Tortilla Soup Broth, Cilantro/Onion, Green Cabbage, Guacamole, Jalapenos, Mexican Rice, Red & Green Cabbage, Sour Cream, and Spring Mix

Ruby Tuesday
[www.rubytuesday.com]

Brunch

Food	Cal.	Total Fat	Sat. Fat	Chol.	Carb.	Fiber	Sug.	Prot.	Sod.
Berry Good Yogurt Parfait (no granola, no Garlic Cheese Biscuits, and no brunch potatoes)	162	3	NA	NA	28	1	NA	5	127
Mini Benedicts – Steak (no Garlic Cheese Biscuits, no brunch potatoes, no bun)	934	54	NA	NA	72	7	NA	40	1447
Steak & Eggs	1100	39	NA	NA	7	2	NA	72	1241
Western Omelet	1381	65	NA	NA	18	1	NA	55	2172

Desserts

Food	Cal.	Total Fat	Sat. Fat	Chol.	Carb.	Fiber	Sug.	Prot.	Sod.
Berry Good Yogurt Parfait (no granola)	162	3	NA	NA	28	1	NA	5	127

Fork-Tender Ribs

Food	Cal.	Total Fat	Sat. Fat	Chol.	Carb.	Fiber	Sug.	Prot.	Sod.
Jumbo Skewered Shrimp Add-On (No Garlic Cheese Biscuits, no Louisiana Fried Shrimp add-on) 1 skewer	81	6	NA	NA	0	0	NA	6	348
Jumbo Skewered Shrimp Add-On (No Garlic Cheese Biscuits, no Louisiana Fried Shrimp add-on) 2 skewers	161	13	NA	NA	0	0	NA	12	695
Memphis Dry Rub Baby-Back Ribs (No Garlic Cheese Biscuits, no Louisiana Fried Shrimp add-on) full rack	460	29	NA	NA	6	0	NA	44	150

Fresh All-Natural Chicken

Food	Cal.	Total Fat	Sat. Fat	Chol.	Carb.	Fiber	Sug.	Prot.	Sod.
Barbecue Grilled Chicken (No Garlic Cheese Biscuits and no Boston barbecue sauce)	250	4	NA	NA	14	1	NA	40	500

Food Serving size	Cal.	Total Fat (g)	Sat. Fat (g)	Chol. (mg)	Carb. (g)	Fiber (g)	Sug. (g)	Prot. (g)	Sod. (mg)
Chicken Bella (No Garlic Cheese Biscuits and no parmesan cream sauce)	360	17	NA	NA	6	3	NA	46	775
Chicken Fresco (No Garlic Cheese Biscuits and no lemon-butter sauce)	352	19	NA	NA	8	0	NA	41	739
Chicken Three Ways (No Garlic Cheese Biscuits, no lemon-butter sauce on the Chicken Fresco, no Parmesan cream sauce on the Chicken Bella, no brown-rice pilaf)	979	40	NA	NA	84	8	NA	74	2983

Fresh Handcrafted Burgers

Food Serving size	Cal.	Total Fat (g)	Sat. Fat (g)	Chol. (mg)	Carb. (g)	Fiber (g)	Sug. (g)	Prot. (g)	Sod. (mg)
Alpine Swiss Burger (No Garlic Cheese Biscuits, no bun, no french fries)	1017	65	NA	NA	60	6	NA	50	1246
Avocado Grilled Chicken Sandwich	891	47	NA	NA	54	5	NA	64	1185
Avocado Turkey Burger	968	61	NA	NA	57	5	NA	50	1601
Bacon Cheeseburger (No Garlic Cheese Biscuits, no bun, no french fries)	1007	67	NA	NA	58	4	NA	49	1426
Boston Blue Burger (no Garlic Cheese Biscuits, no bun, no french fries, no onion rings, no Boston barbecue sauce)	1165	72	NA	NA	82	6	NA	51	1913
Classic Cheeseburger (No Garlic Cheese Biscuits, no bun, no french fries)	947	61	NA	NA	58	4	NA	46	1216
Ruby's Classic Burger (No Garlic Cheese Biscuits, no bun, no french fries)	877	55	NA	NA	57	4	NA	42	976
Smokehouse Burger (no Garlic Cheese Biscuits, no bun, no french fries, no onion rings, no barbecue sauce)	1175	73	NA	NA	82	4	NA	51	1749
Triple Prime Bacon Cheddar Burger	1136	82	NA	NA	47	4	NA	54	1247
Triple Prime Burger	916	63	NA	NA	47	4	NA	41	757
Triple Prime Cheddar Burger	1076	77	NA	NA	47	4	NA	51	1037
Turkey Burger	801	48	NA	NA	56	4	NA	41	1349

Food Serving size	Cal.	(g) Total Fat	(g) Sat. Fat	(mg) Chol.	(g) Carb.	(g) Fiber	(g) Sug.	(g) Prot.	(mg) Sod.
Fresh, Fresh, Sides									
Diced Apples (kids' menu)	59	0	NA	NA	16	3	NA	0	1
Fresh Baked Potato	259	2	NA	NA	52	10	NA	9	103
Fresh Grilled Asparagus	78	5	NA	NA	5	3	NA	3	218
Fresh Grilled Green Beans	45	2	NA	NA	5	2	NA	2	145
Fresh Grilled Zucchini	41	2	NA	NA	4	1	NA	1	321
Fresh Steamed Broccoli	53	2	NA	NA	7	3	NA	3	82
Grapes (kids' menu)	27	0	NA	NA	7	0	NA	0	0
Loaded Baked Potato	568	28	NA	NA	54	10	NA	19	536
Roasted Spaghetti Squash	54	3	NA	NA	6	2	NA	1	69
Sliced Tomatoes with Balsamic Vinaigrette	52	1	NA	NA	15	0	NA	2	293
Sugar Snap Peas	113	6	NA	NA	8	3	NA	3	164
White Cheddar Mashed Potatoes	223	14	NA	NA	21	2	NA	3	430

Garden Fresh Salads

(no croutons or Garlic Cheese Biscuits.) *Gluten/Wheat Free Dressings: Thousand Island, Balsamic Vinaigrette, Zesty Italian, Ranch, Lite Ranch, Blue Cheese, Honey Mustard, Olive Oil & Vinegar) *You may include gluten/wheat free toppings: sliced tomatoes, edamame, green peas, diced eggs, shredded cheddar cheese, Parmesan cheese, bacon bits, diced ham, black olives, sunflower seeds.

Food Serving size	Cal.	(g) Total Fat	(g) Sat. Fat	(mg) Chol.	(g) Carb.	(g) Fiber	(g) Sug.	(g) Prot.	(mg) Sod.
Grilled Chicken Salad (no croutons)	1066	90	NA	NA	28	2	NA	25	2318
Phillipsburg Broccoli Salad	786	28	NA	NA	48	7	NA	24	1057

Food Serving size	Cal.	(g) Total Fat	(g) Sat. Fat	(mg) Chol.	(g) Carb.	(g) Fiber	(g) Sug.	(g) Prot.	(mg) Sod.
Kids' Brunch									
Eggscellent Combo (No Garlic Cheese Biscuits, no brunch potatoes)	541	35	NA	NA	33	4	NA	24	999
Kids' Menu									
Beef Mini Burgers (No Garlic Cheese Bisuits and no bun)	779	46	NA	NA	58	6	NA	33	1037
Chop Steak (No Garlic Cheese Bisuits)	464	33	NA	NA	18	4	NA	25	417
Grilled Chicken (No Garlic Cheese Bisuits)	259	10	NA	NA	18	4	NA	25	407
Pasta Classics									
Spaghetti Squash Marinara (order without Garlic Cheese Biscuits)	257	12	NA	NA	29	9	NA	7	836
Petite Lunch Plates									
Chicken Fresco (no Garlic Cheese Biscuits or lemon-butter sauce)	374	21	NA	NA	24	4	NA	25	843
Creole Catch	284	14	NA	NA	18	4	NA	25	397
Grilled Chicken Salad (no Garlic Cheese Biscuits or croutons)	372	10	NA	NA	23	4	NA	9	346
Jumbo Shrimp Scampi (no Garlic Cheese Biscuits)	279	16	NA	NA	18	4	NA	17	944
Sliced Sirloin	398	21	NA	NA	20	4	NA	32	657
Spaghetti Squash Marinara (no Garlic Cheese Biscuits)	177	9	NA	NA	17	5	NA	5	667
Premium Seafood									
Creole Catch (no Garlic Cheese Biscuits)	240	10	NA	NA	0	0	NA	40	200
Jumbo Skewered Shrimp (no Garlic Cheese Biscuits)	242	19	NA	NA	0	0	NA	18	1043

Food Serving size	Cal.	(g) Total Fat	(g) Sat. Fat	(mg) Chol.	(g) Carb.	(g) Fiber	(g) Sug.	(g) Prot.	(mg) Sod.
New Orleans Seafood (no Garlic Cheese Biscuits or Parmesan cream sauce)									
	365	19	NA	NA	2	0	NA	66	472

Steakhouse Steaks

	Cal.	Total Fat	Sat. Fat	Chol.	Carb.	Fiber	Sug.	Prot.	Sod.
Asiago Peppercorn Sirloin (no Parmesan cream sauce)									
	401	20	NA	NA	3	0	NA	52	1023
Chef's Cut Sirloin									
	564	29	NA	NA	5	0	NA	69	881
Petite Sirloin									
	476	27	NA	NA	12	3	NA	45	967
Petite Sirloin & Jumbo Skewered Shrimp									
	462	28	NA	NA	3	0	NA	48	925
Rib Eye									
	912	71	NA	NA	7	0	NA	61	1040
Top Sirloin									
	562	31	NA	NA	13	3	NA	57	1110

Additional Gluten-Free Menu Items
(nutritional information was not available)

Blue Cheese Iceberg Tower (no croutons), Lobster Tail Add-On, Veggie Trio & Garden Bar

SONIC, America's Drive-In
[www.sonicdrivein.com]

Add-In Flavors & Toppings

	Cal.	Total Fat	Sat. Fat	Chol.	Carb.	Fiber	Sug.	Prot.	Sod.
Blue Coconut – Large 1 serving	60	0	0	0	14	0	11	0	10
Blue Coconut – Medium 1 serving	35	0	0	0	9	0	7	0	5
Blue Coconut – Rt 44 1 serving	70	0	0	0	18	0	15	0	10
Blue Coconut – Small 1 serving	20	0	0	0	5	0	4	0	0

Food Serving size	Cal.	(g) Total Fat	(g) Sat. Fat	(mg) Chol.	(g) Carb.	(g) Fiber	(g) Sug.	(g) Prot.	(mg) Sod.
Blue Coconut – Wacky Pack 1 serving	20	0	0	0	5	0	4	0	0
Caramel Topping – Large 1 serving	180	2.5	1.5	5	38	0	24	0	180
Caramel Topping – Medium 1 serving	120	1.5	1	5	25	0	16	0	120
Caramel Topping – Rt 44 1 serving	240	3	2	10	50	0	32	0	240
Caramel Topping – Small 1 serving	60	1	0.5	0	13	0	8	0	60
Caramel Topping – Wacky Pack 1 serving	60	1	0.5	0	13	0	8	0	60
Cherry – Large 1 serving	70	0	0	0	20	0	19	0	10
Cherry – Medium 1 serving	50	0	0	0	14	0	13	0	5
Cherry – Rt 44 1 serving	100	0	0	0	26	0	25	0	10
Cherry – Small 1 serving	30	0	0	0	8	0	7	0	0
Cherry – Wacky Pack 1 serving	30	0	0	0	8	0	7	0	0
Chocolate Topping – Large 1 serving	160	0	0	0	38	0	0	0	60
Chocolate Topping – Medium 1 serving	110	0	0	0	25	0	0	0	40
Chocolate Topping – Rt 44 1 serving	210	0	0	0	51	0	0	0	80
Chocolate Topping – Small 1 serving	50	0	0	0	13	0	0	0	20
Chocolate Topping – Wacky Pack 1 serving	50	0	0	0	13	0	0	0	20
Fresh Lemon – Large 1 serving	5	0	0	0	2	0	1	0	0

Food Serving size	Cal.	(g) Total Fat	(g) Sat. Fat	(mg) Chol.	(g) Carb.	(g) Fiber	(g) Sug.	(g) Prot.	(mg) Sod.
Fresh Lemon – Medium 1 serving	5	0	0	0	2	0	0	0	0
Fresh Lemon – Rt 44 1 serving	10	0	0	0	3	0	1	0	0
Fresh Lemon – Small 1 serving	0	0	0	0	1	0	0	0	0
Fresh Lemon – Wacky Pack 1 serving	0	0	0	0	1	0	0	0	0
Fresh Lime – Large 1 serving	5	0	0	0	2	0	0	0	0
Fresh Lime – Medium 1 serving	5	0	0	0	1	0	0	0	0
Fresh Lime – Rt 44 1 serving	5	0	0	0	2	0	0	0	0
Fresh Lime – Small 1 serving	0	0	0	0	1	0	0	0	0
Fresh Lime – Wacky Pack 1 serving	0	0	0	0	1	0	0	0	0
Grape – Large 1 serving	60	0	0	0	14	0	14	0	15
Grape – Medium 1 serving	40	0	0	0	9	0	9	0	10
Grape – Rt 44 1 serving	80	0	0	0	19	0	18	0	25
Grape – Small 1 serving	20	0	0	0	5	0	5	0	5
Grape – Wacky Pack 1 serving	20	0	0	0	5	0	5	0	5
Green Apple – Large 1 serving	90	0	0	0	22	0	17	0	10
Green Apple – Medium 1 serving	60	0	0	0	15	0	11	0	5
Green Apple – Rt 44 1 serving	120	0	0	0	29	0	22	0	15

Food Serving size	Cal.	(g) Total Fat	(g) Sat. Fat	(mg) Chol.	(g) Carb.	(g) Fiber	(g) Sug.	(g) Prot.	(mg) Sod.
Green Apple – Small 1 serving	30	0	0	0	7	0	6	0	0
Green Apple – Wacky Pack 1 serving	30	0	0	0	7	0	6	0	0
Hot Fudge Topping – Large 1 serving	200	7	6	0	32	2	25	2	90
Hot Fudge Topping – Medium 1 serving	130	4.5	4	0	22	1	16	1	60
Hot Fudge Topping – Rt 44 1 serving	270	9	8	0	43	2	33	2	125
Hot Fudge Topping – Small 1 serving	70	2.5	2	0	11	1	8	1	30
Hot Fudge Topping – Wacky Pack 1 serving	70	2.5	2	0	11	1	8	1	30
LowCal Diet Cherry – Large 1 serving	10	0	0	0	2	0	1	0	5
LowCal Diet Cherry – Medium 1 serving	10	0	0	0	2	0	1	0	5
LowCal Diet Cherry – Rt 44 1 serving	10	0	0	0	2	0	1	0	10
LowCal Diet Cherry – Small 1 serving	5	0	0	0	2	0	1	0	0
LowCal Diet Cherry – Wacky Pack 1 serving	5	0	0	0	2	0	1	0	0
Minute Maid Cranberry – Large 1 serving	60	0	0	0	15	0	15	0	5
Minute Maid Cranberry – Medium 1 serving	40	0	0	0	10	0	10	0	0
Minute Maid Cranberry – Rt 44 1 serving	80	0	0	0	20	0	19	0	10
Minute Maid Cranberry – Small 1 serving	20	0	0	0	5	0	5	0	0
Minute Maid Cranberry – Wacky Pack 1 serving	20	0	0	0	5	0	5	0	0

Food Serving size	Cal.	(g) Total Fat	(g) Sat. Fat	(mg) Chol.	(g) Carb.	(g) Fiber	(g) Sug.	(g) Prot.	(mg) Sod.
Orange – Large 1 serving	60	0	0	0	15	0	13	0	10
Orange – Medium 1 serving	40	0	0	0	10	0	8	0	5
Orange – Rt 44 1 serving	80	0	0	0	20	0	17	0	15
Orange – Small 1 serving	20	0	0	0	5	0	4	0	0
Orange – Wacky Pack 1 serving	20	0	0	0	5	0	4	0	0
Peach – Large 1 serving	0	0	0	0	1	0	0	0	20
Peach – Medium 1 serving	0	0	0	0	0	0	0	0	15
Peach – Rt 44 1 serving	5	0	0	0	1	0	0	0	30
Peach – Small 1 serving	0	0	0	0	0	0	0	0	5
Peach – Wacky Pack 1 serving	0	0	0	0	0	0	0	0	5
Pineapple Topping – Large 1 serving	70	0	0	0	17	0	15	0	10
Pineapple Topping – Medium 1 serving	45	0	0	0	11	0	10	0	5
Pineapple Topping – Rt 44 1 serving	90	0	0	0	22	0	20	0	10
Pineapple Topping – Small 1 serving	25	0	0	0	6	0	5	0	0
Pineapple Topping – Wacky Pack 1 serving	25	0	0	0	6	0	5	0	0
Powerade Mountain Blast – Large 1 serving	70	0	0	0	19	0	19	0	60
Powerade Mountain Blast – Medium 1 serving	50	0	0	0	13	0	13	0	40

Food Serving size	Cal.	(g) Total Fat	(g) Sat. Fat	(mg) Chol.	(g) Carb.	(g) Fiber	(g) Sug.	(g) Prot.	(mg) Sod.
Powerade Mountain Blast – Rt 44 1 serving	100	0	0	0	26	0	26	0	80
Powerade Mountain Blast – Small 1 serving	25	0	0	0	6	0	6	0	20
Powerade Mountain Blast – Wacky Pack 1 serving	25	0	0	0	6	0	6	0	20
Raspberry – Large 1 serving	0	0	0	0	0	0	0	0	20
Raspberry – Medium 1 serving	0	0	0	0	0	0	0	0	15
Raspberry – Rt 44 1 serving	0	0	0	0	0	1	0	0	25
Raspberry – Small 1 serving	0	0	0	0	0	0	0	0	5
Raspberry – Wacky Pack 1 serving	0	0	0	0	0	0	0	0	5
Strawberry Topping – Large 1 serving	60	0	0	0	14	1	13	0	10
Strawberry Topping – Medium 1 serving	40	0	0	0	10	1	9	0	10
Strawberry Topping – Rt 44 1 serving	80	0	0	0	19	2	18	0	15
Strawberry Topping – Small 1 serving	20	0	0	0	5	0	4	0	0
Strawberry Topping – Wacky Pack 1 serving	20	0	0	0	5	0	4	0	0
Vanilla – Large 1 serving	60	0	0	0	16	0	16	0	0
Vanilla – Medium 1 serving	40	0	0	0	11	0	11	0	0
Vanilla – Rt 44 1 serving	80	0	0	0	21	0	21	0	5
Vanilla – Small 1 serving	20	0	0	0	5	0	5	0	0

Food Serving size	Cal.	(g) Total Fat	(g) Sat. Fat	(mg) Chol.	(g) Carb.	(g) Fiber	(g) Sug.	(g) Prot.	(mg) Sod.
Vanilla – Wacky Pack 1 serving	20	0	0	0	5	0	5	0	0
Watermelon – Large 1 serving	70	0	0	0	17	0	13	0	10
Watermelon – Medium 1 serving	45	0	0	0	12	0	8	0	5
Watermelon – Rt 44 1 serving	90	0	0	0	23	0	17	0	15
Watermelon – Small 1 serving	25	0	0	0	6	0	4	0	0
Watermelon – Wacky Pack 1 serving	25	0	0	0	6	0	4	0	0

Bottled Water

Sonic Wave 16.9 oz	0	0	0	0	0	0	0	0	0

Cheese

American Cheese 1 slice	70	6	3	20	1	0	0	4	330
Shredded Cheddar Cheese 1 oz	100	9	6	25	1	0	0	6	490
Shredded White American Cheese 1 oz	100	9	5	25	1	0	0	6	460
Sliced Cheddar Cheese 1 slice	70	6	3	20	1	0	0	4	330
Sliced Monterey Jack Cheese 1 slice	60	5	3	15	0	0	0	3	300
Sliced Pepperjack Cheese 1 slice	60	6	3	15	0	0	0	3	330
Sliced Swiss Cheese 1 slice	60	4.5	2.5	15	1	0	0	4	280

Food Serving size	Cal.	(g) Total Fat	(g) Sat. Fat	(mg) Chol.	(g) Carb.	(g) Fiber	(g) Sug.	(g) Prot.	(mg) Sod.
Creamslush Treats									
Blue Coconut Creamslush Treat – Large									
32 oz	1100	52	37	185	150	0	142	14	540
Blue Coconut Creamslush Treat – Medium									
20 oz	610	28	21	90	84	0	80	7	280
Blue Coconut Creamslush Treat – Mini									
10 oz	380	18	13	50	55	0	52	4	150
Blue Coconut Creamslush Treat – Small									
14 oz	420	20	15	55	59	0	56	5	180
Cherry Creamslush Treat – Large									
32 oz	1110	52	37	185	152	0	146	14	540
Cherry Creamslush Treat – Medium									
20 oz	610	28	21	90	86	0	82	7	280
Cherry Creamslush Treat – Mini									
10 oz	390	18	13	50	55	0	53	4	150
Cherry Creamslush Treat – Small									
14 oz	420	20	15	55	60	0	58	5	180
Grape Creamslush Treat – Large									
32 oz	1100	52	37	185	150	0	144	14	550
Grape Creamslush Treat – Medium									
20 oz	610	28	21	90	84	0	79	7	280
Grape Creamslush Treat – Mini									
10 oz	380	18	13	50	55	0	53	4	160
Grape Creamslush Treat – Small									
14 oz	420	20	15	55	59	0	57	5	180
Lemon Creamslush Treat – Large									
32 oz	1100	52	37	185	152	0	141	14	540
Lemon Creamslush Treat – Medium									
20 oz	610	28	21	90	86	0	79	7	270
Lemon Creamslush Treat – Mini									
10 oz	390	18	13	50	55	0	52	4	150
Lemon Creamslush Treat – Small									
14 oz	420	20	15	55	60	0	56	5	180

Food Serving size	Cal.	(g) Total Fat	(g) Sat. Fat	(mg) Chol.	(g) Carb.	(g) Fiber	(g) Sug.	(g) Prot.	(mg) Sod.
Lemonberry Creamslush Treat – Large 32 oz	1150	52	37	185	164	2	155	15	560
Lemonberry Creamslush Treat – Medium 20 oz	640	28	21	90	94	1	89	7	280
Lemonberry Creamslush Treat – Mini 10 oz	400	18	13	50	59	1	56	4	160
Lemonberry Creamslush Treat – Small 14 oz	440	20	15	55	64	1	61	5	180
Lime Creamslush Treat – Large 32 oz	1100	52	37	185	152	0	141	14	540
Lime Creamslush Treat – Medium 20 oz	610	28	21	90	86	0	79	7	270
Lime Creamslush Treat – Mini 10 oz	390	18	13	50	55	0	52	4	150
Lime Creamslush Treat – Small 14 oz	420	20	15	55	60	0	56	5	180
Orange Creamslush Treat – Large 32 oz	1100	52	37	185	151	0	143	14	550
Orange Creamslush Treat – Medium 20 oz	610	28	21	90	85	0	80	7	280
Orange Creamslush Treat – Mini 10 oz	390	18	13	50	55	0	52	4	150
Orange Creamslush Treat – Small 14 oz	420	20	15	55	60	0	57	5	180
Strawberry Creamslush Treat – Large 32 oz	1150	52	37	185	162	2	155	15	560
Strawberry Creamslush Treat – Medium 20 oz	640	28	21	90	93	1	88	7	280
Strawberry Creamslush Treat – Mini 10 oz	400	18	13	50	59	1	56	4	160
Strawberry Creamslush Treat – Small 14 oz	440	20	15	55	63	1	61	5	180
Watermelon Creamslush Treat – Large 32 oz	1110	52	37	185	152	0	143	14	550

Food Serving size	Cal.	(g) Total Fat	(g) Sat. Fat	(mg) Chol.	(g) Carb.	(g) Fiber	(g) Sug.	(g) Prot.	(mg) Sod.
Watermelon Creamslush Treat – Medium 20 oz	610	28	21	90	86	0	80	7	280
Watermelon Creamslush Treat – Mini 10 oz	390	18	13	50	55	0	52	4	150
Watermelon Creamslush Treat – Small 14 oz	420	20	15	55	60	0	57	5	180

Dessert

Banana Split 1 serving	490	18	13	70	76	2	53	6	210

Dish

Vanilla Dish 1 serving	240	13	9	55	26	0	25	4	140

Famous Slushes

Blue Coconut Slush – Large 32 oz	450	0	0	0	119	0	116	0	70
Blue Coconut Slush – Medium 20 oz	280	0	0	0	75	0	73	0	45
Blue Coconut Slush – Rt 44 44 oz	610	0	0	0	163	0	160	0	95
Blue Coconut Slush – Small 14 oz	190	0	0	0	51	0	50	0	30
Blue Coconut Slush – Wacky Pack 12 oz	170	0	0	0	44	0	43	0	25
Cherry Slush – Large 32 oz	460	0	0	0	122	0	122	0	70
Cherry Slush – Medium 20 oz	290	0	0	0	77	0	77	0	45
Cherry Slush – Rt 44 44 oz	630	0	0	0	168	0	167	0	100
Cherry Slush – Small 14 oz	190	0	0	0	52	0	52	0	30

Food Serving size	Cal.	(g) Total Fat	(g) Sat. Fat	(mg) Chol.	(g) Carb.	(g) Fiber	(g) Sug.	(g) Prot.	(mg) Sod.
Cherry Slush – Wacky Pack 12 oz	170	0	0	0	45	0	45	0	25
Grape Slush – Large 32 oz	450	0	0	0	119	0	119	0	80
Grape Slush – Medium 20 oz	280	0	0	0	75	0	75	0	50
Grape Slush – Rt 44 44 oz	610	0	0	0	163	0	163	0	110
Grape Slush – Small 14 oz	190	0	0	0	51	0	51	0	35
Grape Slush – Wacky Pack 12 oz	170	0	0	0	44	0	44	0	30
Green Apple Slush – Large 32 oz	480	0	0	0	127	0	122	0	75
Green Apple Slush – Medium 20 oz	300	0	0	0	80	0	77	0	45
Green Apple Slush – Rt 44 44 oz	660	0	0	0	174	0	167	0	100
Green Apple Slush – Small 14 oz	200	0	0	0	54	0	52	0	30
Green Apple Slush – Wacky Pack 12 oz	180	0	0	0	47	0	45	0	25
Minute Maid Cranberry Slush – Large 32 oz	450	0	0	0	121	0	120	0	70
Minute Maid Cranberry Slush – Medium 20 oz	280	0	0	0	76	0	76	0	45
Minute Maid Cranberry Slush – Rt 44 44 oz	620	0	0	0	165	0	165	0	95
Minute Maid Cranberry Slush – Small 14 oz	190	0	0	0	51	0	51	0	30
Minute Maid Cranberry Slush – Wacky Pack 12 oz	170	0	0	0	45	0	45	0	25
Orange Slush – Large 32 oz	450	0	0	0	120	0	120	0	75

Food Serving size	Cal.	(g) Total Fat	(g) Sat. Fat	(mg) Chol.	(g) Carb.	(g) Fiber	(g) Sug.	(g) Prot.	(mg) Sod.
Orange Slush – Medium 20 oz	290	0	0	0	76	0	76	0	45
Orange Slush – Rt 44 44 oz	620	0	0	0	165	0	165	0	100
Orange Slush – Small 14 oz	190	0	0	0	51	0	51	0	30
Orange Slush – Wacky Pack 12 oz	170	0	0	0	45	0	45	0	25
Watermelon Slush – Large 32 oz	460	0	0	0	122	0	122	0	75
Watermelon Slush – Medium 20 oz	290	0	0	0	77	0	77	0	45
Watermelon Slush – Rt 44 44 oz	630	0	0	0	168	0	168	0	100
Watermelon Slush – Small 14 oz	190	0	0	0	52	0	52	0	30
Watermelon Slush – Wacky Pack 12 oz	170	0	0	0	45	0	45	0	25

Fresh Brewed Iced Teas

(Flavored Syrups Are Added to Flavored Teas)

Food Serving size	Cal.	Total Fat	Sat. Fat	Chol.	Carb.	Fiber	Sug.	Prot.	Sod.
Cranberry Tea – Large 32 oz	60	0	0	0	17	0	15	0	25
Cranberry Tea – Medium 20 oz	40	0	0	0	11	0	10	0	15
Cranberry Tea – Rt 44 44 oz	80	0	0	0	23	0	19	0	35
Cranberry Tea – Small 14 oz	20	0	0	0	6	0	5	0	10
Cranberry Tea – Wacky Pack 12 oz	20	0	0	0	6	0	5	0	10
Iced Tea – Large 32 oz	5	0	0	0	2	0	0	0	20
Iced Tea – Medium 20 oz	5	0	0	0	1	0	0	0	10

Food Serving size	Cal.	(g) Total Fat	(g) Sat. Fat	(mg) Chol.	(g) Carb.	(g) Fiber	(g) Sug.	(g) Prot.	(mg) Sod.
Iced Tea – Rt 44 44 oz	10	0	0	0	3	0	0	0	25
Iced Tea – Small 14 oz	5	0	0	0	1	0	0	0	10
Iced Tea – Wacky Pack 12 oz	5	0	0	0	1	0	0	0	10
Peach Iced Tea – Large 32 oz	10	0	0	0	2	0	0	0	40
Peach Iced Tea – Medium 20 oz	5	0	0	0	1	0	0	0	25
Peach Iced Tea – Rt 44 44 oz	10	0	0	0	3	0	0	0	55
Peach Iced Tea – Small 14 oz	5	0	0	0	1	0	0	0	15
Peach Iced Tea – Wacky Pack 12 oz	5	0	0	0	1	0	0	0	15
Raspberry Iced Tea – Large 32 oz	10	0	0	0	2	0	0	0	40
Raspberry Iced Tea – Medium 20 oz	5	0	0	0	2	0	0	0	25
Raspberry Iced Tea – Rt 44 44 oz	10	0	0	0	3	1	0	0	50
Raspberry Iced Tea – Small 14 oz	5	0	0	0	1	0	0	0	15
Raspberry Iced Tea – Wacky Pack 12 oz	5	0	0	0	1	0	0	0	15
Sweet Iced Tea – Large 32 oz	290	0	0	0	75	0	73	0	20
Sweet Iced Tea – Medium 20 oz	180	0	0	0	48	0	47	0	10
Sweet Iced Tea – Rt 44 44 oz	400	0	0	0	103	0	100	0	25
Sweet Iced Tea – Small 14 oz	150	0	0	0	39	0	38	0	10

Food Serving size	Cal.	(g) Total Fat	(g) Sat. Fat	(mg) Chol.	(g) Carb.	(g) Fiber	(g) Sug.	(g) Prot.	(mg) Sod.
Sweet Iced Tea – Wacky Pack 12 oz	120	0	0	0	31	0	30	0	5

Grilled Meat Only
(Bread, Cheese, and Condiments not included)

Food Serving size	Cal.	Total Fat	Sat. Fat	Chol.	Carb.	Fiber	Sug.	Prot.	Sod.
Beef Patty Only (1) 2 oz, approx pre-cooked weight	130	10	4.5	35	0	0	0	9	50
Beef Patty Only (1) 4 oz, approx pre-cooked weight	350	28	12	100	0	0	0	25	100
Breakfast Sausage Patty 1 patty	190	18	6	40	1	0	0	7	330
Crispy Bacon 2 slices	70	5	2	15	0	0	0	4	260
Egg approx 2.5 oz cooked	70	8	2.5	285	1	0	0	10	420
Grilled Onions approx 1 oz	25	2	0	0	2	1	1	0	30
Philly Steak – approx 4 oz precooked 1 steak	280	17	7	85	0	0	0	30	230
Pork and Beef Hot Dog Frank – approx 12 inches precooked 1 frank	380	35	14	70	3	0	2	13	830
Premium Beef Hot Dog – approx 6 inches precooked 1 frank	170	15	6	40	2	0	0	7	620
Red and Green Peppers approx 1.2 oz	70	7	1	0	2	1	1	0	0
Sliced Ham (Ham only) 4 slices	60	2	0.5	15	1	0	1	8	590

Iced Teas

Food Serving size	Cal.	Total Fat	Sat. Fat	Chol.	Carb.	Fiber	Sug.	Prot.	Sod.
Diet Green Tea – Large 32 oz	5	0	0	0	1	0	1	0	20
Diet Green Tea – Medium 20 oz	5	0	0	0	0	0	0	0	10
Diet Green Tea – Rt 44 44 oz	10	0	0	0	1	0	1	0	25

Food Serving size	Cal.	(g) Total Fat	(g) Sat. Fat	(mg) Chol.	(g) Carb.	(g) Fiber	(g) Sug.	(g) Prot.	(mg) Sod.
Diet Green Tea – Small 14 oz	5	0	0	0	0	0	0	0	10
Diet Green Tea – Wacky Pack 12 oz	0	0	0	0	0	0	0	0	5
Green Tea – Large 32 oz	210	0	0	0	59	0	56	0	20
Green Tea – Medium 20 oz	140	0	0	0	37	0	36	0	10
Green Tea – Rt 44 44 oz	290	0	0	0	80	0	77	0	25
Green Tea – Small 14 oz	110	0	0	0	32	0	30	0	10
Green Tea – Wacky Pack 12 oz	90	0	0	0	24	0	23	0	10

Kids' Meals

Food Serving size	Cal.	(g) Total Fat	(g) Sat. Fat	(mg) Chol.	(g) Carb.	(g) Fiber	(g) Sug.	(g) Prot.	(mg) Sod.
Apple Slices 1 serving	35	0	0	0	9	2	7	0	0
Apple Slices with Fat-Free Caramel Dipping Sauce 1 serving	110	0	0	0	28	2	15	0	60
Beef Patty Only (1) 2 oz, approx pre-cooked weight	340	17	6	35	34	1	6	15	640
French Fries small serving	200	8	1.5	0	30	2	0	2	270
Hi–C Fruit Punch – Wacky Pack 12 oz	120	0	0	0	31	0	31	0	10
Milk (1 %) 1 serving	110	2.5	1.5	10	13	0	12	8	130
Milk, Chocolate (1%) 1 serving	160	2.5	1.5	10	27	0	25	8	210
Minute Maid Apple Juice Box 1 serving	100	0	0	0	23	0	21	0	15
Premium Beef Hot Dog (1) approx 6 inches pre-cooked	170	15	6	40	2	0	0	7	620

Food Serving size	Cal.	(g) Total Fat	(g) Sat. Fat	(mg) Chol.	(g) Carb.	(g) Fiber	(g) Sug.	(g) Prot.	(mg) Sod.
Tots small serving	220	12	2	0	27	2	0	2	560

Limeades

Cherry Limeade – Large 32 oz	340	0	0	0	91	0	88	0	65
Cherry Limeade – Medium 20 oz	220	0	0	0	59	0	57	0	45
Cherry Limeade – Rt 44 44 oz	460	0	0	0	122	0	120	0	90
Cherry Limeade – Small 14 oz	170	0	0	0	45	0	44	0	35
Cherry Limeade – Wacky Pack 12 oz	140	0	0	0	37	0	36	0	30
Limeade – Large 32 oz	270	0	0	0	73	0	72	0	60
Limeade – Medium 20 oz	170	0	0	0	47	0	46	0	40
Limeade – Rt 44 44 oz	370	0	0	0	100	0	98	0	85
Limeade – Small 14 oz	140	0	0	0	38	0	37	0	30
Limeade – Wacky Pack 12 oz	110	0	0	0	30	0	29	0	25
LowCal Diet Cherry Limeade – Large 32 oz	20	0	0	0	4	0	1	0	25
LowCal Diet Cherry Limeade – Medium 20 oz	15	0	0	0	3	0	1	0	15
LowCal Diet Cherry Limeade – Rt 44 44 oz	25	0	0	0	4	0	1	0	30
LowCal Diet Cherry Limeade – Small 14 oz	10	0	0	0	2	0	1	0	10
LowCal Diet Cherry Limeade – Wacky Pack 12 oz	10	0	0	0	2	0	1	0	10

Food Serving size	Cal.	(g) Total Fat	(g) Sat. Fat	(mg) Chol.	(g) Carb.	(g) Fiber	(g) Sug.	(g) Prot.	(mg) Sod.
LowCal Diet Lime Limeade – Large 32 oz	10	0	0	0	1	0	0	0	15
LowCal Diet Lime Limeade – Medium 20 oz	10	0	0	0	1	0	0	0	10
LowCal Diet Lime Limeade – Rt 44 44 oz	15	0	0	0	2	0	0	0	25
LowCal Diet Lime Limeade – Small 14 oz	5	0	0	0	1	0	0	0	10
LowCal Diet Lime Limeade – Wacky Pack 12 oz	5	0	0	0	1	0	0	0	5
Minute Maid Cranberry Limeade – Large 32 oz	310	0	0	0	83	0	81	0	65
Minute Maid Cranberry Limeade – Medium 20 oz	200	0	0	0	53	0	52	0	40
Minute Maid Cranberry Limeade – Rt 44 44 oz	420	0	0	0	113	0	110	0	90
Minute Maid Cranberry Limeade – Small 14 oz	150	0	0	0	41	0	41	0	35
Minute Maid Cranberry Limeade – Wacky Pack 12 oz	120	0	0	0	33	0	32	0	25
Strawberry Limeade – Large 32 oz	310	0	0	0	83	1	80	1	70
Strawberry Limeade – Medium 20 oz	200	0	0	0	53	1	51	1	45
Strawberry Limeade – Rt 44 44 oz	420	0	0	0	112	2	109	1	95
Strawberry Limeade – Small 14 oz	150	0	0	0	41	0	40	0	35
Strawberry Limeade – Wacky Pack 12 oz	120	0	0	0	33	0	32	0	25

Minute Maid Juices

Food Serving size	Cal.	(g) Total Fat	(g) Sat. Fat	(mg) Chol.	(g) Carb.	(g) Fiber	(g) Sug.	(g) Prot.	(mg) Sod.
Minute Maid Apple Juice Box 1 box	100	0	0	0	23	0	21	0	15

Food Serving size	Cal.	(g) Total Fat	(g) Sat. Fat	(mg) Chol.	(g) Carb.	(g) Fiber	(g) Sug.	(g) Prot.	(mg) Sod.
Minute Maid Cranberry – Large 20 oz	210	0	0	0	56	0	54	0	25
Minute Maid Cranberry – Regular 14 oz	150	0	0	0	40	0	39	0	20
Minute Maid Cranberry – Wacky Pack 12 oz	130	0	0	0	36	0	35	0	15
Minute Maid Orange Juice – Large 20 oz	200	0	0	0	48	0	42	3	30
Minute Maid Orange Juice – Regular 14 oz	140	0	0	0	33	0	29	2	20
Minute Maid Orange Juice – Wacky Pack 12 oz	130	0	0	0	30	0	27	2	20

Ocean Water

Food Serving size	Cal.	(g) Total Fat	(g) Sat. Fat	(mg) Chol.	(g) Carb.	(g) Fiber	(g) Sug.	(g) Prot.	(mg) Sod.
Ocean Water – Large 32 oz	310	0	0	0	81	0	78	0	65
Ocean Water – Medium 20 oz	200	0	0	0	53	0	51	0	40
Ocean Water – Rt 44 44 oz	430	0	0	0	112	0	109	0	90
Ocean Water – Small 14 oz	150	0	0	0	41	0	40	0	35
Ocean Water – Wacky Pack 12 oz	120	0	0	0	33	0	32	0	25

Old School Floats

Food Serving size	Cal.	(g) Total Fat	(g) Sat. Fat	(mg) Chol.	(g) Carb.	(g) Fiber	(g) Sug.	(g) Prot.	(mg) Sod.
Barq's Root Beer Float/Blended Float – Large 32 oz	770	35	24	140	109	0	106	10	420
Barq's Root Beer Float/Blended Float – Medium 20 oz	520	23	16	90	75	0	73	7	270
Barq's Root Beer Float/Blended Float – Mini 10 oz	310	13	9	55	46	0	44	4	160
Barq's Root Beer Float/Blended Float – Small 14 oz	340	14	10	55	51	0	50	4	170

Food Serving size	Cal.	(g) Total Fat	(g) Sat. Fat	(mg) Chol.	(g) Carb.	(g) Fiber	(g) Sug.	(g) Prot.	(mg) Sod.
Coca-Cola Float/Blended Float – Large									
32 oz	760	35	24	140	105	0	102	10	390
Coca-Cola Float/Blended Float – Medium									
20 oz	510	23	16	90	72	0	70	7	260
Coca-Cola Float/Blended Float – Mini									
10 oz	300	13	9	55	44	0	42	4	150
Coca-Cola Float/Blended Float – Small									
14 oz	330	14	10	55	49	0	47	4	160
Coke Zero Float/Blended Float – Large									
32 oz	630	35	24	140	70	0	66	10	420
Coke Zero Float/Blended Float – Medium									
20 oz	410	23	16	90	46	0	43	7	280
Coke Zero Float/Blended Float – Mini									
10 oz	240	13	9	55	27	0	25	4	160
Coke Zero Float/Blended Float – Small									
14 oz	260	14	10	55	29	0	27	4	180
Diet Coke Float/Blended Float – Large									
32 oz	630	35	24	140	70	0	66	10	400
Diet Coke Float/Blended Float – Medium									
20 oz	410	23	16	90	46	0	43	7	260
Diet Coke Float/Blended Float – Mini									
10 oz	240	13	9	55	27	0	25	4	150
Diet Coke Float/Blended Float – Small									
14 oz	260	14	10	55	29	0	27	4	160
Diet Dr Pepper Float/Blended Float – Large									
32 oz	630	35	24	140	70	0	66	10	450
Diet Dr Pepper Float/Blended Float – Medium									
20 oz	410	23	16	90	45	0	43	7	300
Diet Dr Pepper Float/Blended Float – Mini									
10 oz	240	13	9	55	27	0	25	4	180
Diet Dr Pepper Float/Blended Float – Small									
14 oz	260	14	10	55	28	0	27	4	190
Dr Pepper Float/Blended Float – Large									
32 oz	750	35	24	140	104	0	100	10	420

Food Serving size	Cal.	(g) Total Fat	(g) Sat. Fat	(mg) Chol.	(g) Carb.	(g) Fiber	(g) Sug.	(g) Prot.	(mg) Sod.
Dr Pepper Float/Blended Float – Medium 20 oz	500	23	16	90	71	0	69	7	280
Dr Pepper Float/Blended Float – Mini 10 oz	300	13	9	55	43	0	42	4	170
Dr Pepper Float/Blended Float – Small 14 oz	320	14	10	55	48	0	46	4	180
Fanta Orange Float/Blended Float – Large 32 oz	770	35	24	140	109	0	106	10	380
Fanta Orange Float/Blended Float – Medium 20 oz	520	23	16	90	75	0	73	7	250
Fanta Orange Float/Blended Float – Mini 10 oz	310	13	9	55	46	0	44	4	150
Fanta Orange Float/Blended Float – Small 14 oz	340	14	10	55	51	0	49	4	160
Sprite Float/Blended Float – Large 32 oz	760	35	24	140	104	0	101	10	410
Sprite Float/Blended Float – Medium 20 oz	510	23	16	90	72	0	69	7	270
Sprite Float/Blended Float – Mini 10 oz	300	13	9	55	43	0	42	4	160
Sprite Float/Blended Float – Small 14 oz	330	14	10	55	48	0	47	4	170
Sprite Zero Float/Blended Float – Large 32 oz	630	35	24	140	70	0	66	10	390
Sprite Zero Float/Blended Float – Medium 20 oz	410	23	16	90	45	0	43	7	260
Sprite Zero Float/Blended Float – Mini 10 oz	240	13	9	55	27	0	25	4	150
Sprite Zero Float/Blended Float – Small 14 oz	260	14	10	55	28	0	27	4	160

Powerade Drinks & Slushes

Powerade Mountain Blast – Large 32 oz	180	0	0	0	47	0	47	0	150

Food Serving size	Cal.	(g) Total Fat	(g) Sat. Fat	(mg) Chol.	(g) Carb.	(g) Fiber	(g) Sug.	(g) Prot.	(mg) Sod.
Powerade Mountain Blast – Medium									
20 oz	110	0	0	0	30	0	30	0	95
Powerade Mountain Blast – Rt 44									
44 oz	240	0	0	0	64	0	64	0	200
Powerade Mountain Blast – Small									
14 oz	90	0	0	0	24	0	24	0	75
Powerade Mountain Blast – Wacky Pack									
12 oz	70	0	0	0	19	0	19	0	60
Powerade Mountain Blast Slush – Large									
32 oz	460	0	0	0	124	0	124	0	120
Powerade Mountain Blast Slush – Medium									
20 oz	290	0	0	0	78	0	78	0	80
Powerade Mountain Blast Slush – Rt 44									
44 oz	630	0	0	0	170	0	170	0	170
Powerade Mountain Blast Slush – Small									
14 oz	200	0	0	0	53	0	53	0	50
Powerade Mountain Blast Slush – Wacky Pack									
12 oz	170	0	0	0	46	0	46	0	45

Premium Roast Coffees

Food Serving size	Cal.	(g) Total Fat	(g) Sat. Fat	(mg) Chol.	(g) Carb.	(g) Fiber	(g) Sug.	(g) Prot.	(mg) Sod.
Coffee – Regular									
14 oz	10	0	0	0	2	1	0	1	35
Coffee – Regular									
20 oz	15	0	0	0	3	1	0	1	50
Java Chiller, Caramel									
10 oz	430	22	16	65	52	0	44	5	250
Java Chiller, Caramel									
14 oz	750	38	28	130	92	0	80	10	470
Java Chiller, Caramel									
20 oz	910	43	31	150	119	0	99	11	600
Java Chiller, Caramel									
32 oz	1210	56	40	200	161	1	133	15	820
Java Chiller, Mocha									
10 oz	460	21	16	65	61	0	35	5	220

Food Serving size	Cal.	(g) Total Fat	(g) Sat. Fat	(mg) Chol.	(g) Carb.	(g) Fiber	(g) Sug.	(g) Prot.	(mg) Sod.
Java Chiller, Mocha 14 oz	780	37	27	125	102	0	65	10	410
Java Chiller, Mocha 20 oz	890	41	29	140	119	0	72	11	470
Java Chiller, Mocha 32 oz	1180	52	37	185	162	1	94	15	630
Java Chiller, Mocha/Caramel 10 oz	570	23	17	70	85	0	50	5	330
Java Chiller, Mocha/Caramel 14 oz	850	38	28	130	116	0	80	10	500
Java Chiller, Mocha/Caramel 20 oz	1090	43	31	150	161	0	99	11	670
Java Chiller, Mocha/Caramel 32 oz	1470	56	40	200	222	1	133	15	920
Sonic Boom Espresso Shot 1 shot	5	0	0	0	1	0	0	0	5

Real Fruit Slushes

Food Serving size	Cal.	(g) Total Fat	(g) Sat. Fat	(mg) Chol.	(g) Carb.	(g) Fiber	(g) Sug.	(g) Prot.	(mg) Sod.
Lemon Real Fruit Slush – Large 32 oz	450	0	0	0	122	0	115	0	70
Lemon Real Fruit Slush – Medium 20 oz	290	0	0	0	77	0	72	0	45
Lemon Real Fruit Slush – Rt 44 44 oz	620	0	0	0	167	1	158	0	95
Lemon Real Fruit Slush – Small 14 oz	190	0	0	0	52	0	50	0	30
Lemon Real Fruit Slush – Wacky Pack 12 oz	170	0	0	0	45	0	43	0	25
Lemonberry Real Fruit Slush – Large 32 oz	440	0	0	0	119	1	116	0	75
Lemonberry Real Fruit Slush – Medium 20 oz	280	0	0	0	75	1	73	1	45
Lemonberry Real Fruit Slush – Rt 44 44 oz	610	0	0	0	163	2	160	1	100

Food Serving size	Cal.	(g) Total Fat	(g) Sat. Fat	(mg) Chol.	(g) Carb.	(g) Fiber	(g) Sug.	(g) Prot.	(mg) Sod.
Lemonberry Real Fruit Slush – Small 14 oz	190	0	0	0	51	0	50	0	30
Lemonberry Real Fruit Slush – Wacky Pack 12 oz	160	0	0	0	44	0	43	0	25
Lime Real Fruit Slush – Large 32 oz	450	0	0	0	121	0	115	0	70
Lime Real Fruit Slush – Medium 20 oz	290	0	0	0	76	0	72	0	45
Lime Real Fruit Slush – Rt 44 44 oz	620	0	0	0	166	1	158	0	95
Lime Real Fruit Slush – Small 14 oz	190	0	0	0	52	0	50	0	30
Lime Real Fruit Slush – Wacky Pack 12 oz	170	0	0	0	45	0	43	0	25
Strawberry Real Fruit Slush – Large 32 oz	440	0	0	0	117	1	116	0	75
Strawberry Real Fruit Slush – Medium 20 oz	280	0	0	0	73	1	73	0	45
Strawberry Real Fruit Slush – Rt 44 44 oz	600	0	0	0	160	2	159	0	100
Strawberry Real Fruit Slush – Small 14 oz	190	0	0	0	50	0	50	0	30
Strawberry Real Fruit Slush – Wacky Pack 12 oz	160	0	0	0	43	0	43	0	25

Sandwich Toppings and Condiments

Food Serving size	Cal.	(g) Total Fat	(g) Sat. Fat	(mg) Chol.	(g) Carb.	(g) Fiber	(g) Sug.	(g) Prot.	(mg) Sod.
Baja Cheese Sauce 1 serving	160	17	3	15	1	0	0	0	270
Caramel Dipping Sauce 1 serving	70	0	0	0	18	0	8	0	60
Carne Asada Sauce 1 serving	50	4	0.5	0	4	0	0	0	190
Celery Salt 1 serving	0	0	0	0	0	0	0	0	310

Food Serving size	Cal.	(g) Total Fat	(g) Sat. Fat	(mg) Chol.	(g) Carb.	(g) Fiber	(g) Sug.	(g) Prot.	(mg) Sod.
Chopped Onions 1 serving	5	0	0	0	1	0	1	0	0
French Fry Sauce 1 serving	45	3.5	0.5	5	3	0	3	0	130
Grape Jelly 1 serving	35	0	0	0	9	0	60	0	0
Green Chiles 1 serving	5	0	0	0	1	0	0	0	5
Hickory BBQ Sauce 1 serving	40	0	0	0	10	0	8	0	450
Honey Mustard Sauce 1 serving	90	7	1	15	7	0	4	0	190
Ketchup 1 serving	15	0	0	0	4	0	3	0	160
Lettuce 1 serving	5	0	0	0	1	0	1	0	0
Light Ranch Dressing 1 serving	70	6	1	10	3	0	2	1	290
Maple Flavored Syrup 1 serving	90	0	0	0	22	0	15	0	0
Marinara Sauce 1 serving	15	0	0	0	4	0	2	0	140
Mayonnaise 1 serving	100	11	1.5	10	1	0	0	0	55
Mustard 1 serving	5	0	0	0	0	0	0	0	55
Philadelphia Cream Cheese 1 serving	70	7	4	20	1	0	1	1	115
Picante Sauce 1 serving	5	0	0	0	1	0	0	0	140
Pickle Spear 1 serving	0	0	0	0	1	0	0	0	320
Ranch Dressing Sauce 1 serving	110	11	2	10	1	0	1	0	230

Food Serving size	Cal.	(g) Total Fat	(g) Sat. Fat	(mg) Chol.	(g) Carb.	(g) Fiber	(g) Sug.	(g) Prot.	(mg) Sod.
Relish 1 serving	40	0	0	0	10	0	10	0	150
Salsa De Sonic 1 serving	0	0	0	0	0	0	0	0	145
Sauerkraut 1 serving	5	0	0	0	1	1	0	1	180
Sliced Pickles 1 serving	0	0	0	0	0	0	0	0	180
Spicy Jalapenos 1 serving	5	0	0	0	1	1	0	0	280
Spicy Mustard 1 serving	15	1	0	0	1	0	0	1	230
Sport Pepper 1 serving	10	0	0	0	2	0	2	0	480
Strawberry Jam 1 serving	35	0	0	0	9	0	6	0	0
Sweet and Sour Sauce 1 serving	50	0	0	0	12	0	7	0	75
Tartar Sauce 1 serving	150	15	2.5	10	3	0	2	0	210
Thousand Island Dressing 1 serving	160	15	2.5	10	4	0	3	0	170
Tomatoes 1 serving	5	0	0	0	1	0	1	0	0

Shakes

Food Serving size	Cal.	(g) Total Fat	(g) Sat. Fat	(mg) Chol.	(g) Carb.	(g) Fiber	(g) Sug.	(g) Prot.	(mg) Sod.
Banana Shake – Large 32 oz	1270	59	42	210	177	7	141	19	590
Banana Shake – Medium 20 oz	860	40	29	135	119	5	94	12	390
Banana Shake – Mini 10 oz	520	26	19	80	69	3	56	7	230
Banana Shake – Small 14 oz	620	31	23	100	80	3	67	9	290

Food Serving size	Cal.	(g) Total Fat	(g) Sat. Fat	(mg) Chol.	(g) Carb.	(g) Fiber	(g) Sug.	(g) Prot.	(mg) Sod.
Caramel Shake – Large 32 oz	1290	61	44	220	168	0	142	16	850
Caramel Shake – Medium 20 oz	870	42	30	145	113	0	95	10	560
Caramel Shake – Mini 10 oz	530	27	19	85	66	0	56	6	320
Caramel Shake – Small 14 oz	630	32	23	105	77	0	67	8	380
Chocolate Shake – Large 32 oz	1410	58	41	210	203	0	106	16	730
Chocolate Shake – Medium 20 oz	850	40	29	135	113	0	71	10	440
Chocolate Shake – Mini 10 oz	570	26	19	80	78	0	45	6	280
Chocolate Shake – Small 14 oz	620	31	23	100	77	0	55	8	320
Hot Fudge Shake – Large 32 oz	1540	79	60	205	187	4	158	16	800
Hot Fudge Shake – Medium 20 oz	890	45	34	135	109	2	93	10	490
Hot Fudge Shake – Mini 10 oz	540	30	22	80	62	1	55	6	270
Hot Fudge Shake – Small 14 oz	610	32	23	100	73	1	64	8	340
Pineapple Shake – Large 32 oz	1130	58	41	210	139	0	130	16	600
Pineapple Shake – Medium 20 oz	760	40	29	135	93	0	87	10	390
Pineapple Shake – Mini 10 oz	480	26	19	80	56	0	53	6	230
Pineapple Shake – Small 14 oz	570	31	23	100	67	0	63	8	290
Strawberry Shake – Large 32 oz	1100	58	41	210	131	2	123	16	600

Food Serving size	Cal.	(g) Total Fat	(g) Sat. Fat	(mg) Chol.	(g) Carb.	(g) Fiber	(g) Sug.	(g) Prot.	(mg) Sod.
Strawberry Shake – Medium 20 oz	750	40	29	135	91	1	85	11	390
Strawberry Shake – Mini 10 oz	470	26	19	80	55	1	52	6	230
Strawberry Shake – Small 14 oz	570	31	23	100	66	1	62	8	300
Vanilla Shake – Large 32 oz	1090	62	44	225	120	0	113	17	630
Vanilla Shake – Medium 20 oz	690	40	29	135	75	0	71	10	380
Vanilla Shake – Mini 10 oz	470	28	20	90	51	0	48	7	250
Vanilla Shake – Small 14 oz	540	31	23	100	58	0	55	9	290

Single Topping Sundaes

Food Serving size	Cal.	(g) Total Fat	(g) Sat. Fat	(mg) Chol.	(g) Carb.	(g) Fiber	(g) Sug.	(g) Prot.	(mg) Sod.
Caramel Sundae 1 serving	510	23	17	85	69	0	57	6	340
Chocolate Sundae 1 serving	500	22	16	80	69	0	41	6	260
Hot Fudge Sundae 1 serving	520	27	20	80	63	1	54	6	280
Nuts Add–On 1 serving	20	1.5	0	0	1	0	0	1	0
Pineapple Sundae 1 serving	440	22	16	80	55	0	51	6	230
Strawberry Sundae 1 serving	410	20	14	80	52	1	48	6	230

Snacks & Sides

Food Serving size	Cal.	(g) Total Fat	(g) Sat. Fat	(mg) Chol.	(g) Carb.	(g) Fiber	(g) Sug.	(g) Prot.	(mg) Sod.
Apple Slices 1 serving	35	0	0	0	9	2	7	0	0
Apple Slices with Fat-Free Caramel Dipping Sauce 1 serving	110	0	0	0	28	2	15	0	60

Food Serving size	Cal.	(g) Total Fat	(g) Sat. Fat	(mg) Chol.	(g) Carb.	(g) Fiber	(g) Sug.	(g) Prot.	(mg) Sod.
French Fries large serving	470	22	4	0	64	5	0	6	490
French Fries medium serving	340	16	3	0	46	4	0	4	360
French Fries small serving	200	8	1.5	0	30	2	0	2	270
French Fries with Cheese large serving	780	41	11	35	88	7	2	15	1330
French Fries with Cheese medium serving	490	26	8	30	53	4	1	10	900
French Fries with Cheese small serving	350	18	5	20	38	3	1	7	620
Fritos Corn Chips 2 oz serving	320	20	3	0	30	2	0	4	340
Tots large serving	580	31	6	0	69	6	1	5	1450
Tots medium serving	360	19	3.5	0	43	4	0	3	890
Tots small serving	220	12	2	0	27	2	0	2	560
Tots with Cheese large serving	840	50	13	40	86	8	2	13	2450
Tots with Cheese medium serving	450	28	8	30	43	4	1	8	1390
Tots with Cheese small serving	290	18	5	20	27	2	1	5	890

Soft Drinks

Food Serving size	Cal.	Total Fat	Sat. Fat	Chol.	Carb.	Fiber	Sug.	Prot.	Sod.
Barq's Root Beer – Large 32 oz	310	0	0	0	82	0	82	0	65
Barq's Root Beer – Medium 20 oz	190	0	0	0	52	0	52	0	40
Barq's Root Beer – Rt 44 44 oz	420	0	0	0	112	0	112	0	90

Food Serving size	Cal.	(g) Total Fat	(g) Sat. Fat	(mg) Chol.	(g) Carb.	(g) Fiber	(g) Sug.	(g) Prot.	(mg) Sod.
Barq's Root Beer – Small 14 oz	160	0	0	0	43	0	43	0	35
Barq's Root Beer – Wacky Pack 12 oz	130	0	0	0	34	0	34	0	25
Coca-Cola – Large 32 oz	270	0	0	0	74	0	74	0	15
Coca-Cola – Medium 20 oz	170	0	0	0	47	0	47	0	10
Coca-Cola – Rt 44 44 oz	370	0	0	0	101	0	101	0	20
Coca-Cola – Small 14 oz	140	0	0	0	39	0	39	0	10
Coca-Cola – Wacky Pack 12 oz	110	0	0	0	30	0	30	0	5
Coke Zero – Large 32 oz	0	0	0	0	0	0	0	0	75
Coke Zero – Medium 20 oz	0	0	0	0	0	0	0	0	50
Coke Zero – Rt 44 44 oz	5	0	0	0	0	0	0	0	105
Coke Zero – Small 14 oz	0	0	0	0	0	0	0	0	40
Coke Zero – Wacky Pack 12 oz	0	0	0	0	0	0	0	0	40
Diet Coke – Large 32 oz	0	0	0	0	0	0	0	0	30
Diet Coke – Medium 20 oz	0	0	0	0	0	0	0	0	20
Diet Coke – Rt 44 44 oz	0	0	0	0	0	0	0	0	40
Diet Coke – Small 14 oz	0	0	0	0	0	0	0	0	15
Diet Coke – Wacky Pack 12 oz	0	0	0	0	0	0	0	0	10

Food Serving size	Cal.	(g) Total Fat	(g) Sat. Fat	(mg) Chol.	(g) Carb.	(g) Fiber	(g) Sug.	(g) Prot.	(mg) Sod.
Diet Dr Pepper – Large 32 oz	0	0	0	0	0	0	0	0	135
Diet Dr Pepper – Medium 20 oz	0	0	0	0	0	0	0	0	85
Diet Dr Pepper – Rt 44 44 oz	0	0	0	0	0	0	0	0	190
Diet Dr Pepper – Small 14 oz	0	0	0	0	0	0	0	0	70
Diet Dr Pepper – Wacky Pack 12 oz	0	0	0	0	0	0	0	0	55
Dr Pepper – Large 32 oz	250	0	0	0	71	0	71	0	80
Dr Pepper – Medium 20 oz	160	0	0	0	45	0	45	0	50
Dr Pepper – Rt 44 44 oz	340	0	0	0	97	0	97	0	110
Dr Pepper – Small 14 oz	130	0	0	0	37	0	37	0	45
Dr Pepper – Wacky Pack 12 oz	100	0	0	0	29	0	29	0	35
Fanta Orange – Large 32 oz	290	0	0	0	80	0	80	0	15
Fanta Orange – Medium 20 oz	190	0	0	0	51	0	51	0	10
Fanta Orange – Rt 44 44 oz	400	0	0	0	109	0	109	0	20
Fanta Orange – Small 14 oz	150	0	0	0	42	0	42	0	10
Fanta Orange – Wacky Pack 12 oz	120	0	0	0	33	0	33	0	5
Hi-C Fruit Punch – Large 32 oz	290	0	0	0	77	0	77	0	25
Hi-C Fruit Punch – Medium 20 oz	180	0	0	0	49	0	49	0	15

Food Serving size	Cal.	(g) Total Fat	(g) Sat. Fat	(mg) Chol.	(g) Carb.	(g) Fiber	(g) Sug.	(g) Prot.	(mg) Sod.
Hi-C Fruit Punch – Rt 44 44 oz	390	0	0	0	105	0	105	0	35
Hi-C Fruit Punch – Small 14 oz	150	0	0	0	40	0	40	0	15
Hi-C Fruit Punch – Wacky Pack 12 oz	120	0	0	0	31	0	31	0	10
Mello Yello – Large 32 oz	290	0	0	0	80	0	80	0	20
Mello Yello – Medium 20 oz	190	0	0	0	51	0	51	0	15
Mello Yello – Rt 44 44 oz	400	0	0	0	109	0	109	0	30
Mello Yello – Small 14 oz	150	0	0	0	42	0	42	0	10
Mello Yello – Wacky Pack 12 oz	120	0	0	0	33	0	33	0	10
Minute Maid Lemonade – Large 32 oz	270	0	0	0	71	0	71	0	115
Minute Maid Lemonade – Medium 20 oz	170	0	0	0	45	0	45	0	70
Minute Maid Lemonade – Rt 44 44 oz	360	0	0	0	97	0	97	0	150
Minute Maid Lemonade – Small 14 oz	140	0	0	0	37	0	37	0	60
Minute Maid Lemonade – Wacky Pack 12 oz	140	0	0	0	36	0	36	0	55
Sprite – Large 32 oz	270	0	0	0	71	0	71	0	60
Sprite – Medium 20 oz	170	0	0	0	45	0	45	0	40
Sprite – Rt 44 44 oz	360	0	0	0	97	0	97	0	80
Sprite – Small 14 oz	140	0	0	0	37	0	37	0	30

Food Serving size	Cal.	(g) Total Fat	(g) Sat. Fat	(mg) Chol.	(g) Carb.	(g) Fiber	(g) Sug.	(g) Prot.	(mg) Sod.
Sprite – Wacky Pack 12 oz	110	0	0	0	29	0	29	0	25
Sprite Zero – Large 32 oz	5	0	0	0	0	0	0	0	15
Sprite Zero – Medium 20 oz	5	0	0	0	0	0	0	0	10
Sprite Zero – Rt 44 44 oz	10	0	0	0	0	0	0	0	20
Sprite Zero – Small 14 oz	5	0	0	0	0	0	0	0	10
Sprite Zero – Wacky Pack 12 oz	5	0	0	0	0	0	0	0	5

Sonic Blast

Food Serving size	Cal.	(g) Total Fat	(g) Sat. Fat	(mg) Chol.	(g) Carb.	(g) Fiber	(g) Sug.	(g) Prot.	(mg) Sod.
M&M's Sonic Blast – Large 32 oz	1800	97	67	290	210	3	197	27	870
M&M's Sonic Blast – Medium 20 oz	1250	68	47	190	146	2	137	18	580
M&M's Sonic Blast – Mini 10 oz	540	29	21	65	62	1	58	7	210
M&M's Sonic Blast – Small 14 oz	910	49	34	130	106	1	99	13	400
Reese's Peanut Butter Cups Sonic Blast – Large 32 oz	1730	83	58	295	219	2	187	31	1020
Reese's Peanut Butter Cups Sonic Blast – Medium 20 oz	1200	57	40	195	153	2	129	22	690
Reese's Peanut Butter Cups Sonic Blast – Mini 10 oz	510	23	17	65	66	1	54	9	270
Reese's Peanut Butter Cups Sonic Blast – Small 14 oz	870	41	29	135	111	1	94	16	490
Snickers Sonic Blast – Large 32 oz	1770	98	63	300	201	2	186	28	1010
Snickers Sonic Blast – Medium 20 oz	1230	68	44	200	139	2	128	19	690

Food Serving size	Cal.	(g) Total Fat	(g) Sat. Fat	(mg) Chol.	(g) Carb.	(g) Fiber	(g) Sug.	(g) Prot.	(mg) Sod.
Snickers Sonic Blast – Mini 10 oz	520	30	19	65	59	1	53	8	270
Snickers Sonic Blast – Small 14 oz	900	50	32	135	101	1	93	14	490

Ted's Montana Grill
[www.tedsmontanagrill.com]

Burgers & Toppings

America's Cup	320	26	13	NA	7	1	NA	19	1569
American Cheese	150	14	9	NA	2	NA	NA	NA	653
Avalon	342	5	12	NA	5	0	NA	8	586
Blue Creek	260	20	10	NA	0	0	NA	19	921
Canyon Creek	298	24	12	NA	2	0	NA	20	840
Cheddar Cheese	170	14	9	NA	0	0	NA	11	264
George's Cadillac	360	24	12	NA	16	1	NA	20	1240
Jack Cheese	160	13	8	NA	0	0	NA	10	228
Kitchen Sink	460	34	15	NA	8	1	NA	33	2104
Montana Breakfast	290	22	11	NA	3	0	NA	24	1187
Naked Beef Burger (order without the bun) 8 oz	334	17	7	NA	0	0	NA	40	1609
Naked Bison Burger (order without the bun) 8 oz	306	15	6	NA	0	0	NA	43	1609

Food Serving size	Cal.	(g) Total Fat	(g) Sat. Fat	(mg) Chol.	(g) Carb.	(g) Fiber	(g) Sug.	(g) Prot.	(mg) Sod.
New Mexico	240	20	9	NA	7	3	NA	11	379
Peppercorn	228	19	8	NA	3	1	NA	13	629
Skinny Dip	90	8	1	NA	5	5	NA	13	4
Swiss & Mushroom	260	20	12	NA	6	1	NA	15	438
Swiss Cheese	160	12	8	NA	2	0	NA	12	82
Ted's Bacon Cheeseburger	320	23	11	NA	7	1	NA	20	827
Vermejo	210	15	9	NA	6	1	NA	12	568

Classics

(order without yeast roll) (Please refer to listing of gluten-free sides when ordering)

Food Serving size	Cal.	(g) Total Fat	(g) Sat. Fat	(mg) Chol.	(g) Carb.	(g) Fiber	(g) Sug.	(g) Prot.	(mg) Sod.
Beef Delmonico Ribeye	1095	73	28	NA	0	0	NA	50	2398
Beef Tenderloin Filet	892	64	20	NA	0	0	NA	40	2330
Bison Delmonico Ribeye	897	58	24	NA	0	0	NA	61	2351
Bison Kansas City Strip Steak	659	38	7	NA	0	0	NA	52	2348
Bison Tenderloin Filet	545	28	5	NA	0	0	NA	53	2307
Cedar Plank Salmon 7 oz	880	48	17	NA	54	7	NA	54	544
Cedar Plank Salmon 9 oz	970	52	17	NA	54	7	NA	67	577
Prime Rib (order without au jus) 12 oz	870	74	30	NA	1	0	NA	47	1087
Prime Rib (order without au jus) 16 oz	1160	98	41	NA	1	0	NA	62	1449

Food Serving size	Cal.	(g) Total Fat	(g) Sat. Fat	(mg) Chol.	(g) Carb.	(g) Fiber	(g) Sug.	(g) Prot.	(mg) Sod.
Roast Turkey (order without dressing and gravy)									
1 serving	866	41	23.1	NA	45	0	NA	67	567
Salt-and-Pepper Trout									
1 serving	653	49	7	NA	15	4	NA	44	1375

Desserts

Coke Float									
1 beverage	540	29	18	NA	60	0	NA	8	118
Haagen-Dazs Ice Cream (Chocolate)									
1 serving	430	29	18	NA	35	2	NA	8	96
Haagen-Dazs Ice Cream (Vanilla)									
1 serving	430	29	18	NA	34	0	NA	8	112
Hand-Made Shakes (Chocolate)									
1 serving	1090	64	39	NA	105	0	NA	19	284
Hand-Made Shakes (Strawberry)									
1 shake	970	64	39	NA	78	1	NA	18	249
Hand-Made Shakes (Vanilla)									
1 shake	1020	64	39	NA	90	0	NA	18	248
IBC Root Beer Float									
1 float	600	29	18	NA	79	0	NA	8	148

Kids' Menu

Bar None Sliders (Beef) (choose gluten-free side and order without roll)									
1 serving	950	57	30	NA	74	8	NA	36	1376
Bar None Sliders (Bison) (choose gluten-free side and order without roll)									
1 serving	920	48	25	NA	74	5	NA	43	1376
Cedar Plank Salmon (choose gluten-free side)									
1 serving	500	22	8	NA	36	4	NA	38	1404
Steak and Fries (choose gluten-free side)									
1 serving	576	30	8	NA	18	2	NA	36	1844

Salads

(Eggless Caesar, Honey Mustard, Basil Vinaigrette, Bleu Cheese, Olive Oil & Red Wine Vinegar and Thousand Island Dressings. Also order salad without croutons)

Balsamic Bleu Steak (order without crispy fried onion straws)									
1 serving	703	29	9	NA	32	3	NA	41	1653

Food Serving size	Cal.	(g) Total Fat	(g) Sat. Fat	(mg) Chol.	(g) Carb.	(g) Fiber	(g) Sug.	(g) Prot.	(mg) Sod.
Grilled Chicken Caesar Salad 1 serving	1380	115	37	NA	31	6	NA	54	1752
Ted's Chopped Salad (Full) 1 serving	670	53	12	NA	40	3	NA	16	1279
Cedar Plank Salmon Caesar Salad 1 serving	1280	109	35	NA	32	6	NA	47	1445
House Salad (no dressing) 1 serving	140	9	7	NA	13	2	NA	3	128
Wedge Salad (no dressing) 1 serving	100	6	2	NA	5	2	NA	7	342

Sides

Food Serving size	Cal.	(g) Total Fat	(g) Sat. Fat	(mg) Chol.	(g) Carb.	(g) Fiber	(g) Sug.	(g) Prot.	(mg) Sod.
Asparagus 1 serving	60	5	0	NA	3	2	NA	2	155
Baked Potato (Plain) 1 potato	310	2	1	NA	64	7	NA	8	3
Buttered Broccoli 1 serving	50	2	1	NA	6	NA	NA	NA	417
Cole Slaw 1 serving	330	31	4	NA	12	2	NA	2	379
French Cut Fries 1 serving	300	18	1	NA	30	3	NA	3	490
Garlic Mashed Potatoes (order without gravy) 1 serving	240	13	10	NA	25	2	NA	4	1
Sweet Potato (Plain) 1 potato	170	0	0	NA	39	6	NA	4	68
Vine-Ripened Tomatoes 1 serving	15	0	0	NA	3	1	NA	1	4

Starters

Food Serving size	Cal.	(g) Total Fat	(g) Sat. Fat	(mg) Chol.	(g) Carb.	(g) Fiber	(g) Sug.	(g) Prot.	(mg) Sod.
Grilled Shrimp 1 serving	497	43	12	NA	25	1	NA	25	948

Food Serving size	Cal.	(g) Total Fat	(g) Sat. Fat	(mg) Chol.	(g) Carb.	(g) Fiber	(g) Sug.	(g) Prot.	(mg) Sod.

Additional Gluten-Free Menu Items
(nutritional information was not available)

Classic Caesar Salad (with Plank Salmon), Classic Caesar Salad (with Grilled Shrimp), Big Sky Grilled Salad (with Chicken), Big Sky Grilled Salad (with Beef Burger), Big Sky Grilled Salad (with Bison Burger), Classic Caesar Side Salad

Uno Chicago Grill
[www.unos.com]

Burgers & Sandwiches

Bring Home the Bacon Burger									
1 burger	1040	76	30	265	29	2	6	60	1440
Cheddar Burger									
1 burger	890	62	25	235	29	2	6	51	1000
Kid's Cheeseburger									
1 burger	370	23	10	75	20	1	2	21	480
The Uno Burger									
1 burger	780	53	19	205	28	2	6	44	820

Chicken

Baked Stuffed Chicken									
1 serving	360	14	7	130	10	2	1	50	1420
Chicken Tikka Masala									
1 serving	550	21	6	115	52	5	13	42	1710
Herb-Rubbed Breast of Chicken									
1 serving	490	37	6	100	6	1	0	36	1360

Desserts

Bananas Foster									
1 serving	1280	64	36	185	163	4	129	16	530
Mini Bananas Foster									
1 serving	350	17	9	45	46	1	36	4	140

Food Serving size	Cal.	(g) Total Fat	(g) Sat. Fat	(mg) Chol.	(g) Carb.	(g) Fiber	(g) Sug.	(g) Prot.	(mg) Sod.
Salads									
Caesar Side Salad 1 salad	250	22	5	25	8	2	2	7	430
Classic Cobb Salad 1 salad	880	66	20	420	27	11	9	50	1940
House Side Salad 1 salad	90	5	1	0	10	2	3	2	95
Sides									
Red Bliss Mashed Potato 1 serving	270	14	3.5	5	34	3	3	4	650
Roasted Seasonal Vegetables 1 serving	80	4.5	0	0	10	3	5	2	160
Steamed Broccoli 1 serving	70	6	1	0	5	3	0	3	360
Steamed Seasonal Vegetables 1 serving	100	7	1.5	0	9	3	4	2	90
Whole Grain Brown Rice with Craisins 1 serving	180	6	0.5	0	32	1	4	3	100
Soup									
Chili 1 serving	410	54	6	45	54	10	10	21	1250
Cuban Black Bean & Lentil 1 serving	220	4.5	0	5	34	9	6	12	1230
Steak & Seafood									
Lemon Basil Salmon 1 serving	490	34	4.5	120	0	0	0	43	740
Top Sirloin Steak 8 oz	410	14	5	105	0	0	0	66	132
Thin Crust Pizza									
Gluten-Free Cheese Thin Crust Pizza 1 serving	870	32	11	40	124	5	11	27	1860

Food Serving size	Cal.	(g) Total Fat	(g) Sat. Fat	(mg) Chol.	(g) Carb.	(g) Fiber	(g) Sug.	(g) Prot.	(mg) Sod.
Gluten-Free Pepperoni Thin Crust Pizza									
13 oz	1010	45	16	70	124	5	11	32	2400
Gluten-Free Veggie Thin Crust Pizza									
16.2 oz	960	37	13	50	130	6	15	33	1990

Additional Gluten-Free Menu Items
(nutritional information was not available)

New York Strip Steak, Grilled Shrimp and Sirloin, Ice Cream Sundae

Wendy's®
[www.wendys.com]

Beverages

All Natural Lemonade									
1 serving	190	0	0	0	49	0	46	0	5
Barq's Root Beer									
small	180	0	0	0	50	0	50	0	40
Brewed Sweetened Iced Tea									
1 serving	110	0	0	0	29	0	28	0	10
Brewed Unsweetened Iced Tea									
1 serving	5	0	0	0	1	0	0	0	10
Caramel Apple Frosty Parfait (no granola)									
206g	340	8	4	25	60	1	47	7	140
Caramel Frosty Shake									
352g	650	14	9	50	121	0	97	10	310
Chocolate Frosty									
212g	300	8	5	30	49	0	42	7	140
Chocolate Frosty Shake									
342g	580	13	8	45	104	2	93	11	250

Wendy's® ingredient information is based on standard product formulations. Variations may occur due to differences in suppliers, ingredient substitutions, recipe revisions, product assembly at the restaurant level, and/or season of the year. Certain menu items may not be available at all locations. Temporary products are not included. This information is effective as of June 2012.

Visit www.wendys.com <http://www.wendys.com> for the most comprehensive and up-to-date information. © 2012 Oldemark LLC. Reprinted with permission. The Wendy's name, design and logo are registered trademarks of Oldemark LLC and are licensed to Wendy's International, Inc.

Food Serving size	Cal.	(g) Total Fat	(g) Sat. Fat	(mg) Chol.	(g) Carb.	(g) Fiber	(g) Sug.	(g) Prot.	(mg) Sod.
Coca-Cola small	160	0	0	0	44	0	44	0	0
Coffee small	0	0	0	0	0	0	0	0	0
Coffee Creamer 1 serving	20	2	1	10	0	0	0	0	10
Coke Zero small	0	0	0	0	0	0	0	0	5
Diet Coke small	0	0	0	0	0	0	0	0	15
Dr Pepper small	160	0	0	0	43	0	43	0	40
Fanta Orange small	180	0	0	0	49	0	49	0	25
Hi-C Flashin Fruit Punch small	170	0	0	0	46	0	46	0	15
Hot Tea small	0	0	0	0	1	0	0	0	0
Iced Tea small	0	0	0	0	1	0	0	0	0
Juicy Juice Apple Juice 1 serving	90	0	0	0	22	0	20	0	5
Minute Maid Light Lemonade 1 serving	5	0	0	0	1	0	0	0	5
Nestle Pure Life Bottled Water 1 bottle	0	0	0	0	0	0	0	0	0
Pibb Xtra 1 serving	160	0	0	0	43	0	43	0	25
Sprite 1 serving	160	0	0	0	43	0	43	0	35
Strawberry Frosty Shake 341g	550	13	8	45	99	1	90	9	170
TruMoo Lowfat Chocolate Milk 1 container	140	2.5	1.5	10	22	0	20	7	170

Food Serving size	Cal.	(g) Total Fat	(g) Sat. Fat	(mg) Chol.	(g) Carb.	(g) Fiber	(g) Sug.	(g) Prot.	(mg) Sod.
TruMoo Lowfat White Milk 1 container	100	2.5	1.5	10	12	0	11	8	125
Vanilla Bean Frosty Shake 347g	590	13	8	45	109	0	78	9	430
Vanilla Frosty 204g	280	7	4.5	30	47	0	40	7	135
Wild Berry Frosty Shake 1 serving	520	13	8	45	90	1	79	10	180
Wild Berry Lemonade small	230	0	0	0	58	1	54	0	10
Wild Berry Tea small	70	0	0	0	16	1	14	0	10

Condiments

Food Serving size	Cal.	(g) Total Fat	(g) Sat. Fat	(mg) Chol.	(g) Carb.	(g) Fiber	(g) Sug.	(g) Prot.	(mg) Sod.
American Cheese 1 slice	40	3.5	2	10	0	0	0	2	200
Buttery Best Spread 1 serving	50	5	1	0	0	0	0	0	95
Cheddar & Pepper Jack Cheese Blend 30g serving	120	9	6	30	1	0	0	7	230
Cheddar Cheese, Shredded 1 serving	70	6	3.5	15	1	0	0	4	110
Dill Pickles 3 slices	0	0	0	0	0	0	0	0	110
Guacamole 1 serving	90	9	1.5	0	5	3	0	1	200
Heinz Dip & Squeeze Ketchup 1 packet	10	0	0	0	3	0	2	0	95
Honey Mustard Sauce 1 serving	40	3.5	0	5	3	0	2	0	75
Hot Chili Seasoning Packet 1 packet	5	0	0	0	1	0	1	0	270
Lettuce 1 leaf	0	0	0	0	0	0	0	0	0

Food Serving size	Cal.	(g) Total Fat	(g) Sat. Fat	(mg) Chol.	(g) Carb.	(g) Fiber	(g) Sug.	(g) Prot.	(mg) Sod.
Mayonnaise 1 serving	50	5	1	5	0	0	0	0	30
Monterey Jack 1 serving	40	3.5	2	10	0	0	0	2	200
Mustard 1 serving	5	0	0	0	0	0	0	0	50
Natural Asiago Cheese 1 serving	50	4	2.5	15	1	0	0	3	100
Ranch Sauce 1 serving	40	4	0.5	5	1	0	0	0	55
Red Onion 2 rings	0	0	0	0	0	0	0	0	0
Reduced Fat Sour Cream 1 serving	45	3.5	2	10	2	0	1	1	50
Signature Sauce 1 serving	45	4.5	0.5	5	1	0	1	0	105
Tartar Sauce 1 serving	110	12	2	10	0	0	0	0	150
Tomato 1 slice	5	0	0	0	1	0	1	0	0

Meats

Food Serving size	Cal.	(g) Total Fat	(g) Sat. Fat	(mg) Chol.	(g) Carb.	(g) Fiber	(g) Sug.	(g) Prot.	(mg) Sod.
Applewood Smoked Bacon 1 strip	30	2.5	1	5	0	0	0	2	100
Hamburger Patty 1/4 lb	220	15	7	70	0	0	0	19	290
Ultimate Grilled Chicken Fillet 1 filet	130	1.5	0	90	3	0	0	27	470

Salads & Dressings

Food Serving size	Cal.	(g) Total Fat	(g) Sat. Fat	(mg) Chol.	(g) Carb.	(g) Fiber	(g) Sug.	(g) Prot.	(mg) Sod.
Apple Pecan Chicken Salad (no pecans) 1 serving	350	11	7	115	30	5	20	35	950
Avocado Ranch Dressing 1 serving	100	10	2	10	2	0	1	1	210

Food Serving size	Cal.	(g) Total Fat	(g) Sat. Fat	(mg) Chol.	(g) Carb.	(g) Fiber	(g) Sug.	(g) Prot.	(mg) Sod.
Baja Salad 1 serving	540	32	14	90	34	12	10	32	1600
BLT Cobb Salad 1 serving	460	25	11	290	10	3	5	47	1410
Caesar Side Salad (no croutons) 1 serving	60	3.5	2.5	10	5	2	2	4	115
Classic Ranch Dressing 1 serving	100	10	1.5	10	2	0	1	1	150
Creamy Red Jalapeno Dressing 1 serving	100	10	2	10	2	0	1	1	270
Fat Free French Dressing 1 serving	40	0	0	0	9	0	8	0	95
Garden Side Salad (no croutons) 1 serving	25	0	0	0	5	2	3	1	30
Italian Vinaigrette Dressing 1 serving	70	6	1	0	4	0	3	0	180
Lemon Garlic Caesar Dressing 1 serving	110	11	2	10	2	0	1	2	180
Light Classic Ranch Dressing 1 serving	50	4.5	1	10	2	0	1	1	150
Pomegranate Vinaigrette Dressing 1 serving	60	3	0	0	8	0	7	0	160
Seasoned Tortilla Strips 1 serving	80	4.5	1.5	0	11	1	0	1	105
Thousand Island Dressing 1 serving	160	15	2.5	15	5	0	4	0	290

Sides & Baked Potatoes

Food Serving size	Cal.	(g) Total Fat	(g) Sat. Fat	(mg) Chol.	(g) Carb.	(g) Fiber	(g) Sug.	(g) Prot.	(mg) Sod.
Apple Slices 1 serving	40	0	0	0	9	2	7	0	0
Bacon & Cheese Baked Potato 1 potato	580	25	12	65	67	7	5	21	1080
Broccoli & Cheese Baked Potato 1 potato	470	15	8	40	69	8	5	16	690

Food Serving size	Cal.	(g) Total Fat	(g) Sat. Fat	(mg) Chol.	(g) Carb.	(g) Fiber	(g) Sug.	(g) Prot.	(mg) Sod.
Cheese Baked Potato 1 potato	580	25	14	75	68	7	5	22	880
Chili small serving	210	6	2.5	40	21	6	6	17	880
Chili & Cheese Baked Potato 1 potato	660	27	15	90	76	10	7	28	1210
Plain Baked Potato avg. wgt. 10 oz	270	0	0	0	61	7	3	7	25
Sour Cream & Chives Baked Potato 1 potato	320	3.5	2	10	63	7	4	8	50

Restaurant Chains

Additional restaurants with gluten-free menu items include:

Arby's [www.arbys.com]

Austin Grill [www.austingrill.com]

BJ's Restaurant & Brewhouse [www.bjsrestaurants.com]

Biaggi's [www.biaggis.com]

Bonefish Grill [www.bonefishgrill.com]

Buca di Beppo [www.bucadibeppo.com]

Carino's Italian Restaurant [www.carinos.com]

Carrabba's Italian Grill [www.carrabbas.com/menu/gluten-free]

Charlie Brown's Steakhouse [www.charliebrowns.com]

Cheeseburger in Paradise [www.cheeseburgerinparadise.com]

Domino's Pizza [www.dominos.com]

Elephant Bar [www.elephantbar.com]

Fleming's Prime Steakhouse & Wine Bar [www.flemingssteakhouse.com]

Garlic Jim's [www.garlicjims.com]

Glory Days Grill [www.glorydaysgrill.com]

Godfather's Pizza [www.godfathers.com]

Hobee's California Restaurants [www.hobees.com]

Lee Roy Selmon's [www.leeroyselmons.com]

Legal Seafoods [www.legalseafoods.com]

Mellow Mushroom [www.mellowmushroom.com]

The Melting Pot [www.meltingpot.com]

Mighty Taco [www.mightytaco.com/gluten.php]

Mitchell's Fish Market Seafood Restaurant & Bar [www.mitchellsfishmarket.com]

Morton's, The Steakhouse [www.mortons.com]

Passport Pizza 'n' Ribs [www.passportpizza.com]

Pasta Pomadoro [www.pastapomodoro.com]

Pizza Fusion [www.pizzafusion.com]

Pizza Ranch [www.pizzaranch.com]

Redstone American Grill [www.redstonegrill.com]

Rusty Bucket Restaurant and Tavern [www.myrustybucket.com]

Shane's Rib Shack [www.shanesribshack.com]

Skyline Chili [www.skylinechili.com]

Wildfire Restaurant [www.wildfirerestaurant.com]

Winger's Bar & Grill [www.wingers.info]

Appendix

PRODUCT MANUFACTURERS

1-2-3 Gluten Free
125 Orange Tree Drive
Orange, OH 44022
Phone: (216) 378-9233
www.123glutenfree.com

8th Continent
Stremicks Heritage Foods
4002 Westminster Avenue
Santa Ana, CA 92703
Phone: (800) 247-6458
Company has an online e-mail
contact form
www.8thcontinent.com

505 Southwestern
(a division of Treasure Valley Food Group)
P.O. Box 7067
Boise, ID 83616
Phone: (800) 292-9900
Fax: (208) 383-0757
Email: contact@treasurevalley.com
www.505chile.com

Against the Grain Gourmet
22 Browne Court, Unit 119
Brattleboro, VT 05301
Phone: (802) 258-3838
Email:
info@againstthegraingourmet.com
www.againstthegraingourmet.com

Aidell's Sausage Company
2411 Baumann Avenue
San Lorenzo, CA 94580
Phone: (877) 243-3557
Email: info@aidells.com
www.aidells.com

Aleia's Gluten Free Bakery
4 Pin Oak Drive
Branford, CT 06405
Phone: (203) 488-5556
Email: contact@aleias.com
www.aleias.com

Amazing Grass
220 Newport Center Drive, Suite 22
Newport Beach, CA 92660
Phone: (866) 472-7711
Email: info@amazinggrass.com
www.amazinggrass.com

Amy's
P.O. Box 449
Petaluma, CA 94953
Phone: (707) 781-7535;
(707) 568-4500
Email: amy@amyskitchen.net
www.amys.com

**Ancient Harvest Quinoa /
Quinoa Corporation**
P.O. Box 279
Gardena, CA 90248-0279
Phone: (310) 217-8125
(8am-4pm PT)
Email: quinoacorp@quinoa.net
www.quinoa.net

Andean Dream, LLC.
P.O. Box 411404
Los Angeles, CA 90041
Phone: (310) 281-6036
Email: info@andeandream.com
www.andeandream.com

**Annie Chun's All Natural Asian
Cuisine**
P.O. Box 911170
Los Angeles, CA 90091
Phone: (866) 595-8917 (6am-3pm PT)
Email: info@anniechun.com
www.anniehun.com

Annie's
1610 Fifth Street
Berkeley, CA 94710
Phone: (510) 558-7500;
(800) 288-1089 (Consumer Relations)
www.annies.com

Applegate Farms
750 Rt. 202 South, Suite 300
Bridgewater, NJ 08807-5530
Phone: (866) 587-5858
(Mon-Fri, 8am-5pm ET)
Fax: (800) 358-8289
Email: help@applegate.com
www.applegatefarms.com

Arrowhead Mills
The Hain Celestial Group, Inc.
4600 Sleepytime Drive
Boulder, CO 80301
Phone: (800) 434-4246
(Mon-Fri, 9am-7pm ET)
www.arrowheadmills.com

Attune Foods
535 Pacific Avenue, 3rd Floor
San Francisco, CA 94133
Phone: (800) 641-4508
Toll-Free: (866) 972-6879
Email:
customerservice@worldpantry.com
www.attunefoods.com

Bakery on Main
375 Park Avenue
East Hartford, CT 06108
Phone: (860) 895-6622
Fax: 860-895-6624
Email: info@bakeryonmain.com
www.bakeryonmain.com

Barbara's Bakery, Inc.
300 Nickerson Road
Marlborough, MA 01752
Phone: (800) 343-0590
www.barbarasbakery.com

Bard's Beer
P.O. Box 24835
Minneapolis, MN 55424-0835
Phone: (877) 440-2337
Fax: (816) 222-0413
Email: info@bardsbeer.com
www.bardsbeer.com

Beanitos, Inc.
3006 Bee Caves Road (RM 2244)
Suite A-315
Austin, TX 78746
Phone: (512) 609-8017
Email: customers@Beanitos.com
or info@Beanitos.com
www.beanitos.com

Betty Crocker
P.O. Box 9452
Minneapolis, MN 55440
Phone: (800) 446-1898
(Mon-Fri, 7:30am-5:30pm CT)
Fax: (763) 764-8330
www.bettycrocker.com

Bhuja
1187 Wilmette Avenue, Suite 319
Wilmette, IL 60091
Phone: (847) 307-5216
Fax: (847) 441-3469
www.bhuja.com

Bigelow Teas
201 Black Rock Turnpike
Fairfield, CT 06825
Phone: (888) 244-3569
(Mon-Fri, 9am-5pm ET)
www.bigelowtea.com

BiProUSA
11000 West 78th Street, Suite 210
Eden Prairie, MN 55344
Phone: (877) 692-4776
Email: customerservice@biprousa.com
www.biprousa.com

Birkett Mills
P.O. Box 440
Penn Yan, NY 14527
Phone: (315) 536-3311
Fax: (315) 536-6740
Email: contact@thebirkettmills.com
www.thebirkettmills.com

Bisquick
P.O. Box 9452
Minneapolis, MN 55440
Phone: (800) 446-1898
(Mon-Fri, 7:30am-5:30pm CT)
Fax: (763) 764-8330
Company has an online email
contact form
www.bettycrocker.com

Blue Diamond
Phone: (800) 987-2329
Company has an online email
contact form
www.almondbreeze.com

Blue Diamond Almonds
Phone: (800) 987-2329
Company has an online
email contact form
www.bluediamond.com

Boar's Head
Phone: (800) 352-6277
www.boarshead.com

Bob's Red Mill
13521 SE Pheasant Court
Milwaukie, OR 97222
Phone: (503) 654-3215 or
(800) 349-2173
www.bobsredmill.com

BOLD Organic
Company has an online email
contact form
www.bold-organics.com

BOOST
Nestlé HealthCare Nutrition
Consumer & Product Support
445 State Street
Fremont, MI 49412
Phone: (800) 247-7893
(Mon-Sat, 8am-4:30pm CT)
www.boost.com

Bora Bora
1050 17th Street, Suite 1000
Denver, CO 80265
Phone: (888) 552-8926
Email: customerservice
@boraborafoods.com
www.boraborafoods.com

Boulder Canyon Natural Foods
Phone: (866) 890-1004
www.bouldercanyonfoods.com

Brown Cow Farm
3810 Delta Fair Blvd.
Antioch, CA 94509
Phone: (888) 429-5459
(Mon-Fri, 6am-3pm PT)
www.browncowfarm.com

Buddig Organic
950 West 175 Street
Homewood, IL 60430
Phone: (888) 633-5684
www.buddig.com

Bumble Bar Organic Sesame Bar
3808 North Sullivan Road
Building 12, Suite P
Spokane Valley, WA 99216
Phone: (509) 924-2080
Email: info@bumblebar.com
www.bumblebar.com

Campbell's Soup Company
1 Campbell Place
Camden, NJ 08103-1701
Phone: (800) 257-8443
(Mon-Fri, 9am-7pm ET)
www.campbellsoup.com

The Candy Tree
Bay C
2828 – 54 Avenue SE
Calgary, Alberta Canada
Phone: (800) 668-7677
Fax: (403) 272-9558
Email: info@thecandytree.ca
www.thecandytree.ca

Canyon Bakehouse
Company has an online email
contact form
www.canyonbakehouse.com

Cause You're Special, Inc.
P.O. Box 316
Phillips, WI 54555
Phone: (715) 339-6959
Fax: (603) 218-6374
Email: info@causeyourespecial.com
www.causeyourespecial.com

Celestial Seasonings
The Hain Celestial Group, Inc.
4600 Sleepytime Drive
Boulder, CO 80301
Phone: (800) 351-8175
(Mon-Fri, 7am-5pm MT)
www.celestialseasonings.com

Chatila's Bakery
The Breckinridge Plaza
254 North Broadway
Salem, NH 03079
Phone: (603) 898-5459
Toll-Free: (877) 619-5398
Fax: (603) 893-1586
Email:
customercare@chatilasbakery.com
Company has an online email
contact form
www.chatilasbakery.com

Chebe
1840 Lundberg Drive
Spirit Lake, IA 51360
Phone: (800) 217-9510
(Mon-Fri, 8am-5pm CT)
Company has an online email
contact form
www.chebe.com

Cherrybrook Kitchen
P.O. Box 335
Haverhill, MA 01831
Phone: (866) I-LUV-CBK
www.cherrybrookkitchen.com

Chex
General Mills, Inc.
P.O. Box 9452
Minneapolis, MN 55440
Phone: (800) 328-1144
(Mon-Fri, 7:30am-5:30pm CT)
Fax: (763) 764-8330
www.chex.com

Classico
Company has an online email
contact form
www.classico.com

Conrad Rice Mill
P.O. Box 10640
New Iberia, LA 70562-0640
Phone: (337) 364-7242
Fax: (337) 365-5806
Toll-Free: (800) 551-3245
www.conradricemill.com

Conte's Pasta
310 East Wheat Road
Vineland, NJ 08360
Phone: (856) 697-3400
Fax: (856) 697-1757
Toll-Free: (800) 211-6607
Email: customer_service
@contespasta.com
www.contespasta.com

Cravings Place LLC., The
1020 SE Paiute Way #1
Bend, OR 97701
Phone: (541) 388-2253
Fax: (541) 388-7553
Email: queenofthekitchen
@thecravingsplace.com
www.thecravingsplace.com

Crunchmaster
Phone: (800) 896-2396
www.crunchmaster.com

DeBoles
The Hain Celestial Group, Inc.
4600 Sleepytime Drive
Boulder, CO 80301
Phone: (800) 434-4246
(Mon-Fri, 9am-7pm ET)
www.deboles.com

Earth Balance
A division of GFA Brands, Inc.
7102 LaVista Place, Suite 200
Niwot, CO 80503
Phone: (201) 421-3970
www.earthbalancenatural.com

Earthbound Farm
1721 San Juan Highway
San Juan Bautista, CA 95045
Phone: (800) 690-3200
www.ebfarm.com

Eden Foods, Inc.
701 Tecumseh Road
Clinton, Michigan 49236
Phone: (888) 424-3336
(Mon-Fri, 8am-5:15pm)
(Toll-free US and Canada)
Email: info@edenfoods.com
www.edenfoods.com

Edward & Sons
*(product family encompasses
Edward & Sons, Native Forest,
Let's Do...Organic, The Wizards,
Premier Japan, Let's Do...,
and Road's End Organics)*
P.O. Box 1326
Carpinteria, CA 93014
Phone: (805) 684-8500
Fax: (805) 684-8220
www.edwardandsons.com

El's Kitchen
P.O. Box 1014
Weston, CT 06883
Phone: (203) 454-7013
Email: glutenfree@elskitchen.com
www.elskitchen.com

**Elisabeth Hasselbeck's NoGii
No Gluten Bars**
Email: info@sbibrands.com
www.nogiidiet.com

Ella's Kitchen
Phone: (800) 685-7799
www.ellaskitchen.com

Ener-G Foods, Inc.
5960 First Avenue South
Seattle, WA 98124-5787
Phone: (206) 767-3928
Toll-Free: (800) 331-5222
Fax: (206) 764-3398
Email: customerservice@ener-g.com
www.ener-g.com

Enjoy Life Foods
3810 River Road
Schiller Park, IL 60176
Phone: (847) 260-0300
Fax: (847) 260-0306
www.enjoylifefoods.com

Ensure
Phone: (800) 986-8501
www.ensure.com

Everybody Eats, Inc.
294 Third Avenue
Brooklyn, NY 11215
Phone: (718) 369-7444
www.everybodyeats-inc.com

FAGE USA Dairy Industry Inc.
Customer Relations
1 Opportunity Drive
Johnstown Industrial Park
Johnstown, NY 12095
Phone: (866) 962-5912
(Mon-Fri, 9am-5pm ET)
Fax: (518) 762-5918
www.fageusa.com

Feel Good Foods
11706 Darlington Avenue, Suite 102
Los Angeles, CA 90049
Phone: (800) 638-8949
Email: info@feelgf.com
www.feel-good-foods.com

Food for Life
www.foodforlife.com

Food Should Taste Good
P.O. Box 9452
Minneapolis, MN 55440
Phone: (877) 588-3784
(Mon-Fri, 7:30am-5:30pm CT)
www.foodshouldtastegood.com

French Meadow Bakery
127 Airport Road
St. Simons Island, GA 31522
Company has an online email
contact form
www.frenchmeadow.com

Friedas
4465 Corporate Center Drive
Los Alamitos, CA 90720
Phone: (800) 241-1771
www.friedas.com

Frito-Lay
P.O. Box 660634
Dallas, TX 75266-0634
Phone: (800) 352-4477
(Mon-Fri, 9am-4:30pm CT)
www.fritolay.com

Full Flavor Foods
Company has an online
email contact form
www.forfullflavor.com

Galaxy Nutritional Foods
Company has an online
email contact form
www.galaxyfoods.com

Garden Lites
165-35 145th Drive
Jamaica, NY 11434
Phone: (718) 439-0200, ext. 627
Email: info@garden-lites.com
www.garden-lites.com

General Mills, Inc.
P.O. Box 9452
Minneapolis, MN 55440
Phone: (800) 248-7310
(Mon-Fri, 7:30am-5:30pm CT)
www.generalmills.com
www.glutenfreely.com

Get Fresh Bakehouse
4 Edison Place
Fairfield, NJ 07004
Phone: (855) 438-3774
Email: info@getfreshbakehouse.com
www.getfreshbakehouse.com

GFL Foods, Inc.
2012 Sans Avenue
Merrick, NY 11566
Phone: (516) 223-1865
Email: info@gflfoods.com
www.gflfoods.com
www.glutenfreepitas.com

Gilbert's Gourmet Goodies
Phone: (203) 733-8217
Email: liz@gilbertsgourmetgoodies.com
Company has an online
email contact form
www.gilbertsgourmetgoodies.com

Gillian's Foods
82 Sanderson Avenue
Lynn, MA 01902
Phone: (781) 586-0086
www.gilliansfoodsglutenfree.com

Gluten Free Café
The Hain Celestial Group, Inc.
4600 Sleepytime Drive
Boulder, CO 80301
Phone: (800) 434-4246
(Mon-Fri, 9am-7pm ET)
www.myglutenfreecafe.com

GlutenFreeda
P.O. Box 1364
Glenwood Springs, CO 81602-1364
Phone: (970) 319-0382
www.glutenfreeda.com

Gluten Free Naturals Products
P.O. Box 1626
Cranford, NJ 07016
Phone: (866) 761-6147
Email: info@gfnfoods.com
www.gfnfoods.com
www.glutenfreenaturals.com

Glutino Food Group
115 West Century Road, Suite 260
Paramus, NJ 07652
Phone: (201) 421-3970
Toll-Free: (800) 363-3438
Fax: (201) 568-6374
www.glutino.com

Goldbaum's Natural Foods
54 Freeman Street
Newark, NJ 07105
Phone: (973) 854-0688
Fax: (973) 854-0689
Email: info@goldbaums.com
www.goldbaums.com

Good Karma
755 17th Street
Prairie du Sac, WI 53578
Phone: (800) 550-6731
Fax: (608) 370-7374
www.GoodKarmaFoods.com

**Hain Celestial Group, Inc. /
Hain Pure Foods**
The Hain Celestial Group, Inc.
4600 Sleepytime Drive
Boulder, CO 80301
(800) 434-4246
(Mon-Fri, 9am-7pm ET)
www.hain-celestial.com

**Hansen Beverage Company /
Hansen's Natural**
550 Monica Circle, Suite 201
Corona, CA 92880
Phone: (800) 426-7367
(Mon-Fri, 9am-5pm)
Email: info@hansens.com
www.hansens.com

Hodgson Mill, Inc.
1100 Stevens Avenue
Effingham, IL 62401
Phone: (800) 347-0105
Fax: 217-347-0198
Email:
CustomerService@HodgsonMill.com
www.hodgsonmill.com

Homestead Gluten Free, LLC
P.O. Box 896
Nanuet, NY 10954-0896
Phone: (845) 709-9287
Email: info@HomesteadGlutenFree.com
www.homesteadglutenfree.com

Honest Tea/Honest Ade
4827 Bethesda Avenue
Bethesda, MD 20814
Phone: (301) 652-3556 or
(800) 865-4736
www.honestea.com

Hormel Foods Corporation
1 Hormel Place, Austin, MN 55912
Phone: (800) 523-4635
(Mon-Fri, 8am-4pm CT;
summer hours vary)
Company has an online
email contact form
www.hormelnatural.com

I.M. Healthy,
The SoyNut Butter Company
4220 Commercial Way
Glenview, IL 60025
Phone: (800) 288-1012
Fax: (847) 635-6801
Company has an online
email contact form
www.soynutbutter.com

Ian's Natural Foods
190 Fountain Street
Framingham, MA 01702
Phone: (800) 543-6637
Fax: (508) 283-1175
Email: customerservice
@iansnaturalfoods.com
www.iansnaturalfoods.com

Idahoan Foods, LLC
357 Constitution Way
Idaho Falls, ID 83402-3538
Phone: (208) 754-4686
Company has an online
email contact form
www.idahoan.com

Joan's GF Great Bakes
90 East Merrick Road
Freeport, NY 11520
Phone: (516) 804-5600
Fax: (516) 804-5602
Email: gfgreatbakes@yahoo.com
www.gfgreatbakes.com

Jones Dairy Farms
800 Jones Avenue
P.O. Box 808
Port Atkinson, WI 53538-0808
Phone: (800) 563-1004
www.jonesdairyfarm.com

Jo-sefs Gluten Free
8 Hoover Street
Inwood, NY 11096
Phone: (516) 837-8700
Fax: (516) 837-8737
Email: info@josefsglutenfree.com
www.josefsglutenfree.com

Jovial Foods, Inc.
5 Tyler Drive
North Franklin, CT 06254
Phone: (877) 642-0644
(Mon-Fri, 8:30am-4:30pm ET)
Company has an online
email contact form
www.jovialfoods.com

Justin's
2434 30th Street
Boulder, CO 80301
Phone: (303) 449-9559
Fax: (303) 442-0881
Email: comments@justinsnutbutter.com
http://justinsnutbutter.com

Kay's Naturals, Inc.
P.O. Box 669
100 First Ave, SE
Clara City, MN 56222
Phone: (320) 847-3220
Fax: (320) 847-3110
www.kaysnaturals.com

Kettle Cuisine
270 Second Street
Chelsea, MA 02150
Phone: (617) 884-1219
Email: sales@kettlecuisine.com
www.kettlecuisine.com

KIND Healthy Snacks
Phone: (855) 884-5463
Email:
customerservice@kindsnacks.com
www.kindsnacks.com

King Arthur Flour
135 US Route 5 South
Norwich, VT 05055
Phone: (800) 827-6836 (Mon-Fri,
8am-9pm; Sat & Sun, 9am-5pm ET)
Email:
customercare@kingarthurflour.com
www.kingarthurflour.com

Kinnikinnick Foods Inc.
10940-120 Street
Edmonton, Alberta
Canada T5H 3P7
Toll-Free: (877) 503-4466
Local: (780) 424-2900
(Mon-Fri, 9am-4:30pm)
Fax: (780) 421-0456
Email: info@kinnikinnick.com
www.kinnikinnick.com

The Kitchen Table Baker's
41 Princeton Drive
Syosset, NY 11793
Phone: (516) 931-5113
Toll Free: (800) 486-4582
Fax: (516) 932-5467
Email: Info@KitchenTableBakers.com
www.kitchentablebakers.com

Kozy Shack
83 Ludy Street
Hicksville, NY 11801
Company has an online
email contact form
www.kozyshack.com

La Tortilla Factory
Phone: (800) 446-1516
Company has an online
email contact form
www.latortillafactory.com

Larabar
P.O. Box 18932
Denver, CO 80218
Phone: (720) 945-1155
Customer Feedback: (800) 543-2147
Fax: (720) 941-1158
Company has an online
email contact form
www.larabar.com

Lifeway Foods, Inc.
6431 West Oakton Street
Morton Grove, IL 60053
Phone: (877) 281-3874
Fax: (847) 967-6558
Company has an online
email contact form
www.lifeway.net

Lisanatti Foods
1815 Red Soils Court
Oregon City, OR 97045
Toll-Free: (866) 864-3922
Local: (503) 652-1988
Fax: (503) 653-1979
www.lisanatti.com

Little Soya
Company has an online
email contact form
www.littlesoya.com

Living Harvest Foods, Inc.
P.O. Box 1131
Weston, CT 06883
Toll-Free: (888) 690-3958
(Mon-Wed, 8am-5pm PT)
Email:
customerservice@livingharvest.com
www.livingharvest.com

Lotus Foods, Inc.
5210 Wall Avenue
Richmond, CA 94804
Phone: (510) 525-3137
Toll-Free: (866) 972-6879
Email: info@lotusfoods.com
customerservice@worldpantry.com

Lucini
Phone: (888) 558-2464
Email: info@lucini.com
www.lucini.com

Lucy's Gluten Free
930 Denison Avenue, Suite 101-A
Norfolk, VA 23513
Phone: (757) 233-9495
Email: info@drlucys.com
www.drlucys.com

Luna Protein Bars
Clif Bar & Company
1451 66th Street
Emeryville, CA 94608-1004
Phone: (800) 586-2227
(Mon-Fri, 8am-5pm PT)
www.lunabar.com

Lundberg Family Farms
5311 Midway
P.O. Box 369
Richvale, CA 95974
Phone: (530) 538-3500
(Mon-Fri, 8:30am-5pm PT)
Fax: (530) 882-4500
Email: info@lundberg.com
www.lundberg.com

Maple Grove Farms
Company has an online
email contact form
www.maplegrove.com

Maplegrove Gluten Free Foods
(Pastariso, Pastato, Celifibr)
13112 Santa Ana Avenue, Unit A2-A3
Fontana, CA 92337
Phone: (909) 823-8230
Fax: (909) 823-2708
Company has an online
email contact form
www.maplegrovefoods.com

MaraNatha Nut Butters
Company has an online
email contact form
www.maranathafoods.com

Mariani Premium Fruit
500 Crocker Drive
Vacaville, CA 95688-8706
Phone: (707) 452-2800
Fax: (707) 452-2973
Email: productinfo@mariani.com
www.marianifruit.com

Mary's Gone Crackers
P.O. Box 965
Gridley, CA 95948
Phone: (888) 258-1250
Email: info@marysgonecrackers.com
www.marysgonecrackers.com

G.L. Mezzetta, Inc.
105 Mezzetta Court
American Canyon, CA 94503
Phone: (707) 648-1050
Toll-Free: (800) 941-7044
(Mon-Fri, 7:30am-4:30pm PT)
Fax: (707) 648-1060
www.mezzetta.com

Mrs. Leepers
Company has an online
email contact form
www.mrsleepers.com

Nana's Cookies Company
4901 Morena Blvd., Suite 401
San Diego, CA 92117
Phone: (800) 836-7534
Company has an online
email contact form
www.nanascookiecompany.com

Nature Factor
(See Edward & Sons)

Nature's Path Foods
9100 Van Horne Way
Richmond, BC Canada V6X 1W3
Toll-Free: (888) 808-9505
(Mon-Fri, 12pm-8pm ET)
www.naturespath.com

Nestlé USA
Phone: (800) 225-2270
(Mon-Fri, 8am-8pm ET)
Company has an online
email contact form
www.nestleusa.com

Newman's Own
Online contact form
www.newmansown.com

Noosa Yoghurt
P.O. Box 403
Bellvue, CO 80512
Phone: (970) 493-0949
Email: info@noosayoghurt.com
www.noosayoghurt.com

The Organic Bistro
1882 Mcgaw Avenue, Suite A
Irvine, CA 92614
Toll-Free: (866) 328-8638
Fax: (949) 648-5943
Email: contactus@theorganicbistro.com
www.theorganicbistro.com

Orgran (Australia)
47-53 Aster Avenue
Carrum Downs
VICTORIA 3201 AUSTRALIA
Phone: +61 3 9776 9044
Fax: +61 3 9776 9055
Company has an online
email contact form
www.orgran.com

Pace
Campbell Soup Company
1 Campbell Place
Camden, NJ 08103-1701
Phone: (800) 257-8443
(Mon-Fri, 9am-7pm ET)
www.pacefoods.com

Pacific Foods of Oregon
19480 SW 97th Avenue
Tualatin, OR 97062
Phone: (503) 692-9666
Fax: (503) 692-9610
Consumer inquiries: (503) 924-4570
www.pacificfoods.com

Pamela's Products, Inc.
1 Carousel Lane, Suite D
Ukiah, CA 95482
Phone: (707) 462-6605
Fax: (707) 462-6642
Email: info@pamelasproducts.com
www.pamelasproducts.com

Perdue
(800) 473-7383
(Mon-Fri, 9:30am-6pm ET)
www.perdue.com

Pirate Brands
100 Roslyn Avenue
Sea Cliff, NY 11579
Phone: (516) 656-4545
Email: info@piratebrands.com
www.piratebrands.com

PopChips
550 Montgomery Street, Suite 925
San Francisco, CA 94111
Phone: (866) 217-9327
Email: snackers@popchips.com
www.popchips.com

Popcorn Indiana
1 Cedar Lane
Englewood, NJ 07631
Phone: (800) 707-4444
(Mon-Fri, 9am-4:30pm ET)
www.popcornindiana.com

Post Cereals
275 Cliff Street
Battle Creek, MI 49014
Phone: (800) 431-7678
(Mon-Fri, 9am-5pm ET)
Company has an online
email contact form
www.postfoods.com

Power of Fruit
www.poweroffruit.com

Dr. Praeger's Sensible Foods
9 Boumar Place
Elmwood Park, NJ 07407
Phone: (877) 772-3437 or
(201) 703-1300
www.drpraegers.com

Prego
(See Campbell's Soup Company)

Progresso
General Mills, Inc.
P.O. Box 9452
Minneapolis, MN 55440
Phone: (800) 200-9377
(Mon-Fri, 7:30am-5:30pm CT)
Fax: (763) 764-8330
Company has an online
email contact form
www.progresso.com

Promax Energy Bar
100 Bayview Circle, Suite 200
Newport Beach, CA 92660
Phone: (888) 728-8962
Fax: (949) 502-4847
www.promaxnutrition.com

Purefit Nutrition Bars
216 Technology, Suite E
Irvine, CA 92618
Phone: (866) 787-3348 or
(949) 679-7997
Fax: (949) 679-7998
Email: info@purefit.com
www.purefit.com

The Quaker Oats Company
P.O. Box 049003
Chicago, IL 60604-9003
Phone: (800) 367-6287
(Mon-Fri, 7:30am-5pm CT)
www.quakeroats.com

Quest Nutrition
Phone: (888) 212-0601
Company has an online
email contact form
www.questproteinbar.com

The Really Great Food Company
P.O. Box 2239
St. James, NY 11780
Phone: (800) 593-5377
General Inquiries: (631) 361-3553
Fax: (631) 361-6920
Email: support@reallygreatfood.com
www.reallygreatfood.com

Redbridge Beer
www.redbridgebeer.com

Rice Krispies
Phone: (800) 962-1413
www.ricekrispies.com

Riceworks Gourmet Brown Rice Chips
Phone: (888) GREAT-CHIPS
www.riceworks.com

Rise Bar
16752 Millikan Avenue
Irvine, CA 92606
Phone: (800) 440-6476
Fax: (949) 407-6425
Email: sales@risebar.com
www.risebar.com

Road's End Organics
(See Edward & Sons)

Rudi's Gluten Free Bakery
3300 Walnut Street, Unit C
Boulder, CO 80301
Phone: (877) 293-0876 or
(303) 447-0495
Fax: (303) 447-0516
www.rudisglutenfree.com

RW Garcia Premium Corn-Based Snacks
521 Parrott Street
San Jose, CA 95112
Phone: (408) 287-4616
Company has an online
email contact form
www.rwgarcia.com

Sabra
P.O. Box 660634
Dallas, TX 75266-0634
Phone: (888) 957-2272
(Mon-Fri, 9am-4:30pm CT)
Company has an online
email contact form
www.sabra.com

San-J International Inc.
2880 Sprouse Drive
Richmond, VA 23231
Phone: (804) 226-8333
Toll-Free: (800) 446-5500
Fax: (804) 226-8383
Email: info@san-j.com
www.san-j.com

Savory Choice
2121 South El Camino Real,
Suite C-210
San Mateo, CA 94403
Toll Free: (866) 472-8679
Phone: (650) 638-1024
Fax: (650) 638-1178
Email: info@savorychoice.com
www.savorychoice.com

Schar
1050 Wall Street West, Suite 370
Lyndhurst, NJ 07071
Email: info@schar.com
www.schar.com

Seeds of Change
P.O. Box 4908
Rancho Dominguez, CA 90220
Phone: (888) 762-4240
(24 hours a day, 7 days a week)
www.seedsofchange.com

**Sharkies Organic Fruit Chews /
Sharkies Kids**
401 York Avenue
Duryea, PA 18642
Phone: (800) 489-9149
Email: web@sharkiesinc.com
www.sharkiesinc.com

Simply Fruit Roll-Up
(See General Mills)

Simply Organic Foods
Phone: (800) 437-3301
(Mon-Fri, 7am-6pm CT)
Fax: (800) 717-4372
Email:
customercare@simplyorganic.com
www.simpleorganic.com

Smart Balance, Inc.
115 West Century Road, Suite 260
Paramus, NJ 07652-1432
Phone: (201) 421-3970
Company has an online
email contact form
www.smartbalance.com

Snapple
Phone: (800) 696-5891
Company has an online
email contact form
www.snapple.com

Snikiddy
Phone: (866) 892-5365
Company has an online
email contact form
www.snikiddy.com

Snyder's of Hanover
Company has an online
email contact form
www.snydersofhanover.com

So Delicious
Turtle Mountain, LLC
P.O. Box 21938
Eugene, OR 97402
Phone: (866) 388-7853
(Mon-Fri, 8am-5pm PT)
Fax: (541) 388-9401
www.sodeliciousdairyfree.com

Soyjoy Natural Fruit & Soy Bar
P.O. Box 9606
Mission Hills, CA 91346
Phone: (888) 676-9569
Company has an online
email contact form
www.soyjoy.com

Stonyfield Organic
10 Burton Drive
Londonderry, NH 03053
Phone: (800) 776-2697
(Mon-Fri, 9am-6pm ET)
Company has an online
email contact form
www.stonyfield.com

Sunbutter Sunflower Seed Spread
Red River Commodities, Inc.
501 42nd Street
North Fargo, ND 58102
Phone: (800) 437-5539
Fax: (701) 282-5325
Email: info@sunbutter.com
www.sunbutter.com

Svelte Energy Protein Drinks
Phone: (877) 941-9311
(Mon-Fri, 8am-5pm PT)
Email: contactus@sveltebrand.com
www.sveltebrand.com

Swanson
Phone: (800) 442-7684
Company has an online
email contact form
www.swansonbroth.com

Tasty Bite
c/o WorldPantry.com, Inc.
1192 Illinois Street
San Francisco, CA 94107
Toll-Free: (866) 972-6879
Fax: (415) 401-0087
www.tastybite.com

Thai Kitchen
Simply Asia Foods, LLC.
P.O. Box 13242
Berkeley, CA 94712-4242
Phone: (800) 967-8424
Company has an online
email contact form
www.thaikitchen.com

Thumann's
670 Dell Road
Carlstadt, NJ 07072
Phone: (201) 935-3636
Email:
customer.service@thumanns.com
www.thumanns.com

Tinkyada Gluten Free
120 Melford Drive, Unit 8
Scarborough, Ontario, Canada
M1B 2X5
Phone: (416) 609-0016
Fax: (416) 609-1316
Email: iris@tinkyada.com
www.tinkyada.com

Udi's Gluten Free
12000 East 47th Avenue, Suite 400
Denver, CO 80239
Phone: (303) 657-6366
Email: mail@udisglutenfree.com
www.udisglutenfree.com

V8 V-Fusion/V8 Splash
Company has an online
email contact form
www.v8juice.com

Van's Natural Foods
3285 East Vernon Avenue
Vernon, CA 90058
Phone: (323) 585-8923
Fax: (323) 585-4084
Email: info@vansfoods.com
Company has an online
email contact form
www.vansfoods.com

Vitacoco
Company has an online
email contact form
www.vitacoco.com

Welch's
Phone: (800) 340-6870
(Mon-Fri, 9am-4pm ET)
Company has an online
email contact form
www.welchs.com

Wellaby's Gluten Free
a subsidiary of
InterNatural Foods
1455 Broad Street, 4th Floor
Bloomfield, NJ 07003
Phone: (973) 338-1499
Fax: (973) 338-1485
Email: info@worldfiner.com
www.wellabys.com
www.internaturalfoods.com

Wholesome Sweeteners
8016 Highway 90-A
Sugar Land, TX 77478
Phone: (800) 680-1896
Fax: (281) 275-3170
Email: CS@OrganicSugars.biz
www.wholesomesweetners.com

Wholly Guacamole
Company has an online
email contact form
www.eatwholly.com

The Wizard's Organic
(See Edward & Sons)

Woodchuck Hard Cider
The Woodchuck Cidery
153 Pond Lane
Middlebury, VT 05753
Phone: (802) 388-0700
Company has an online
email contact form
www.woodchuck.com

Yoplait
General Mills, Inc.
P.O. Box 9452
Minneapolis, MN 55440
Phone: (800) 248-7310
(Mon-Fri, 7:30am-5:30pm CT)
Fax: (763) 764-8330
www.yoplait.com

ZenSoy
Company has an online
email contact form
www.zensoy.com

WHERE TO FIND GLUTEN-FREE PRODUCTS

NORTH AMERICAN SUPERMARKETS

Bashas
www.bashas.com
Barbara Ruhs, MS, RD, LDN oversees a gluten-free program that includes a list of gluten-free products, shelf tags, and Eat Smart Nutrition Card on gluten-free eating.

Dierberg's Markets
www.dierbergs.com
Find a list of gluten-free products and recipes and look for gluten-free shelf tags.

Fred Meyer
www.fredmeyer.com
Find a gluten-free section under the Healthy Living tag that provides a gluten-free product list, recipes, a gluten-free guide and frequently asked questions.

Giant Eagle
www.gianteagle.com
Access a list of gluten-free products.

Hannaford
www.hannaford.com
The Hannaford website provides a brochure that lists the gluten-free items for sale in their stores along with gluten-free recipes.

HEB/Central Market
www.heb.com
Look for a gluten-free product list and gluten-free shelf tags. HEB also develops gluten-free products.

Hy-Vee
www.hy-vee.com
Provides a downloadable list of gluten-free foods as well as gluten-free recipes.

Ingles
www.ingles-markets.com
Leah McGrath, MS, RD provides gluten-free support in the form of a gluten-free product list, gluten-free fairs and presentations, and an Ask Leah feature.

Jewell-Osco
www.jewelosco.com
Create a shopping list with their Gluten-Free Food Finder.

Kroger's Supermarkets

On the top of the home page of each of the Kroger supermarkets, *follow the "Pharmacy and Health" link* for a downloadable list of gluten-free products sold in their stores. Kroger's registered dietitians can be reached at (866) 632-6900.

Kroger
www.kroger.com

Fred Meyer
www.fredmeyer.com

Ralphs
www.ralphs.com

King Soopers
www.kingsoopers.com

Dillons
www.dillons.com

Quality Food Centers
www.qfc.com

City Market
www.citymarket.com

Owen's Market
www.owensmarket.com

Jay C Foods
www.jaycfoods.com

Gerbes
www.gerbes.com

Lowes Food Stores

www.lowesfoods.com
Cindy Silver, MS, RD, LDN, corporate dietitian, developed gluten-free shelf talkers and provides a list of private label gluten-free foods.

Meijer

www.meijermealbox.com
Shari Steinbach, MS, RD, leads a team of dietitians who provide gluten-free resources along with a gluten-free list of available products.

Publix

www.publix.com/rightfoods
The Publix list of gluten-free items is available online.

Safeway

Provides gluten-free shelf tags.

Safeway
www.safeway.com

Randalls
www.randalls.com

Tom Thumb
www.tomthumb.com

Genuardi's
www.genuardis.com

Carrs
www.carrsqc.com

Shaws

www.shaws.com
Utilize their Gluten-Free Food Finder and find tips for gluten-free baking.

Shoprite

www.shoprite.com
Provides a list of gluten-free items and displays gluten-free shelf tags. Contact Natalie Menza, RD, corporate dietitian with questions.

Stop and Shop
www.stopandshop.com
Look for gluten-free shelf tags.

Trader Joe's
www.traderjoes.com
Offers a downloadable product list of their gluten-free items.

United & Market Street
www.marketstreetunited.com
Robin Hawkins, MS, RD, LD leads gluten-free tours. Find gluten-free shelf tags and a dedicated gluten-free aisle along with a gluten-free product list and guide.

Wegmans
www.wegmans.com
Wegmans' team of dietitians led by Jane Andrews, MS, RD, provides gluten-free shelf tags, a list of gluten-free products, a Shopping Gluten-Free with Wegmans' brochure, a Gluten-Free with Ease video, and a dedicated gluten-free aisle.

Whole Foods
Provides store-specific lists of gluten-free items.
www.wholefoodsmarkets.com

OUTSIDE NORTH AMERICA

Sainsbury's (U.K.)
www.sainsburys.co.uk
In addition to a list of gluten-free products, find gluten-free recipes and a gluten-free diet plan.

Delhaize (Belgium)
www.delhaize.be
Find a gluten-free product section and an assortment of gluten-free specialty foods. A list of gluten-free items (in French) is available on their website.

www.GlutenFree.co.il (Israel)
This is the largest store in Israel for Kosher gluten-free products. They ship worldwide.

GLUTEN-FREE PRODUCTS BY MAIL

The Gluten-Free Mall
www.celiac.com/glutenfreemall
Offers a wide selection of gluten-free, wheat-free, casein-free and other allergy-related health foods and special dietary products.

GlutenFree.com
www.glutenfree.com
Founded by professional chef and food writer Beth Hillson, this site offers not only gluten-free groceries but also ideas to help readers thrive on a gluten-free diet.

Free From Market
www.freefrommarket.com
This specialty food store has an extensive collection of close to 3,000 gluten-free items.

SafelyGlutenFree
www.safelyglutenfree.com
Visit this site to shop and browse for recipes, baking tips, and articles.

RESOURCES / ORGANIZATIONS

NATIONAL SUPPORT GROUPS

Academy of Nutrition and Dietetics

Headquarters
120 South Riverside Plaza, Suite 2000
Chicago, Illinois 60606-6995
Phone: (800) 877-1600
Phone: (312) 899-0040

Washington, D.C. Office
Academy of Nutrition and Dietetics
1120 Connecticut Avenue NW,
Suite 480
Washington, D.C. 20036
Phone: (800) 877-0877
Phone: (202) 775-8277
www.eatright.org

American Celiac Disease Alliance

2504 Duxbury Place
Alexandria, VA 22308
Phone: (703) 622-3331
Email: info@americanceliac.org
www.americanceliac.org

Canadian Celiac Association

5025 Orbitor Drive
Building 1, Suite 400
Mississauga, ON, L4W 4Y5
Phone: (905) 507-6208
Toll-Free: (800) 363-7296
Email: info@celiac.ca
www.celiac.ca

Celiac Disease Awareness Campaign of the National Institutes of Health

c/o National Digestive Diseases
Information Clearinghouse
2 Information Way
Bethesda, MD 20892-3570
Phone: (800) 891-5389
Fax: (703) 738-4929
Email: celiac@info.niddk.nih.gov
www.celiac.nih.gov

Celiac Disease Center at Columbia University

Harkness Pavilion
180 Fort Washington Avenue,
Suite 934
New York, NY 10032
Phone: (212) 342-4529
Fax: (212) 342-0447
Email: celiac@columbia.edu
www.celiacdiseasecenter.org

Celiac Disease Foundation

20350 Ventura Blvd, Suite 240
Woodland Hills CA 91364
Phone: (818) 716-1513
Fax: (818) 267-5577
www.celiac.org

Celiac Sprue Association/USA

1941 South 42nd Street, Suite 522
Omaha, NE 68105
Phone: (402) 558-0600
(Mon-Fri, 9am-4pm CT)
www.csaceliacs.org

Children's Digestive Health and Nutrition Foundation (CDHNF)
1501 Bethlehem Pike
P.O. Box 6
Flourtown, PA 19031
Phone: (215) 233-0808
Email: cdhnf@cdhnf.org
https://www.cdhnf.org

Gluten Intolerance Group
31214 124th Avenue SE
Auburn, WA 98092
Phone: (253) 833-6655
Fax: (253) 833-6675
www.gluten.net

Kids with Food Allergies, Inc.
73 Old Dublin Pike, Suite 10, #163
Doylestown, PA 18901
Phone: (215) 230-5394
Fax: (215) 340-7674
www.KidsWithFoodAllergies.org

National Foundation for Celiac Awareness (NFCA)
124 South Maple Street
Ambler, PA 19002
Phone: (215) 325-1306
Fax: (215) 643-1707
Mailing Address:
P.O. Box 544
Ambler, PA 19002-0544
www.celiacawareness.org

North American Society for Pediatric Gastroenterology, Hepatology and Nutrition (NASPGHAN) / NASPGHAN Foundation for Children's Digestive Health & Nutrition
P.O. Box 6
Flourtown, PA 19031
Phone: (215) 233-0808
Fax: (215) 233-3918
Email: naspghan@naspghan.org
www.naspghan.org

The University of Maryland School of Medicine Center for Celiac Research
20 Penn Street, Room S303B
Baltimore, MD 21201
Phone: (410) 706-5516
Email:
celiaccenter@peds.umaryland.edu
www.celiaccenter.org

Celiac Disease and Gluten-free Resource
www.celiac.com

Celiac Frequently Asked Questions (FAQ)
www.enabling.org/ia/celiac/faq.html

Gluten-Free On the Go
www.glutenfreeonthego.com

Gluten-Free Passport
www.glutenfreepassport.com

Gluten-Free Restaurant Awareness Program
www.glutenfreerestaurants.org

National Institutes of Health
http://digestive.niddk.nih.gov/ddiseases/pubs/celiac

R.O.C.K. (Raising Our Celiac Kids)
www.celiackids.com

University of Chicago, Celiac Disease Program
http://www.uchospitals.edu/specialties/celiac/index.php

Easy, Gluten-Free
Expert Nutrition Advice with More than 100 Recipes
by Tricia Thompson MS, RD, and Marlisa Brown
http://www.glutenfreeeasy.com

Gluten-Free Diet
A Comprehensive Resource Guide
by Shelley Case, B.Sc., RD
www.glutenfreediet.ca

Gluten-Free Friends
An Activity Book for Kids
by Nancy Patin Falini, MA, RD, LDN
www.amazon.com

Gluten-Free, Hassle Free
A Simple, Sane, Dietitian-Approved Program for Eating Your Way Back to Health
by Marlisa Brown, MS, RD, CDE, CDN
http://www.glutenfreeeasy.com

Gluten-Free Living
National Newsletter for People with Gluten Sensitivity
www.glutenfreeliving.com

Gluten-Free Online Cooking Magazine
www.glutenfreeda.com

Living Without Magazine
www.livingwithout.com

Your Guide to Healthful Eating and Wise Food Shopping

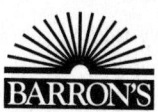

"... a comprehensive reference ... with tips and knowledge to keep in mind when dining out ... a much recommended read."
—*The Midwest Book Review*

Quick Check Food Facts
Third Edition

This pocket guide is packed with U.S. Department of Agriculture charts listing nutrient values of every food type under these headings:

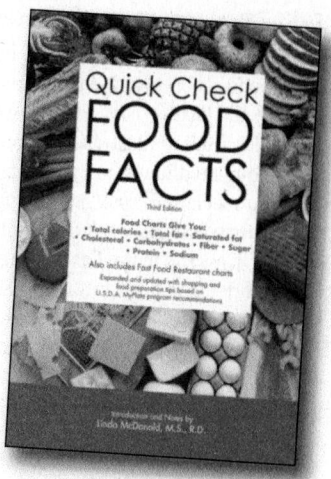

- Calories • Total Fat • Saturated Fat
- Cholesterol • Carbohydrates • Fiber
- Sugar • Protein • Sodium

You'll also find nutritional values for restaurant foods plus tips for grocery shopping and preparing foods, based on the U.S.D.A. ChooseMyPlate program recommendations for Daily Goals and Portion Sizes.

Introduction and Notes by Linda McDonald, M.S., R.D., a noted dietitian and the operator of SUPERMARKET SAVVY, a resource for consumers and health professionals on shopping healthy.

Paperback, 978-1-4380-0010-7, $6.99, *Can$7.99*   Prices subject to change without notice.

Available at your local book store or visit **www.barronseduc.com**

Barron's Educational Series, Inc.
250 Wireless Boulevard
Hauppauge, NY 11788
Order toll-free: 1-800-645-3476
Order by fax: 1-631-434-3217

In Canada:
Georgetown Book Warehouse
34 Armstrong Avenue
Georgetown, Ontario L7G 4R9
Canadian orders: 1-800-247-7160
Order by fax: 1-800-887-1594

(#272) R 10/12

Here's what leading food writers have said . . .

BARRON'S

"As thick and as satisfying as a well-stuffed sandwich."
—*The New York Times*

"Essential for anyone who talks, eats, or thinks about food."
—*Bev Bennett, Chicago Sun-Times*

"... one of the best reference books we've seen, a must for every cook's library."
—*Bon Appétit magazine*

The Deluxe Food Lover's Companion

Sharon Tyler Herbst and Ron Herbst

More than 6,700 alphabetically arranged entries
describe foods of every kind, preparation techniques,
cooking and baking tools, serving suggestions, and
more. Hundreds of illustrations show all kinds of foods
and food-related items, ranging from beef-cut dia-
grams to specialized cooking utensils. Separate glos-
saries throughout the book cover pork, fish, cheese,
bread, spices, and more. Fascinating sidebar features
include brief food preparation tips and pithy quota-
tions about food. The deluxe hardcover binding with
dust jacket comes with a ribbon place-marker and
golden-tipped page edges.

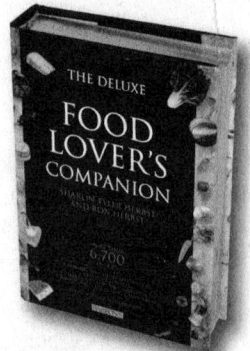

Hardcover w/jacket, ISBN 978-0-7641-6241-1, $29.99, *Can$35.99*

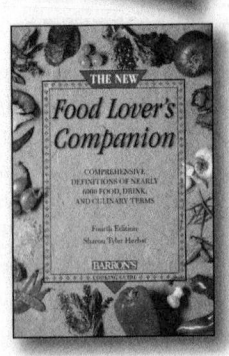

The New Food Lover's Companion,
4th Edition   *Sharon Tyler Herbst*

This widely praised reference guide is a smaller, paperback version of *The Deluxe Food Lover's Companion*, and
contains many of the features found in the larger book.
Alphabetically arranged entries describe fruits, vegeta-
bles, meats, fish, shellfish, breads, pastas, herbs and spices, cheeses, international
foods, cooking tools and techniques, and much more. This practical volume is not a
cookbook—but it includes hundreds of cooking tips, a bibliography of cookbooks and
food-related literature, food preparation and serving tips, and much more.

Paperback, ISBN 978-0-7641-3577-4, $16.99, *Can$19.99*

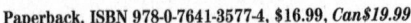

Prices subject to change without notice.

Available at your local book store
or visit **www.barronseduc.com**

#106 R 12/12

Barron's Educational Series, Inc.
250 Wireless Boulevard • Hauppauge, NY 11788
Order toll-free: 1-800-645-3476
Order by fax: 1-631-434-3217
In Canada: Georgetown Book Warehouse
34 Armstrong Avenue • Georgetown, Ontario L7G 4R9
Canadian orders: 1-800-247-7160
Fax in Canada: 1-800-887-1594